RADIATION UNITS

Quantity	SI Unit	Conventional Unit	Relationship
intensity (I)	$W/m^2 = J/m^2/s$		
exposure (X)	C/kg	roentgen (R)	$1\ R = 2.58 \times 10^{-4}\ C/kg$
air kerma (K)	gray (Gy)		
dose (D)	gray (Gy)	rad	1 Gy = 100 rad
	1 Gy = 1 J/kg		
dose equivalent	sievert (Sv)	rem	1 Sv = 100 rem
activity	becquerel (Bq)	curie (Ci)	$1\ Ci = 3.7 \times 10^{10}\ Bq$
	1 Bq = 1 decay/s		

RADIATION SAFETY ACTIONS AND PRINCIPLES

Actions	Principles
minimize exposure time	justification
maximize distance	optimization (ALARA)
adequate shielding	limitation

STANDARD DOSE LIMITS

Exposed Individual	Annual Limit
Occupational	
adult worker	50 mSv/y (5 rem/y) EDE
	150 mSv/y to lens of eye
	500 mSv/y any other organ
minor	5 mSv/y (0.5 rem/y)
pregnant	5 mSv (0.5 rem) to fetus
Member of public	1 mSv/y (100 mrem/y)

PHYSICS OF
RADIOLOGY

PHYSICS OF RADIOLOGY

Anthony Brinton Wolbarst, PhD
Formerly Instructor
Harvard Medical School
Boston, MA, and
Staff Medical Physicist
National Cancer Institute
Bethesda, MD

With Illustrations by Gordon Cook
NYU Medical Center
A. J. Lanzo Laboratory
Tuxedo, NY

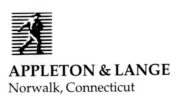

APPLETON & LANGE
Norwalk, Connecticut

Author's disclaimer: Since 1986 I have been an employee of the US Environmental
Protection Agency. This book is solely my own responsibility, however, and its
production is unrelated to my activities at the EPA. It has not been reviewed by
the Agency, and it does not necessarily reflect Agency policy. I did not work on
the book during business hours, nor did I receive any financial or other support
from the Federal government for it.

Copyright © 1993 by Appleton & Lange
Simon & Schuster Business and Professional Group

93 94 95 96 97 / 10 9 8 7 6 5 4 3 2 1

Prentice Hall International (UK) Limited, *London*
Prentice Hall of Australia Pty. Limited, *Sydney*
Prentice Hall Canada, Inc., *Toronto*
Prentice Hall Hispanoamericana, S.A., *Mexico*
Prentice Hall of India Private Limited, *New Delhi*
Prentice Hall of Japan, Inc. *Tokyo*
Simon & Schuster Asia Pte. Ltd., *Singapore*
Editora Prentice Hall do Brasil Ltda., *Rio de Janeiro*
Prentice Hall, *Englewood Cliffs, New Jersey*

Library of Congress Cataloging-in-Publication Data

Wolbarst, Anthony Brinton
    Physics of radiology / Anthony Brinton Wolbarst ; with illustrations by
Gordon Cook.
        p. cm.
    ISBN 0-8385-5769-4
    1. Diagnostic imaging. 2. Medical physics. I. Title.
    [DNLM: 1. Diagnostic Imaging. 2. Health Physics. WN 110 W848m
1993]
    RC78.7.D53W65 1993
    616.07'54—dc20
    DNLM/DLC
    for Library of Congress   92–48557

ISBN 0-8385-5769-4
90000
9 780838 557693

Production Editor: Elizabeth Ryan

For Eleanor
"At the still point of the turning world."

T. S. Eliot
Burnt Norton

Contents

Preface

This is a textbook on the science and technology that underlie the creation of diagnostic medical images. It is written primarily for radiology residents and medical students in courses on the physics of radiology, and for other interested physicians. I hope that it will also be helpful to scientists and engineers seeking a qualitative introduction to the field of medical imaging.

Medical images can be produced in a number of ways: with x-ray tubes and photographic film; with a radiopharmaceutical injected into a patient and a gamma camera; with the magnetic and radio frequency fields of a magnetic resonance imager; and even with high frequency sound. At first these approaches may seem quite disparate; but there is, in fact, a core of basic physical science that is common to all of them. A primary aim of *Physics of Radiology* is to leave the reader with a clear and comfortable overview of how, for each of the principal modalities, the basic science pieces fit together to form a coherent and integrated whole. Such an overview is indispensible to anyone seeking a solid introduction to this complex and rapidly evolving field or attempting to stay abreast of the latest developments.

Physics of Radiology is also intended to provide a considerable amount of practical and detailed information on how imaging technologies actually work. A physician needs this to ensure that equipment and staff are generating diagnostic information of high quality and are doing so in a safe manner. He or she must also communicate effectively and confidently with medical physicists, engineers, and salespeople, all of whom play important roles in the operations of a modern imaging department. Then, too, there is the personal satisfaction that comes with the mastery of a discipline: the more you understand the scientific foundations and technological tools of your field, the more intellectual pleasure you will derive from *all* aspects of it.

A radiology resident who has digested this material and has had a year or so of hands-on experience should run into little difficulty with the radiological physics part of the American Board of Radiology certification examination. Passing the ABR examination commonly involves the memorization of hundreds of equations and a zillion facts, all of which decay away after the exam with an astonishingly short half-life. This book attempts to present the principles and details as parts of an integrated, coherent whole in such a way that they will be with you, and remain useful, long after the trauma of exams is past. As such, it takes a cyclic approach: important ideas are introduced in simple terms and presented again one or several times in increasingly sophisticated form, as the necessary language skills develop and as the frame of reference becomes firmer and broader. My experience has been that when a large volume of complex information must be absorbed and placed in context, some intentional repetition of the central concepts can greatly help.

A cursory thumbing through will reveal a sprinkling of mathematical formulae. Although the book could have been written without them, I believe that they generally serve to *simplify* arguments by presenting them in purest form. A closer examination, moreover, should convince even the most math-averse reader that the algebra is very elementary. Nearly all of the equations involve no more than proportionalities or the occasional exponential. The properties of such functions, and the elementary ideas about probability and statistics that are needed, are reviewed in appendices to the appropriate chapters. The meanings of many of the equations are illustrated in the Exercises.

Medical imaging is surely one of the most exciting fields in which anyone could work—combining a dazzling, cutting edge technology with the challenges and rewards of clinical practice. I hope that your association with imaging will be gratifying, and I trust that your understanding of the science and technology behind it will make it all the more stimulating for you and beneficial for your patients.

On the Structure of the Book

Physics of Radiology is comprised of four segments. The first consists of two chapters—one, an introduction, covers the different types of imaging modalities, and the other provides a basic introduction to radiography. The second segment deals with the scientific foundations of imaging. It consists largely of a review of the relevant properties of matter and of electromagnetic radiation (x-ray and light energy, in particular), and an exploration of the ways in which the two can interact—in the intensifying screens of a radiographic cassette, in film, in the sodium iodide crystals of a gamma camera, and in people.

The third segment, on analog x-ray imaging, combines these somewhat abstract concepts to explain in detail the workings of one very concrete imaging technique: conventional screen/film radiography. Once it is clear how the underlying physical ideas work together in this paradigm, it becomes a fairly straightforward matter to apply them to more complex imaging technologies. This segment also addresses the nature of the evidence concerning the risks from ionizing radiation and describes professionally acceptable radiation safety practices.

The fourth segment of the book deals with computer-based imaging. Over the past two decades, the computer has extended the capabilities of some modalities, such as conventional nuclear medicine and ultrasound, almost beyond recognition. Others, such as CT, MRI, SPECT, and PET, could not exist without the ability of machines to perform large numbers of calculations extremely quickly. Computer-based Picture Archiving and Communication Systems (PACS), moreover, can greatly increase the speed and reliability with which images can be retrieved from storage, displayed, and transported down the hall or around the world.

Physics of Radiology covers more topics than are presented in the typical residents' course in medical physics. The instructor can thus employ the outline and main ideas of the text to provide a general framework, and pick and choose for more in-depth study, according to particular interests and needs. There should also be enough material to satisfy the initial needs of the reader who wishes to dig deeper.

A REQUEST FROM THE AUTHOR

Finally, a request for assistance from you, the reader or instructor. My primary objective has been to find ways of presenting the central ideas of medical imaging in as clear, interesting, and professionally useful a fashion as possible. Please do let me have your suggestions for things that should be added, or deleted, or corrected, or simply put better, care of the publisher. If a second edition is destined to appear, you could be an important part of it. In advance, I thank you.

Acknowledgments

Each chapter in *Physics of Radiology* has been examined by at least two reviewers knowledgable in the area—mostly medical physicists, engineers, and physicians, but some others, as well. Their comments have helped me to clean up unclear arguments, and to avoid a few significant faux pas. Whatever successes this book may achieve are largely attributable to their suggestions, and it is with great appreciation that I extend my thanks to Jack Abarbanel, Steve Bacharach, Ed Barnes, Harrison Barrett, Bengt Bjarngard, Andre Bruwer, Alan Brodsky, Gordon Burley, Stuart Bushong, Penny Butler, John Cameron, Burton Conway, Bruce Curran, Jim Deye, Bob Dyer, Don Elliott, Fred Fahey, Tom Fearon, Marie Foley Kijewski, Bill Hendee, Doreen Hill, Steve Horii, David Hoult, Ken Kase, Michael King, Rick Lee, Hector Lopez, Wendell Lutz, Charlie Marwick, Charles Metz, Charles Miller, Rick Morin, Sun Ki Mun, the Nelson twins (Chris and Neal), Ali Parsa, Hal Peterson, Lowell Ralston, Frank Ranallo, Allan Richardson, Jim Rogers, Tim Schultheiss, Bob Siddon, Ned Sternick, Andy Wallo, Michael Wood, Ray Wu, Jim Zagzebski, Robert Zamenhof, Sandra Zink, and Bob Zwicker. These people have taken of their very precious time, and put energy and thought—in some cases, a great deal of effort—into assisting me. I can only hope that they understand how very real is my sense of indebtedness to each of them.

A few went far above and beyond the call of duty. John Cameron offered invaluable early encouragement and some advice that led me to alter considerably the book's overall aims and structure. Rick Morin commented at length on a variety of chapters and provided moral support at a difficult time. Harrison Barrett and Charles Metz worked carefully through the seven chapters of Part 4, "The Formation of A Radiographic Image" which, I feel, form the core of the book, and they helped to straighten out my thinking on a number of points. Finally, Robert Zamenhof, in addition to having taught me much of what I know about radiology, reviewed about a third of the book with unfailingly good sense and good humor, and was nearly a second author on several chapters. My special thanks to them.

The graphics of Gordon Cook speak most eloquently for themselves. Still, I must say, that I, for one, think they're grand. I would like to add that beyond being a fine draftsman and clever fellow, he is also one of the most pleasant and helpful people I have ever worked with. He turned what could have been a long and stressful process, the transformation of my scratches into fine illustrations, into a genuine pleasure.

I believe that I have given proper credit when borrowing ideas for pictures that are not already in wide circulation, and any failures along that line are unintentional.

I gratefully acknowledge the help of many people and corporations, as cited in the captions, in acquiring photographs. In particular, I wish to thank the American College of Radiology for use of films from their excellent teaching file, and Robert Irving for his fine photography work. In selecting photographs from among those provided by manufacturers, I have attempted to achieve a fair and representative balance—weighted somewhat, I admit, by the degree to which the suppliers made serious efforts to provide images appropriate for a textbook. But most importantly, I have chosen the photos that I feel have greatest value for teaching purposes. *In no case should the use of a photograph or diagram be interpreted as an endorsement of a product.*

Others have helped in other ways. My thanks especially to the various members, of all sizes, shapes, and ages, of the Wolbarst and Nealon families for their interest, and for being there. And next time, Kate, I *will* drive you to the airport!

I would never have undertaken (much less completed) *Physics of Radiology* had it not been for the support and intelligent advice of my closest friend and favorite companion, my wife Eleanor Nealon. A book is extraordinarily consuming of time and attention, and she has remained encouraging, unselfish, and wise throughout the whole process. As but a small indication of my appreciation, I dedicate this book, with my love, to her.

Introduction

I

Sketches of the Imaging Modalities

For three quarters of a century following Roentgen's discovery of x-rays in 1895, improvements in radiology came slowly but steadily, culminating in the invention of the image intensifying tube. The past few decades, by contrast, have seen changes as revolutionary as the computers that have made them possible: computerized tomography, magnetic resonance imaging, and the totally digital department. These developments are turning imaging into one of the most exciting, but technologically demanding, fields of medicine.

This chapter and the next provide initial, very brief sketches of the major imaging modalities that are currently being employed to examine the structure and functioning of the body. The meanings of some of the terms and ideas used freely here, such as "photon" and "radioisotope," may not be completely clear, but they should become so in the chapters that soon follow.

1. RADIOGRAPHY

A medical image is created by detecting the effects that the patient's body has on a suitable probe (Fig. 1–1).

For **transmission** imaging, the body must be *partially transparent* to the probe. If the probe passes through all tissues without interacting with any of them, like light through clear glass, no differences among the tissues can be visualized. Similarly, if the probe is completely blocked, nothing of interest can be observed. But if the probe is only partially absorbed, scattered, or reflected by the body, we may be able to detect small differences in its interactions with the various tissues. And from such information, it may be possible to create diagnostically useful images.

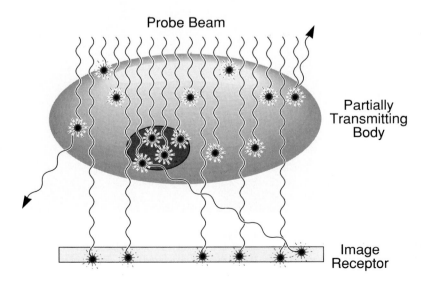

Probe Beam

Partially Transmitting Body

Image Receptor

Figure 1–1. In transmission imaging, probes are directed into the part of the body of interest. Where above-average numbers of these probes are absorbed or scattered or otherwise affected by nonuniformities in the body tissues, there will be a reduction in the numbers that reach the image receptor. With conventional x-ray imaging, the probes are x-ray photons, and the image receptor is a cassette containing a sheet of photographic film.

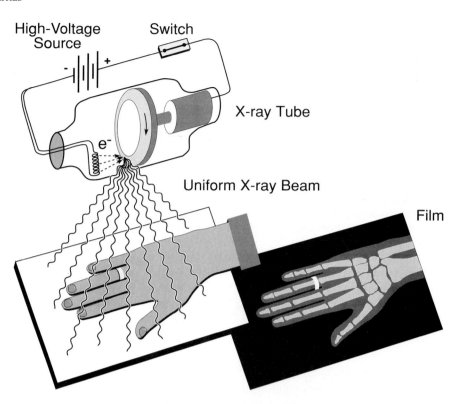

Figure 1–2. To produce an x-ray image, you need a uniform x-ray beam (produced by a high-voltage source and an x-ray tube) and an image receptor (cassette and film). Within the evacuated x-ray tube, negatively charged electrons (indicated by the *e⁻*) boil off from the heated cathode filament, at the left. During the fraction of a second that an exposure is being made, these electrons are accelerated by a strong electric field toward the anode target. In colliding with the anode, they produce x-ray energy (and much heat—the anode is made to rotate rapidly to spread out the heat over a large area, to prevent the overheating of any one spot). A bone attenuates the x-ray beam more effectively than does soft tissue, and produces a deeper x-ray shadow. Less x-ray energy reaches the film, and less silver is laid down in it during the development process. That portion of film ends up more transparent, and the bone appears lighter on the view box.

A beam of x-ray photons is such a probe (a **photon** is a localized bundle of electromagnetic energy). In conventional **radiography,** a nearly uniform x-ray beam exposes the anatomic region of interest for a fraction of a second, and the transmitted x-ray shadow is captured on radiographic film. The various body tissues **attenuate** different parts of the beam by different amounts. The more a tissue **absorbs** or **scatters** x-ray photons, the smaller the amount of x-ray energy that passes through to darken the film, and the clearer or lighter the developed film will appear.

X-ray photons are created when electrons are accelerated to high velocity within an x-ray tube, and made to collide with its metal target (Fig. 1–2). A nearly *uniform x-ray beam* produced in this fashion might then enter a patient's hand. Bone and the various soft tissues absorb and scatter the x-rays by different amounts, and the depth of the shadow cast in the exiting beam varies over the area being imaged. The emerging beam, which is no longer uniform, exposes a sheet of film in a cassette. The resultant pattern is distilled into a permanent visible record, through the **development** of the film, and placed on a view box for inspection (Fig. 1–3).

What is of interest, and what is ultimately responsible for the patterns of clear and dark in the radiograph, is the distribution of the tissues *within* the body. What is recorded and available for diagnostic purposes is a representation on film of the spatially varying x-ray intensity transmitted *through* the body. The radiographic process is thus a mapping, a condensation, if you will, from patient anatomy in three dimensions to a visual image in two.

The image's usefulness depends on the **contrast** it displays among the various tissues, on its **resolution** and **sharpness** (the ability to capture fine detail), and on the level of interfering **noise** of various sorts that might be present. An important aspect of the job of the physician and his or her staff is to ensure (by way of a quality assurance program) that the

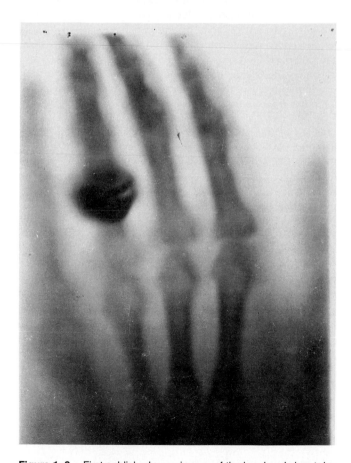

Figure 1–3. First published x-ray image, of the hand and signet ring of Professor Roentgen's wife, was produced December 22, 1895. *(Courtesy of the Deutsches Roentgen-Museum, Remscheid-Lennep, Germany.)*

technique factors (such as the peak kilovoltage, tube current, and exposure duration) for any particular study and the performance characteristics of the imaging system in general are such as to yield films with clinically adequate contrast, resolution, and noise level, and at minimal cost in radiation **dose** to patient and medical personnel.

2. FLUOROSCOPY

Late in the evening of November 8, 1895, Wilhelm Conrad Roentgen noted that when he caused an electric discharge to occur in a partially evacuated glass tube, a nearby piece of paper coated with barium platinocyanide glowed in the dark.

He thereby discovered x-ray radiation by observing the emission of light that it induced in a nearby **fluorescent** material.

If an x-ray tube is left on, so as to produce a continuous beam rather than a short pulse, the light emitted from a fluorescent screen can be viewed directly by eye (Fig. 1–4A). Indeed, because of the unreliability of both films and x-ray tubes in the early days, this technique of **fluoroscopy** initially played nearly as important a role as did film-based radiography. It offered the added advantage that the physician could observe moving anatomy; fractures could be reduced under direct observation, and foreign objects removed or put in place. The images produced in this fashion were extremely faint, however, and required dark adaptation of the eye, which wasted a considerable amount of time. So with the steady flow of improve-

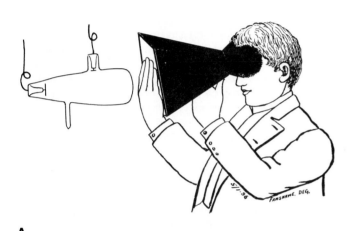

A

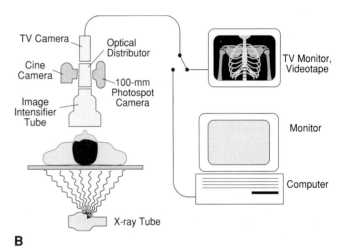

B

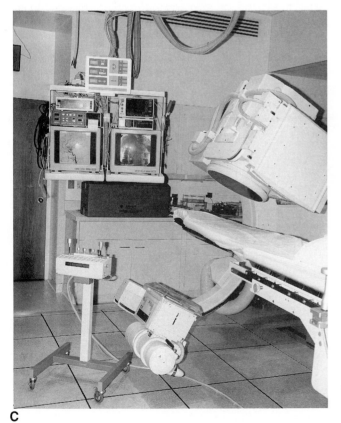

C

Figure 1–4. **A.** An early fluorographic system, as used before the need for radiation safety procedures became apparent. This illustration is reproduced from a book published in 1896, less than a year after the discovery of x-rays. **B.** Schematic of a typical modern fluoroscopic system. The image receptor is an image intensifier tube that transforms a life-sized x-ray image into a small, bright optical image. This, in turn, is routed to a spot film, cine, or television camera by means of the optical distributor. The video signal from the TV camera can either be fed directly into a TV monitor and videotape or be digitized for entry into a computer. **C.** The x-ray tube (below the table) and imaging tower (upper right) of this digital fluoroscopic system, at opposite ends of the C-arm, can be rotated about the patient table. The square device on the near side of the image intensifier is a film changer, which may be swung down into the beam path (in front of the image intensifier tube) to produce high-resolution radiographic film images. (**A** *courtesy of Trevert, E.* Something about X-rays for Everyone. *Madison, WI: Medical Physics Publishing Company, 1896.)*

ments to conventional radiography over the first half of this century, fluorography largely fell by the wayside.

The development of the x-ray **image intensifier** (II) tube in the 1950s led to a renaissance of fluoroscopy. An II is an electronic vacuum tube device that can transform a life-sized pattern of x-ray energy emerging from a patient into a small, very bright corresponding pattern of visible light. The output of the II tube may be photographed directly with a still or cine camera or viewed with a television camera (Fig. 1–4B and C). An image picked up by TV can, in turn, be seen directly on a nearby or remote TV monitor, and perhaps stored on videotape. Alternatively, it can be sampled and **digitized** (put in digital electronic form) and fed into a computer for electronic image processing before display, as in digital subtraction angiography.

3. DIGITAL SUBTRACTION ANGIOGRAPHY

Digitizing an image is like the converse of painting by numbers. A computer partitions the image into many small square **pixel**s, each with its unique location, or spatial **address** (Fig. 1–5A). It then represents the shade of gray (or color) at every address by means of a numerical **pixel value**. The entire image can then be represented as a long string of the addresses and corresponding pixel value numbers (Fig. 1–5B). If the fineness of a two-dimensional image is 1024 × 1024 pixels, which may be the case for digital radiography, then there will be about one million pixels. One million numbers, representing the shades of gray of the million pixels, are therefore used for a complete digital encoding. (For computerized tomography or magnetic resonance imaging, the pixel matrix is more likely to be something like 256 × 256, and much less **computer memory** is required to store the image.)

There can be advantages to digitizing and computer processing fluoroscopic images, most notably in **digital subtraction angiography** (DSA). Suppose, for example, that an obstruction in a carotid artery is suspected. A conventional angiographic approach is to thread a guidewire and catheter percutaneously into the femoral artery, through the abdominal aorta and thoracic aorta, and into the carotid, to a point below the region of interest (ROI), all under fluoroscopy. Iodine-based contrast agent, which strongly attenuates x-rays, is injected. The result, as seen immediately under conventional fluoroscopy or on a set of rapidly, sequentially exposed x-ray films, will be an image of the vessels that contain contrast material, superimposed on a background of patterns caused by soft tissues and bones. The irrelevant background gives rise to a good deal of visual interference, and the image of importance may easily be lost in the confusion. The invasive procedure itself, moreover, can be somewhat risky—there is a possibility of patient reaction to the contrast agent.

With digital subtraction angiography, the catheter normally follows the same route into the carotid artery. The study begins with the digitization of a fluoroscopic image of the ROI, before administration of contrast agent, (Fig. 1–6A) and its storage in computer memory. Contrast agent is then injected and, a short while later, a second fluoroscopic image is obtained, digitized, and stored (Fig. 1–6B). The two images should differ only where the contrast material is present. Therefore, subtracting the two from one another point by point (i.e., pixel by pixel) will generate a "difference" image that shows only the contrast agent-containing vessels (Fig. 1–6C). Almost all the distracting background information is canceled out, and the contrast of the blood vessels in the final image is high. Because the difference image is in digital form, it can be "windowed" and, in other ways, computer processed to enhance its clinical utility, and the physician can view the results

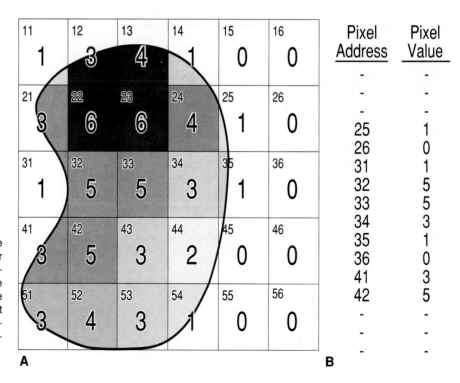

Figure 1–5. Digitization of an image. **A.** The number in the upper left corner of each pixel, or picture element, is its address. The larger, central number represents the pixel value, i.e., the degree of "brightness," as averaged over the entire pixel, where (in this example) 0 is lightest and 7 is darkest. **B.** The image can be represented as a string of pixel addresses and corresponding pixel values.

Pixel Address	Pixel Value
-	-
-	-
-	-
25	1
26	0
31	1
32	5
33	5
34	3
35	1
36	0
41	3
42	5
-	-
-	-
-	-

A   B

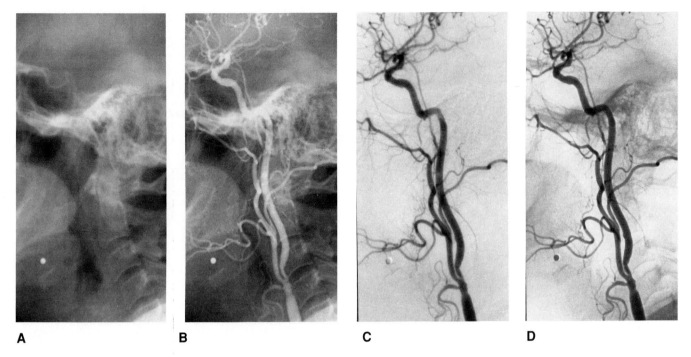

A   B   C   D

Figure 1–6. Digital subtraction angiography (DSA) images are made before and after contrast medium fills the blood vessels of interest, and the two images are subtracted from one another. Lateral view of the carotid artery: **A.** Mask image. **B.** Angio image, with iodine in the vessels. **C.** Difference image, highlighting those areas where a change has occurred. **D.** Difference image after edge enhancement and the addition of some anatomic backgrounding. *(Courtesy of Siemens Medical Systems, Inc.)*

immediately, in real time. Finally, less contrast agent is normally required.

4. COMPUTED TOMOGRAPHY

Imagine the body as consisting of thin, flat, longitudinal slices of tissue (Fig. 1–7A). Looking at a conventional radiograph is like filming the tissue slices individually, but viewing the films when all are stacked in a pile. With this superpositioning of slice images, overlapping structures obscure one another, and the three-dimensional aspect of the anatomy is lost. **Computed tomography** (CT) is capable of preserving and extracting the different images corresponding to separate (transverse) slices (Fig. 1–7B).

A mother suspects that her baby has swallowed some objects. You radiograph the infant from several different angles, and hope to make sense of the films. What entities (and in what configuration) could possibly give rise to this particular *set* of radiographs? After a modicum of head scratching, you deduce that the patient ate two small coins and a paperclip. Images obtained at a few additional angles support your initial hypothesis. Objects of more complex shapes would require a greater number of views for an unequivocal determination.

That, in essence, is how CT works. It creates, digitizes, and stores in a computer the radiologic images from a large number (typically 720 to 1440) of different perspectives. The computer then works backward to *reconstruct* the spatial distribution of the materials (or, more precisely, the spatial distribution of the x-ray attenuation properties of the materials) that must have been responsible for this particular set of 720 to 1440 images. The necessary mathematical manipulations are complex and must be carried out on a relatively powerful computer, but the basic idea is a simple one.

Computed tomography uses an x-ray "fan" beam as wide as the patient but only a few millimeters high. The reconstructed image therefore corresponds to a single transverse pancake of tissue several millimeters thick. As with DSA, the CT image does away with the visual interference of the optical patterns arising from over- and underlying organs, and it thereby provides much better image contrast between different soft tissues than does radiography or conventional fluoroscopy (Fig. 1–8). The spatial resolution is poorer, however, and the procedure can be more time consuming and costly.

Three-dimensional display may be obtained by generating multiple adjacent transverse slice images, one at a time, and combining the results. Much current CT research involves the development of lifelike, three-dimensional images that can

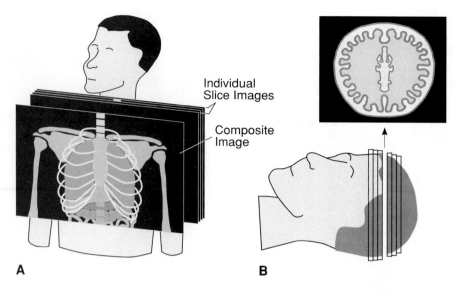

A   **B**

Figure 1–7.   Imagine a patient as being composed of many thin slices. A separate image is made of the tissues of each slice. **A.** An ordinary x-ray film (shown as the front film, here) is like the composite that would result from the superpositioning of the set of separate films of the individual (longitudinal) slices. **B.** With CT, it is possible to obtain the individual (transverse) slice images separately.

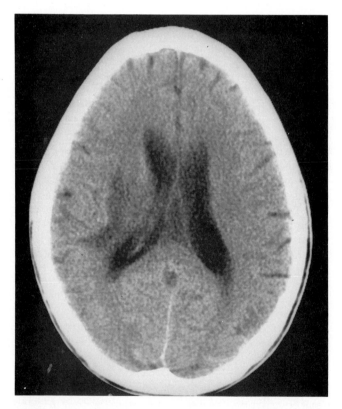

Figure 1–8.   Computed tomography image of a transverse slice of the brain, providing information on its anatomy. *(Photo courtesy of GE Medical Systems.)*

be rotated, dissected, and otherwise manipulated in real time by the physician. Some of these, in the near future, may employ *holographic* and *virtual reality* display technologies.

5. NUCLEAR MEDICINE, SINGLE-PHOTON EMISSION COMPUTED TOMOGRAPHY, AND POSITRON EMISSION TOMOGRAPHY

Nuclear medicine makes use of a radioactive material that both concentrates in a particular physiologic or anatomic compartment and emits **gamma rays.** (Gamma rays are identical to x-rays, but are of different origin: They are emitted by the nuclei of some radioactive atoms, rather than created in the collisions of high-velocity electrons with the target of an X-ray tube.) Ingested or injected iodine concentrates in the thyroid, for example. And just as a hot fire poker glows in a dark room, so also a thyroid containing the radioisotope iodine-123 (commonly written ^{123}I) "glows" gamma rays. The same is true for a liver whose Kupffer cells filter out and collect injected sulfur colloid tagged with the radionuclide technetium-99m. Or for a lung, the capillaries of which have briefly trapped microscopic clumps of ^{99m}Tc-tagged albumin. Or normal myocardium that has taken up the radioactive isotope ^{201}Tl of thallium, a potassium analog.

The organ emitting gamma rays is imaged by means of a **gamma camera** (Fig. 1–9), which works somewhat like an eye. Gamma rays, unlike light, cannot be focused, so the role of the lens is played by a collimator, a 1 in.-thick, highly attenuating lead plate through which run numerous, closely spaced paral-

GAMMA CAMERA

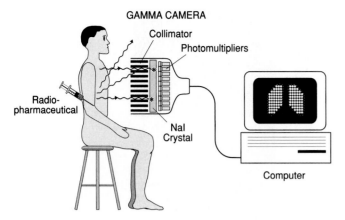

Figure 1–9. Nuclear medicine lung scan: An injected radiopharmaceutical concentrates in the lungs and "glows" gamma rays. Although invisible to the eye, gamma rays can be imaged by a gamma camera.

lel (or nearly parallel) channels. Behind the collimator is a large (40 cm or more in diameter) but thin single *fluorescent* sodium iodide crystal and an array of photomultiplier tubes and associated electronic circuitry. Together, these serve as a retinal photoreceptor and neural network. Any gamma ray that passes along a channel of the collimator and then interacts with the crystal triggers the production of a scintillation (burst of light). The photomultiplier system senses this event and determines its location in the crystal. With an older gamma camera, a pinpoint of light immediately appears at the corresponding point on the display screen of a cathode ray tube. With a modern system, the scintillation information is digitized and entered into a computer, and the processed image is displayed on a TV monitor.

The resulting nuclear medicine image is of relatively low spatial resolution, and reveals only the rough shape and size of the organ or tissue under consideration. But any part of the organ that takes up an excessive amount of radiopharmaceutical will glow especially brightly on the display. If a portion of the organ fails to take up the radiopharmaceutical (Fig. 1–10), or is missing, or is obscured by overlying tissues, the corresponding region of the image appears dark. A nuclear medicine image thus provides information largely on the physiology and pathology of an organ, rather than on the details of its anatomy.

Three aspects of nuclear medicine are currently generating much interest:

- The binding of radionuclides to specific antibodies may greatly refine the selection of tissues to be imaged.
- In single-photon emission computerized tomography (SPECT), one or several gamma camera heads are rotated around the patient, and the accumulated data are used to generate a set of CT-like slice images or a three-dimensional image (Fig. 1–11).
- Positron emission tomography (PET) scanning makes use of special radionuclides that emit **positrons** (positively charged electrons). A positron travels less than a millimeter or so in tissue before colliding with an ordinary atomic electron. The positron and electron "anni-

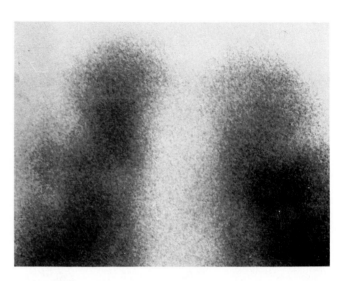

Figure 1–10. Nuclear medicine provides information that is primarily physiologic, rather than anatomic, in nature. The dark areas in this lung scan, indicating regions that fail to take up radiopharmaceutical, are caused by pulmonary emboli.

hilate" one another, and a pair of high-energy annihilation photons come into existence, traveling in opposite directions. Sometimes, both photons of the pair will be detected simultaneously (Fig. 1–12A) by independent detectors. Detection of many such pairs of annihilation photons leads to localization of their region of origin within the body.

Some of the elements that have radionuclides suitable for use in PET (carbon, nitrogen, oxygen, and fluorine) can be fully incorporated into physiologically important biomolecules, such as glucose. The technique can then be employed to spatially map some clinically

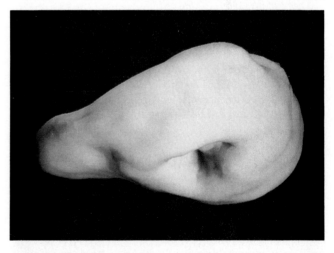

Figure 1–11. Three-dimensional rendering of a SPECT liver study, clearly demonstrating a space-occupying lesion. The imaging process involved 120 views of the region, took 15 minutes, and reconstructed the individual slice images with a 128 × 128 matrix. *(Courtesy of Picker International.)*

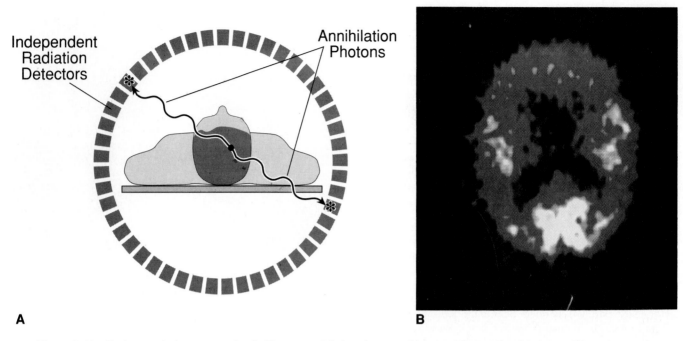

A

B

Figure 1–12. Positron emission tomography. **A.** The two annihilation photons, which travel in opposite directions, originated at a point somewhere along the line between the two triggered detectors. By keeping track of many such pairs, the spatial distribution of radiopharmaceutical in the brain can be imaged. **B.** PET image of a transverse slice of the brain. The spatial pattern of the metabolism of radiolabeled glucose indicates that the patient suffers from Alzheimer's disease. The clinical utility of PET (and of some other medical) images may be enhanced through the use of color display.

revealing metabolic processes (Fig. 1–12B). (Color display may significantly enhance the diagnostic utility of PET, and of some other medical, images.)

But a cyclotron is needed on-site to produce the short-lived radionuclides (the half-lives of ^{11}C, ^{13}N, and ^{15}O are 20, 10, and 2 minutes, respectively—the half-life of a radioactive material being the time it takes for half of any sample of it to decay away spontaneously), along with a "hot lab" for incorporating the isotope immediately into the metabolite of interest. Also, the PET scanner itself is expensive, as are the highly specialized technical personnel required to support the whole process. PET is an exciting and valuable research instrument, and there appear to be some diagnostic situations (e.g., focal epilepsy) where PET is especially helpful. As with all other major high-tech devices, the extent of its success as a clinical tool will be determined by a balancing of such benefits against the costs.

6. MAGNETIC RESONANCE IMAGING

Computerized tomography provides superb information on the distribution of the densities of tissues within the body, that is, on anatomy. Nuclear medicine reveals much about the physiology and pathology of the organs being examined. **Magnetic resonance imaging** does both! And it poses no radiation risk to the patient, as no gamma or x-ray energy is involved. MRI makes use, rather, of magnetic fields and radio waves.

A fundamental characteristic of a magnetic field is that it exerts a force on a *moving* charge. The interaction between moving charges (e.g., a current in a wire) and a magnetic field

underlies the operation of an electric motor. Another manifestation of this phenomenon is the tendency of a spinning charged body to orient its spin axis along an externally applied magnetic field (Fig. 1–13A). The nucleus of a hydrogen atom, in particular, behaves like a spinning charged particle. So when a patient lies within the hollow core of an MRI magnet, the hydrogen nuclei **(protons)** of the molecules in her or his cells tend to align along the field that the magnet produces, like compass needles.

In your mind's eye, twist a compass needle through 180 degrees, so that it points South. After being released, it will oscillate a few times about the North (Fig. 1–13B) and eventually settle back along it. The time this process takes is called a **relaxation time.** Somewhat analogous (but essentially different, as we shall see) relaxation processes occur for protons in a magnetic field, and it is primarily the spatial variations in such proton relaxation times (called $T1$ and $T2$) that MRI images.

A magnetic resonance imaging device assesses, point by point throughout the body, the local concentration of hydrogen nuclei in cellular water and lipid molecules. It also maps out variations in the associated proton relaxation times $T1$ and $T2$. The relaxation time for our oscillating compass was affected by the frictional forces occurring at the mechanical contact points where the needle is supported. The proton relaxation times in a tissue are determined by (and are highly sensitive to the detailed nature of) frictionlike and other interactions of the local water and lipid molecules with various intracellular biomolecules. The concentrations and biophysical characteristics of these biomolecules, in turn, depend on the type and physiologic status of the cells they inhabit. MRI may therefore be able to distinguish not only between histologically

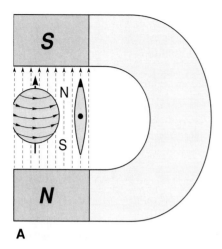 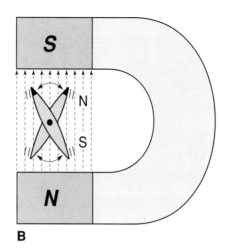

A   B

Figure 1–13. Magnetic resonance imaging. **A.** Protons and most other atomic nuclei will, like compass needles, tend to align in an external magnetic field. **B.** The settling down of a compass needle oscillating in an external magnetic field—analogous to (but different from) nuclear spin relaxation.

different tissues (Fig. 1–14), but even between healthy and pathologic forms of the same tissue.

Magnetic resonance imaging exploded onto the scene in the early 1980s, and its clinical potentials are still being rapidly developed. Resolution has improved steadily (and is now better than 1 mm), as has the modality's capability of performing different sorts of in vivo pathology studies. MRI even supports a form of angiography. At first, data acquisition was slow, requiring tens of minutes per patient. But imaging time has been

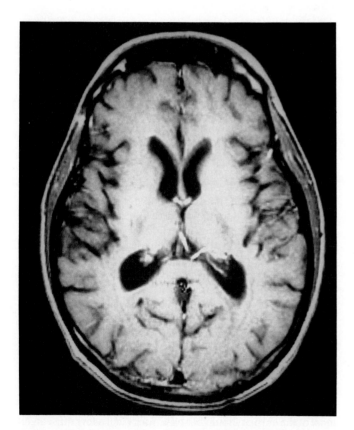

Figure 1–14. Magnetic resonance image of the brain, in the same patient and at approximately the same location as in Figure 1–8, providing information on both anatomy and physiology. *(Photo courtesy of GE Medical Systems.)*

driven down dramatically and is no longer a major limiting factor. Purchase and maintenance costs, however, remain significant.

7. ULTRASOUND

Sound is a mechanical disturbance that propagates through a medium. Normal audible sounds consist of waves of compression and rarefaction, of frequencies in the range of 20 to 20,000 cycles per second, that propagate through air. When a drum is struck, for example, the vibrating drum head alternately increases and reduces the pressure in the air directly adjacent to it, which pushes and pulls on the next "layer" of air, and so on. The disturbance radiates outward and eventually causes the displacement of the tympanic membrane of your ear, resulting in the sensation of a sound.

Clinical **ultrasound** (US) involves oscillations of from 1 to 10 million cycles per second propagating in a similar fashion through soft tissues and fluids. US imaging produces information about organs, blood vessels, and other structures within the body by creating pictures out of the **echoes** that are **reflected** back from them. Unlike x-ray imaging, it makes no use of the signal transmitted through them.

The US system and process are similar to those of SONAR, developed during World War II for the detection of submarines. A transmitter produces a train of short pulses of high-frequency electrical oscillations (Fig. 1–15). Like a loudspeaker, a **transducer** transforms the electronic signal into pulses of high-frequency mechanical vibrations that enter the body. In a homogeneous material, such as water (or the fluid contents of a cyst), a US beam simply dissipates its energy as it penetrates to greater depths. But if a beam passes through different tissues, energy is reflected back at interfaces among them. The time of return of an echo is proportional to the depth within the patient of the interface that produced it. The echo's intensity depends on the degree of difference in physical properties of the materials on the two sides of the interface, as well as on its depth.

Echoes are detected by the transducer, now acting as a microphone, and transformed back into electrical signals. The signals are processed by the receiver, and may be sent to a com-

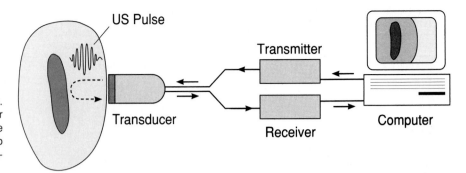

Figure 1–15. B-Mode ultrasound system. Electrical pulses produced by the transmitter are converted into sound by the transducer. The transducer also picks up any subsequent echo signals, and feeds them into the receiver, computer, and display.

puter, which keeps track of the return times and amplitudes of the various echoes. From this information, the computer creates an image (Fig. 1–16). Sophisticated US systems display the anatomy as CT-like images in real time.

Ultrasound is most useful in the study of soft tissues and organs that are too similar radiologically to provide adequate x-ray image contrast. Also, if a diagnostic question can be resolved by any of several modalities, then US may be preferable because of both low cost and the absence of ionizing radiation. The modality is widely used for obstetric/gynecologic, cardiac, and general abdominal imaging. Ultrasound energy does not pass readily across tissue/air or tissue/bone interfaces, however, so US is of limited use for the study of the lung or of the intracranium.

The US images of certain tissues, such as the liver, display distinctive spatial characteristics, or "textures." An exciting area of research involves the use of computers to recognize irregularities in such textural patterns and relate them to the presence of various diseases.

At the intensities normally used for imaging, there are no known deleterious biologic effects from US, even to a fetus. Higher-intensity beams, however, can be destructive of tissues. It is therefore important always to ensure that the equipment is functioning properly, being operated correctly, and being used for a medically good reason, especially when imaging the fetus.

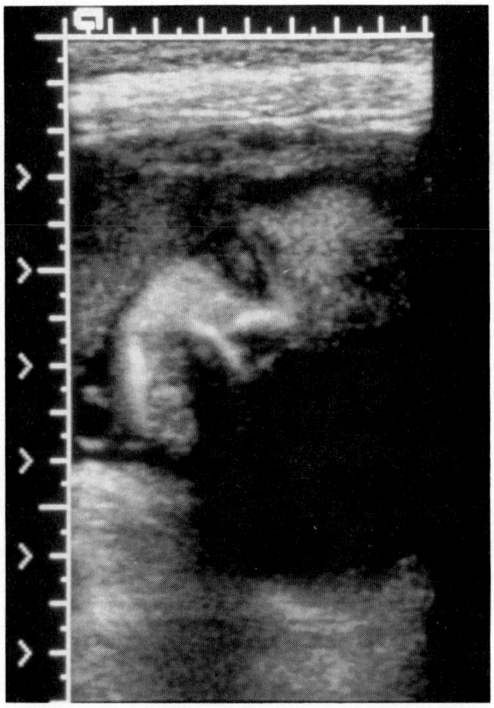

8. A PRELIMINARY COMPARISON OF THE MODALITIES

We have seen that different kinds of diagnostic probes may interact with different kinds of matter in dissimilar ways. And the different interaction mechanisms of the various imaging modalities may allow us to obtain different kinds of information on biologic structures. Two tissues that have the same effect on one probe may influence another probe in radically different ways. Differences among soft tissues that are not at all apparent to x-ray photons, for example, may be clearly distinguished with the sound waves of ultrasound or the radio waves of magnetic resonance imaging. Likewise, microcalcifications in the breast that could be missed by CT, US, and MRI might easily be seen with mammographic radiography. Thus, the various modalities may well provide pieces of information that complement one another.

Before we explore in more detail the ways in which energy and matter interact, and how those interactions may be exploited to generate images, it may be helpful to compare a few of the important imaging characteristics for the principal modalities. Table 1–1 lists typical values for some of these for conventional screen–film radiography (X), fluoroscopy (Fl) with an image intensifier tube, DSA, CT, conventional nuclear medicine (NM), SPECT, PET, MRI, and US. The explanations of most of the entries should be self-evident, but a few must await discussion in the coming chapters. The entries are typical, again, and may differ quite a bit from those of specific imaging systems and situations.

Figure 1–16.   B-Mode US image of a fetal face. *(Courtesy of Acuson Corporation.)*

TABLE 1–1. TYPICAL CHARACTERISTICS AND CAPABILITIES OF SOME OF THE PRINCIPAL IMAGING MODALITIES (ENTRIES FOR A PARTICULAR IMAGING SYSTEM OR STUDY MAY BE QUITE DIFFERENT)

	X	FI	DSA	CT	NM	SPECT	PET	MRI	US
What is detected?	transmitted x-rays				Emitted γ-rays			[a]	[b]
Signal detector	S/F	II	II	[c]	NaI	NaI	[c]	rf coil	[d]
What is imaged?	Electron density of tissue				Radionuclide uptake			[e]	[f]
Primarily reveals anatomy (A) physiology (P)	A	A	A	A	P	P	P	A&P	A
Spatial resolution (mm)	0.1	1	1	1	5	5	5	1	2
Soft tissue contrast high (1), lower (3)	3	3	1	2	2	1	1	1	2
Computer not used (N), advantageous (A), essential (E)	N	N	E	E	A	E	E	E	A

Abbreviations: S/F, Screen–film system; II, Image intensifier.
[a]Radio frequency voltage induced by precessing magnetization.
[b]Reflected ultrasound energy.
[c]Numerous small scintillation detectors or ionization chambers.
[d]Piezo-electric crystal.
[e]Nuclear magnetization.
[f]Discontinuities in tissue elasticity or density.

9. THE DIGITAL DEPARTMENT

Computers are absolutely essential for image generation with some diagnostic modalities (e.g., CT, MRI, SPECT, PET) and invaluable for image processing or enhancement with others (NM, US).

Image digitization also allows the entry of image information from all imaging devices into a computer-based picture archiving and communications system (*PACS*) (Fig. 1–17). Digitized images from all modalities can then be stored inexpensively, retrieved by any system workstation in seconds, and transmitted across the continent at the speed of light **(teleradiology).** Image and alphanumeric (text) information obtained from different but compatible systems, moreover, can be presented in composite, integrated form. And images can be massaged electronically to enhance contrast, to correct distortions, and to diminish the effects of various kinds of "noise."

Perhaps most significantly of all, in the long term, computers are growing ever more capable of *analyzing*, and even interpreting, information. The science of **artificial intelligence** is in its embryonic state, yet computer-based **expert systems**

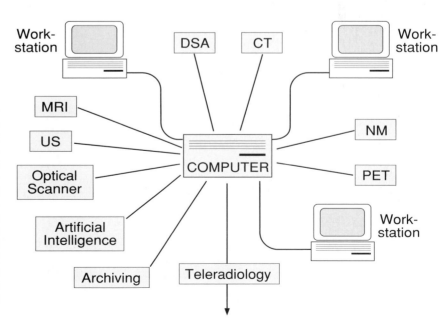

Figure 1–17. A picture archiving and communications system. A computer (or system of computers) is fed information from various imaging devices and workstations, including the computer-based hospital information system that holds patient records and other data. The system illustrated here accepts images generated by digital subtraction angiography (DSA), computed tomography (CT), nuclear medicine (NM), positron emission tomography (PET), magnetic resonance imaging (MRI), ultrasound (US), and an optical scanner that digitizes ordinary radiographs. All of this information can be processed, analyzed with the aid of artificial intelligence, stored in archives and retrieved rapidly, and transmitted over long distances (teleradiology).

and **neural networks** are already augmenting certain roles of the physician as diagnostician. Some expert systems are growing quite adept at pattern recognition. They can analyze electrocardiograms, for example, with success rates comparable to those of experienced cardiologists, and are used routinely to scan Halter tapes for cardiac irregularities. The application of computer analysis to two-dimensional radiologic images is orders of magnitude more difficult, and will be much slower in coming. But the handwriting is on the display monitor.

The diagnostic physician is not about to be replaced by an expert system, at least not in the foreseeable future. Without question, however, the computer will continue to bring about major, rapid changes in medical imaging—indeed, in all aspects of the practice of medicine—over the next few decades. And the physicians who fare best in dealing with these changes, and who can take fullest advantage of them, will be those who understand the basics of the science and revolutionary technologies that underlie them.

An Introduction to Radiography

This chapter tells, in more detail than the last, the story of the taking of an x-ray film. For it *is* a story, with a beginning (the generation of an x-ray beam), a thickening of the plot (the interaction of the beam with the bones and soft tissues of the patient, and then with the image receptor), and a possibly life-and-death denouement (the formation of a radiographic image that may, or may not, be capable of resolving a crucial clinical question).

The success of the effort may depend critically on aspects of image quality, such as image contrast, resolution, and noise content. Those factors, in turn, may be determined largely by the effectiveness of the operator's quality control program. There is a small risk associated with the diagnostic process itself, moreover, and before the x-ray is taken, this risk must be weighed against the probable medical benefits.

Despite the rapid growth of the other imaging modalities, screen-film radiography remains the most widely employed means of obtaining medical images. It is also, in many respects, the easiest to describe. A significant part of this book will therefore be devoted to the science and technology underlying conventional radiography, because of its importance in its own right and because of its usefulness as a steppingstone for explaining the other modalities.

1. THE FOUR PROCESSES OF RADIOGRAPHY

In standard radiography, a uniform x-ray beam exposes a portion of the body, and the transmitted, nonuniform x-ray "shadow" exiting the body is captured on film. The less material there is in the path of any part of the beam, the greater the amount of x-ray energy that passes through the body to expose the corresponding part of the film and the more opaque it is

after development. Where the body absorbs or scatters the beam more, conversely, the developed film's optical density is less; that is, it ends up more transparent.

Radiographic imaging may be thought of as involving four separate processes (Fig. 2–1):

- *Generation* of a relatively *uniform beam* of penetrating x-rays. These emanate from a point and travel in straight lines which, as they reach the patient, diverge only slowly.
- *Differential attenuation* of the beam by the tissues and organs being imaged. Different parts of the patient's body *absorb* and *scatter* different amounts of energy, and thereby sculpt the *primary x-ray image* out of the formerly uniform beam.
- *Detection* of the radiation exiting the body by film in a cassette. Any *spatial nonuniformities* in the emerging beam recorded on film are revealed, on its development, as spatially varying shades of gray (or, more precisely, as variations in film opacity) which forms the final visual x-ray image.
- *Analysis* and interpretation of the image. This depends on the quality of the final image, the viewing conditions, and the skills of the physician.

2. PRODUCING A UNIFORM BEAM OF PENETRATING RAYS

Our story begins with the production of a uniform beam* of x-rays by means of an **x-ray tube** and a **generator** of nearly

---

*This is something of an idealization. As will be seen in Chapter 11, the beam produced by a real x-ray tube is not completely "flat."

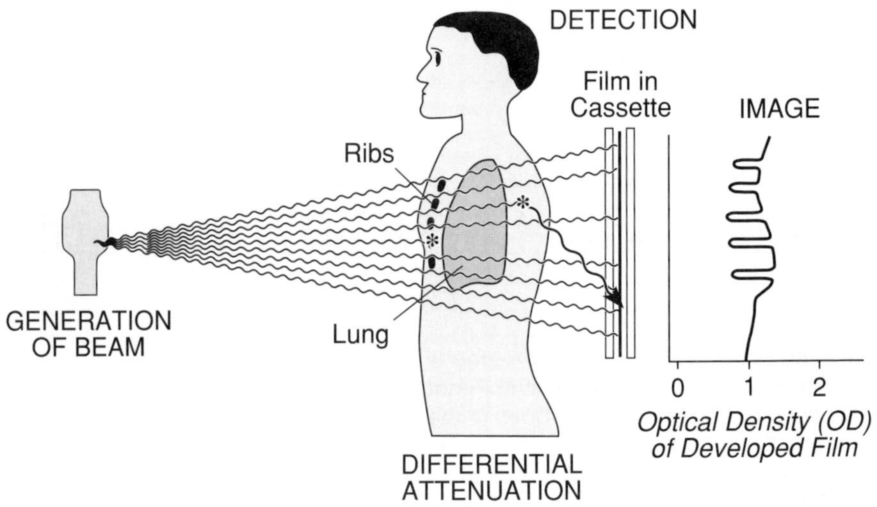

Figure 2–1. The standard radiographic process consists of the generation of a uniform x-ray beam, the introduction of information into the beam through its interaction with the patient's body tissues, the capture of that information by means of photographic film in a cassette, and the inspection of the visual patterns by the physician. Typical values of optical density (OD) of developed film range from near 0, where the film is nearly perfectly transparent, to 2 or 3, where it is highly opaque.

steady direct current (DC) **high voltage** or **potential** (Fig. 2–2). The tube itself consists of two metal electrodes, a **cathode** and an **anode** (or *target*), within an evacuated glass envelope. The cathode is attached to the negative pole of the generator, and the anode to its positive pole. The circuit is made complete for short periods (typically tens of milliseconds, as determined by a **timer**) by briefly closing an **exposure switch.** The magnitude of the potential produced by the generator, and applied across the tube when the exposure switch is closed, is selected by means of the **peak kilovoltage (kVp) control.**

The cathode is a coil of resistive wire, or **filament**, that is heated when a **filament current** is forced through it by means of the **filament power supply.** (In some kinds of vacuum tubes, the heating filament and the cathode are two separate electrodes.) When the cathode is sufficiently hot (2000°C or more), it "boils off" electrons. On those occasions that the exposure switch is closed, these electrons are drawn from the cathode to the anode. The size of this **tube current** depends mainly on the rate at which electrons boil off the cathode, and that, in turn, is determined by its temperature; thus the **tube current control,** or

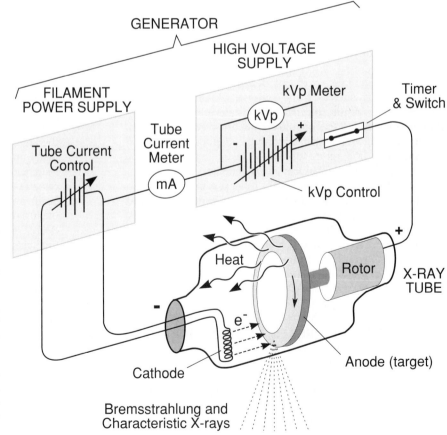

Figure 2–2. Simplified schematic of an x-ray tube and power source. Within the tube, electrons "boil off" the cathode. When the switch is closed, these electrons are attracted to the anode, which is attached to the positive pole of a source of high voltage. (A set of alternating long and short lines, the standard symbol for a battery, will be used in this book to denote any kind of DC voltage source. The arrow means that the voltage is adjustable.) When electrons collide with the anode, some of their kinetic energy is transformed into bremsstrahlung and characteristic x-ray energy, but more than 99% of it becomes heat. The power of penetration of the x-ray beam into and through the patient is controlled largely by the potential (peak kilovoltage, or kVp) applied across the tube, as measured by the kVp meter. The quantity of x-ray energy generated during an exposure (and the resulting darkening of film) depends also on the current (milliamperes, or mA) through the tube and on the duration (seconds) of the exposure.

milliampere (mA) control, actually works primarily by adjusting the filament temperature. The final velocity and kinetic energy of the electrons just before they crash into the anode, by contrast, are determined entirely by the x-ray tube potential, or kVp.

Two things happen as the high-velocity electrons from the cathode collide with the anode, and both are critically significant in the operation of the tube. First, as with the flow of electric current through a resistor, the motion of these electrons into and through the metal of the anode generates *heat.* Ninety-nine percent or more of the energy of the stream of electrons is wasted in this fashion, in fact, and if the heat is not somehow quickly dissipated, the anode can be irreparably damaged in seconds. In most modern diagnostic tubes, the anode is made to rotate rapidly about an axis, so as to reduce the instantaneous rate of heating of any one point on its surface.

The other 1% or less of the energy of the electrons is transformed directly into x-ray energy through two distinct processes: the production of bremsstrahlung radiation and the production of characteristic x-rays.

Bremsstrahlung may be translated from the German as "braking radiation," as in hitting the brakes of an automobile, and it refers to a particular energy conversion process: Whenever a charged particle experiences a rapid change of speed or direction, a portion of its energy of motion is transformed into electromagnetic radiation. Energy is not created or destroyed in the event, it simply changes form. In an x-ray tube, in particular, bremsstrahlung is produced when a high-velocity electron passes close by the nucleus of an atom in the anode and undergoes a sharp change in its trajectory.

Characteristic x-rays are created in a different fashion. When an outer-orbital electron of an atom is somehow excited into a higher-energy state, it usually returns to the ground state with the emission of visible light. When an *inner* electron of an atom of the anode material is ejected by a passing high-velocity electron, the atom may return to its ground state by giving off a characteristic (also known as fluorescence) x-ray photon, typically tens of thousands of times more energetic than a visible light photon. Although the characteristic x-ray contribution to a standard diagnostic beam intensity is usually under about 20%, in mammography it is dominant.

Thus, as a stream of electrons accelerated through an x-ray tube crashes into the anode, a small fraction of their energy ends up as a beam of bremsstrahlung and characteristic x-ray energy. As we shall see, the more energetic the electrons incident on the anode (i.e., the higher the voltage between cathode and anode), the more energetic and penetrating will be the resultant beam.

The tube potential, the tube current, and the exposure time are chosen (by means of the kVp, mA, and timer controls, respectively) by the radiologic technologist. These three parameters, known collectively as **technique factors** for the exposure, largely determine the ability of the beam to penetrate the patient's body, the capability of the imaging system to distinguish among the different tissues, and the overall average level of brightness of the end-product image on film. Optimal technique factors are chosen clinically for any procedure and patient so as to maximize the diagnostic utility of the image while minimizing the patient dose.

3. WHAT THE PATIENT'S BODY DOES TO THE X-RAY BEAM: DIFFERENTIAL ATTENUATION AND FORMATION OF THE PRIMARY X-RAY IMAGE

The beam of radiation produced by the x-ray tube and incident on a patient is nearly uniform. The beam emerging from the patient's body is spatially modulated; the various parts of the beam pass through different types and thicknesses of tissues, and are attenuated by different amounts.

Imagine the x-ray beam as consisting of a bundle of separate geometric rays, as was shown in Figure 2–1, traveling in straight, slowly diverging lines. Every one of these lines will encounter a unique set of tissues along its path. The properties of each such set of tissues, in turn, determine how much of the transiting x-ray energy will be lost before emerging from the body to strike the film cassette.

It is the pattern of x-rays that have *not* interacted with the body's tissues, the **primary x-ray image,** that exposes the cassette and film and (after development of the film) gives rise to the visual image.

Because the beam is diverging, the image of an anatomic region of interest will be somewhat larger than life size. The size of the image of any particular entity in the body, moreover, depends on its distance from the film cassette system; this can cause image **distortion**, which may occasionally lead to confusion unless standardized patient setups are used.

4. ATTENUATION BY A TISSUE DEPENDS ON ITS THICKNESS, DENSITY, AND EFFECTIVE ATOMIC NUMBER, AND ON THE kVp OF THE BEAM

The issue of central importance, then, is the relationship between the rate of **attenuation** of the x-ray beam and the properties of the tissues traversed.

The attenuation of an x-ray beam by any kind of matter may be studied by means of the type of experiment shown in Figure 2–3. X-ray energy is emitted from a tube at a constant rate, and a narrow beam is produced by means of a **collimator.** The intensity of the beam reaching a **detector** some distance away is monitored as different amounts of the material are inserted into the beam path.

It is found that as the **thickness** or **density** of a homogeneous piece of material *increases,* the *attenuation increases;* because the *transmission* through the material decreases, the reading of the *detector* goes *down.* No surprise there. It also happens (although it may be less obvious why) that the *attenuation* also *increases* with an *increase* in the average **atomic number** of the material, and almost always with a *lowering* of the **tube kilovoltage** (Fig. 2–4).

In Figure 2–5, for example, the amount of transmission and the reading of the detector are related to attenuator thickness for two materials, lung and muscle. Lung is chemically similar to muscle, but only about a third as dense. Consequently it attenuates x-rays a third as effectively. With a tube potential of 70 kVp say, the intensity of the beam falls by a factor of a half after passing through about 6 cm of lung, but after only 2 cm of muscle.

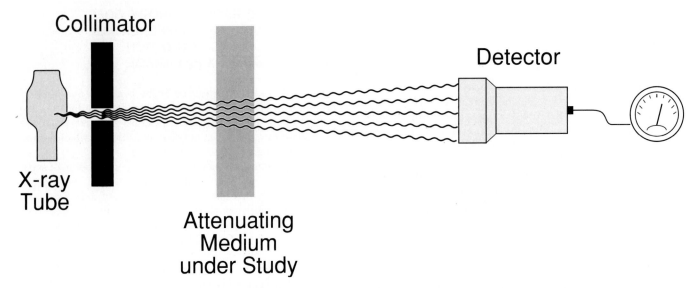

Figure 2–3. Experimental setup for the study of the interaction of an x-ray beam with matter. Variables of interest are the thickness, density, and chemical makeup of the attenuating material and the kVp applied across the tube.

Similarly, the attenuation in compact bone is considerably faster than in muscle. Compact bone is 1.7 times denser than muscle, but even more importantly, its effective atomic number is much greater (12 vs. 7.6).

Finally, as a general rule (with important exceptions): In any medium, the higher the tube potential (kVp), the less the beam will be attenuated. Figure 2–5 compares the intensities of 70- and 120-kVp beams transmitted through different thicknesses of muscle.

In summary, attenuation along a geometric ray path depends on the thicknesses, densities, and chemical compositions (in particular, the effective atomic numbers) of the media encountered and on the x-ray photon energy. For this reason, the x-ray beam emerging from a patient carries information on the spatial distribution of the various attenuating materials within. And one of the most important *controllable* parameters that affect the quality of that information is the tube kilovoltage.

5. THE PRINCIPAL PHOTON–ELECTRON INTERACTION MECHANISMS: PHOTOELECTRIC AND COMPTON EFFECTS

The last section described the attenuation of an x-ray beam in passing through thick amounts of tissue. It is possible to ex-

plain this behavior in terms of the interaction of x-ray energy with individual atoms of the irradiated body.

In some ways, an x-ray beam acts like a stream of hard, compact particles moving at the speed of light. Such x-ray **photons** can collide with atomic electrons, ejecting them from their orbits. There are several qualitatively different mechanisms by which such atomic **ionization** events can occur.

In the simplest of these (Fig. 2–6A), all the energy of the incident photon is imparted to the atomic electron. Some goes into overcoming the electron's attachment to its nucleus. The rest ends up, after the electron has been set free, as its kinetic energy of motion. The probability of occurrence of this **photoelectric** event increases rapidly with the atomic number of the parent atom and (usually) with decreasing x-ray photon energy. Both of these behaviors are consistent with what was said, earlier, about the dependence of beam attenuation on the effective atomic number of the irradiated medium and on the x-ray tube voltage. In diagnostic radiology, most interactions between x-ray photons and bones, and between x-ray photons and the image receptor (intensifying screens and film in the cassette), are by means of the photoelectric effect.

The other photon interaction mechanism of importance to radiography is the **Compton** effect (Fig. 2–6B). Here, only some of the x-ray photon's energy is used in liberating an atomic electron. The rest leaves the scene of the collision as a Compton scatter pho-

Figure 2–4. Attenuation of an x-ray beam by a block of matter increases with its thickness and density and, in general, with its average atomic number. Attenuation usually decreases with an increase in the kVp. The greater the attenuation (i.e., the less the transmission), the lower the reading of a radiation detector, or the optical density (OD) of exposed film.

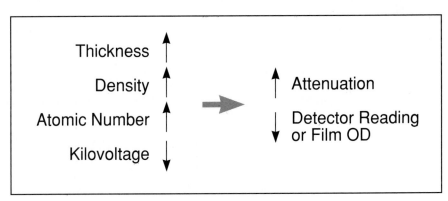

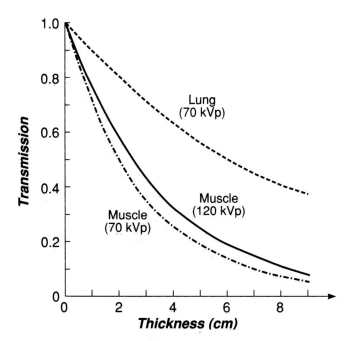

Figure 2–5.   Transmission through a block of soft tissue as a function of its thickness. The curves record measurements made on muscle and lung (with one-third the density of muscle) at 70 kVp and on muscle at 120 kVp. Beam penetration is greater with less dense tissue and with higher kVp.

ton of lower energy. Most interactions between diagnostic x-ray photons and soft tissue are Compton events.

These photoelectric and Compton interactions, occurring within the various tissues of the patient in differing amounts, give rise to shadow patterns in the transmitted x-ray beam. They also underlie the functioning of the image receptor. And finally, in tissues they cause cellular chemical changes that may, very rarely, lead to serious health effects.

6. CAPTURING THE IMAGE ON FILM

The intensity of the x-ray beam emerging from the patient is spatially modulated, containing an x-ray (as opposed to visible light) image of the attenuating materials within the body. This x-ray image may be used to expose film directly, as is sometimes done when especially fine detail is required.

Radiographic film is relatively insensitive to x-ray energy, however, and the x-ray image is usually converted into a usable visual record in a two-step process within a **film cassette:** It is first transformed into a pattern of visible light by the cassette's intensifying screens, and this visible image is then captured permanently on the film (Fig. 2–7).

A cassette consists of two fluorescent **intensifying screens,** between which the film is sandwiched. A *fluorescent* substance emits a pinpoint of visible light wherever an incident x-ray photon undergoes a photoelectric or Compton collision with one of its atoms. It is almost always this fluorescence light that actually exposes the film, rather than the incident x-ray itself. The fluorescent material in a screen is fairly thick, densely packed, and of high atomic number. An x-ray photon is therefore a good deal more likely to interact with the screen (and with the film only indirectly, via the resultant fluorescence light) than with the film itself. Thus, much less x-ray exposure is required to bring about a given level of film darkening when a cassette is used (Fig. 2–8), and the dose to a patient may be tens or even hundreds of times lower.

Radiographic film is a thin sheet of inert plastic coated on both sides with **emulsion.** The emulsion consists of a suspension of microscopic silver iodobromide crystals in a gelatin. During an exposure, visible light photons from the intensifying screens of the cassette strike some of these photosensitive microcrystals. In the subsequent chemical **development** of the film, the crystals thus affected lose all their halide component, becoming specks of metallic silver. In a region of film subject to a higher level of x-irradiation (or, more precisely, to more light

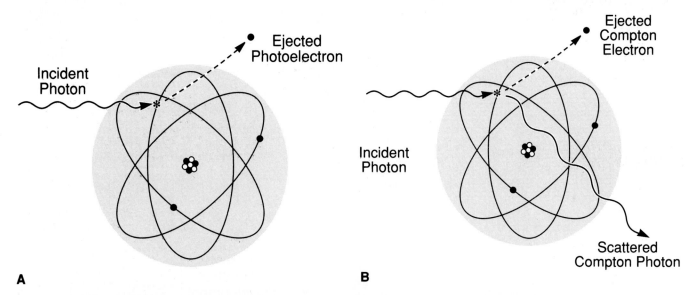

A   **B**

Figure 2–6.   The two principal mechanisms by which diagnostic x-ray photons (of relatively low energies) interact with matter: **A.** In a photoelectric event, all the energy of the incident x-ray photon is expended in ejecting an electron (the photoelectron) from its atomic orbit. **B.** With a Compton event, some of the energy of the incident x-ray photon is used to liberate an electron (the Compton electron) from an atom; the rest reappears in the form of a (reduced energy) Compton scatter x-ray photon.

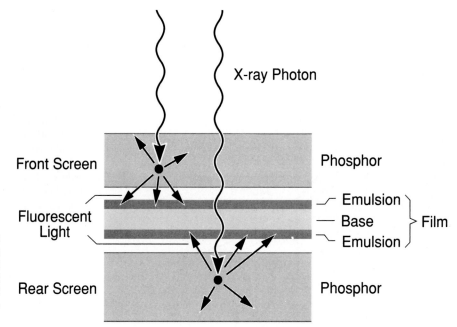

Figure 2–7. In standard radiography, the film is held between the two fluorescent screens of a cassette. An x-ray photon interacts with and stimulates a screen, and the resulting pinpoint of light exposes the film; during development of the film, a tiny cluster of silver grains is deposited there.

from the intensifying screens), a greater fraction of the silver halide microcrystals are converted into colloidal silver during development. The developed film will be more opaque to light, and appear darker to the eye.

7. THE QUALITY OF THE IMAGE: CONTRAST, RESOLUTION, AND NOISE

Any medical imaging system must be judged on its ability to deliver diagnostically useful images. The value of the images depends, in turn, on the contrast and resolution they display and on the presence of interfering noise, distortions, and artifacts.

Radiographic **contrast** refers to the extent to which the various different tissue structures within the body are displayed as different shades of gray in the image (Fig. 2–9). Contrast is determined in part by the inherent properties of the tissues, such as their thickness, density (lung vs. muscle), and chemical composition (bone vs. soft tissue). It is also affected by controllable aspects of the imaging process, such as the technique factors employed and the purity, concentration, and temperature of the film developer fluid.

In some situations, contrast can be enhanced by artificially altering the radiologic properties of the tissues of interest with **contrast agents.** Because of the high atomic number of iodine, intravenously injected iodine compounds, for example, allow

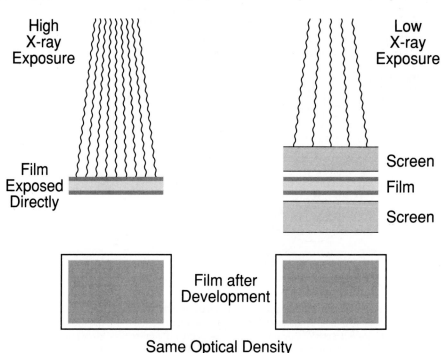

Figure 2–8. A cassette "amplifies" the effect of the x-rays—much less exposure (and radiation dose to the patient) is needed, for film in a cassette, to reach any particular optical density. The level of image sharpness and detail, however, may be less.

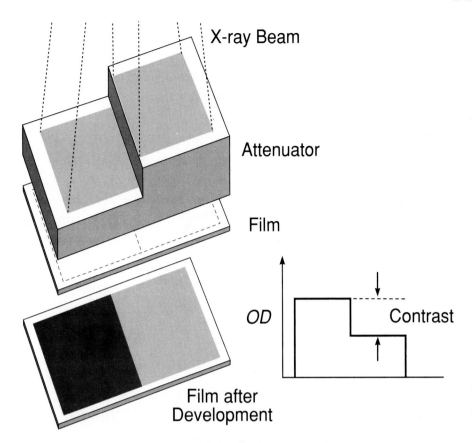

X-ray Beam

Attenuator

Film

OD Contrast

Film after
Development

Figure 2–9. Contrast refers to a relative difference (between two regions) in the level of optical density, radiation intensity, or some other relevant parameter.

the display of blood vessels that would otherwise be indistinguishable from the surrounding soft tissues. Barium finds similar application for the alimentary tract.

The x-ray photons that make it through a body and reach the cassette fall into two general categories. *Primary* photons have undergone no interactions whatsoever within the body. *Scattered* photons, on the other hand, leave the scatter points heading in random, new directions. Image information is carried by the primary photons (or, equivalently, by the absence of primary photons, indicating that interactions have taken place). But the primary x-ray image is degraded, and its contrast diminished, by any scatter x-rays that manage to arrive at the image receptor. (Exactly the same loss of contrast occurs when you see objects through cloudy water [Fig. 2–10].) Keeping the area of the beam as small as possible and placing an **antiscatter grid** between the patient and the image receptor can effectively remove much scatter radiation (Fig. 2–11) and improve contrast.

The **resolution** or *resolving power* of a system is a measure of its proficiency at revealing fine detail. Resolution usually refers specifically to the system's ability to determine that small, high-contrast objects that lie close to one another are, in fact,

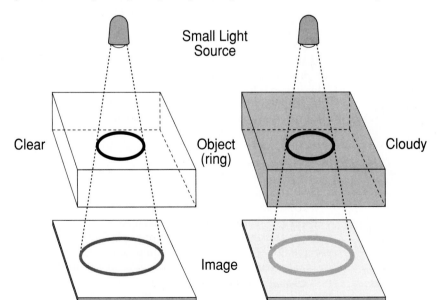

Small Light Source

Clear Object (ring) Cloudy

Image

Figure 2–10. Shadow of a ring in a glass tank that holds clear or cloudy water: an example of a reduction, caused by scatter, in the contrast in an image.

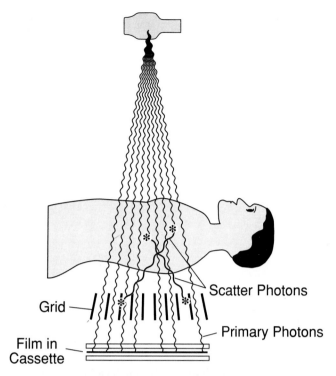

Figure 2–11. Compton scatter photons produced within the patient's body degrade contrast. A grid reduces this loss of contrast: Most of the primary image x-ray photons run parallel to and between the lead leaves of the grid, and reach the film; most Compton scatter photons enter the grid at an angle and are absorbed by the leaves. With a "focused" grid, such as this, the lead sheets are aligned to account for the natural divergence of the x-ray beam.

spatially separate. Resolution is commonly measured by means of a test pattern composed of narrow lead strips, such as that in Figure 2–12 and reported in terms of the number of line pairs per millimeter (lp/mm) that can just barely be distinguished in the image. *Sharpness* refers to the closely related issue of an image's ability to represent sharp edges, for example, at bone surfaces.

As with optical systems (Fig. 2–13), an important determinant of the achievable resolution of a radiographic system is the size of the **focal spot** (the region on the x-ray tube anode's surface where the x-ray beam is actually produced). Diffusion of light within the intensifying screens of the film cassette also contributes to radiographic unsharpness. So may motion of the

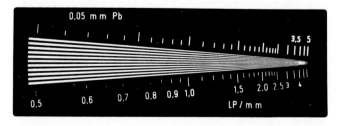

Figure 2–12. The resolving power of an x-ray imaging system is commonly measured by means of a test pattern. Resolution may then be reported as the closeness of the lead lines (expressed in line pairs per millimeter, lp/mm) that are just barely distinguishable in an image. Radiographic images of a test pattern like this one may be seen in Figure 18–6. *(Photo courtesy of Radiation Measurements, Inc. [RMI], Middleton, WI.)*

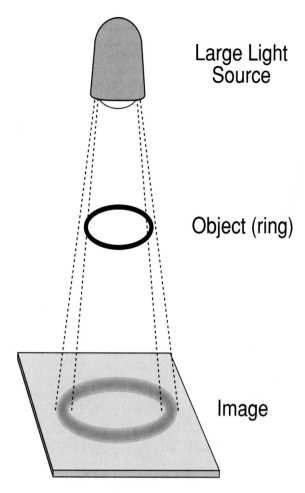

Figure 2–13. As suggested by comparison with Figure 12–10, a smaller source of light leads to sharper shadow patterns. In radiography, a smaller x-ray tube focal spot yields higher-resolution radiographs.

patient, or of the imaging equipment, unless the exposure time is sufficiently short.

Another important characteristic of an image is the **noise** level. The most important form of radiographic noise, **quantum mottle,** is illustrated in the simulated radiographic images of a contrast-detail test device (Fig. 2–14). As fewer x-ray photons are employed in generating the image (but with each photon producing correspondingly more darkening), less image information is transferred to the film and the image quality diminishes—low-contrast and small objects disappear from view. The amount of mottle that occurs depends on the types of film and cassette used and on the technique factors selected. An unacceptably mottled, noisy appearance, as in Figure 2–14B, where each x-ray photon has left a distinct calling card, would normally indicate too fast a screen–film combination coupled with too low an x-ray exposure.

To summarize, the ability of a radiographic system to reveal clinical abnormalities is determined by all three quantities—contrast, resolution, and noise level (Fig. 2–15). It is important to ensure that the equipment and procedures constantly perform at their peak levels, so that contrast and resolution will remain high, and noise and patient dose low. Hence the need for a quality assurance program.

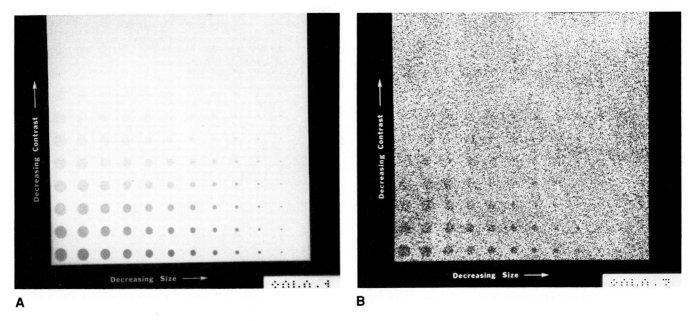

Figure 2–14. A radiograph displays *quantum mottle* if too few x-ray photons are employed in its creation. **A.** This is a simulation of a radiograph (of a contrast-detail quality assurance test device) in which thousands of x-ray photons expose each square millimeter of film. Each photon contributes only slightly to the overall film density, and its effect is not discernible. **B.** "Noise" similar to quantum mottle is displayed. A much smaller number of x-ray photons go into generating the image, but each photon is caused to produce more darkening of the film, and has a noticeable individual impact. Why is there noise in the "background" region in **B** while there is none in **A**? *(Photos from the American College of Radiology Learning File, courtesy of the ACR.)*

8. QUALITY ASSURANCE: OPTIMIZING THE PERFORMANCE OF THE SYSTEM

The quality of an imaging system's performance will depend on the inherent capabilities designed into the equipment, on the skill of the technologists in selecting the best operating parameters for it, and on the care and competence with which it is installed, maintained, and fine-tuned.

Specific diagnostic studies should be carried out, of course, only with suitable imaging systems. A conventional radiographic unit normally will not show soft-tissue malignancies within the cranium, for example, nor will CT generally reveal a fine hairline fracture in bone. And the technique factors

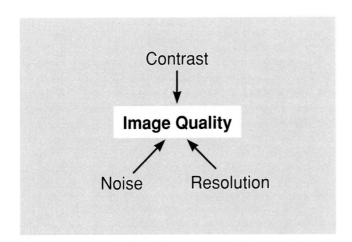

Figure 2–15. Three principal determinants of image quality are contrast, resolution or sharpness, and the noise level.

selected must be appropriate for the particular study and the individual patient. Technique factors that are optimal for chest radiography are radically different from those that should be used for mammography.

But even for the right kind of study and with the best possible technique factors, the images produced may not be as sharp and clear as they should and could be, if the equipment is not working properly. It is the function of a **quality assurance (QA)** or quality control program to assess the constituent parts of the imaging chain objectively and quantitatively and to ensure that all of them are functioning optimally. Quality assurance involves the verification of the accuracy of the timer setting, the high-voltage setting for the generator, and the like. It also addresses seemingly mundane issues like the purity of the film developer chemicals and the uniformity of the light output of view boxes. The weakest link in the imaging chain is not necessarily complicated and high-tech.

Some quality assurance tests involve the formation of images under specific test conditions. Resolution can be ascertained, for example, by means of a *test pattern* imaged in lieu of a patient (see Fig. 2–12). The blurring in the image actually becomes significant somewhat gradually, rather than abruptly at a particular separation of the lead strips, and it is possible and useful to describe and interpret this continuous loss of detail quantitatively, as we shall see. Other tests allow assessment of contrast, noise, and other image characteristics.

One final, but critical, aspect of quality assurance is the determination and control of the levels of dose delivered to the patient and to the staff under various operating conditions. Although the risks associated with the clinical uses of radiation are *extremely* small, they are nonetheless finite. A proper **radiation safety** program can ensure that they are kept to the absolute minimum consistent with good image quality and medical care.

9. WHAT THE X-RAY BEAM DOES TO THE PATIENT'S BODY: BIOLOGIC EFFECTS OF DOSE AND THE NEED FOR A RADIATION SAFETY PROGRAM

X-ray images are formed when high energy *photons* are differentially absorbed or scattered by various tissues of the body. This occurs via photoelectric and Compton events, and, in both processes, atomic electrons are liberated and sent coursing through the tissues. That, unfortunately, is not the end of the story for the *electrons.*

Each of these high-velocity electrons is itself capable of ionizing hundreds or thousands of other molecules. Some of these will be DNA molecules. Others will be molecules (in particular, water) that, once ionized, transform into chemically reactive "free radicals" which can attack DNA. Either way, the net effect is that DNA may be damaged. In nearly all cases the harm is either reparable or insignificant. But occasionally it can lead to carcinogenesis, or to genetic effects manifesting in one's progeny, or, in the case of the irradiation of the fetus, to mental retardation and other congenital abnormalities.

It is therefore clearly necessary to be able to quantify radiation. In the United States, the standard measures of radiation delivered to tissues are the **rad** and the **rem.** The corresponding units in the metric International System (SI) of units, used in much of the world (and increasingly so in the United States), are the **gray (Gy)** and the **sievert (Sv),** which are 100 times greater than the rad and the rem, respectively (Table 2–1). The precise meanings of the gray and the sievert (and of the rad and the rem) are somewhat different, as we shall see, but for virtually all radiologic imaging purposes, they are *numerically* exactly equal (Table 2–2). A third common measure of the quantity of radiation, the **roentgen (R),** is nearly equal numerically to the rad and rem.

Because of their numerical closeness, the rad, the rem, and the roentgen are commonly used interchangeably in clinic situations, and all are referred to loosely as "dose" or "exposure." Later in the book, we shall find advantage in defining all of these terms more carefully.

EXERCISE 2–1.

The entrance skin exposure from a chest radiograph is typically 25 mR. What are the corresponding dose in centigray (cGy) and the dose equivalent in millisieverts (mSv)? Centi- (c) = 1/100, and milli- (m) = 1/1000.

SOLUTION: Numerically, $25 \text{ mR} = 25 \times 10^{-3} \text{ cGy} = 25 \text{ mrad} = 0.25 \text{ mSv} = 25 \text{ mrem}$. Some of these units may seem rather awkward, but they are what people are using.

TABLE 2–1. SI RADIATION UNITS[a]

Measure	United States	SI	Relationship
Dose	rad	Gy	1 Gy = 100 rad
Dose equivalent	rem	Sv	1 Sv = 100 rem
Exposure	R	C/kg	1 R = 2.58×10^{-4} C/kg

[a]The International System (SI) is replacing the system of units commonly used in the United States. The differences among these units will be discussed in later chapters.

TABLE 2–2. WHAT ONE HAS TO REMEMBER, FOR IMAGING PURPOSES, ABOUT THE RADIATION UNITS

The centigray (1 cGy = 1 rad) of dose is commonly used to describe the deposition of ionizing radiation in matter. The millisievert (1mSv = 0.1 rem) of dose equivalent is employed in consideration of the health risks associated with radiation. The roentgen (R) is a measure of the output of an x-ray tube.

For x-ray and gamma ray energy, the rad and the rem are *numerically* identical, and the roentgen is nearly the same as the rad and the rem.

$$1 \text{ rad} = 1 \text{ rem} \sim 1 \text{ R}$$
$$(1 \text{ cGy}) \quad (10 \text{ mSv})$$

When a patient is exposed to x-rays, the deposited dose varies significantly from place to place within the body. Skin exposed directly to the beam receives more dose than do tissues either beneath the surface or outside the beam (which may receive a small amount of scatter radiation). The midline doses from a typical chest examination are mapped out in millisieverts in Figure 2–16. Dose equivalent to skin where the beam enters is 0.25 mSv (25 mrem), but only a few percent of that where the beam leaves the body (and enters the film cassette). From this, it should be apparent that the statement "the dose from a chest film is 25 mrem" would be more correct as "the dose equivalent to skin at beam entrance is 0.25 mSv."

How much radiation does a centigray or a millisievert represent? The following figures may provide some perspective. The average American receives the equivalent of 3 mSv (300 mrem) to the whole body over the course of a year from natural sources such as cosmic rays, radioactive materials in the soil, radioactive materials occurring naturally in the body, and radon gas that seeps from the ground into homes and is inhaled. A dose of 100 mSv (10 rem) to the entire blood pool leads to a detectable increase in the number of chromosomal aberrations. An acute (rapidly delivered) 1-Sv (100-rem) dose of whole body irradiation may produce mild sensations of sickness, which soon pass. Roughly half of all people exposed to 4.5 Sv (450 rem) of whole-body irradiation will die within weeks from loss of critical blood-forming tissues. Finally, a typical course of 20 radiotherapy treatment may involve the total delivery of 50 to 60 Gy (5000 to 6000 rad), but only to a rather small part of the body.

In radiology, skin doses are typically of the order of only 1 mSv (100 mrem), give or take a factor of 2 or 4. For the nonpregnant patient, the radiation issue of greatest concern is cancer. The risk of a cancer being caused by a carefully executed procedure is very small. The likelihood of dying of cancer from a chest x-ray, for example, is less than one in a million—perhaps much less than the risk associated with *not* having the radiograph, when need for it is indicated. If everyone in the country had an annual chest film, however, and if our risk estimates are correct, then several tens or hundreds of us would die each year because of it. And yet, lives might be saved through such a screening program, by virtue of the early discovery of unsuspected cases of cancer and cardiovascular disease. All of this raises interesting and important societal, as well as ethical, cost/benefit questions.

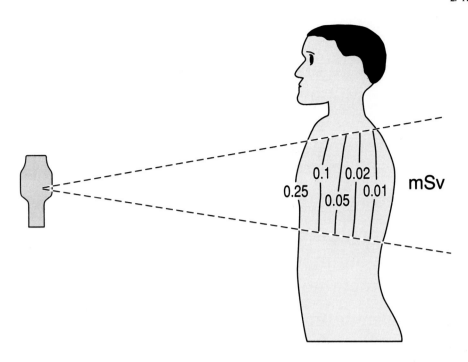

Figure 2–16. Midline doses, at different depths in the body, from a typical chest examination. It is incorrect to say that the dose from the procedure is 0.25 mSv (25 mrem).

A *uniform* dose of 1 mSv (100 mrem) to the *whole body* will increase the probability of eventual death by cancer, we believe, by about 4 parts in 100,000. That is, our current estimate of the risk rate is about 4×10^{-5} per mSv: If 100,000 people each were to receive a 1 mSv whole-body exposure, about 4 of them would be expected to die prematurely from cancer because of the exposure. This is in addition to the 20,000 of them who would die of cancer anyway, an observation that is irrelevant if you are concerned about the *increment* in risk brought about by the additional exposure from a procedure. If only a portion of the body is irradiated, as in any form of radiography, the risks are correspondingly smaller.

Radiologists and their support personnel are allowed by law an annual work-related, whole-body exposure of at most 50 mSv (5 rem). Most medical radiation workers actually receive less than a fiftieth of the limit. If you received an annual occupational dose of 1 mSv (100 mrem) over a professional life of 30 years, then the probability of your eventually dying from a radiation-induced cancer would be on the order of 1 in 1000. You face about the same 0.1% lifetime risk of dying in a natural catastrophe, such as a tornado, flood, or earthquake, and the odds of being killed in an auto accident are more than an order of magnitude (factor of ten) greater than that.

The moral of the story of dose is simple: For both patients and medical staff the risks are very low *if* one is intelligent and careful in the use of radiation.

II

Scientific Foundation

Part 1

Energy and Matter

Chapter 3

Motion and Force

1. **Velocity and the Rate at Which It Changes**
2. **Units: A Matter of Convention and Convenience**
3. **The Acceleration of an Object Is Proportional to the Force Acting on It**
4. **Newton's Apple: Constant Acceleration in a Uniform Gravitational Field**
   Appendix 3–1. Keeping Track of How Things Change: A Brief Review of Functions and Graphs

X-ray tubes, TV cameras and monitor tubes, and image intensifiers all make critical use of electrons accelerating through vacuums. To appreciate how such equipment operates, it is necessary to understand the behavior of an electron in an electric field. As a guide, we shall first explore briefly the similar, but perhaps more familiar, situation of an apple falling in a uniform gravitational field.

This chapter and the next should serve to refresh your memory on some basic and relevant concepts about motions, forces, fields, and waves—all of which play significant roles in what follows. Happily, the level at which we shall need to consider these ideas is very elementary. You may wish to go over the review material in the Appendix at the end of this chapter before proceeding.

1. VELOCITY AND THE RATE AT WHICH IT CHANGES

It is often possible to describe the interesting aspects of a physical entity in terms of its motions.

Imagine that as you sit, an object moves past you in a straight line and at constant speed. In this case, it is easy to calculate the magnitude $v_{constant}$ of the velocity. If over the period of time t the object moves the distance x, then the speed is just $v_{constant} = x/t$. The standard International System (SI) units of distance and time are the meter (m) and the second (s), respectively, so the unit of velocity is the meter per second (m/s or $m \cdot s^{-1}$). In Figure 3–1A, our object's distance x from some reference point is displayed as a function of the time t. The velocity x/t appears as the *slope* of this curve.

Velocity is a meaningful and useful concept, of course, even when the speed is not constant. The *average speed* is ob-

tained by dividing the total distance traveled by the total time it took. But we can be much more precise than that, and describe the *instantaneous speed* at any particular time. To emphasize this point, we can express the velocity at time t as the function $v(t)$. And if an object moves through the small distance Δx over the short time span Δt, then its instantaneous speed is $v(t) = \Delta x/\Delta t$. In Figure 3–1B, the velocity at time t' is shown as the slope of the curve at that time. The symbol Δ will be used throughout this book to represent a small amount of, or increment in, something.

In the limiting case in which Δx and Δt are simultaneously allowed to become extremely small, their ratio is called the "derivative of x with respect to t" and written dx/dt. The ideas in this book will be presented, however, without making use of calculus.

The velocity of a moving object refers not only to its speed, but also to the direction of its motion. Velocity is therefore said to be a **vector** quantity, and may be represented by an arrow (Fig. 3–2). The arrow points in the direction of the motion, and its length is proportional to the magnitude of the velocity, or speed. For the time being, we shall be concerned with processes that can be represented, at least approximately, in one dimension. That is, we shall arrange for the motions and forces in any problem all to lie along the same straight line. It will therefore not be necessary to use vector notation, and we can simply add or subtract velocities (or other vector quantities, such as accelerations and forces), depending on whether they point in the same or opposite direction.

EXERCISE 3–1.

Traveling at nearly constant speed on the freeway from Washington, DC, to Annapolis, MD, a car covers a distance of 40 miles in 50 minutes. What was its velocity?

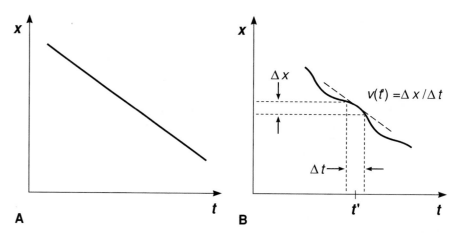

Figure 3–1. Velocity, shown as the relationship between distance traveled, x, and time, t.
A. For constant velocity, the speed is simply x/t.
B. The velocity at time t' is indicated by the slope, $\Delta x/\Delta t$, of $v(t)$ at that time.

SOLUTION: The *average* speed was $v = x/t = 40$ miles$/50$ min $= 0.8$ mile$/$min $= 48$ miles$/$h.

___ **EXERCISE 3–2.** _____

In passing another vehicle, the car of Exercise 3–1 briefly speeded up to 70 miles$/$h. How many feet did it travel in 2 seconds when it was going about 60 miles$/$h?

SOLUTION: 60 miles$/$h $=$ (60 miles$/$h)(5280 ft$/$mile) $\times$ (1/3600 h$/$s) $= 88$ ft$/$s. The distance travelled in two seconds was $\Delta x = v(t) \cdot \Delta t = (88$ ft$/$s)(2 seconds) $= 176$ feet.

An object that is not traveling with constant velocity is said to be accelerating. The **acceleration,** denoted a, is defined as the *rate at which the velocity is changing*. Suppose that at time t, and over a brief interval of duration Δt, the speed changes from v m$/$s to the slightly greater speed $v + \Delta v$ m$/$s. The acceleration at that moment is $a(t) = \Delta v/\Delta t$. If the speed of an object increases from 6.98 to 7.04 m$/$s over $\Delta t = 0.004$ s, for example, then the acceleration is $(7.04 - 6.98$ m$/$s$)/(0.004$ s$) = 15$ m$/$s^2. Because the SI units of velocity are meters per second, m$/$s, the rate at which velocity is changing with time should be expressed in meters per second per second, and abbreviated m$/$s^2 or m $\cdot$ s^{-2}.

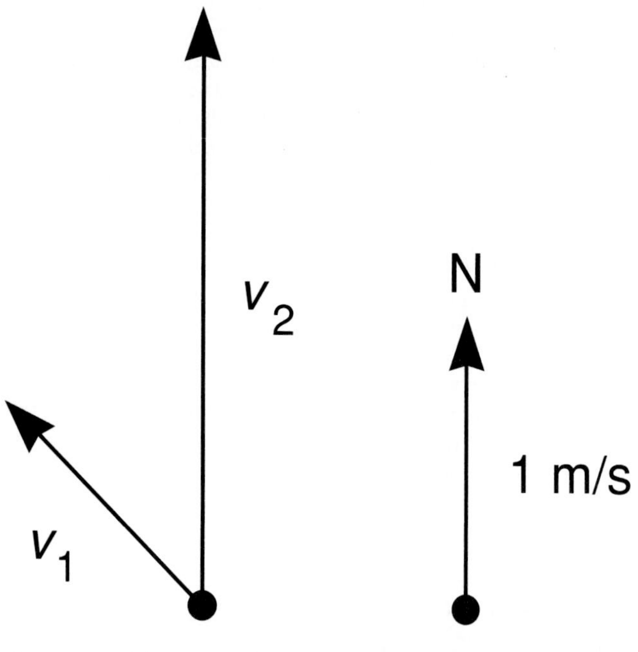

___ **EXERCISE 3–3.** _____

An apple is falling to Earth. Its velocity is 4.200 m$/$s at some time of observation, 4.494 m$/$s 30 milliseconds after that, 4.788 m$/$s after another 30 milliseconds, and so on. What is its rate of acceleration? Plot its acceleration, its velocity, and its distance $x(t)$ above the ground as functions of time.

SOLUTION: The velocity increases by 0.294 m$/$s every 0.03 second, and its rate of change with time is thus downward and of magnitude $a = 9.8$ m$/$s^2. The acceleration is constant, in this example. Because the rate of increase velocity is constant, the velocity is *linear* in (directly proportional to) elapsed time.

2. UNITS: A MATTER OF CONVENTION AND CONVENIENCE

People don't count for the sake of counting. We count apples or patients. Minutes or hours. Kilometers or miles to go before we sleep. We count to keep track of *amounts* of things. And it is obviously every bit as important to be aware of the *units* in which the things are being counted (inches vs. feet vs. kilometers vs. . . .) as it is to know the final tally itself.

The kilometer is no more or less natural a unit of length than the inch, nor is the liter a better measure of volume than the gallon. The choice of units is determined solely by convention and convenience. It greatly simplifies complex calculations, however, if a unified, internally consistent set of units is adopted.

In 1791 the **meter (m)** was defined by the Paris Academy of Sciences as one ten-millionth of the distance from the equator to the North Pole, and the **second (s)** as the time for a pendulum 1m long to make a single swing. With some refinement, these units, together with the **kilogram (kg)** of mass, the **ampere (A)** of electric current, the **mole (mol)** of molecules, the **kelvin (K)** of thermodynamic temperature, and the **candela (cd)** of luminous intensity form the basis for the standard **Interna-**

Figure 3–2. Vector quantities may be represented by arrows. The reference arrow on the right indicates North, and its length corresponds to a velocity of 1 m/s. Object 1 is moving Northwest at 1 m/s. Object 2 is traveling twice as fast, due North.

tional System (SI) of units, also known as the **MKS** or **metric system** (Table 3–1). These seven entities are the so-called SI Base Units, and all other measurables can be expressed in terms of them or combinations of them. Speed, for example, is reported in the units m/s, and the "derived unit" of energy, the *joule* (*J*), is just a shorthand notation for kg · m²/s².

In some situations, more convenience is gained than lost in employing non-SI units. In dealing with atomic phenomena, for example, the **electron volt (eV)** of energy is frequently easier to use than the joule, where 1 eV = 1.6×10^{-19} J. And the derived unit of dose of ionizing radiation in common usage in the United States is still the rad, even though the corresponding SI unit, the gray (Gy), which is exactly 100 times larger, is rapidly gaining widespread acceptance. With a few exceptions (in particular, the electron volt), we shall stick with the SI system, but from time to time we shall include the conventional units in parentheses.

Some prefixes used with metric quantities are listed in Table 3–2. For example, 5×10^{-7} m, the wavelength of green light, can be expressed also as 500 nm or 0.5 μm. The energies involved in chemical reactions tend to be of the order of electron volts per molecule; x-ray energies are typically tens of kilo-electron volts; and nuclear reactions involve mega-electron volts per nucleus.

3. THE ACCELERATION OF AN OBJECT IS PROPORTIONAL TO THE FORCE ACTING ON IT

Physics may be thought of as the systematic study of the most fundamental cause-and-effect relationships underlying physical phenomena in the material world. One of its primary objectives is to explain the complexity of physical reality in terms of a few, relatively simple "laws." Among the best known and most useful of these laws are the three that bear Isaac Newton's name. Indeed, the publication of his *Philosophiae Naturalis Principia Mathematica* in 1687 marked, as much as any other single event, the beginnings of modern science.

Newton's First Law observes that the state of motion of a body does not change unless something is done to change it, that is, unless a force is applied to it. For example, the velocity of an isolated body (with no forces at all acting on it) remains constant over time. The First Law implies that a rocket moving toward the Andromeda Galaxy at 7000 m/s, relative to the Solar System, will remain in that state as long as it experiences negligible gravitational or frictional forces, and keeps its engines turned off. Similarly, a hockey puck will slide forever at a constant speed and in a straight line on an "ideal" frictionless horizontal table. The real world may seem to be at variance with this (things do slow down), but only because we are usually unaware of the frictional forces at play.

Newton's Second Law describes what happens when a force *is* applied to an object: Its rate of acceleration (or deceleration), *a*, will be directly proportional to the net **force,** *F*, acting on it, and inversely proportional to its mass, *m*. That is, *a* = *F*/*m*, or equivalently,

$$F = m \cdot a \qquad (3.1)$$

The SI unit of mass is the kilogram (kg), so Equation 3.1 reveals that the SI unit of force is the kg · m/s². The unit of force is used so widely that it has been given a special name, the newton (N), where 1 N = 1 kg · m/s².

Let us accept, as the meaning of the term "force," the intuitive notion of a push or pull; the harder the push, the greater the force. The response of an object to any such force is then

TABLE 3–1. THE SEVEN BASIC SI UNITS AND SOME DERIVED SI UNITS

SI Basic Units		SI Derived Units	
Quantity	*SI Unit*	*Quantity*	*SI unit*
Length	meter (m)	Frequency	hertz (Hz = s⁻¹, cycle/s)
Mass	kilogram (kg)	Force	newton (N = kg · m/s²)
Time	second (s)	Pressure	pascal (Pa = N/m²)
Electric current	ampere (A)	Work, energy	joule (J = N · m)
Temperature	kelvin (K)	Power	watt (W = J/s)
Amount of substance	mole (mol)	Electric charge	coulomb (C = A · s)
Luminous intensity	candela (cd)	Electric potential	volt (V = J/C)
		Resistance	ohm (Ω = V/A)
1 in. = 2.54 cm		Capacitance	farad (F = C/V)
1 pound = ~0.454 kg		Magnetic flux density	tesla (T)
		Temperature	degree Celsius (°C)

electron volt: 1 eV = 1.6×10^{-19} J

SI Radiation Units

Quantity	*SI Unit*	*Conventional Unit*	*Relationship*
Intensity	J/m² · s = W/m²		
Exposure	C/kg	roentgen (R)	$1 R = 2.58 \times 10^{-4}$ C/kg
Dose, kerma	gray (Gy = J/kg)	rad	1 Gy = 100 rad
Dose equivalent	sievert (Sv = J/kg)	rem	1 Sv = 100 rem
Activity	becquerel (Bq = s⁻¹)	curie (Ci)	$1 Ci = 3.7 \times 10^{10}$ Bq

TABLE 3–2. SOME PREFIXES TO UNITS

Prefix	Abbreviation	Power of Ten
pico-	p	10^{-12}
nano-	n	10^{-9}
micro-	μ	10^{-6}
milli-	m	10^{-3}
centi-	c	10^{-2}
kilo-	k	10^{3}
mega-	M	10^{6}
giga-	G	10^{9}

described by Equation 3.1. The maximum rate of acceleration of a small taxi increases with the power of its engine, for example, but decreases with the number of radiologists in the back seat. The force F to be used in Equation 3.1 should be the (vector) sum of *all* the forces acting on the object, including that of friction.

EXERCISE 3–4.

Suppose a 5-kg basket of apples experiences a constant gravitational force of 49 N. At what rate will it accelerate?

SOLUTION: By Equation 3.1, $a = F/m = (49 \text{ kg} \cdot \text{m/s}^2)/(5 \text{ kg}) = 9.8 \text{ m} \cdot \text{s}^{-2}$.

4. NEWTON'S APPLE: CONSTANT ACCELERATION IN A UNIFORM GRAVITATIONAL FIELD

Equation 3.1 reveals how the motion of an object is affected by the application of any kind of force whatsoever. By positing a particular functional form for the gravitational force and calling upon the Second Law, Newton was able to describe quantitatively the parabolic trajectory of a thrown object, the elliptic paths of the planets around the Sun, and the swinging of a pendulum.

Consider the particularly simple and familiar situation of an apple hanging from a tree. The gravitational force on the apple is proportional to its mass m, a claim that can be expressed more compactly as

$$F_{grav} = m \cdot g \qquad (3.2)$$

The more massive the apple (which depends on how many atoms it contains and what kinds), the more the Earth pulls downward on it. The constant of proportionality g is measured to be 9.8 m/s². (The units of the other terms in Equation 3.2 reveal that the units of g must be m · s⁻², even if it is not yet obvious why.) The apple does not fall because the tree pulls *upward* on it with exactly the same force, so that the net force on it is zero.

It is useful to couch this in slightly different language: Because of its mass, the Earth gives rise to a gravitational **field.** Near any point at the Earth's surface, the gravitational field is **uniform,** that is, everywhere of the same magnitude and pulling in the same direction (downward). The gravitational field strength, or force per unit mass on any object in the field, is of magnitude $g = F_{grav}/m$. The value of g is determined entirely by

the mass and radius of the Earth, and is independent of the mass, shape, position, or state of motion of any small object moving through its gravitational field.

EXERCISE 3–5.

A 3-kg basket is sitting on the ground. How much force is the Earth exerting on it? How much force must you apply to lift it?

SOLUTION: By Equation 3.2, the Earth pulls the basket down with a force of (3 kg)(9.8 m/s²) = 29.4 kg · m/s² = 29.4 N. The surface of the Earth must be pushing up on it with exactly the same amount of force. To lift the basket, you must apply a tiny bit more force than that.

EXERCISE 3–6.

On the smaller planet Mars, the gravitational field is much weaker, and g is only 3.7 m · s⁻². What is the pull on a 3-kg mass?

SOLUTION: $F_{grav} = m \cdot g = (3 \text{ kg})(3.7 \text{ m/s}^2) = 11.1 \text{ N}$.

What happens when the stem of our hanging apple snaps? The Second Law of motion, Equation 3.1, is a general relationship for the rate of change of velocity of an object in response to the net force acting on it. Equation 3.2, on the other hand, describes one particular kind of force. When an apple falls in a gravitational field (Fig. 3–3), both relationships apply. The dynamics of the situation may then be determined by using the expression for gravitational force, $F_{grav} = m \cdot g$, di-

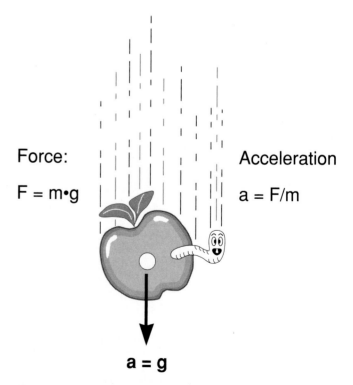

Force:

$F = m \cdot g$

Acceleration

$a = F/m$

$a = g$

Figure 3–3. The acceleration of a falling apple is determined both by the magnitude of the force acting on it (F = m · g) and by its mass (since a = F/m). In a gravitational field, a = g.

rectly in the equation of motion, $F = m \cdot a$. The result of this synthesis

$$m \cdot g = m \cdot a \qquad (3.3)$$

leads immediately to the value of the acceleration: $a = g$. That is, the acceleration of a body is (in the absence of frictional forces) independent of its mass. This may be a bit puzzling and, indeed, until the time of Galileo, everybody accepted Aristotle's assurance that heavier bodies do fall faster. Not so. According to Equation 3.3, the more massive the apple, the greater the gravitational force ($m \cdot g$) acting on it. But also the greater its inertia, and the greater the force needed to accelerate it ($m \cdot a$). The two effects cancel, and the apple's acceleration ends up being independent of its mass.

APPENDIX 3–1. Keeping Track of How Things Change: A Brief Review of Functions and Graphs

Suppose you wish to monitor the height and speed of your freshman physics text as it drops from a high balcony. Its height above the ground, y, at any instant, will be a function of the time, t, elapsed since the beginning of its fall. This connection may be written in mathematical shorthand as $y(t)$. y and t are said to be the "dependent" and "independent" **variables,** respectively, of the **function** $y(t)$.

There are three common ways to represent a functional dependence of one variable on another, that is, to demonstrate the manner in which something varies in response to changes in something else: a table, a graph, and a mathematical formula.

For the falling book, the dependence of y on t, $y(t)$, could be determined experimentally by photographing the event with a strobe light flashing every half-second. The timer starts at $t = 0$ as the book begins its descent from a height of, say, 20 meters: $y(0) = 20$ m. Values of y obtained at the flashes and the times t to which they correspond are recorded in **tabular** form in Table 3–3. The use of decimal points for both variables serves as a reminder that their values are determined experimentally, and subject to experimental error, as does the subscript "expt."

The pairs of numbers (t, y_{expt}), with representative error bars, can also be displayed as a *graph*, as in Figure 3–4. By convention, the independent variable is usually plotted along the abscissa (horizontal axis) and the dependent along the ordinate. Note that the meanings of both axes in Figure 3–4 are clearly identified, as are the units employed. An effective way to create problems for yourself, and for your readers when you publish, is to fail to define and indicate clearly your variables and the axes of your graphs.

The preceding experimental results are consistent with theory. As revealed within the plummeting text itself, the instantaneous height above the floor of a falling object is related to the time elapsed since release by means of a mathematical **formula,** $y_{\text{theo}}(t) = y(0) - \frac{1}{2}g \cdot t^2$. The constant $g = 9.8$ m/s^2 is a measure of the strength of the gravitational field at the Earth's surface. The minus sign occurs because "up" corresponds to positive values of y, while the acceleration is downward. This formula may be graphed by calculating a table of values $y_{\text{theo}}(t)$

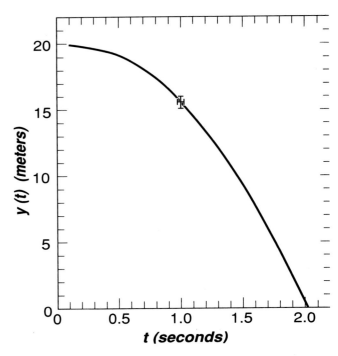

Figure 3–4. Experimental study of a physics book falling from a shelf. Measurements are made every half-second (±0.05 s) with an accuracy of ±0.5 m. Note that the axes are clearly labeled with the appropriate variables and units, and that error bars provide estimates of experimental accuracy.

for representative values of t (Table 3–3). Plotting then yields a diagram similar to Figure 3–4.

It is often helpful to classify functions according to the way in which the dependent variable varies with the independent variable. Consider the expression for the instantaneous velocity of a body in free fall: $v(t) = -g \cdot t$. The independent variable is raised only to the first power ($t^1 = t$), and a graph of $v(t)$ against t is a straight line. The function $v(t)$ is therefore said to be directly proportional to t, or **linear** in t. By comparison, the function $y_{\text{theo}}(t) = y(0) - \frac{1}{2}g \cdot t^2$ contains the independent variable raised to the second power, t^2, and is said to be quadratic in t.

Finally, you should bear in mind that any measurement or statistical estimation is subject to error, and that a graph or function is only an approximate representation of reality. It is therefore every bit as important to assess and report on the reliability of a number (e.g., the **error bars** on a graph) as it is to

TABLE 3–3. EXAMPLE OF THE FALLING BOOK: DISTANCE ABOVE THE FLOOR AS A FUNCTION OF TIME

Measured		Calculated	
t (s)	$y_{\text{expt}}(t)$ (m)	t (s)	$y_{\text{theo}}(t)$ (m)
0.0	20.0	0	20
0.5	18.9	$\frac{1}{2}$	18.78
1.0	15.0	1	15.10
1.5	8.8	$1\frac{1}{2}$	8.98
2.0	0.0	2	0.40

determine "the number" (the location of the data point) in the first place.

Likewise, you should include no more digits in a number than are truly significant. Consider, for example, the second entry in Table 3–3 in the $y_{expt}(t)$ column. This number reflects an average of the readings reported by three separate measuring devices: 18.9321, 18.8622, and 18.9162. But presenting it as 18.9035 would have implied a very high degree of accuracy, which is not warranted. The number 18.9 gives a much better idea of how trustworthy the reported measurement really is.

We have just plotted a well-known formula with well-known values for the constants involved. Much of science involves the converse process, in which a researcher attempts to find formulas and constants that can be fitted closely to experimentally obtained data sets. That can happen in three quite different ways.

In the ideal case, the functional forms of the relevant formulas are known in advance from a basic understanding of nature, as are the numerical parameters. The new data might then serve to confirm a novel aspect of the theory.

Much more commonly, a problem is partially understood, and the experimental data allow one to fill in some of the missing pieces. It is known with assurance, for example, that the activity (number of decays per second) of a pure sample of any radioisotope will decrease exponentially with time, but the half-life of a particular radionuclide is obtained by curve fitting.

In the worst-case scenario, the true functional relationship between dependent and independent variables is not known. A cleverly guessed-at formula with the right general shape and several fitted constants may be useful, however, for storing and concisely expressing the results of an experiment, even if the formula cannot (yet) be derived from more basic ideas.

It is suggested that whenever you see a new formula or graph, you should determine which of these three situations is occurring.

Electric and Magnetic Fields
and Electromagnetic Waves

The preceding last chapter described the motion of an apple in a gravitational field. An electron in an electric field, such as that of an x-ray tube or TV monitor, behaves much the same. But electrons are more interesting in other ways.

A moving charged body, such as an electron traveling through a wire or a nucleus spinning on an axis, produces a magnetic field. Such a moving charge also experiences a force when in the presence of an applied magnetic field. These two related but separate phenomena have important practical implications. The first, for example, is responsible for the operation of an electromagnet. The second underlies magnetic resonance imaging.

Electric and magnetic fields are both involved in the creation and propagation of light and x-ray energy, and in their interactions with matter. Much of the science and technology of medical imaging is concerned precisely with those phenomena.

Finally, waves will appear on a number of occasions in this book, in a variety of guises. Electromagnetic radiation, ultrasound, even the electrons whirling about within atoms all display wavelike properties. We shall even explore the ways that entire images can be represented as combinations of waves. Hence the chapter concludes with a brief introduction to wave phenomena.

You can produce such a field by attaching the terminals of a battery to two parallel, closely spaced metal plates. Some electrons are drawn away from one plate, leaving it with a net positive charge, and an equal number of electrons are forced onto the other. This creates a nearly uniform electric field in the region between them.

Chapter 3, Section 4, defined the strength of the gravitational field as the force per unit mass. In direct analogy, the *electric field strength*, $\mathcal{E}$, at a point in space is defined to be the electric force F_ε per unit charge that any charged body would experience there:

$$\mathcal{E} = F_\varepsilon \, / \, q \qquad (4.1)$$

As the charge q increases, so also does the force, but their ratio remains the same. So the field strength has a unique meaning, independent of the magnitudes or kinds of charges that happen to be within the field. The SI unit for electric charge is the Coulomb (C); from Equation 4.1, the SI unit for electric field must be the newton per coulomb (N/C), or $kg \cdot m/s^2 \cdot C$.

By Equation 4.1, the force on an electric charge is proportional to the strength of the local electric field, $F_\varepsilon = \mathcal{E} \cdot q$. Doubling $\mathcal{E}$ would have the same effect on a "free falling" charge as would doubling the gravitational field strength g for a falling apple: Both the force on the object and its rate of acceleration would increase by a factor of 2.

1. A CHARGE PRODUCES AN ELECTRIC FIELD, AND A CHARGE SITUATED IN AN ELECTRIC FIELD EXPERIENCES A FORCE

Chapter 3 ended with a discussion of an apple falling in a uniform gravitational field. Similar arguments apply to the motion of a charged particle in a uniform electric field (Fig. 4–1).

2. ELECTRONS ACCELERATING IN THE ELECTRIC FIELDS OF X-RAY TUBES, IMAGE INTENSIFIERS, AND TV MONITOR TUBES

We shall be very concerned with the motions of *electrons*, in particular, in various electric fields, such as within an x-ray tube or within an atom. Because of its importance in science,

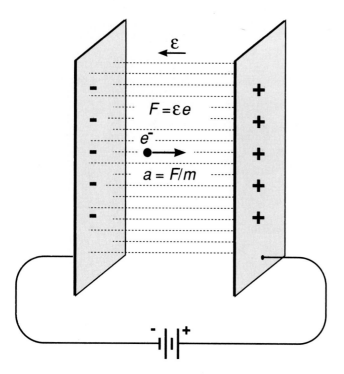

Figure 4–1. An electric field of strength ε has been created between a pair of parallel metal plates by connecting them to a battery. An electron of charge e "falls freely" in this electric field with an acceleration of $a = \varepsilon \cdot e/m$.

the charge on an electron, 1.6×10^{-19} C, has been honored with its own special symbol, e (Table 4–1). The force on an electron in a field of strength ε is then $\varepsilon \cdot e$. The acceleration of an electron in a vacuum in a uniform electric field may be determined by combining this particular expression for the force with the Second Law of motion, $F = m_e \cdot a$; then

$$\varepsilon \cdot e = m_e \cdot a \qquad (4.2)$$

from which $a = \varepsilon \cdot e/m_e$. The rate of acceleration is thus proportional to the electric field strength. Unlike the case of the apple in the gravitational field (Equation 3.3), here the mass of the electron, m_e, does not drop out of the picture.

EXERCISE 4–1.

Suppose that the electric field between the cathode and anode of an x-ray tube is approximately uniform (in reality, it is not). With a certain applied tube voltage, the field strength is 10,000 N/C. What is the acceleration of an electron in this field?

SOLUTION: From Equation 4.2, $a = \varepsilon \cdot e/m_e = (10,000 \text{ kg} \cdot m/s^2 \cdot \text{C})(1.6 \times 10^{-19} \text{ C})/(9.11 \times 10^{-31} \text{ kg}) = 1.8 \times 10^{15} \text{ m/s}^2$.

TABLE 4–1. SOME IMPORTANT PHYSICAL CONSTANTS

Quantity	Symbol	Value
Charge on electron	e	1.602×10^{-19} C
Mass of electron	m_e	9.110×10^{-31} kg
Speed of light	c	2.9979×10^{8} m/s
Planck's constant	h	6.626×10^{-34} J $\cdot$ s
Avogadro's number	N_a	6.022×10^{23} molecules/mol
Absolute zero	$0°K$	$-273.15°C$

EXERCISE 4–2.

A car that goes from 0 to 28 m/s (100 km/h) in 10 seconds accelerates at the average of 2.8 m/s². What electric field strength is required to accelerate an electron by that amount?

SOLUTION: With $a = 2.8$ m/s² in Equation 4.2, and e and m_e from Table 4–1, $\varepsilon = 1.6 \times 10^{-11}$ N/C.

Falling apples and electrons in the electric field of a diagnostic x-ray tube obey Newton's laws, and are said to be described by "classical" physics. Classical physics provides a powerful mathematical formalism for dealing with these, and much more complex, problems. The basic question it answers is this: If we know the initial positions and velocities of all the constituent parts of a physical system, and the forces among them, what will be their positions and velocities at a later time? One of the great insights of Galileo and Newton was that acceleration is the quantity of central importance. The more abstract ideas of mass and force are intimately related to it, and follow from it. The other characteristics of the system, such as its shape, are usually of secondary or no importance.

For electrons bound to atoms, or moving through matter, or accelerated by strong fields up to velocities near that of light, the simple rules break down. The concepts of position, velocity, mass, and time lose their ordinary meanings, and classical physics no longer applies. Instead, the radically different approaches of quantum mechanics and relativity theory must be employed. More about that in Chapters 6 and 7.

3. THE INVERSE SQUARE (COULOMBIC) ELECTROSTATIC FIELD

Until now we have been concerned with force fields that are uniform—the force on an object is independent of its position in the field. Although easy to discuss, such fields are rarely encountered in the real world.

The *Coulombic* or electrostatic force between two small charged bodies, for example, is proportional to the charge on each, as you would expect. Its strength is not independent of their relative positions, however, but rather decreases with the square of the distance, r, between them, that is, as $1/r^2$.

Consider, for example, the Coulombic force that binds an electron to an atomic nucleus. It is sometimes useful (albeit an oversimplification, for many purposes) to view an atom as consisting of a massive, positively charged nucleus surrounded by orbiting, negative electrons. The nucleus of the hydrogen atom, for example, consists of one proton, bearing a charge of magnitude equal to the electron charge, but of positive sign ($+e$). The Coulombic force of attraction between the proton and a single electron (charge $= -e$) in an orbit of radius r is

$$F_\varepsilon = k \cdot e^2/r^2 \qquad (4.3)$$

(Fig. 4–2). Because of the form of the dependence on r, this is said to be an *inverse square* force. The electric *field* produced by the nucleus, and experienced by the electron, is of magnitude $\varepsilon = k \cdot e/r^2$. The constant k is found experimentally to have the value 9×10^9 N $\cdot$ m²/C².

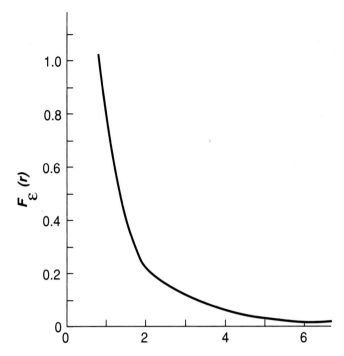

Figure 4–2. The Coulombic electric force between two point charges decreases with the square of the distance between them, that is, as $1/r^2$. For convenience, the units of this diagram have been adjusted so that $F_\varepsilon(1) = 1$.

4. A MOVING CHARGE PRODUCES A MAGNETIC FIELD, AND A CHARGE MOVING THROUGH A MAGNETIC FIELD EXPERIENCES A FORCE

In 1820, Hans Christian Oersted found that an **electric current** (flow of charge) in a wire generates a **magnetic field,** in which a compass needle will align (Fig. 4–3).

A diagnostic modality, *magnetoencephalography* (MEG), is being developed to monitor the very weak magnetic fields produced by electric currents within the body. The exquisitely sensitive superconducting quantum interference device (SQUID) is used to measure the biomagnetism arising from electrical activity in the brain, the heart, and elsewhere. Although still in an early stage of development, MEG has already indicated some clinical promise, as in the noninvasive study of epilepsy.

Soon after Oersted's discovery, André Marie Ampère found a quite different relationship between moving charges and magnetism: Any charged body passing through a region in which there is already a magnetic field will experience a force because of that field. Figure 4–4, which shows the paths of some high velocity electrons and positrons in a magnetic field, provides a modern demonstration of this.

In Figure 4–4, high-energy photons enter from the right. A Compton interaction between an incident photon and some lucky atomic electron at point C is indicated by the path of the resulting Compton electron (the trail of the Compton scatter photon being invisible). As noted in Chapter 2, nearly all interactions between diagnostic beam x-ray photons and matter (both in the patient and in the image receptor) occur by way of Compton and photoelectric mechanisms.

There is a strong magnetic field pointing into the page. A magnetic field exerts a deflecting force on any moving charged particle (unless the particle happens to be moving parallel to the field); the negatively charged electron released at point C therefore spirals upward, clockwise. A positron, which is a positively charged electron, would circle in the opposite direction.

Another incident high-energy photon interacts with the field of an atomic nucleus at point A in such a way that its energy is transformed into mass, in the form of an electron and a positron, each with high initial kinetic energy. The same thing happens at point B. (In sharp contrast to the situation shown here, the photons of a diagnostic x-ray beam are not sufficiently energetic for the production of electron–positron pairs.)

The electron created at point A collides with an atomic nucleus at point D, and loses much of its energy (revealed by the abrupt change in the curvature of its path) through the creation of a *bremsstrahlung* photon. (Nearly all the x-ray en-

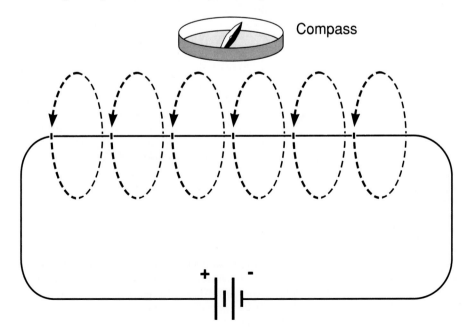

Compass

Figure 4–3. An electric current creates a magnetic field. If you bring a compass close to a long wire attached to a battery, the needle will align across the wire. This suggests the presence of a magnetic field curling around the wire.

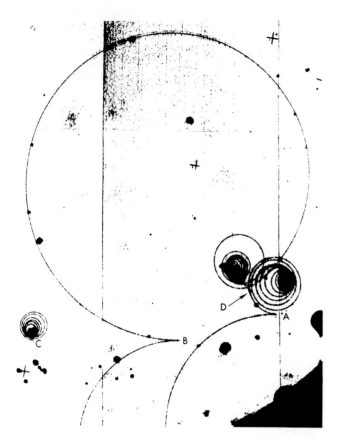

Figure 4–4. This bubble chamber record of the production of electron–positron pairs by the Stanford Linear Accelerator illustrates a number of interesting points, a few of which will be described in more detail later. Most noticeable, however, is the curvature of the trajectories of moving charged particles in a magnetic field. *(Photograph and interpretation courtesy of Ken Kase, SLAC.)*

ergy produced by a standard, nonmammographic, x-ray tube is generated through bremsstrahlung events that occur when high-velocity electrons interact strongly with the nuclei of the tungsten atoms of the tube's target.)

The positron created at point A (curving downward) will eventually collide with an atomic electron, with their mutual annihilation and the creation of a pair of 511-keV annihilation photons. The positrons used in PET scanning are not produced in this fashion, but rather appear during the decay of certain kinds of radioactive nuclei.

This photograph illustrates not only the effect of a magnetic field on a moving charge, but also photon–electron (Compton), photon–nuclear (pair production), electron–nuclear (bremsstrahlung), and electron–positron (annihilation) interactions. All of these but pair production play important roles in medical imaging.

There is an even simpler way to demonstrate the magnetic force on moving charges. Suppose electric current flows in a small, rigid loop of wire. When the loop is inserted into a magnetic field, the magnetic forces on the flowing electrons will tend to twist the loop around, until its plane becomes perpendicular to the field. It is this kind of twisting force that underlies the working of an electric motor.

This suggests an explanation of the behavior of the compass needle. A bar magnet (such as a compass needle) may be thought of as being made up of many atom-sized current

loops. All these will attempt to align in an external magnetic field, with the result that the whole needle does, too.

Finally, an atomic nucleus acts somewhat like a charged ball (or stack of charged hoops) rotating about an axis. The nucleus therefore creates a magnetic field itself, and also experiences a twisting force when placed in an external magnetic field. Both of these phenomena play critically important roles in magnetic resonance imaging.

5. A CHANGING MAGNETIC FIELD PRODUCES AN ELECTRIC FIELD, AND A CHANGING ELECTRIC FIELD PRODUCES A MAGNETIC FIELD

In 1831, Michael Faraday reported yet another process linking electricity and magnetism: When the current in one wire is abruptly changed, a brief current is induced in another, nearby conductor.

More generally, a changing magnetic field gives rise to a transient electric field in the surrounding space, a phenomenon known as electromagnetic induction. The classic demonstration of magnetic induction is to drop a bar magnet through a loop of wire that includes a voltmeter (Fig. 4–5). As the mag-

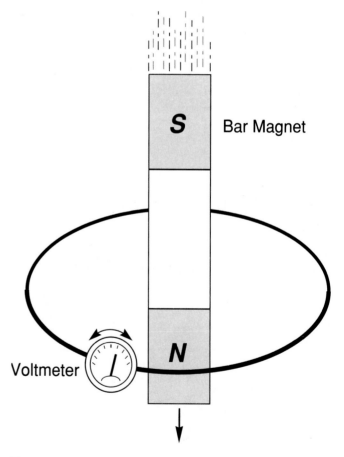

Figure 4–5. Magnetic induction. A changing magnetic field creates an electric field. As the bar magnet falls through the loop of wire, the voltmeter responds. A voltage is produced by an electric generator in a similar fashion. The converse is also true: A changing electric field gives rise to a (changing) magnetic field.

net passes through the loop, the resulting brief electric field drives a pulse of current around it, and the meter registers. The world's simplest electric generator.

Guided by the discovery of electromagnetic induction, James Clerk Maxwell postulated the existence of the converse phenomenon, in which a changing electric field gives rise to a transient magnetic field. The reality of this effect, too, can be demonstrated by experiment

6. PUTTING IT ALL TOGETHER: ELECTROMAGNETIC WAVES

In 1864, Maxwell combined all of the preceding ideas to produce a single, unified theory of electromagnetism. What Newton had done for gravitational forces and motions, Maxwell did for electricity, magnetism, and **electromagnetic radiation.**

Maxwell's mathematical formalism implied the creation and propagation through space of electromagnetic (em) waves. It revealed that electromagnetic radiation is emitted any time electric charges (and in particular, electrons) are made to accelerate. The metal antenna of a radio station generates electromagnetic radiation, for example, when the transmitter drives electrons back and forth along it. The more powerful the transmitter, and the greater the numbers of electrons involved and the more accelerated their motions, the greater the rate at which electromagnetic energy is radiated.

Once an electromagnetic wave is under way, a changing electric field creates a changing magnetic field a short distance away, which in turn generates a changing electric field a bit beyond that, which produces a changing magnetic field still further along, and so on. The electric and magnetic fields point in directions perpendicular to one another, and the wave propagates in the direction perpendicular to both of them. Maxwell was even able to calculate the speed of propagation of these waves, and it turned out to be remarkably close to the experimentally measured speed of light.

Figure 4–6A captures the sinusoidal spatial dependence of the electric (ε) and magnetic (B) fields of an electromagnetic wave, moving in the x direction, at a single instant of time, as if in a snapshot. The separation between adjacent peaks is called the **wavelength,** and is commonly designated λ.

In Figure 4–6B, the electric field at one point in space (like the vertical position of a buoy at sea) is followed over time. The number of peaks per second observed as the wave passes by is called the **frequency,** f, of the wave. The SI unit of frequency is the *Hertz (Hz)*, where 1 Hz = 1 cycle per second = 1 s^{-1}.

As the peaks are λ apart and pass a point at the rate of f per second, the velocity v of the wave must be

$$\lambda \cdot f = v \qquad (4.4)$$

This is a general expression valid for any kind of traveling wave. But the speed of electromagnetic radiation plays so central a role in modern physical theory that it has been distinguished with its own symbol, c. Hence for electromagnetic radiation, $\lambda \cdot f = c$, where $c = 3.00 \times 10^8$ m/s.

___ **EXERCISE 4–3.** _____

A snapshot of the ocean reveals that a typical wave is 12 m from crest to crest. At the same time, a buoy is observed to fall and rise again every 10 seconds. How fast are the waves traveling?

SOLUTION: By Equation 4.4, $v = (12$ m$)(0.1$ Hz$) = 1.2$ m/s.

___ **EXERCISE 4–4.** _____

A person takes 1.8 strides per second, each 0.9 m in length. What is his velocity? What stride length would be required to walk at the same velocity, but with 2.2 steps per second?

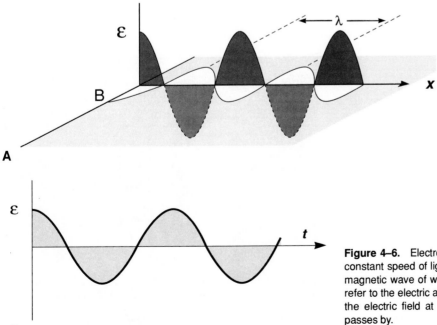

Figure 4–6. Electromagnetic waves propagate in free space at the constant speed of light, $c = 3 \times 10^8$ m/s. **A.** "Snapshot" of an electromagnetic wave of wavelength λ traveling in the x direction. (ε and B refer to the electric and magnetic fields, respectively.) **B.** Magnitude of the electric field at a point over time, as an electromagnetic wave passes by.

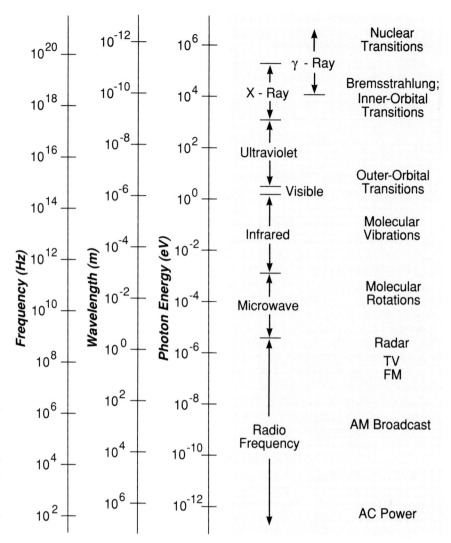

Figure 4–7. Electromagnetic spectrum. The frequency f and wavelength λ are inversely related to one another through $\lambda \cdot f = c$. As will be discussed in Chapter 6, the energy of a photon of frequency f is hf, where h is Planck's constant. Electromagnetic energy in the range 20 to 150 keV is employed in x-ray and gamma ray (nuclear medicine) imaging. Radiofrequency energy is used in magnetic resonance imaging. Ultrasound, by contrast, is not a form of electromagnetic radiation, but rather a mechanical disturbance propagating through tissue.

SOLUTION: By Equation 4.4, the velocity is $(0.9 \text{ m})(1.8 \text{ s}^{-1})$ $= 1.62$ m/s. With a step frequency of 2.2 s^{-1} and the same velocity, stride length would be 0.74 m.

___ **EXERCISE 4–5.** ___

The wavelengths of visible light range from 4×10^{-7} m (violet) to 7×10^{-7} m (red). What are the corresponding frequencies?

SOLUTION: By $\lambda \cdot f = c$, the frequency of violet light is $f = (3 \times 10^8 \text{ m/s})/(4 \times 10^{-7} \text{ m}) = 8 \times 10^{14} \text{ s}^{-1}$. Similarly, that of red light is 4×10^{14} Hz.

___ **EXERCISE 4–6.** ___

A typical diagnostic x-ray has a frequency of 1.5×10^{19} Hz. What is its wavelength?

SOLUTION: $\lambda = (3 \times 10^8 \text{ m/s})/(1.5 \times 10^{19} \text{ s}^{-1}) = 0.2 \times 10^{-10}$ m.

Radio waves, microwave energy, infrared light, light of all colors, ultraviolet light, gamma rays, and x-rays are all forms

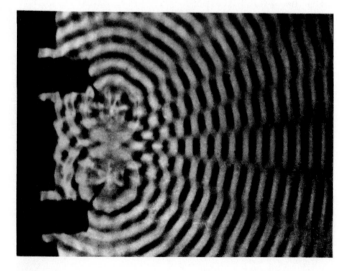

Figure 4–8. Ripple tank displaying interference patterns, which are characteristic of wave phenomena.

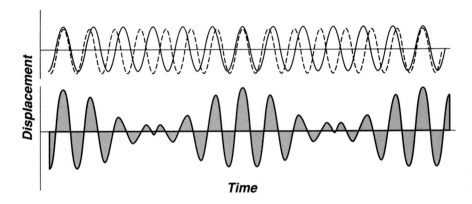

Figure 4–9. "Beat" interference pattern of two waves of slightly different wavelengths traveling together through space.

of electromagnetic radiation. Like the tones from a violin, they differ in their frequency and wavelength (Fig. 4–7), but in other respects they are inherently the same. The manner in which the radiation is produced, the amount of energy it transports, and the ways in which it interacts with matter may depend very strongly on the frequency (or, equivalently, on the wavelength), however, as will be seen in later chapters.

In 1905, Albert Einstein published the Special Theory of Relativity. Along with much else, this finally revealed that electric and magnetic fields, which had previously seemed so closely intertwined, are in fact two faces of a single entity, the electromagnetic field. It was thus not until the twentieth century that the fundamental unity of all electric and magnetic phenomena was fully appreciated.

7. WAVE INTERFERENCE

Waves are fundamentally different from particles, or solid bodies. Drop two pebbles near each other into a lake. The ripples from the two do not bounce off one another like pool balls; rather, they pass through one another without interacting. But for the brief moment that waves from the two sources intersect, they are superimposed, on top of one another. That is, the total vertical displacement of the water surface above or below normal is the sum of the displacements brought about by the two waves separately. This *superpositioning* that occurs when several waveforms occupy the same place at the same time is an important characteristic of wave phenomena.

The phenomenon of wave **interference** is a direct consequence of wave superpositioning. Figure 4–8 illustrates interference in two dimensions. Two sticks are tapping a water surface with the same steady frequency. Some points on the surface are exactly one-half wavelength farther from one stick than from the other; whenever a crest from one stick reaches such a *node*, a trough from the other will always be arriving there. Nodal lines, where such destructive interference occurs and the surface is disturbed relatively little, are clearly visible in the figure. At the places where the waves from the two sources are always in phase, and a crest from one arrives together with a crest from the other, *constructive interference* is said to occur. Similar interference effects, known as *diffraction*, may occur when a wave from a single source passes through a slit or small hole or by a sharp edge.

In Figure 4–9, two waves of slightly different wavelengths are traveling through the same region. The *beating* in their combined waveform is directly attributable to constructive and destructive interference. If the two original waves are of frequencies f_1 and f_2, the composite wave displays beats of frequency = $f_1 - f_2$.

Because of their propagation, the em wave of Figure 4–6 and the water waves of Figure 4–8 are known as *traveling waves*. By contrast, a piano string, fixed at both ends and vibrating at its resonant frequency, is supporting *standing waves* that do not go anywhere. A standing wave will result, however, if two traveling waves of the same frequency, wavelength, and amplitude pass through one another in opposite directions.

Energy

Energy was mentioned on a number of occasions in the first two chapters—the kinetic energy of electrons accelerating toward the anode (target) of an x-ray tube, the conversion of this into x-ray energy by means of the bremsstrahlung process, and the transformation of x-ray into light energy in the intensifying screen of a radiographic cassette; the energy required to flip over a proton in a magnetic field during magnetic resonance imaging; and the vibrational energy reflected from a tissue interface and contributing to an ultrasound image. The list is long and interesting.

This chapter and the next few will explore some of the varied roles that energy plays in the behavior of electrons, molecules, x-ray film, and everything else. An appreciation of the central role of energy is essential for a real understanding of the physical processes underlying each and every one of the imaging modalities.

1. ENERGY COMES IN MANY FORMS

As seen in the last two chapters, the behavior of some simple systems can be described adequately in terms of the way that masses respond, in space and over time, to applied forces. This is nice, when it happens, because the meanings of time and space are intuitively clear (unless you worry about what they did on Saturday nights before the Big Bang or where they did it). Force, too, is the kind of thing with which we have direct, everyday experience as a quantifiable entity. Often you can easily feel, for example, that one force is roughly twice as great as another.

A concept that is essential for a deeper understanding of physical reality, but that is somewhat less intuitive, is that of

energy. Instead of trying to provide a formal definition of energy, it is perhaps more helpful to begin by describing some of the guises in which it appears.

A falling apple has **kinetic energy** associated with its motion. This kinetic energy is clearly a function of both the apple's mass and its instantaneous speed, but how it depends on each of these is not self-evident. It also possesses **potential energy** attributable to its position in the gravitational field, its distance above the ground. The bigger the apple and the higher up it is at any moment, the greater its potential energy. But which, if either, is the dominant factor?

The situation is complicated by the ability of energy to change its forms. As the apple falls, its potential energy is converted into kinetic energy. And on impact, this kinetic energy becomes sound energy and heat energy. Similarly, the kinetic and potential energy of the water molecules in a river may be transformed into the rotational kinetic energy of a turbine, which is converted by a generator into **electrical energy**; electrical current imparts **heat energy** to the filament of a bulb that, in turn, radiates **visible light energy**, which induces the retinal **chemical energy** transformations by which you read this page. And so on.

2. POTENTIAL ENERGY OF AN ELECTRON IN A UNIFORM ELECTRIC FIELD

Despite its radically different manifestations, energy can be quantified. The simplest example of this involves the application of a constant net force F to a body, thereby causing it to move the distance Δx in the direction of the force. This activity requires the expenditure of the amount

$$\text{work energy} = F \cdot \Delta x \tag{5.1}$$

of **work** energy. The amount of work involved is proportional to how hard you push and how far. It is apparent from Equation 5.1 that the SI unit of energy is the newton-meter or, in more rudimentary terms, the kg · m²/s². This derived SI unit of energy is called the joule (J), and 1 J = 1 N · m = 1 kg · m²/s².

_____ EXERCISE 5–1. _____

How much work does an elevator expend in lifting a 3-kg sack of apples through 150 m?

SOLUTION: The Earth's gravitational field exerts a 29.4-N downward force on a 3-kg sack of apples. In addition to having to overcome frictional forces, the elevator must impart (29.4-N)(150 m) = 4410 J of energy to the sack simply to push it through 150 m against the force of gravity.

Suppose you apply just enough force to an object in a gravitational force field to lift it slowly through the vertical distance Δx (Fig. 5–1). The work you do on it is transformed into **potential energy** (**PE**) of the system consisting of the object and the gravitational field. And the change in potential energy, ΔPE, is numerically equal to $m \cdot g \cdot \Delta x$. In Exercise 5–1, for ex-

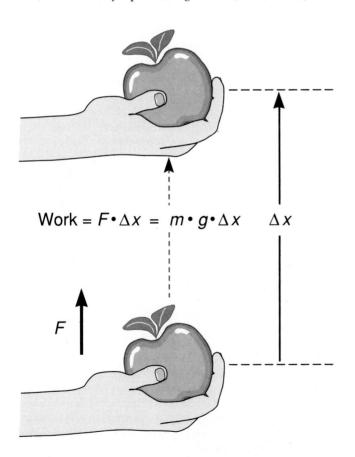

$$\text{Work} = F \cdot \Delta x = m \cdot g \cdot \Delta x \qquad \Delta x$$

F

Figure 5–1. The work required to lift an apple of mass m through distance Δx against the force of gravity: work = $F \cdot \Delta x = m \cdot g \cdot \Delta x$. This is also the increase in the apple's potential energy. Should the apple fall, $m \cdot g \cdot \Delta x$ is the amount of kinetic energy it would acquire.

ample, the increase in PE for the apples in the gravitational field was 4410 J.

So also for electrons in a uniform electric field of strength $\mathcal{E}$. The force exerted on an electron is $\mathcal{E} \cdot e$. The work required to grab hold of an electron somehow and push it through the distance Δx "upstream" against the field is $\mathcal{E} \cdot e \cdot \Delta x$. As a consequence of the move, the electron (or, more correctly, the electron-plus-electric field system) has acquired that same amount of potential energy:

$$\Delta PE = \mathcal{E} \cdot e \cdot \Delta x \tag{5.2}$$

It is sometimes helpful, for bookkeeping purposes, to establish a "zero" reference position in an electric field, $x = 0$, where the PE is also defined to be zero. This causes no problems, as the things invariably of interest are a _change_ in an electron's position in the field and the associated _change_ in its energy. Likewise, for a hanging apple, what determines its total change in potential energy when it falls is only the height of the limb above ground, not the location of the tree—on a high plateau or at sea level. Then even a negative energy is meaningful; it indicates simply that the apple is below the reference point, which you might have chosen to be at the top of the tree, or anywhere else that is convenient. But the choice of reference point and the "zero of energy" have no effect on the _changes_ in energy that occur during an event, and it is only these changes that are relevant.

3. KINETIC ENERGY OF MOTION

Suppose that our electron in the electric field is now released and allowed to accelerate freely back downfield. Over the distance Δx, the field performs $\mathcal{E} \cdot e \cdot \Delta x$ work on it, according to equation 5.1. That amount of potential energy is thereby transformed into **kinetic energy (KE)** of motion.

The kinetic energy of an object clearly must increase both with its speed and with its mass. One might initially suspect KE to be of the form $m \cdot v$. But $m \cdot v$ cannot be right, because it has the units kg · m/s, rather than the kg · m²/s² required of energy, as indicated by the units in Equation 5.1. The correct relationship turns out to be, for our purposes, KE = $\frac{1}{2}m \cdot v^2$.

_____ EXERCISE 5–2. _____

After falling through 150 m, the velocity of a 3-kg sack of apples is 54.22 m/s. What is its KE?

SOLUTION: KE = $\frac{1}{2}$(2 kg) (54.22 m/s)² = 4410 J. See Exercise 5.1.

First our electron was lifted through an electric field, during which process work was performed on it, and it gained potential energy. Then it was released, and lost potential energy but acquired kinetic energy. Eventually it crashes into something, such as the target of an x-ray tube, whereupon the kinetic energy is transformed into heat and radiant electromagnetic energy. In each and every one of these events, a most remarkable phenomenon occurs: All the energy of any one kind that is lost will reappear in another form.

4. THE INVIOLATE LAW OF CONSERVATION OF ENERGY

The extraordinary usefulness of the concept of *energy* rests on a single observation: Regardless of how many times and ways that energy changes form in a series of transformations, there is always as much of it remaining in the universe at the end as there existed in the first place. This assertion has been verified countless times in many types of experiments, and is codified as the fundamental and inviolate *Law of the Conservation of Energy*: The total amount of energy in existence is constant. Energy cannot be created or destroyed; it can only change form and place.

Of course, you must learn the necessary prescriptions for quantifying work, potential energy, kinetic energy, and heat, light, x-ray, chemical, and every other kind of energy. You must follow what happens to every bit of it meticulously and carry out your bookkeeping impeccably. But if you do all that, you will find that no matter what transpires during a process of interest, the sum total of energy remains unchanged.

> It is rarely necessary, however, to follow what is going on throughout the entire universe. A "closed" system usually will do. A closed system is one into or out of which no energy flows, to a good enough approximation for the problem at hand. To apply the Law of Conservation of Energy, then, you determine what most likely constitutes the relevant closed system and then worry only about those energy transformations that occur within it.
>
> During the free fall of an apple, for example, the total energy of the closed apple/gravitational field system, consisting of the KE and the PE, is constant: PE + KE = constant. Thus, the increase in KE comes about at the expense of lost PE. To account for what happens when the apple strikes the ground, a wider closed universe is required.

_____ EXERCISE 5–3. _____

A 10-kg basket of apples drops from a height of 20 m. What is its speed just before hitting the ground?

SOLUTION: The change in PE is $-m \cdot g \cdot \Delta x$. Assuming the basket was initially at rest, the acquired KE is $\frac{1}{2}m \cdot v^2$, where v refers to the terminal velocity. Equate these and cancel out the mass, yielding $v = \sqrt{2g \cdot \Delta x} = 19.8$ m/s, independent of the mass.

_____ EXERCISE 5–4. _____

An electron accelerates through a distance of 0.1 m in a 10,000 N/C electric field. What is its final velocity? The mass and charge of an electron in SI units are 9.11×10^{-31} kg and 1.6×10^{-19} C.

SOLUTION: The closed system consists of the electron and the electric field. The loss in potential energy, by Equation 5.2, is $\mathcal{E} \cdot e \cdot \Delta x = (10^4 \text{ N/C})(1.6 \times 10^{-19} \text{ C})(0.1 \text{ m}) = 1.6 \times 10^{-16}$ J. If this amount of PE is transformed completely into KE, and KE = $\frac{1}{2}m \cdot v^2$, then the final velocity can be obtained from 1.6×10^{-16} J $= \frac{1}{2}(9.11 \times 10^{-31} \text{ kg}) \cdot v^2$. From this, $v = 1.9 \times 10^7$ m/s. If we are interested in what happens after the electron strikes the anode,

the closed system must be expanded so as to account for thermal energy and radiation, as well.

5. VOLTS OF POTENTIAL DIFFERENCE VERSUS ELECTRON VOLTS OF ENERGY

On numerous occasions, we shall be concerned with the behavior of electrons in electric fields. Instead of having to keep track of the potential energy of every electron in a system, it is usually simpler to make use of a more general construct, the **voltage difference,** also called the **potential difference** (not to be confused with potential energy). The voltage difference between any two points in an electric field, denoted ΔV, or simply V, is defined to be the difference in potential energy per unit charge:

$$V = \Delta PE / \text{unit charge} \qquad (5.3)$$

Like the electric field strength, the voltage difference is independent of the amount of charge on any object that happens to be in the field. The SI unit for voltage difference is the joule per coulomb (J/C), which has a special name, **volt** (V). (The potential and the unit in which it is measured share the same symbol.) The kilovolt (kV) is a thousand times larger.

_____ EXERCISE 5–5. _____

One point is 2 cm upfield of another in a uniform electric field of strength 5,000,000 N/C. What is the potential difference between the points?

SOLUTION: Over a distance Δx in a uniform electric field of strength $\mathcal{E}$, the difference in potential energy for an electron, by Equation 5.2, is $\mathcal{E} \cdot e \cdot \Delta x$. By Equation 5.3, ΔPE can also be written $V \cdot e$. Then, $V = \Delta PE / e = \mathcal{E} \cdot \Delta x$. That is, the voltage difference between two points is proportional to the field strength and to their separation. In the present example, $V = (5 \times 10^6$ N/C)(0.02 m) = 100,000 V, or 100 kV. This is a typical value for the potential difference between the cathode and anode of an x-ray tube.

_____ EXERCISE 5–6. _____

Two metal plates are 1.5 cm apart, and attached to the poles of a generator that produces a steady 120,000-V potential difference. What is the electric field strength between the plates?

SOLUTION: From Exercise 5–5, $\mathcal{E} = V/\Delta x = (120,000 \text{ V})/(1.5 \text{ cm}) = 80 \text{ kV/cm} = 8 \times 10^6$ N/C.

The gain in PE of an electron transported across a potential difference of V volts (or the increase in KE of an electron that free-falls through that potential difference) is $V \cdot e$. (This is true even when the electric field is nonuniform.) The energy involved in moving one electron through a 1-V potential difference, in particular, is (1 V)(1.6 × 10^{-19} C) = (1.6 × 10^{-19} J) (Fig. 5–2). This is comparable to the energies involved in many atomic processes, such as the emission of light and the formation or breaking of chemical bonds, so it, too, has been singled out for a special designation. Movement of one electron

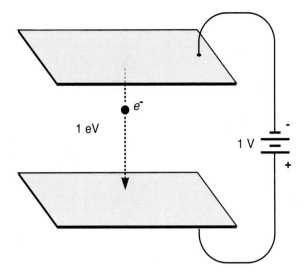

Figure 5–2. One electron volt (eV) of energy is involved in moving an electron between two points that differ in voltage by 1 V. If the electron is somehow forced "upstream" against the electric field, it gains 1 eV of potential energy. If it subsequently "free-falls" back again, it loses 1 eV of PE but acquires 1 eV of kinetic energy.

through 1 V of potential difference involves the transformation of one **electron volt (eV)** of energy, Table 5–1.

When accelerating through the vacuum of an x-ray tube or a TV monitor tube, electrons acquire typically tens of thousands of electron volts of kinetic energy. It is therefore convenient also to introduce a larger unit of energy, the **keV**, which is 1000 times larger than the electron volt. Nuclear transformations may involve the release of millions of electron volts, where 1 MeV = 10^6 eV.

_____ **EXERCISE 5–7.** _____

A steady potential difference of 70 kV (70,000 V) is applied across an x-ray tube. What is the kinetic energy of each of the electrons arriving at the anode?

SOLUTION: One electron accelerating through 70 kV of potential difference acquires $V \cdot e$ = 70 keV of KE.

6. THE ENERGY SPECTRUM AND CURRENT OF AN ELECTRON BEAM

In Exercise 5–7, each of the electrons accelerated from the cathode to the anode of an x-ray tube ends up with 70 keV of kinetic energy. The **energy spectrum** of the electron beam, the dashed line in Figure 5–3, shows the relative number of electrons that have any particular final kinetic energy, and consists (for our example) of a single sharp line. Because the spectrum

TABLE 5–1. THE ELECTRON VOLT OF ENERGY

1 ev	=	1.6×10^{-19} J
1 keV	=	10^3 eV
1 MeV	=	10^6 eV

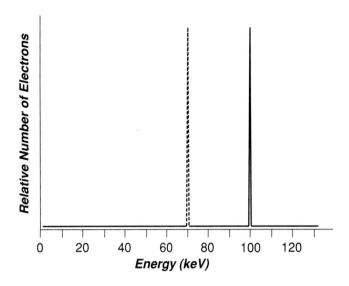

Figure 5–3. The discrete energy spectrum of a monochromatic beam of electrons, each of which has 70 keV of kinetic energy just before colliding with an anode, is shown as the dashed line. The solid line applies to another, 100-keV electron beam.

is sharply peaked, rather than a continuous band, it is said to be *discrete*. As there is only one such peak, moreover, the beam is *monochromatic*. Also shown in the figure, as the solid line, is the spectrum of a 100-keV electron beam.

Totally distinct from the energy per electron is the issue of the electron **current**—the rate at which electrons flow past a point.* The SI unit of electric current is the **ampere**, defined as the flow of 1 C of charge per second (Fig. 5–4). The **milliampere (mA)** is 1000 times less.

_____ **EXERCISE 5–8.** _____

What flow, in electrons per second, gives rise to a current of 100 mA?

SOLUTION: If the charge on one electron is 1.6×10^{-19} C, then 1 C consists of 6.25×10^{18} electrons. 100 mA = 0.1 A is the flow of 6.25×10^{17} electrons per second.

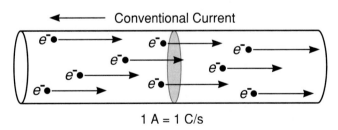

Figure 5–4. Electric current, denoted *I*, refers to the number of electrons that pass by a point in 1 second. One ampere (A) corresponds to a flow of 1 coulomb (C) of electrons (6.25×10^{18} electrons) per second. A milliampere (mA) is smaller by a factor of 1000. "Conventional current" was defined, in the early days, as the flow of positive charges; electrons flow in the opposite direction.

_____

*For historical reasons, "conventional current" is defined to flow in the opposite direction. In this book, arrows signify the direction of electron flow.

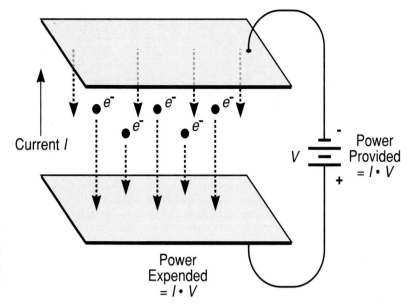

Figure 5–5. One way of expending power: Two electrodes are attached to a source of potential *V* volts. A current *I* of electrons liberated somehow from the cathode flows to the anode. Energy will be deposited in the anode (almost entirely as heat) at the rate power = *I · V*. The source must provide energy at the same rate.

7. POWER IS THE RATE AT WHICH ENERGY IS TRANSFERRED OR TRANSFORMED

When electrons accelerate through an x-ray tube and crash into the anode, electron kinetic energy is transformed into heat and x-ray energy at a rate that depends on the number of electrons arriving each second and on the kinetic energy that each electron bears. It is critically important to control the rate at which energy is being delivered, both to generate the correct x-ray beam intensity and to prevent the anode from overheating.

The rate at which energy is delivered to the anode depends on the current through the tube and on the voltage drop across it. If the current through an x-ray tube is *I* amperes, electrons from the cathode reach the anode at the rate of *I/e* per second. With a constant tube potential of *V* volts, then each electron acquires *V · e* of kinetic energy in the process. Therefore, when the electrons are brought rapidly to a halt at the anode, their kinetic energy is converted into other energy forms (heat and x-rays) at the rate $(I/e)(V \cdot e)$, or

$$\text{power} = \text{energy}/\text{time} = I \cdot V \qquad (5.4)$$

(Fig. 5–5). This rate of energy expenditure or conversion per unit time is called **power.** The SI unit for power is the joule/second, or **watt (W).** Note that if you multiply *milli*amps by *kilo*volts in Equation 5.4, the factors of 1/000 and 1000 cancel, and you end up with ordinary watts.

Similarly, when a potential difference *V* across a resistive metal wire produces a current *I* through it, the rate at which energy is dissipated in it as heat is *I · V*, for essentially the same reason (Fig. 5–6).

EXERCISE 5–9.

With a tube potential of 70 kV and a tube current of 100 mA, at what rate is energy being deposited in the anode?

SOLUTION: By Equation 5.4, the power is $(0.1 \text{ A})(7 \times 10^4 \text{ V})$ = 7000 W = 7 kW.

8. ENERGY TRANSFERRED TO THE ANODE OF AN X-RAY TUBE . . .

It is often sufficient, when dealing with an infinitesimally small particle like an electron, to consider only its potential and kinetic energies. Until now, in fact, we have even treated apples as if they, too, are such particles. But condensed matter, which is made up of many individual atoms, contains additional forms of energy as a result of the interactions of the constituent atoms with one another and because of their relative motions.

The most obvious of these forms is **heat energy.** The atoms of a solid are attached to one another by springlike electrical forces, and the addition of heat energy causes the atoms to vibrate more violently about their equilibrium positions. This manifests as a rise in the material's *temperature.* Under ordi-

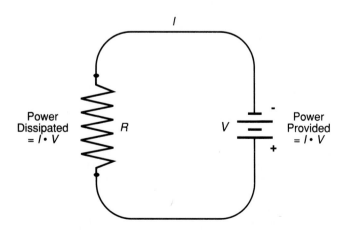

Figure 5–6. Another way of expending power: A resistor of resistance *R* is attached to a potential of *V* volts, and a current *I* flows. Heat is produced in the resistor at the rate *I · V.*

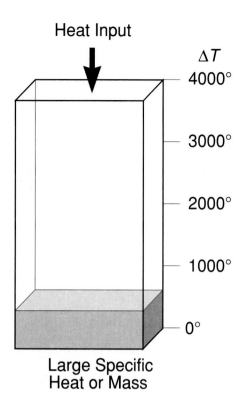

Heat Input

ΔT
4000°

3000°

2000°

1000°

0°

Large Specific
Heat or Mass

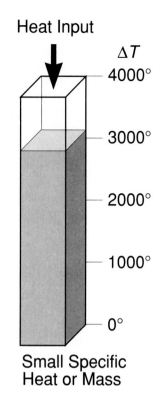

Heat Input

ΔT
4000°

3000°

2000°

1000°

0°

Small Specific
Heat or Mass

Figure 5–7. The smaller the heat capacity, the greater the temperature changes, ΔT, of Equation 5.5. Think of heat as being analogous to water, the product ($m \cdot c$) as corresponding to the cross-sectional area of a container, and the temperature as being like the water level. Pour the same amount of water (heat) into various containers (pieces of material); the final water level (temperature) will be greatest for the container of smallest area (value of $m \cdot c$).

nary, everyday circumstances, the increase ΔT in temperature is simply proportional to the amount dQ of heat added

$$\Delta T = \Delta Q / m \cdot c \qquad (5.5)$$

where m is the mass of the object being heated, and the constant of proportionality c is called the *specific heat*. (The same symbol happens to be used for the speed of light.) The specific heat of water (and, approximately, of soft tissue) at normal temperatures is about 4200 J/kg · °C. Tungsten metal, with a specific heat of 130 J/kg · °C, warms up much more readily, and this has important implications for the design of x-ray tube anodes (Fig. 5–7).

_____ **EXERCISE 5–10.** _____

Ten joules of energy is imparted to 10 kg of water as heat. How much will its temperature rise?

SOLUTION: By Equation 5.5, ΔT = (10 J)/(10 kg)(4200 J/kg · °C) = 1/4200°C ~ 2×10^{-4} °C.

9. ... IS CONDUCTED AWAY AND RADIATED AWAY AS THERMAL ELECTROMAGNETIC ENERGY ...

A hot object in direct physical contact with a cooler body will transfer heat energy to it by means of **thermal conduction.** Similarly, heat can be passed on to circulating air or oil, and carried away by **convection.**

But even when there are no other bodies around, when it

is alone and isolated in a vacuum, a relatively hot object will thermally radiate away its energy as **electromagnetic radiation.** The rate $\Delta E/\Delta t$ at which this electromagnetic energy is radiated away is proportional to the fourth power of the temperature T above "absolute zero" (–273°C = –460°F):

$$\Delta E/\Delta t = \text{constant} \cdot T^4 \qquad (5.6)$$

This is the principal means by which heat leaves the metal anode of a rotating-anode x-ray tube. An anode, or the filament of an ordinary light bulb, glows because this emission occurs primarily as visible light and infrared electromagnetic energy.

_____ **EXERCISE 5–11.** _____

The anode of an x-ray tube may reach temperatures near the melting point of tungsten, 3380°C. How much more rapidly would it radiate heat there than at room temperature (22°C)?

SOLUTION: $(3380 + 273)^4/(22 + 273)^4 = 2.4 \times 10^4$ times more rapidly.

10. ... OR AS BREMSSTRAHLUNG AND CHARACTERISTIC X-RAY ELECTROMAGNETIC ENERGY ...

When high-velocity electrons collide with the solid target of an x-ray tube, most of their kinetic energy is expended in heating it. (All of that heat energy will subsequently be conducted off through the metal backing of the target or radiated away thermally.) A small fraction of the electron kinetic energy is trans-

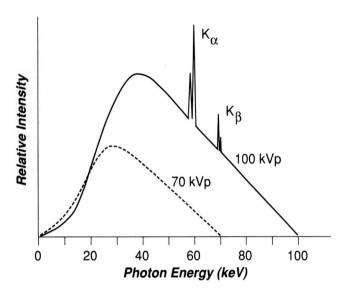

Figure 5–8. The continuous energy spectrum of bremsstrahlung radiation produced by 70-keV electrons is shown as the dashed curve. The solid curve, for 100-keV electrons, also displays discrete peaks corresponding to tungsten characteristic x-rays. The labeling of the peaks will be explained in the next chapter. (Compare with Figure 5–3.)

formed directly into x-rays instead, however, by means of the x-ray fluorescence and bremsstrahlung processes.

The next chapter will argue that electromagnetic energy sometimes acts as if it comes in the form of highly localized bundles of energy, or *photons*, instead of as extensive waves. In the bremsstrahlung process, in particular, x-ray photons with all energies between zero and the energy of the bombarding electrons are created. That is, the spectrum of bremsstrahlung radiation (unlike that of the beam of high-velocity electrons that produced it, see Fig. 5–3) is neither discrete nor monochromatic, but rather *continuous*. With an applied voltage of 70 kV,

for example, each electron strikes the anode with 70 keV of kinetic energy. X-ray photons are generated with all energies up to, but not exceeding, 70 keV, as with the dashed curve in Figure 5–8. The shape of this bremsstrahlung curve (and in particular, the energy at which the x-ray intensity drops to zero) is determined mainly by the energy of the incident electrons. It does not depend, in particular, on the nature of the target material. (The efficiency with which bremsstrahlung radiation is produced, hence the overall intensity of an x-ray beam, does depend on the target material, as we shall see.)

With a tungsten-target tube, the use of tube potentials above about 70 kV leads to the occurrence of an additional phenomenon. X-ray photons with a few very specific energies are produced. Correspondingly, discrete **emission peaks** appear superimposed on the continuous bremsstrahlung beam spectrum. The solid line in Figure 5–8 was obtained, for example, with an applied voltage of 100 kVp. In contrast with the case of the bremsstrahlung spectrum, the energies of the discrete emission peaks are characteristic of the type of atoms out of which the target is made. For this reason, the x-rays involved are known as *characteristic x-rays*. The next chapter discusses the origin of characteristic x-rays.

Figure 5–9 provides a general summary of the most significant energy transformation processes that occur in an x-ray generator and x-ray tube. The next important issue is what happens to the x-ray energy when it enters a patient's body.

11. ... WHICH MAY BE DEPOSITED IN MATTER: DOSE

As suggested in Chapter 2, x-ray energy can interact with matter via the photoelectric and Compton mechanisms. The response of a piece of x-ray-sensitive material, such as the fluorescent screen of a radiographic film cassette, almost inevitably

Figure 5–9. Overview of the energy transformation processes taking place in an x-ray generator and tube. The analogy of a man-made waterfall may be useful: An electric pump (the generator) forces water to the top of the falls. Water droplets (electrons), initially with high potential energy, plummet to the lake, giving up their energy as sound (x-ray photons) and heat, whereupon they are ready to be pumped to the top again.

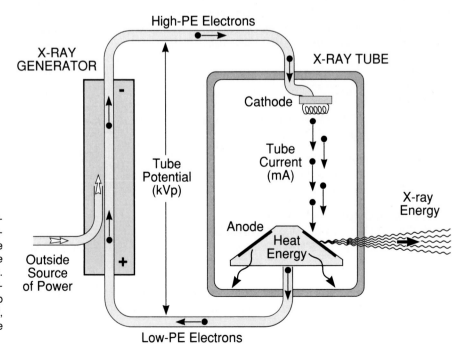

increases with the amount of x-ray energy deposited in it via these mechanisms. Similarly, it is usually assumed that the hazard to health associated with a radiologic procedure is proportional to the quantity of ionizing radiation energy deposited in the body's tissues.

The amount of ionizing radiant energy absorbed by matter per unit mass, or the density of ionizing energy, is called the *dose*. The SI unit of dose is the *gray* (*Gy*): One gray is defined as 1 J of ionizing energy absorbed per kilogram of material irradiated (Table 2–1). The unit in conventional use in the United States, the rad, is 100 times smaller. To simplify the transition to SI units, it is now common practice to refer to a rad as a centigray (cGy).

How much energy density does a gray represent? By the results of Exercise 5–10, depositing 1 Gy uniformly throughout any volume of water (whether it be 1 cc or a swimming pool) will, like pumping 1 J of ordinary heat into each kilogram of it, raise its temperature by about 2×10^{-4} °C. (A fundamental way of calibrating radiation sources, in fact, is to follow the radiation-induced change in temperature of a known mass of water with a calorimeter. This requires extremely sensitive temperature measurement and precise heat flow regulation.)

_____ **EXERCISE 5–12.** _____

Confirm that the mechanical energy equivalent of 1 rad is sufficient to lift any object through 0.001 m, or to give it a velocity of 0.14 m/s.

SOLUTION: 1 rad = 1 cGy is equivalent to 0.01 J/kg. By Equation 5.1, raising a 1-kg mass through 0.001 m does require $(1 \text{ kg})(9.8 \text{ m/s}^2)(0.001 \text{ m}) = 0.01$ J. Since KE $= \frac{1}{2}mv^2$, a 1-kg mass moving at 0.14 m/s does possess $\frac{1}{2}(1 \text{ kg})(0.14 \text{ m/s})^2 = 0.01$ J of kinetic energy.

Depositing a dose of 5 Gy (500 rad) uniformly throughout a person's entire body will raise his or her temperature only by about 0.001°C, less than what is caused by drinking a cup of hot tea. There is, however, about a 50% chance that the 5 Gy will kill the person. Why the biologic difference between x-ray energy and heat?

Ionizing radiation is radically different from heat energy in one all-important respect: It comes in the form of localized individual bundles of energy known as *photons*, as will be discussed in the next chapter. By analogy, an air gun pellet may carry no more energy than does a basketball, but the effect on your hand is notably different. And although an extra 5 J of heat per kilogram may raise a person's temperature immeasurably, a whole-body dose of 5 Gy delivered by highly energetic photons can be lethal. More about that later.

12. THE LAWS OF CONSERVATION OF LINEAR AND ANGULAR MOMENTUM ARE LIKE, BUT SEPARATE FROM, THAT FOR ENERGY

The Law of Conservation of Energy reflects a certain kind of orderliness that underlies physical reality. Indeed, the search for physical laws often goes hand in hand with the awareness that some things in Nature, such as total energy, simply do not change, or are *conserved*. To date, a dozen or so fundamental invariants have been identified, in addition to the total energy in the universe.

Another conserved quantity is the total electric charge. In every kind of event that we have ever observed, the *total electric charge* (where one positive electron charge balances one negative one) has been conserved. In a positron annihilation event, for example, an electron and a positron come together and destroy one another, with the production of a pair of high-energy photons (see Fig. 1–12). The total charge of the system before the interaction, $(-1) + (+1) = 0$, is the same as that after.

The wheel of an overturned tricycle may continue to rotate long after its owner has wiped away his or her tears. Without the slight frictional forces exerted by the bearings and the air, the wheel would spin at constant speed forever. This inclination of a system to maintain its rotational status quo is an example of the Law of Conservation of *Angular Momentum*. Were it not for the angular momenta of the nuclei of hydrogen and other atoms, there would be no magnetic resonance imaging.

Likewise, the tendency of an object to continue to move at constant speed and along a straight line, in the absence of applied forces, reflects the Law of Conservation of *Linear Momentum*. As with angular momentum, this is like, but inherently separate from, the Law of Conservation of Energy. The Law of Conservation of Momentum, which is as fundamental and inviolate as that for energy, requires that the sum of the momenta of all the particles involved in an interaction remain constant.

> If a body of mass m is moving with a speed v (significantly less than the speed of light, so that there are no relativistic effects), its momentum is of magnitude $m \cdot v$. Unlike kinetic energy, linear momentum is a vector quantity.

In a collision of billiard balls, both energy and linear momentum must be conserved (and angular momentum, too). This composite requirement places severe constraints on the possible outcomes of the event. On impact, the balls do not fly off in random directions. Their motions are uniquely determined by the parameters of the collision, rather, and by the several relevant conservation laws that simultaneously obtain. Were this not so, pool would be a game of chance rather than of skill.

Chapter 6

Atoms and Photons

The production of characteristic x-rays for use in mammographic imaging; the creation of a flash of light when an x-ray photon strikes a fluorescent screen; the spin relaxation of a proton in a magnetic field during magnetic resonance imaging—all of these are described most fruitfully in terms of transitions among quantum states. Hence this qualitative introduction to such states and to the photons commonly involved in the transitions among them.

Quantum systems behave in strange, nonintuitive ways. An atom functions somewhat like a microscopic solar system, but the orbiting electrons act as much like waves as like particles. Similarly, electromagnetic radiation sometimes is fully describable as a wavelike phenomenon, but it also sometimes displays particle-like attributes instead.

The fundamental link between the two halves of this wave–particle duality is the Einstein relation, $E = hf$, which relates the energy, E, of a (particle-like) photon or electron with its (wavelike) frequency, f. This expression, along with the rest of quantum mechanics, allows us to predict and describe the physical behavior of atoms, and of everything built out of them, with remarkable accuracy and in great detail.

1. THE PLANETARY ATOM

Unlike a falling apple near the Earth's surface, an orbiting satellite moves in a direction perpendicular to that of the force acting on it. It continuously "falls" toward the center of the Earth, but it has enough lateral motion (by definition of its being "in orbit") for its path to follow the Earth's curvature. So its altitude remains (nearly) constant (Fig. 6–1). The planets orbit the Sun in a like fashion.

The *planetary* model of the atom is similar, with light, negatively charged electrons (planets) orbiting a massive, positively charged nucleus (the Sun). The atom is held together by the inverse square Coulombic force, rather than by the inverse square gravitational force, but otherwise the two systems would seem much alike. Naturally, there were early attempts by theorists to calculate the properties of such planetary atoms.

The results of these theoretical efforts, however, did not even begin to resemble what the experimentalists were clearly finding.

2. PROBLEMS WITH CLASSICAL ATOMIC ORBITALS

The wavelike properties of electromagnetic radiation were well understood by the turn of the century. According to the Maxwell theory, electromagnetic waves are emitted by any charge that is caused to undergo an acceleration. Circular motion is a kind of acceleration, involving the change of direction of motion rather than of speed. If an atom is like a tiny solar system, then why do the orbiting electrons not radiate away their energy and spiral into the nucleus? And when atoms are heated in a flame or excited by an electric discharge (as in a neon tube), why is light emitted at specific, discrete energies, rather than over a continuous range? It was found experimentally that visible light is produced by excited hydrogen gas, for example, only at certain wavelengths (Fig. 6–2).

These and other findings indicated serious problems with the application of classical mechanics and electromagnetic theory to atomic processes.

3. THE WAVE–PARTICLE DUALITY AND THE EINSTEIN RELATION: *E = hf*

Max Planck's study in 1900 of the spectrum of thermal radiation emitted by a hot body (see Chapter 5, Section 9) and Einstein's explanation in 1905 of the photoelectric effect (see Chapter 2, Section 5) each led separately to the same revolutionary conclusion: Electromagnetic radiation displays not only wavelike properties, but also corpuscular, particle-like behavior. That is, in certain kinds of experiments, light and x-rays appear to be diffuse, to have wavelength and frequency, and to undergo interference (see Chapter 4, Section 7) as only waves can. In others, however, electromagnetic energy is absorbed

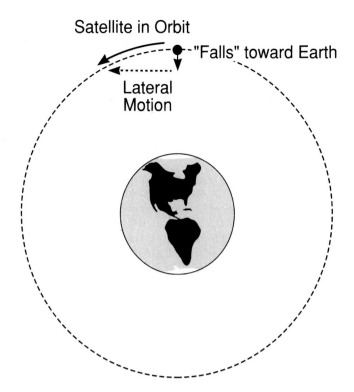

Figure 6–1. A satellite moves far enough laterally, as it "falls" toward the Earth, to remain in orbit.

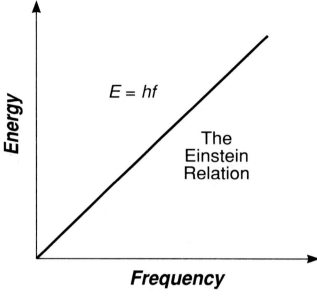

Figure 6–3. The energy of a photon (a particle-like concept) is proportional to its (wavelike) frequency—a critically important idea sometimes known as the Einstein relation. Units were intentionally omitted from this diagram to emphasize the validity of the relationship for *all* photon frequencies, in the radiofrequency range (kilo- and megahertz) as well as for x-ray and gamma ray photons (10^{20} Hz and higher). Like the speed of light, Planck's constant, *h*, is one of the fundamental constants of nature. This expression also relates the frequency of the "probability wave" associated with a "particle," such as an electron, to its energy.

and emitted in discrete, localized bundles, and acts somewhat like particles, now known as **photons.** Nothing with which we have everyday experience displays such a dichotomy. This rather schizophrenic behavior of electromagnetic radiation is an example of the *wave–particle duality* that underlies quantum physics.

The crucially important *Einstein relation*

$$E = hf \qquad (6.1)$$

Figure 6–3 provides the essential link between the wavelike and particle-like aspects of electromagnetic (em) radiation. *f* is

the frequency of the radiation (wave picture), and *E* is the energy of the corresponding photons (particle picture). The constant of proportionality linking them, $h = 6.626 \times 10^{-34}$ J · s, is known as *Planck's constant.* The reason we normally are totally unaware of the quantum nature of radio waves or light is that each photon carries so little energy, and there are so many of them, that we can experience only their collective effect.

Figure 4–7, a chart of the electromagnetic spectrum, in-

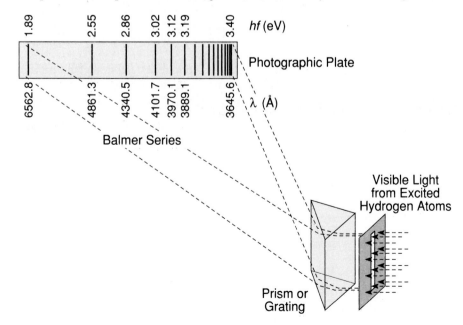

Figure 6–2. An electric discharge passes through hydrogen gas, and the resulting light is separated by means of a prism: The amount of refraction of light depends on its wavelength, λ. Wavelengths are presented in angstroms, where 1 Å = 10^{-10} m. It is found that hydrogen produces light only of certain, specific wavelengths. The spectrum is *discrete,* rather than *continuous.* This phenomenon could not be explained by prequantum physics.

cludes photon energies in electron volts. It also notes some of the mechanisms by which em radiation of various energies comes into being.

EXERCISE 6–1.

Visible light ranges in wavelength from about 700 nm (red) to about 400 nm (violet) in wavelength. What are the frequency and energy (in eV) of orange light photons of 600 nm wavelength?

SOLUTION: This takes three steps: (1) By Equation 4.4, $f = c/\lambda = (3 \times 10^8 \text{ m/s})/(6 \times 10^{-7} \text{ m}) = (5 \times 10^{14} \text{ Hz})$. (2) By the Einstein relation, $E = (6.626 \times 10^{-34} \text{ J} \cdot \text{s})(5 \times 10^{14} \text{ Hz}) = (3.3 \times 10^{-19}\text{J})$. (3) This can be expressed in electron volts as $(3.3 \times 10^{-19} \text{ J})/(1.6 \times 10^{-19} \text{ J/eV}) = 2.1 \text{ eV}$. A moral of this little story is that visible light photons are of the order of a few electron volts in energy.

EXERCISE 6–2.

How many photons per second are produced by a 100-W source of orange light? At what rate do they strike your eye when you are 10 m away?

SOLUTION: By Exercise 6–1, the energy of one photon is 3.3×10^{-19} J. To produce 100 J/s of energy, the source must emit 3×10^{20} photons per second. Imagine the light source at the center of a sphere of radius $r = 10$ m. The total surface area of the sphere is $4\pi r^2 = 4\pi (10 \text{ m})^2$, or about 1000 m². The area of the front of your eye is about 1 cm², so only 1 in 10^7 of the photons emitted from the source enter it. But that's still 3×10^{13} photons per second, which is why you do not sense them one at a time.

Photons act like waves traveling with the speed of light c, and their frequency and wavelength λ are related according to $f = c/\lambda$ (Equation 4.4). The Einstein relation can therefore be presented in the fully equivalent form $E = h \cdot c/\lambda$. It is common practice to express the wavelength of x-ray energy in a unit called the *Ångstrom* (Å), where $1 \text{ Å} = 10^{-10}$ m. With photon energy in kilo-electron volts, then, this reduces to

$$E \text{ [keV]} = 12.4/\lambda \text{ [Å]} \qquad (6.2)$$

where the units are shown in square brackets. This combines the three steps of Exercise 6–1 into a single expression. The units are convenient, as the wavelengths of the x-rays encountered in imaging are typically of the order of an angstrom, and their energies are usually presented in kilo-electron volts (keV).

EXERCISE 6–3.

Demonstrate the validity of Equation 6.2.

SOLUTION: Expressing $E = h \cdot c/\lambda$ in SI units, $E \text{ [J]} = (6.626 \times 10^{-34} \text{ J} \cdot \text{s})(3 \times 10^8 \text{ m/s})/\lambda = 1.99 \times 10^{-25}/(\lambda \text{ [m]})$. Multiply the right-hand side by 10^{10} Å/m, and divide it by 1.6×10^{-16} J/keV.

EXERCISE 6–4.

An x-ray generator is set at 100 kVp, and the tube produces photons of energies up to 100 keV. What is the wavelength of the most energetic x-ray photon thus generated?

SOLUTION: By Equation 6.2, the wavelength (in Å) and energy (in keV) of the most energetic photons are related through $100 = 12.4/\lambda$, from which $\lambda = 0.124$ Å. All the other x-ray photons are of longer wavelength and lower frequency.

Not only do electromagnetic waves possess particle-like characteristics, but also "particles" such as electrons display wavelike characteristics. A moving electron, in particular, has a kind of wavelength, λ, and frequency, f, associated with its motion. A beam of electrons impinging on the surface of a crystal, for example, produces interference patterns that can be explained only if the individual electrons possess some sort of wavelike attribute.

Physicists have been scratching their heads for three quarters of a century wondering what it is that is actually waving. The generally agreed-on answer, "the probability amplitude function," will not make much sense unless one has studied quantum mechanics, and perhaps not even then. The only real reason for putting much credence in such a ridiculous notion as a "probability amplitude wave" is that the approach works. Perfectly. Always and everywhere.

4. THE BOHR ATOM: A MIXTURE OF CLASSICAL AND QUANTUM IDEAS

In 1913, Niels Bohr used the idea of wavelike electrons to explain, after a fashion, both the stability of atoms and the discrete nature of atomic emission spectra.

The simplest atom is normal hydrogen, consisting of one proton and one electron. Bohr proposed that the electron is in an orbit of radius r about its nucleus, held by the Coulombic force (Equation 4.3). The total energy (potential plus kinetic) of the orbiting electron is easily found to be $-k \cdot e^2/2r$. Exactly the same kind of expression describes the total gravitational energy of a planet as a function of its distance from the center of the Sun, and Bohr's system is commonly called the *planetary model* of the hydrogen atom.

So far everything is completely classical. But the constraints of the wave–particle duality now enter the picture with a very nonclassical postulate: The particle wave associated with an electron in a stable orbital is a standing wave. That is, the wave must undergo an integral number of cycles, and close upon itself, as the electron undergoes one orbit (Fig. 6–4). If the electron's wavelength is λ, as determined by its energy, and if the circumference of the orbit is $2\pi r$, then $2\pi r = n\lambda$, where n, the so-called **principal quantum number**, *must be an integer: $n = 1$, 2, 3, ...* This postulate and the otherwise classical expression for the electron's energy together imply that the *energy of the hydrogen atom is quantized:* The electron can only have total energies with the discrete values

$$E_n \text{ [eV]} = -13.6/n^2, \qquad n = 1, 2, 3, \ldots \qquad (6.3)$$

The 13.6 materialized after multiplying and dividing a plethora of constants such as the mass and charge of the electron,

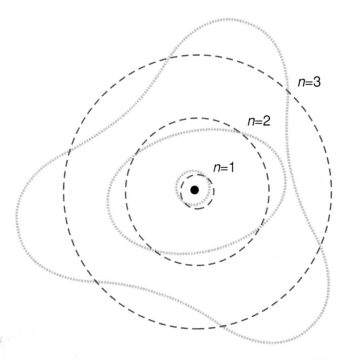

Simple plausibility argument for the quantization of the possible energies of the hydrogen atom. An atomic orbital is stable only if the probability density wave associated with the orbiting electron closes upon itself as it circles the nucleus, that is, forms a standing wave. That constraint, together with the Einstein relation and the classical planetary model, yields the energy levels of the Bohr atom.

Planck's constant, and the speed of light. (This important result was first obtained by Bohr via somewhat different reasoning.

The total energy is defined to be zero for the $n = \infty$ orbital, in which the electron is infinitely far away from its nucleus but devoid of kinetic energy, only barely moving. An electron bound to an atom has negative total energy, whereas a free electron (such as one accelerating across an x-ray tube) has a positive total energy, $E > 0$.

The energy levels of hydrogen are shown in Figure 6–5. The atom is most stable in its *ground state*, with its electron in the lowest ($n = 1$) level. But just as it is possible to boost an orbiting rocket into higher orbit by turning on its engines briefly, so also an outside source may provide the right amount of energy to *excite* the electron to a higher level, where it may stay for a while. Such energy could be provided by a passing high-velocity photoelectron or Compton electron. Or it might come with the absorption of a photon whose energy, hf, happens to equal the difference between the energies of the atomic levels:

$$hf_{\text{photon}} = E_{\text{higher}} - E_{\text{lower}} \qquad (6.4)$$

_____ **EXERCISE 6–5.** _____

Show that a photon with an energy of 10.2 eV would be required to kick the electron from the hydrogen ground level, $n = 1$, up to the first excited level, $n = 2$. How much energy would a second photon then need to excite this $n = 2$ electron further, into the $n = 4$ level?

SOLUTION: By Equation 6.3, the ground ($n = 1$) and first excited ($n = 2$) levels are of energy –13.6 and –3.4 eV, respectively. By Equation 6.4, a photon of energy (–3.4 eV) – (–13.6 eV) = 10.2 eV could bring about the transition. Subsequent ex-

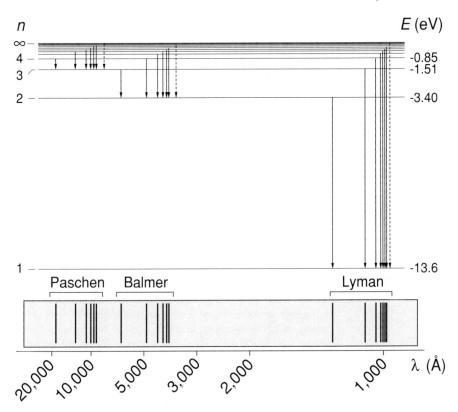

Figure 6–5. Energy levels of the hydrogen atom, in agreement with Equation 6.3. The principal quantum number (n) is noted to the left, and the energy in eV of the corresponding level (E_n) is to the right. A Balmer series photon is emitted if the electron of an excited hydrogen atom drops down (in energy) into the $n = 2$ shell from any higher shell. (Compare with Fig. 6–2.) The dashed vertical line for any level indicates the ionization energy.

citation from the $n = 2$ to $n = 4$ state would take an additional $(-0.85 \text{ eV}) - (-3.4 \text{ eV}) = 2.55 \text{ eV}$.

An excited atom can relax to a state of lower energy by emitting a photon of the appropriate energy. Thus, the transition of the electron from the $n = 4$ orbital of an excited hydrogen atom to the ground level would result in the *emission* of a 12.8-eV photon. The possible transitions of the electron among the various hydrogen orbitals are indicated in Figure 6–5.

_____ **EXERCISE 6–6.** _____

Show that the experimental "Balmer series" emission spectrum of Figures 6–2 and 6–5 agrees with the predictions of the Bohr model, for electrons that drop from upper excited states into the first excited state ($n = 2$).

SOLUTION: The least energetic photon in the series, of 1.89-eV energy, corresponds to a transition from the $n = 3$ to the $n = 2$ orbital. The $n = 4$ to $n = 2$ emission line is at 2.55 eV (see Exercise 6–5), and the next is at 2.86 eV.

If more than 13.6 eV of energy is imparted to a ground-state hydrogen atom, the electron will be removed from it altogether, in an **ionization** event. This leaves the atom with an excess positive charge (or, equivalently, with a deficiency in negative charge), and may impart to the ejected electron a significant amount of kinetic energy of its own. Much of the study of the physics of radiology is concerned with the useful (and sometimes harmful) things that such ionized atoms and high-velocity electrons do.

5. THE MODERN QUANTUM MECHANICAL PICTURE OF THE ATOM

The Bohr model was, in essence, a classical model with a quantum constraint tacked on. It was capable of providing one critically important result, the energy levels of the hydrogen atom, but not much else. And even for hydrogen, the agreement of its predictions with experiment was not perfect in the details.

The fundamental problem is that the laws of "classical" physics simply break down when the system of interest is very small. Werner Heisenberg's *Uncertainty Principle* demonstrated, in particular, that it is impossible to know precisely the position and velocity (momentum) of an electron simultaneously. But the whole purpose of Newton's laws is to relate these two quantities, and at the same moment of time. Newton's laws, therefore, cannot be applied reliably to atom-sized systems.

Despite the notable successes of a few patch-up jobs, such as the Bohr atom, it became apparent that further real progress would require the invention of a substantially more general and powerful approach. This challenge led to a spectacular explosion of intellectual creativity in the mid-1920s, as Heisenberg, Erwin Schroedinger, Paul Dirac, and others gave birth to "modern" quantum mechanics. Quantum mechanics is an abstract, mathematically complex theory that is capable of explaining virtually all the observable physical phenomena (excepting perceptions and thoughts) of everyday life.

A cornerstone of this subtle and all-encompassing theory

is the axiom that at any instant, an atomic system is "in" a **quantum** *state*. The various possible orbitals of a one-electron atom, for example, correspond to different states. The formalism of quantum mechanics provides ways of obtaining mathematical functions that represent the various quantum states in which a system can exist. And knowledge of these state functions then allows one to extract information on all physical characteristics of the system and their changes over time.

Analysis of the hydrogen atom with the heavy mathematical machinery of modern quantum mechanics reveals that there are, in fact, two distinct states with an energy corresponding to the $n = 1$ *energy level* of the Bohr atom. These two, which are denoted "*s* states," happen to have exactly the same energy (except when the atom is placed in a magnetic field). The $n = 1$ **shell** of an atom is therefore said to be twofold, or doubly, *degenerate*. There are, moreover, eight distinct states with the energy corresponding to the first excited, $n = 2$, level of the simple Bohr atom. These eight states in the second shell actually split, on closer examination, into two *sublevels* that differ slightly in energy. One *subshell* contains a doubly degenerate pair of *s* states, and the other holds six degenerate *p* states. Similarly, of the 18 $n = 3$ states, 2 are a pair of degenerate *s* states, 6 constitute a sixfold degenerate *p* sublevel, and 10 are degenerate *d* states. The designations *s, p, d, f*, . . . , refer to different amounts of electron angular momentum associated with the subshells, a topic we need not consider further here.

To summarize the behavior of the hydrogen atom in quantum mechanical language: Most of the time the atom resides in the ground ($n = 1$) state. But on excitation, with the input of energy from an outside source, it may briefly inhabit one of the higher-lying states, after which it drops back down to the ground state, with the emission of a photon of frequency determined by Equation 6.4.

6. MULTIELECTRON ATOMS

Some, but not all, of the preceding discussion of hydrogen carries over to multielectron atoms.

If $Z - 1$ electrons are removed from an atom of atomic number Z, a one-electron ion is left. For such an ion, the sole electron will orbit the nucleus Z times closer, and will be bound Z^2 times more tightly, than in a hydrogen atom. Equation 6.3 becomes

$$E_n = -13.6 \cdot Z^2/n^2, \quad n = 1, 2, 3, \ldots \quad (6.5)$$

As a result, the energy differences between levels increase Z^2-fold. The binding energy of an electron in the lower-lying orbitals of a high-Z atom can therefore be tens of thousands of electron volts. So also are the energies of the photons involved in electronic transitions among them.

_____ **EXAMPLE 6–7.** _____

Tungsten is the element with atomic number Z = 74. How much energy is released, according to the Bohr model, when an electron in the $n = 2$ level drops down into a vacancy in the $n = 1$ level?

SOLUTION: By Equation 6.5, we would expect an x-ray photon of energy $(74)^2(10.2 \text{ eV}) = 56 \text{ keV}$. The tungsten charac-

TABLE 6–1. DESIGNATION OF THE ATOMIC SHELLS AND SUBSHELLS

Principal Quantum Number, n	Shell	Subshell	Spectroscopic Notation	Maximum Number of Electrons	
1	K	s	1s	2	
2	L	s	2s	2	8
		p	2p	6	
3	M	s	3s	2	
		p	3p	6	18
		d	3d	10	
4	N	s	4s	2	32
		p	4p	6	
			<etc.>		

teristic x-rays corresponding to an $n = 2$ to $n = 1$ transition are within a few percent of that.

A multielectron atom is much more complex an entity, however, than just a hydrogen-type atom with Z protons in the nucleus and Z orbiting electrons. Equation 6.5 is not too wide of the mark for transitions between $n = 2$ and $n = 1$ states, but it fails for electrons more distant from the nucleus. An electron in an outer orbital is attracted by a nucleus shielded by clouds of inner electrons, and thus of diminished apparent positive charge. In dealing with outer electrons, the Z of Equation 6.5 therefore has to be replaced by a much smaller "effective Z." Still, the quantum number n remains somewhat useful for distinguishing orbitals; and the letters $K, L, M, \ldots$, label concentric shells of orbitals corresponding to $n = 1, 2, 3, \ldots$, levels.

One might expect that just as all the apples on a tree can drop to the ground, so also all the electrons in a multielectron system would settle into the two lowest-lying K states. Nature, however, does not operate that way. As described by Wolfgang Pauli's *Exclusion Principle*, no state can hold more than one electron. Thus, at most two electrons can inhabit the $n = 1$ (K) shell, and a third electron would have to go to an $n = 2$ (L) state (Table 6–1). A ground-state lithium atom ($Z = 3$) has exactly that configuration of electrons (Fig. 6–6). This is denoted $(1s)^2(2s)^1$ in the standard shorthand, where the number and letter in parentheses designate a shell and subshell, and the superscript refers to the number of electrons actually inhabiting that subshell.

For nitrogen ($Z = 7$), there are electrons in both $n = 1$ states,

in both $n = 2$ s states, and in three of the six possible $n = 2$ p states, in configuration $(1s)^2(2s)^2(2p)^3$.

The noble gas neon, $Z = 10$, is chemically very inert because it has exactly the right number of electrons to fully populate the K and L shells, $(1s)^2(2s)^2(2p)^6$. Neon tends neither to gain nor to lose electrons, and almost never forms chemical bonds.

Sodium, $Z = 11$, consists of closed K and L shells and a single electron in the $n = 3$ shell, $(1s)^2(2s)^2(2p)^6(3s)^1$. The eleventh electron is much further out than the others, and held quite loosely. Sodium is therefore commonly found in the form of a positively charged *ion*, with only 10 electrons.

Potassium, $Z = 19$, finds it energetically preferable to put its nineteenth electron in a $4s$ state, $(1s)^2(2s)^2(2p)^6(3s)^2(3p)^6(4s)^1$, rather than in a $3d$ state. Things get quite a bit more complicated for heavier atoms. The electron configurations of the 20 lightest elements are displayed in Table 6–2, and the **periodic table** of all the elements is shown on the inside back cover of this book.

It is an oversimplification to think of each electron in a multielectron atom as inhabiting its own hydrogen-like orbital. But it is adequate for our purposes, and a good starting point for more correct quantum mechanical approaches which can describe it all in exquisite detail.

7. CHARACTERISTIC X-RAYS

The chemical properties of an atom are determined overwhelmingly by the electrons in its outermost subshells, which are bound by a few electron volts. That is why chemical reactions are often accompanied by the emission of visible light.

The binding energies of the inner electrons of the heavier atoms are much greater, typically tens of kilo-electron volts, and the photons involved in their transitions are correspondingly more energetic. The energies of the x-rays emitted when an atom's outer electrons drop into empty inner orbitals (left briefly vacant by earlier excitation or ionization events) are characteristic of the atomic number, and thus are known as *characteristic* or *fluorescence x-rays* (to be distinguished from bremsstrahlung x-rays). The symbols K, L, and M label the x-rays emitted when outer electrons drop into vacancies in the K, L, and M shells, respectively (Fig. 6–7). Greek letters and subscripts indicate finer distinctions among the transitions.

The energies of some of the K-series characteristic x-rays

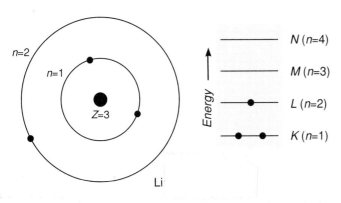

Electron configuration and energy level diagram for the lithium atom, of atomic number $Z = 3$, which has three electrons.

TABLE 6–2. GROUND-STATE ELECTRON CONFIGURATIONS OF THE FIRST 20 ELEMENTS

Element	Symbol	Z	Electron Configuration
Hydrogen	H	1	$(1s)^1$
Helium	He	2	$(1s)^2$
Lithium	Li	3	$(1s)^2(2s)^1$
Beryllium	Be	4	$(1s)^2(2s)^2$
Boron	B	5	$(1s)^2(2s)^2(2p)^1$
Carbon	C	6	$(1s)^2(2s)^2(2p)^2$
Nitrogen	N	7	$(1s)^2(2s)^2(2p)^3$
Oxygen	O	8	$(1s)^2(2s)^2(2p)^4$
Fluorine	F	9	$(1s)^2(2s)^2(2p)^5$
Neon	Ne	10	$(1s)^2(2s)^2(2p)^6$
Sodium	Na	11	$(1s)^2(2s)^2(2p)^6(3s)^1$
Magnesium	Mg	12	$(1s)^2(2s)^2(2p)^6(3s)^2$
Aluminum	Al	13	$(1s)^2(2s)^2(2p)^6(3s)^2(3p)^1$
Silicon	Si	14	$(1s)^2(2s)^2(2p)^6(3s)^2(3p)^2$
Phosphorus	P	15	$(1s)^2(2s)^2(2p)^6(3s)^2(3p)^3$
Sulfur	S	16	$(1s)^2(2s)^2(2p)^6(3s)^2(3p)^4$
Chlorine	Cl	17	$(1s)^2(2s)^2(2p)^6(3s)^2(3p)^5$
Argon	A	18	$(1s)^2(2s)^2(2p)^6(3s)^2(3p)^6$
Potassium	K	19	$(1s)^2(2s)^2(2p)^6(3s)^2(3p)^6(4s)^1$
Calcium	Ca	20	$(1s)^2(2s)^2(2p)^6(3s)^2(3p)^6(4s)^2$

for tungsten, $Z = 74$, are listed in Table 6–3. The radiologically significant lines are shown in Figure 6–7, and were seen earlier in Figure 5–8. The K lines normally do not appear unless a tungsten atom receives a jolt greater than 69.5 keV in energy, as that is the K-shell **binding energy,** i.e., the energy required to eject an electron from the shell, thereby creating a vacancy in it (Table 6–4). The L lines for tungsten occur in the range 8 to 12 keV; they are readily absorbed by an x-ray tube's glass envelope and filters, however, and are usually not seen.

In ordinary radiography, most of the x-ray energy produced at the tungsten anode of the x-ray tube, and used in imaging, is bremsstrahlung radiation. Tungsten characteristic

x-ray photons constitute only a relatively small fraction of the beam's energy. Mammography, on the other hand, uses a molybdenum target tube, and the beam consists almost entirely of molybdenum characteristic x-ray photons, also shown in Table 6–3. The reasons for the difference in the two approaches will become apparent in later chapters.

When an inner electron is somehow ejected from an atom, the vacancy is usually filled within about 10^{-8} second by an outer-orbital electron, and a characteristic x-ray photon is typically emitted in the process. But there are other ways, as well, by which the atom can return to the ground state. In an **Auger** event, an outer-orbital electron drops into the inner-

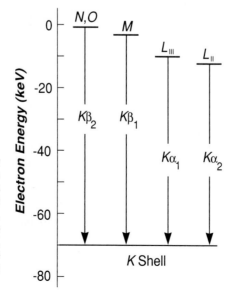

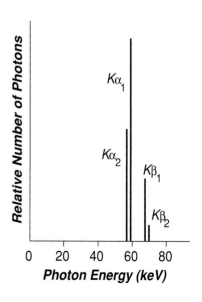

Figure 6–7. When a tungsten-target x-ray tube is operated at a potential greater than about 70 kVp, discrete characteristic x-ray lines appear in the photon spectrum, superimposed on the continuous bremsstrahlung component. The tungsten $K\alpha$ and $K\beta$ lines correspond to transitions from various subshells of the L, M, N, and O levels to vacancies (caused earlier by the bombardment with high-velocity electrons) in the K shell ($n = 1$).

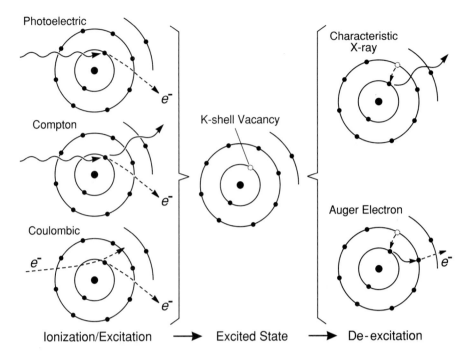

Photoelectric

Compton

Coulombic

Ionization/Excitation ⟶ Excited State ⟶ De-excitation

K-shell Vacancy

Characteristic X-ray

Auger Electron

Figure 6–8. Summary of the atomic excitation and deexcitation processes that occur in the patient's body, in the image receptor, or in both, and are of importance in x-ray imaging. Ejection of an electron from an inner orbital will leave an atom in a highly excited, ionized state. This condition can be brought about by a high-energy photon through a photoelectric or Compton event, or by a high-velocity electron (such as a photoelectron or Compton electron liberated elsewhere) through the Coulombic interaction. (Note that collisions of very energetic electrons with matter can also produce bremsstrahlung radiation—an unrelated issue.) The subsequent filling of the vacancy will result in the emission of a characteristic x-ray or of an Auger electron, and will leave a new vacancy (soon to be filled, somehow) in an outer orbital.

orbital vacancy, and the excess energy is transferred to an outer-orbital *electron* (not to a photon), which comes off in the form of a high velocity *Auger electron*. Immediately following an Auger deexcitation, the atom is left with *two* electron vacancies, both of which are in outer orbitals. The filling of these will involve the emission of lower-energy characteristic x-ray photons.

The spectrum of Auger electrons is discrete, like that of characteristic x-rays. The probability that a particular excited atom will yield a characteristic x-ray (rather than an Auger electron), known as the *fluorescent yield,* is a rapidly increasing function of atomic number: Auger events occur more commonly in atoms of lower atomic number.

The three most important (for radiography) mechanisms by which a high-energy photon or charged particle can ionize or excite an atom are shown in Figure 6–8, along with the two principal mechanisms by which an excited atom or ion can return to the ground state.

TABLE 6–3. Some of the Characteristic X-ray Energies for Tungsten and Molybdenum

Tungsten (W)		Molybdenum (Mo)	
Line	*Energy (keV)*	*Line*	*Energy (keV)*
$K\beta_2$	69.081	$K\beta_{31}$	19.602
$K\beta_1$	67.244	$K\alpha_1$	17.479
$K\beta_3$	66.950	$K\alpha_2$	17.375
$K\alpha_1$	59.321		
$K\alpha_2$	57.984		

From Johns He, Cunningham JR: The Physics of Radiology, 4th ed. Springfield, IL: Charles C Thomas, 1983 (Table 2–3), with permission.

TABLE 6–4. K-Shell Binding Energies (K-Edge) for Some Elements of Radiologic Importance

Z	Element	Energy (keV)
1	Hydrogen (H)	0.0136
6	Carbon (C)	0.28
8	Oxygen (O)	0.53
13	Aluminum (Al)	1.56
20	Calcium (Ca)	4.04
34	Selenium (Se)	12.7
39	Yttrium (Y)	17.0
42	Molybdenum (Mo)	20.0
53	Iodine (I)	33.2
55	Cesium (Cs)	36.0
56	Barium (Ba)	37.4
57	Lanthanum (La)	39.0
64	Gadolinium (Gd)	50.2
67	Holmium (Ho)	56.0
74	Tungsten (W)	69.5
82	Lead (Pb)	88.0

Adapted from Johns HE, Cunningham JR: The Physics of Radiology, 4th ed. Springfield, IL: Charles C Thomas, 1983 (Table 2–2); and Curry TS III, Dowdey JE, Murry RC Jr: Christensen's Physics of Diagnostic Radiology, 4th ed. Philadelphia: Lea & Febiger, 1990 (Table 5–5).

_____ *Chapter 7* _____

The Modern Theory of Matter

1. **Molecular Electron States**
2. **The Energy Bands of a Metal and Ohm's Law**
3. **Superconductors, Insulators, and Semiconductors**
4. **Atomic Nuclei: Elements and Isotopes**
5. **Radioactivity: The Emission of Alpha and Beta Particles and Gamma Rays by Unstable Nuclei**
6. *$E = mc^2$* **and the Interchangeability of Mass and Energy**

It is believed that all the physical phenomena of nature can be explained in terms of four basic forces.

Gravitation holds solar systems and planets together, and ties people to planets, but is of no other relevance here.

The *electromagnetic interaction* is responsible for all the other physical processes of everyday life. The chemical or other properties of the molecules that make up living cells can be described with quantum mechanics and electromagnetic forces, in terms of the behavior of photons and atomic electrons. So, too, can the characteristics of metals, insulators (such as the fluorescent material in a radiographic intensifying screen), semiconductors (of which diode radiation detectors and computer chips are made), and even superconductors (used in the magnets of most magnetic resonance imaging [MRI] devices).

What goes on inside an atomic nucleus, however, is determined largely by the other two forces. The *strong interaction* binds the protons and neutrons to one another. But the *weak interaction* unbalances this situation somewhat. Of the 1500 different naturally occurring or man-made combinations of protons and neutrons, only for 300 or so does the interplay of the strong, weak, and electromagnetic forces result in a stable nuclear balance. The other nuclei are unstable, and radioactive. The magnetic properties of *stable* nuclei are exploited in MRI; it is the gamma rays from *radioactive* nuclei that make possible nuclear medicine.

1. MOLECULAR ELECTRON STATES

Quantum mechanics reveals that the possible "shapes" of the electron orbitals of a molecule, and the energies to which those electron states correspond, are determined largely by the molecule's three-dimensional geometric structure. The less symmetric the molecule, in particular, the smaller the number of states that can be degenerate (isoenergetic).

An isolated atom is the simplest and most symmetric of all "molecular" systems. It possesses the full spherical symmetry of a ball bearing. As noted in Chapter 6, Section 5, the states of

an isolated atom can be doubly (*s* states), sixfold (*p*), tenfold (*d*), or more degenerate.

When an atom is incorporated into a molecule, some of this spherical symmetry is lost. Outer-shell electrons on the atom will now be affected by the presence of other, nearby atoms. The different subshell states of an outer shell may be perturbed in different ways, with the result that they are *no longer degenerate,* no longer all of the same energy. (Inner-shell electrons will still be influenced overwhelmingly by the spherically symmetric potential of their own nucleus; it is only the more loosely bound, outer electrons that are sensitive to their atom's surroundings.)

An isolated nitrogen atom, for example, has a configuration of $(1s)^2(2s)^2(2p)^3$, with three electrons in fully degenerate *atomic 2p states* (Fig. 7–1A). If two nitrogen atoms are brought together to form a diatomic N_2 molecule, which displays rotational symmetry only about the axis linking the two, the six 2p electrons (three from each isolated atom) end up in two groups of *molecular 2p-like states* that differ somewhat in energy (Fig. 7–1B). Figure 7–2 indicates how this energy splitting increases as the separation between the atoms decreases.

2. THE ENERGY BANDS OF A METAL AND OHM'S LAW

Taking this idea one step further: If many identical atoms are brought into close enough proximity, an outer-shell *atomic* level will fan out into an *energy band* of many corresponding *molecular* states that are nearly, but not exactly, degenerate. Figure 7–3 demonstrates this process for sodium (Z = 11). The electronic structure of a free sodium atom is $(1s)^2(2s)^2(2p)^6(3s)^1$. As isolated atoms come together to form solid sodium, the 1s, 2s, and 2p atomic subshells are little affected. But the 3s atomic state splits into a band of many 3s-derived molecular states, each of which now belongs to the solid as a whole (which is, after all, just a very large molecule).

Each state in the band now corresponds to motion of an electron through the entire solid. But there is normally no net

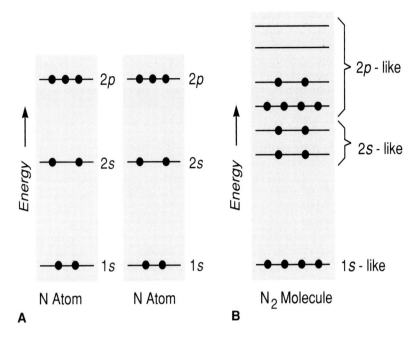

Figure 7–1. Molecular electron states are closely related to the states of the component atoms. **A.** The (identical) energy levels of two widely separated nitrogen atoms. Nitrogen has atomic number $Z = 7$ and the electron configuration $(1s)^2(2s)^2(2p)^3$. The 1s and 2s orbitals are fully occupied, but only three of the six 2p states are filled. **B.** When the two nitrogen atoms are brought close together to form an N_2 molecule, the deeply buried 1s states hardly feel the difference. The four degenerate 2s orbitals (two from each atom) are shifted in energy, however, and split into two groups of molecular states that are predominantly (but not completely) like atomic 2s states. Likewise, the 12-fold degenerate 2p atomic level splits into four molecular levels that are largely 2p-like; two of these are two-fold degenerate, and two are four-fold degenerate. In a neutral N_2 molecule, the 1s-like, 2s-like, and two of the four 2p-like levels are filled with electrons. The ionization energy of the highest-lying electrons is 15.6 eV.

electric current in a piece of sodium metal, as electrons are moving in all different directions at once. That equilibrium is disturbed, however, if an electric field is applied. The (3s)-derived band is only partly filled with electrons, and very little energy is required to elevate some electrons into slightly higher states that correspond to motion in the direction of the field. A metal, such as sodium, is thus a **conductor,** and the partly filled band is known as the *conduction band.*

A potential applied across the ends of a piece of metal wire establishes an electric field within it. Conduction band electrons are prevented from completely free acceleration (which *can* take place within the vacuum of an x-ray tube) primarily

by collisions with the bound, inner electrons of the metal's atoms, and with one another. Such Coulombic interactions deflect the conduction band electrons from their paths, in effect, and, somewhat like a frictional force, hinder their flow. There

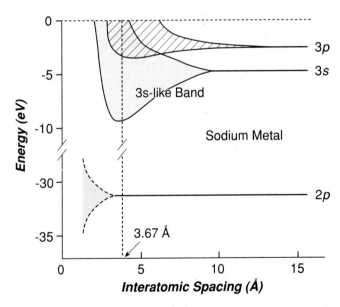

Figure 7–3. The 3s orbital of an isolated sodium atom contains one electron, and the lower-lying shells are filled. When many sodium atoms are brought together, the atomic 3s level splits into a band of many closely spaced 3s-like molecular states. Because the band is only half-filled, electrons in it can respond to an electric field by moving into slightly higher states (in the same band), corresponding to movement in the direction of the field. Hence solid sodium is a conductor of electricity. Also shown is the band created out of (uninhabited) 3p-like states. There are other higher-lying bands, as well, that are not shown here. The interatomic spacing of sodium metal is 3.67 Å. (*After Eisberg R, Resnick R:* Quantum Physics—Of Atoms, Molecules, Solids, Nuclei, and Particles, *2nd ed. New York: Wiley, 1985 [Fig. 13–3].*)

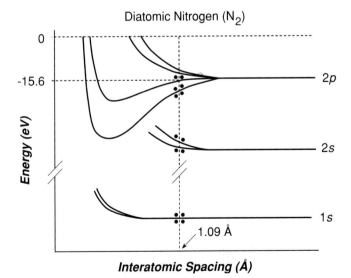

Figure 7–2. The energy splitting of the 2s- and 2p-like molecular states increases as the separation of the nitrogen atoms decreases, and their 2s- and 2p-like nature diminishes. The interatomic spacing for N_2, at equilibrium, is 1.09 Å.

results a balance, in which the current I through the metal is linear in (proportional to) the potential V across it:

$$I = V/R \qquad (7.1)$$

This relationship is known as *Ohm's Law*. The constant of proportionality, R, is called the **resistance** of the wire, the SI unit of which is the *ohm*. It is perhaps helpful to think of the analogy of a pipe partially stopped up with a porous plug, such as a loose rag. The flow of water (current) is proportional to the pressure (voltage) drop across the obstruction, and decreases as the "resistance" of the plug increases.

___ **EXERCISE 7–1.** _____

A 1.5-V dry cell battery is connected across a 1000-ohm resistor (Fig. 7–4). What current will flow, as read by the milliammeter?

SOLUTION: By Equation 7.1, $I = 1.5$ V/1000 ohm = 0.0015 A = 1.5 mA.

___ **EXERCISE 7–2.** _____

A source of potential drives 100 mA through four identical 100-ohm resistors in series. How much potential is developed by the source, and what voltage drop will appear across each resistor?

SOLUTION: By Equation 7.1, the drop across each resistor is 10 V. A 40-V source is required to drive 100 mA through a total resistance of 400 ohm.

Not everything in the world obeys Ohm's Law. The current through an x-ray tube, for example, is far from linear in the high voltage applied across it. So, too, for the current through a superconductor, an insulator, or a semiconductor.

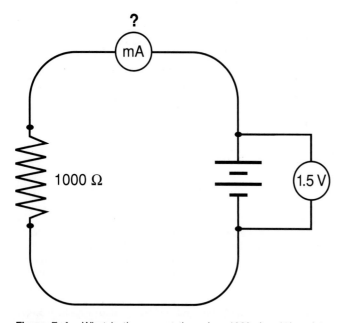

Figure 7–4. What is the current through a 1000-ohm (Ω) resistor (and through the milliammeter) when the voltmeter across the source of potential reads 1.5 V?

3. SUPERCONDUCTORS, INSULATORS, AND SEMICONDUCTORS

The resistance of a piece of normal metal depends on various parameters, in particular, on the temperature: The lower the temperature, the smaller the amplitudes of the vibrations of the atoms constituting the metal, the less they retard the flow of conduction band electrons, and the lower the resistance.

Superconductors

For a metallic **superconductor,** the resistance of the material actually vanishes, completely and abruptly, at its characteristic *critical temperature* (Fig. 7–5). The transition temperatures of metals that become superconducting (not all metals do) lie within a few or a few tens of degrees of absolute zero (−273°C), temperatures that generally can be reached only with the aid of expensive liquid helium and a Dewar vessel to contain it. (A Dewar is a specialized thermos bottle; the double walls are silvered and highly reflective, and the space between them evacuated, so as to minimize heat conduction.) Superconducting materials are used in most MRI magnets, which is one of the many reasons for the great interest in the recent development of ceramics (nonmetallic, claylike substances) and other materials that superconduct at significantly higher (and more easily maintained) temperatures.

Insulators

Energy bands are formed when sodium and iodine ions come together (Fig. 7–6), but the properties of crystalline sodium iodide are quite different from those of sodium metal. Here there are exactly enough electrons in the atomic valence states to completely fill one band, termed the *valence band*, so that there are none left over to go into the next higher-lying one (which is called the conduction band, even though there are no conducting electrons in it). There is an *energy band gap*, typically of the order of 10 eV in width, between valence and conduction bands. An applied electric field normally cannot impart enough en-

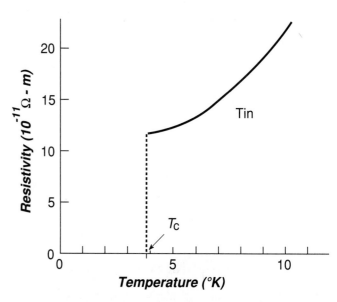

Figure 7–5. Tin is a superconductor (its resistance to electric current totally vanishes) below 3.7°K.

Insulator

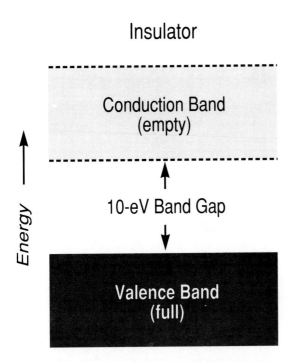

Figure 7–6. In an insulator, such as any alkali halide, the valence energy band is completely filled with electrons. The next-higher (conduction) energy band is empty, and separated from the valence band by a band gap 10 eV or so wide. Neither electric fields nor heat can provide electrons with enough energy to make the transition from valence to conduction band, so no current can flow. What would a diagram of this type, but for a metal, look like (see Fig. 7–3)?

ergy to a valence band electron to kick it into the conduction band, so the solid is an *insulator*. This is another way of saying that all the electrons of an ionic solid are strongly attached to the individual ions, rather than free to roam. Similar considerations apply to covalently bonded crystals such as diamond.

Semiconductors

A **semiconductor** such as silicon, germanium, or gallium arsenide is like an insulator, in that the valence band is nearly full

and the conduction band nearly empty, and the two bands do not overlap (Fig. 7–7). It is also like a metal, however, as the two bands are separated by only 1 eV or so, and a small number of electrons are thermally excited into the conduction band at room temperature. These can then conduct a current, but one that is much smaller than the current through any true metal. Unlike in a metal, the electrical conductivity of a semiconductor increases rapidly with increasing temperature; the amplitudes of the vibrations of the obstructing atoms increase, but that effect is greatly outweighed by the increase in the number of electrons thermally excited into the conduction band.

The presence of impurity atoms or ions can have a profound influence on the properties of a semiconductor. Some of these have been used to advantage in the creation of luminescent materials and other radiation-sensitive materials and of transistors and lasers, as we shall see.

4. ATOMIC NUCLEI: ELEMENTS AND ISOTOPES

The past three sections have dealt with systems consisting of several or many atoms. Here we shall do an about-face and examine the nucleus within a single atom.

The electron cloud of an atom is 2 to 3×10^{-10} m in diameter. Its nucleus is a thousand times smaller and several thousand times more massive. Hence the familiar analogy of the "planetary atom." A nucleus is made up of *protons* and *neutrons*. A *proton* bears a charge of the same magnitude as an electron but of opposite sign, and is 1800 times more massive. A **neutron** is uncharged and slightly more massive than a proton.

The number of protons in a nucleus is called the **atomic number** and is commonly denoted Z. Virtually all the normal chemical, optical, electrical, and mechanical characteristics of an atom are determined solely by Z, that is, by its **element** type.

The properties of the nucleus itself, however, such as its possible nuclear emissions (if it is radioactive, of importance in nuclear medicine) and its magnetic moment (of relevance for MRI), depend on the number of neutrons as well. A nucleus with Z protons also contains typically between Z (for the lighter elements) and $1.6 \cdot Z$ (heavy elements) neutrons. (Nor-

Semiconductor

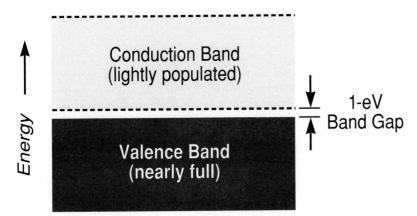

Figure 7–7. In a semiconductor, there are just enough electrons in the valance band to fill it. The band gap is narrow, however, and some electrons are thermally excited across it. These few electrons, now in the conduction band, can readily respond to an applied electric field. In silicon (Si), the band gap is 1.1 eV wide; in germanium (Ge), 0.72 eV; and in gallium arsenide (GaAs), 1.34 eV. The presence of trace amounts of impurities can influence the electrical properties of a piece of semiconductor tremendously.

mal hydrogen, with no neutrons, is an important exception.) The **isotopes** of an element are those nuclear types with the same Z but different numbers of neutrons (Fig. 7–8).

There are several conventional notations for distinguishing the various *isotopes* of an *element*. A common one employs the chemical symbol, with a leading superscript to indicate the mass number, or total number of *nucleons* (protons plus neutrons). The nucleus of ordinary carbon, for example, in which there are six protons and six neutrons, would be written ^{12}C. Occasionally when it is helpful also to note the atomic number, Z will be included as a presubscript, as in $^{12}_{6}C$.

Although the chemical, electrical, mechanical, thermal, and most other characteristics of a collection of atoms of an element are almost entirely independent of the number of neutrons, the *nuclear* properties depend strongly on isotope type.

5. RADIOACTIVITY: THE EMISSION OF ALPHA AND BETA PARTICLES AND GAMMA RAYS BY UNSTABLE NUCLEI

As with an atom, the behavior of a nucleus can be described largely in terms of quantum states. **Radioactivity** is the process whereby an excited, unstable nucleus drops into a state of lower energy and greater (usually) stability. The most important decay pathways by which the various *radionuclides* accomplish this (Fig. 7–9) are gamma ray emission and electron conversion; beta particle emission; positron emission and *K*-electron capture; and alpha particle emission.

Gamma Ray Emission and Conversion Electrons

The nuclear transformation easiest to describe is *gamma emission.* As with an atomic electron, a nucleus can drop from an excited state into one of lower energy through the emission of a photon. Such a **gamma ray** photon differs from an *x-ray photon* in that it originates from a *nuclear transition,* rather than

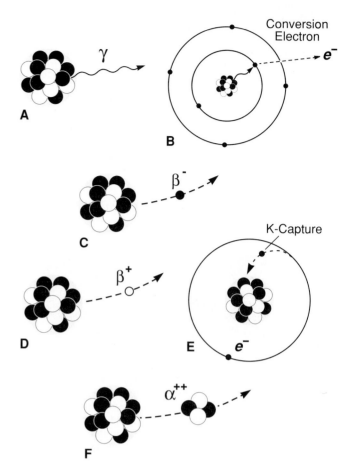

Figure 7–9.   Common modes of nuclear deexcitation. **A.** A nucleus may undergo an isomeric transition (no change in the number of protons or neutrons) by emitting a gamma ray photon. **B.** A nucleus undergoing an isomeric transformation may impart its excess energy to an atomic orbital electron. The ejected electron is called a *conversion electron* (or, if the electron is from the *K* shell, a *K electron*). **C.** With the emission of a beta particle (electron of nuclear origin), the atomic number increases by one, and the number of neutrons decreases by one. **D.** A nucleus can reduce its atomic number by one by emitting a positron, which is identical to a beta particle in every way except for the charge. **E.** Another way a nucleus can reduce its net positive charge is to capture an atomic orbital electron through electron capture (EC). If the orbital electron is from the *K* shell, which lies closest to the nucleus, this is called *K capture*. **F.** Some heavy nuclei emit alpha particles, which are identical to $^{4}_{2}He$ (ordinary helium) nuclei.

Two Isotopes of Carbon

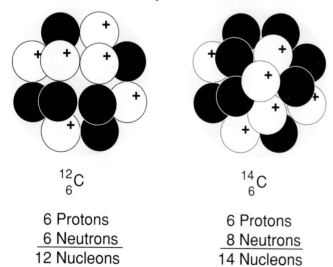

$^{12}_{6}C$	$^{14}_{6}C$
6 Protons	6 Protons
6 Neutrons	8 Neutrons
12 Nucleons	14 Nucleons

Figure 7–8.   Nuclei of the isotopes ^{12}C and ^{14}C of the element carbon contain the same number of protons (6), but different numbers of neutrons.

from an *atomic orbital electron transition* (producing a characteristic x-ray) or a bremsstrahlung event. Gamma rays from radionuclides tend to be (with notable exceptions) more energetic than diagnostic x-ray photons, but they are generally less energetic than some of the x-ray photons produced by the linear accelerators employed for radiotherapy. In other words, it is the source, not the energy, that normally distinguishes gamma ray from x-ray photons.

Technetium-99*m* (^{99m}Tc), the "metastable" excited state of the technetium (Z = 43) isotope that contains 56 neutrons, is the workhorse of the nuclear medicine department. It can deexcite by emitting energy in the form of a single 140-keV gamma ray photon:

$$\ce{^{99m}_{43}Tc -> ^{99}_{43}Tc + gamma} \tag{7.2}$$

(Fig. 7–10). In the decay of $^{99m}_{43}Tc$, the "daughter" nucleus has the same numbers of protons and neutrons as the parent, and this is therefore known as an *isomeric* transformation.

A *conversion electron* is emitted by an atom when, in effect, a gamma ray on the way out of a nucleus interacts with one of the atom's own orbital electrons and ejects it in a sort of "internal photoelectric effect" (Fig. 7–9B). The charge on the nucleus is unchanged, and the vacancy left behind in the atomic cloud will somehow have to be filled later. Most conversion electrons are ejected from the *K* shell, which lies closest to the nucleus, but *L* and *M* conversion events also occur.

> The *coefficient of internal conversion* for an excited nuclear state, commonly written α, is defined as the ratio of the relative numbers of conversion electrons and corresponding gamma rays it emits:
>
> α ≈ conversion electrons/gamma rays

Beta Particle Emission

In contrast to gamma and conversion electron emission, in *beta decay* the charge on the nucleus changes. A nucleus may hold too many neutrons (or, equivalently, not enough protons) for comfort (Fig. 7–11). It may attempt to rectify that awkward situation by transforming one of its neutrons into a proton, which remains within the nucleus, and an electron, which escapes:

$$n \to p + e^- + \bar{\nu} \tag{7.3a}$$

The electron thus created is known as a *beta particle*. Once out of the nucleus, it behaves like any other high-velocity electron, and can ionize the matter through which it happens to pass. (A massless, chargeless antineutrino, $\bar{\nu}$, is also produced, and exits the scene at the speed of light. It hardly ever interacts with anything, however, and is of interest here only in balancing the books for conservation of energy, and the other conservation laws.)

In the case of carbon-14, for example, the beta decay process reads

$$\ce{^{14}_{6}C -> ^{14}_{7}N + e^- + \nu} \tag{7.3b}$$

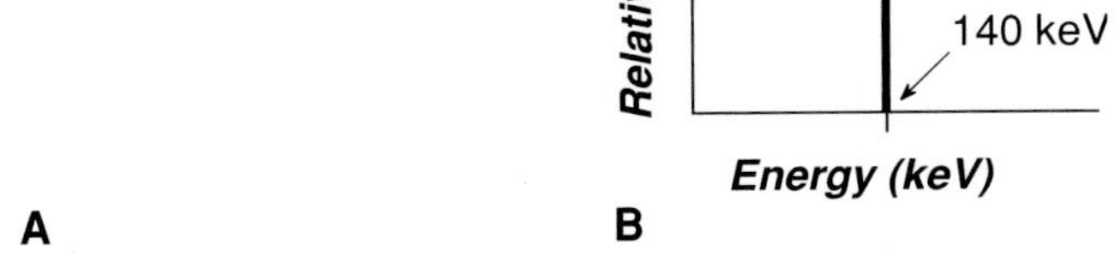

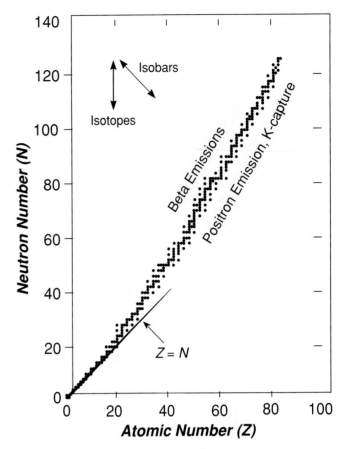

Figure 7–11. Chart of the stable nuclei (black dots). An unstable nucleus with too many neutrons (upper, shaded region) will try to move toward the line of stability, increasing its proton-to-neutron ratio, through beta emission. A neutron-poor nucleus, by contrast, will try to reduce the nuclear charge, through either positron emission or electron capture. *Isotopes* have the same atomic number, *Z*, but different numbers of neutrons, *N*. *Isobars* have the same total number of nucleons, *Z* + *N*. For the lighter elements, the number of neutrons tends to be about the same as the number of protons, *N* = *Z*. The *N/Z* ratio for high-*Z* elements increases to about 1.6.

(Fig. 7–12). The total number of nucleons (protons plus neutrons) in the nucleus is the same (this is therefore said to be an *isobaric transformation*). Also, the overall net charge of the universe is unchanged. But the nucleus is left with one more positive charge than it had before, that is, its atomic number has increased by one, and it is transmuted from carbon into nitrogen. As *Z* has increased, the atom will now have to acquire an additional orbital electron from somewhere.

Positron Emission and *K*-Electron Capture

A nucleus may, by contrast, have too many protons, or not enough neutrons, and seek stability by decreasing the nuclear proton-to-neutron ratio. One of its protons may transform into a neutron, which remains within the nucleus, and a *positron* and a neutrino, which escape it. (The positron is the "antiparticle" to the electron—identical in every respect except that it bears a positive charge.) The overall *positron emission* reaction for fluorine-18, for example, is

$$\ce{^{18}_{9}F -> ^{18}_{8}O + e^+ + \nu} \tag{7.4a}$$

Figure 7–10. A metastable technetium-99 nucleus deexcites by emitting a 140-keV gamma ray photon. A gamma ray photon is identical to an x-ray photon of the same energy, but it is of nuclear (rather than electron orbital or bremsstrahlung) origin. **A.** Energy level diagram for this gamma emission process. **B.** (Discrete) gamma ray emission spectrum.

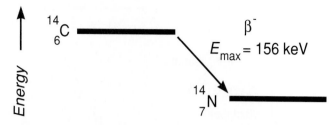

Figure 7–12. Transformation of a carbon-14 nucleus into nitrogen-14 via beta decay. A neutron within the nucleus changes into a proton and an electron, in effect, and the electron is ejected as a beta particle. The beta particle is emitted from this radionuclide with a kinetic energy of up to 156 keV; when the beta particle's kinetic energy is less than 156 keV, the rest of the energy of the nucleus is carried off by a *neutrino* (not shown). What might the beta emission spectrum look like (see Fig. 7–10B)?

A fluorine-18 nucleus can achieve the same end, reducing the nuclear charge, also by means of *K-electron capture*. The nucleus grabs one of its own innermost (*K*-shell) orbital electrons

$$^{18}_{9}F + e^- \rightarrow ^{18}_{8}O + \nu \qquad (7.4b)$$

and thereby neutralizes the charge of one of the protons. The new nucleus may be left in an excited nuclear state, and will have to undergo one or more subsequent transformations to reach stability.

Alpha Particle Emission

Alpha particle emission occurs commonly among the heavier radionuclides, with $Z > 82$. An alpha particle is a tightly bound cluster of two protons and two neutrons (i.e., a helium nucleus), emitted with a relatively large amount of kinetic energy (typically in the range 4 to 9 MeV).

Uranium-238 ($Z = 92$) undergoes alpha decay, leaving behind a thorium-234 ($Z = 90$) nucleus:

$$^{238}_{92}U \rightarrow ^{234}_{90}Th + \alpha \qquad (7.5)$$

The alpha is ejected with 4.2 MeV of kinetic energy. Thorium is itself radioactive, as are its progeny for a number of generations, and the decay of this *series* of radionuclides, down to the stable isotope lead-206, is shown in Figure 7–13.

Alpha particles are doubly charged. Also, because of their great mass, they move relatively slowly, even when they have much kinetic energy. For both reasons, they rapidly expend their energy in ionizing any matter through which they pass. There are two important consequences of that fact: (1) Alpha particles do not travel far in tissue (typically only 50 μm, or 50×10^{-6} m), but (2) because the ionization events they cause are spaced close together, alpha particles are biologically much more efficient (per unit of energy deposited in tissue) in causing cancer than either beta particles or gamma ray photons. Thus, alpha particles incident on skin will be stopped in the epidermis, and can do little harm; but if the radionuclide is inhaled, alpha particles can directly irradiate the tissues of the lung, and that can pose a serious health risk.

Uranium-238 occurs widely in rocks and soils, as does its descendant, radium-226. The radon-222 resulting from the alpha decay of the radium is a noble gas, like helium and

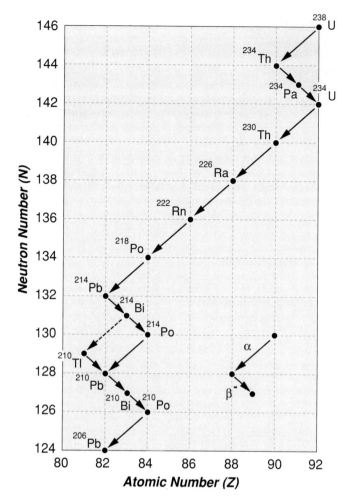

Figure 7–13. The decay scheme, or radioactive series, that begins with the naturally occurring, long-half-life (6.5×10^9 years) radionuclide uranium-238 and ends with the stable isotope lead-206. In the first step, ^{238}U emits an alpha particle; the daughter thorium-234 has four fewer nucleons. In the second step, ^{234}Th emits a beta particle to become protactinium-234; the atomic number increases by one, but the total number of nucleons does not change. (99.96% of all bismuth-214 nuclei decay by way of polonium-214.) There are two other such major, naturally occurring series, beginning with uranium-235 (half-life of 1.0×10^9 years) and with thorium-232 (2×10^{10} years), respectively.

neon. It is chemically nonreactive, not bound up in immobile molecules, and may diffuse from the ground into the basements of houses. There it decays into alpha-emitting isotopes of polonium and lead, individual atoms of which tend to attach to dust. There is strong evidence that where the concentrations of airborne radon and its progeny are high, such as in uranium mines and in some homes and other structures, the hazards of inhalation of such dust are significant.

Alpha emission, beta (electron or positron) emission, *K* capture, and conversion electron emission will invariably disrupt an atom's configuration of *orbital electrons*. The electron cloud will rapidly settle down into its (new) electronic ground state, however, with the release of one or more photons, Auger electrons, or both.

6. *E = mc²* AND THE INTERCHANGEABILITY OF MASS AND ENERGY

Quantum mechanics and the Theory of Relativity are the two pillars on which modern physics is built. An attribute they share is an insistence on predicting phenomena that are totally at variance with normal everyday experience. But an overwhelming body of experimental evidence indicates that both provide correct descriptions of reality.

Relativity says that a clock speeding past you would seem to be ticking more slowly than an identical clock in your hand. It would also weigh more. Suppose you determine the clock's mass to be m when it is not moving relative to you. If you somehow repeat the measurement as it flies by you at velocity v, you will find (correctly) that its mass is increased by the amount indicated in Figure 7–14. The mass would become infinite at $v = c$, implying that material things cannot travel at speeds equal to or greater than that of light.

One of the best known of mathematical equations is Einstein's prescription for extending the Law of Conservation of Energy to cover situations in which matter is converted into radiant energy, and vice versa. If an object is completely transformed into radiation, then its mass and the resulting radiation energy, E, are related as

$$E = m \cdot c^2 \qquad (7.6)$$

The meaning of this is nicely illustrated by the phenomenon of positron annihilation. A positron is the antiparticle of the electron: When the two come into contact, they "annihilate" one another with the production of a pair of 511-keV *annihilation photons* (see Fig. 1–12A). It is such photon pairs, which leave the scene of the collision in nearly opposite directions, that positron emission tomography (PET) uses for imaging.

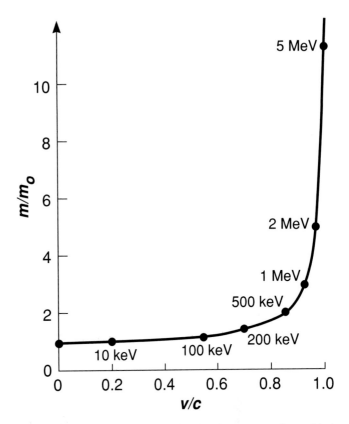

Figure 7–14. By the theory of relativity, the mass m of any object moving at velocity v will be greater than its rest mass m_0 by a factor of $m(v)/m_0 = 1/\sqrt{1 - v^2/c^2}$, where c is the speed of light. The masses and velocities of electrons for several particular energies are noted.

EXERCISE 7–3.

How much energy would be released if the mass of one electron were transformed into radiant energy?

SOLUTION: By Equation 7.6, $(9.11 \times 10^{-31} \text{ kg})(3 \times 10^8 \text{ m/s})^2 = 8.20 \times 10^{-14}$ J = 511 keV.

EXERCISE 7–4.

Under certain conditions, a photon of sufficient energy may be transformed into an electron–positron pair (Fig. 4–4). What is the minimum photon energy required for this process to occur?

SOLUTION: 1022 keV. The positrons used in PET scanning, however, normally come into existence through nuclear decay processes like that of Equation 7.4a.

As everyday objects travel at speeds much less than c, we never observe relativistic effects directly. For particles pushed in accelerators to speeds near that of light, however, the phenomenon in Figure 7–14 can be of great significance. One need not worry much about relativistic effects for 70-keV electrons in a diagnostic x-ray tube, for example, but the situation is quite different at the energies used in radiotherapy. Relativistic effects become apparent when electron kinetic energy is more than a small fraction of the electron rest-mass energy (511 keV).

Part 2

Production of X-rays

Chapter 8

Resistors, Transistors, and All That: The Components of an X-ray Tube Circuit

1. **A Generator Produces Smooth, High-Voltage Direct Current Out of Low-Voltage Alternating Current**
2. **The First Step: Transforming Low-Voltage Alternating Current to High-Voltage Alternating Current**
3. **Rectifying the High-Voltage Alternating Current with a Diode**
4. **The Simplest X-ray Tube Circuit**
5. **Full-Wave Rectification**
6. **Smoothing the Rectified Voltage with a Capacitive Filter; Percentage Ripple**
7. **Timing the Exposure**
8. **Switching the X-ray Beam On and Off**
9. **Triode Valves, and More About Switching**
10. **The Cathode Ray Tube (Another Triode) Is the Heart of the Oscilloscope and of the Television Monitor**
11. **Semiconductor Diodes and Transistors**

Here we begin the discussion of the kinds of equipment, the hardware, used in medical imaging. The approach in this chapter is to build a rudimentary x-ray tube circuit, piece by piece, from its primary constituent parts. Transformers, capacitors, vacuum tube and solid-state diodes, and vacuum tube triodes and solid-state transistors are introduced, and their basic operations are discussed. Much of this material will have application to the other imaging modalities as well.

X-ray tube circuits and the production of x-ray energy were discussed briefly in Chapter 2, Section 2, and you may wish to review that material before continuing.

1. A GENERATOR PRODUCES SMOOTH, HIGH-VOLTAGE DIRECT CURRENT OUT OF LOW-VOLTAGE ALTERNATING CURRENT

Electric current can be driven around a *closed-loop circuit* by a source of electric potential.

Current that flows through a wire in only one direction and with constant magnitude, such as in a flashlight, is known as **direct current (DC)**. A battery is a source of DC voltage and

energy (Fig. 8–1A). Most generators of electric power, however, are of a different sort. It is found to be efficient to transmit energy to homes and hospitals by means of **alternating current (AC)**, in which the amplitude and polarity of the driving voltage and the current vary periodically with time (Fig. 8–1B).

The **analog** audio **signal** that your stereo amplifier delivers to each loudspeaker consists of a voltage and current that vary over time in such a way as to convey information (Fig. 8–1C). Computers and other kinds of digital equipment make use of another approach (Fig. 8–1D)—with a **digital signal**, DC voltage is turned on and off intermittently, as in the transmission of a telegraphic message with Morse code.

Nearly all of the electrical devices in your house or medical department receive AC power through a pair of conducting metal wires (Fig. 8–2). One of these, the *neutral* line, is grounded elsewhere, at a transformer belonging to the power station. The *hot* wire carries a potential that alternates sinusoidally above and below that on the neutral wire 60 times per second, in the United States, with an amplitude typically of 155 to 170 V. (A third, or *ground*, wire is commonly used to reduce the risk of electrical shock from electrical equipment. The third prong of a modern conventional AC plug connects the metal

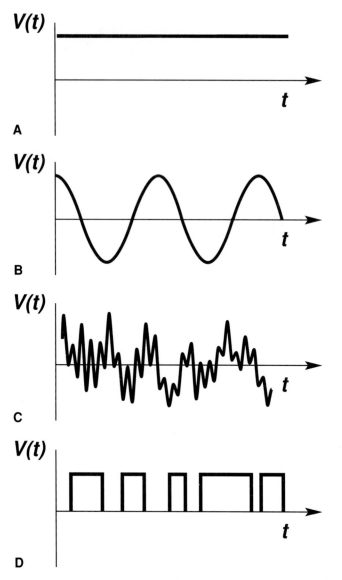

Figure 8–1. Four categories of time-dependent voltages. **A.** Direct current, in which the voltage remains constant. **B.** Alternating current; electricity is commonly provided by the power company in the form of *unchanging*, repetitive alternating current. **C.** Radio frequency and audio frequency electrical signals convey information through *changes* over time in the form of the alternating current. **D.** Digital computers process and transmit information by means of meaningful sequences of intermittent pulses of direct current.

chassis of the equipment to a local ground, such as a buried copper pipe, located somewhere in your building.)

A steady DC voltage will deliver more power to a resistor than does an AC source of the same peak voltage. The amplitude of a sinusoidal AC voltage must be $\sqrt{2}$ times greater than the steady value of DC voltage, in fact, to transform the same amount of electric energy into heat or to perform the same amount of useful work. Thus, AC of 163-V peak voltage corresponds to $163/\sqrt{2}$ = 115 V DC. It is this 115-V *root mean square* (rms), or "effective, DC-equivalent" voltage of an AC source to which one normally refers, and for AC power

$$V_{rms} = V_{peak} / \sqrt{2} \qquad (8.1)$$

EXERCISE 8–1.

A certain machine requires 220 V (rms) power. Over how great a range must the instantaneous voltage change?

SOLUTION: The peak voltage is $220 \cdot \sqrt{2}$ = 310 V. The voltage ranges from –310 to +310 V, relative to neutral.

Although many electrical devices use AC power, an x-ray tube operates best when attached to a source of high, constant voltage. It is a primary function of an x-ray **generator** to transform the low-voltage (several hundred volts) AC supplied by the electric power company to a much higher voltage AC (up to 150,000 V), and then convert that into the desired high-voltage DC. The first of these two steps involves the use of a transformer.

2. THE FIRST STEP: TRANSFORMING LOW-VOLTAGE ALTERNATING CURRENT TO HIGH-VOLTAGE ALTERNATING CURRENT

Recall from Chapter 4, Sections 4 and 5, that a current in a wire will produce a magnetic field around it. Conversely, a *changing* magnetic field at a wire will induce a voltage in it. These complementary phenomena underlie the workings of a *transformer* (Fig. 8–3A). A transformer consists of a *primary* coil of N_1 loops of wire and a *secondary* of N_2 loops. When the primary is attached to a source of AC power, the current through it creates an oscillating magnetic field. The voltage V_2 induced in the secondary coil by this changing magnetic field is related to the driving primary voltage V_1 as

$$V_2/V_1 = N_2/N_1 \qquad (8.2)$$

for a (hypothetical) perfectly efficient transformer. Passage of DC through the primary will *not* give rise to high-voltage DC in the secondary—a transformer works properly only with AC.

The primary and secondary coils are normally wrapped on a ring of iron or some other ferromagnetic material (Fig. 8–3B). This profoundly affects the geometry and strength of the magnetic fields induced by the primary and secondary currents, and leads to more efficient transfer of power between them. But it does not alter Equation 8.2.

Energy is neither created nor destroyed in a transformer. Aside from what is lost in ohmic (resistive) heating, the power coming out of the secondary coil is the same as what is pumped into the primary side. That is, for our ideal transformer,

$$\text{power}_{out} = \text{power}_{in} \qquad (100\% \text{ efficiency}) \qquad (8.3)$$

By the argument that led to Equation 5.4, the power input is the product $V_1 \cdot I_1$ of the voltage drop across the primary and the current through it. So also for the power delivered by the secondary to a *load*, such as a resistor or x-ray tube.

Equations 8.2 and 8.3 together reveal that the currents in the secondary and primary coils depend on the coil turns ratio according to $I_2/I_1 = N_1/N_2$. For a voltage step-up transformer, with N_2/N_1 greater than unity, the current through the secondary and load is (perhaps surprisingly) less than that in the primary circuit.

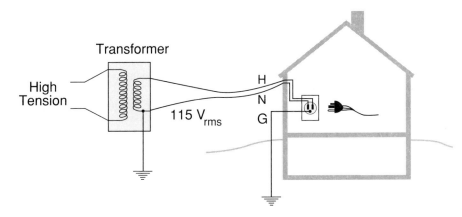

Figure 8–2. A simplified schematic of the way in which electrical power gets to your stereo. Energy is provided on a pair of wires from a power company transformer. The voltage between the "hot" wire and the grounded "neutral" wire varies 60 times per second with a peak amplitude of 163 V. Such AC dissipates energy in a resistor as would a 115-V DC source, and is called "115-V rms AC." The high-tension cables to the power company's transformer carry three-phase power, with voltages typically in the tens of thousands of volts.

_____ EXERCISE 8–2. _____

A transformer with 50 turns in the primary and 25,000 turns in the secondary is attached to a 230-V (rms) AC source. What peak voltage may be obtained from the secondary? What rms voltage?

SOLUTION: Assuming 100% efficiency, the transformer steps up the voltage by a factor of $N_2/N_1 = (25,000/50) = 500$ (Equation 8.2). The rms (effective) voltage in the secondary is $V_{rms} = (500)(230 \text{ V}) = 115,000 \text{ V}$. By Equation 8.1, the peak voltage in the secondary is $V_p = \sqrt{2} \cdot 115,000 \text{ V} = 163 \text{ kV}$.

_____ EXERCISE 8–3. _____

With the transformer and input voltage of Exercise 8–2, an average current of 300 mA is driven through a resistive load on the secondary for 200 milliseconds. What power and energy are delivered to the load? What is its resistance? What is the average power into the primary of the transformer?

SOLUTION: The average power delivered to the load is determined by the rms voltage across it and the average current I_{av} through it: $\text{power}_{av} = V_{rms} \cdot I_{av} = (115,000 \text{ V})(0.3 \text{ A}) = 34.5$ kW. Over 0.2 second, it receives 6,900 J of energy. By Ohm's law (Equation 7.1), the load's resistance is $R = V_{rms}/I_{av} = (115,000 \text{ V})/(0.3 \text{ A}) = 380,000$ ohms. As $I_2/I_1 = N_1/N_2$, current through the primary is $(0.3 \text{ A})(25,000/50) = 150$ A. Energy therefore flows into the transformer at the rate $(230 \text{ V})(150 \text{ A}) = 34.5$ kW.

The numbers in the preceding two exercises are typical of what one might find for the voltage step-up transformer of an

x-ray tube circuit, with a diagnostic tube as the load. As will soon become apparent, however, the value of the voltage applied to the tube and the average current through it depend also on the way the AC power is rectified and smoothed.

3. RECTIFYING THE HIGH-VOLTAGE ALTERNATING CURRENT WITH A DIODE

In an x-ray generator, power supplied by the electric company is converted by a transformer into a high-voltage form which, after rectification and smoothing, is suitable for application across an x-ray tube.

The important characteristic of a rectifier is that it conducts electric current in only one direction. Here will be discussed the use of vacuum tube diodes as rectifiers. Solid state diodes will be considered at the end of the chapter.

Electrons in matter ordinarily have little tendency to fly off into space. But if an isolated piece of metal in a vacuum can be heated to a sufficiently high temperature without vaporizing, a fair number of its electrons may acquire enough thermal energy to "boil off," or undergo _thermionic emission_. The resulting net positive charge on the piece of metal draws electrons back toward it, and causes a cloud of _space charge_ to hover above its surface. The space charge further repels electrons newly emitted from the cathode back toward it, and an equilibrium is established. The size of the cloud of space charge and the number of electrons swarming within it depend on the size, physicochemical properties, and temperature of the metal. An appreciable space charge will form around a piece of tungsten wire, for example, that is heated to above 2200°C.

A vacuum tube diode is an evacuated glass bulb that con-

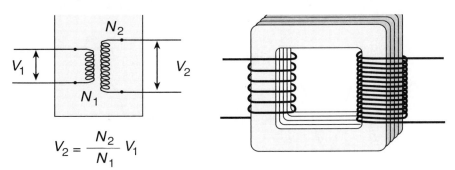

$$V_2 = \frac{N_2}{N_1} V_1$$

A   **B**

Figure 8–3. Use of a transformer to step voltage up or down. **A.** The primary and secondary coils of a perfectly efficient transformer have N_1 and N_2 windings, respectively. With V_1 AC (never DC) applied to the input of the primary, the voltage at the output will be $V_2 = V_1 \cdot (N_2/N_1)$. If the efficiency is less than 100%, the output voltage decreases accordingly. **B.** Transformers are commonly wound on metallic structures (the simplest being an iron ring) to increase their efficiencies.

tains two (hence the "di-") metal *electrodes*, called the **cathode** and **anode** (Fig. 8–4A). The job of the cathode is to produce a cloud of space charge, so it is heated to incandescence, commonly by means of a nearby third element, a coiled *heater* or **filament** of resistive wire through which current is driven by a **filament power supply.** The greater the filament voltage and current, the higher the cathode temperature, and the greater the amount of space charge hovering above it.

EXERCISE 8–4.

The resistance of an x-ray tube filament is 2 ohms, and about 5 A of DC current is required to achieve 2200°C. What voltage must the filament power supply put out?

SOLUTION: By Ohm's law (Equation 7–1), a 10-V DC power supply will do the job.

Suppose a diode is attached across a source of high AC voltage. During the half-cycles that the voltage applied to the cathode is negative relative to the anode (Fig. 8–4B), the space charge equilibrium is disturbed. The electron cloud shifts away from the cathode, and some of it sweeps across to the anode. This creates a current of electrons that flows from cathode to anode, and continues on around the closed loop that includes the high-voltage power supply. (By a convention established

long before people knew about electrons, the direction of the flow of "conventional current" is opposite that of the electrons.) At any instant, the current is exactly the same everywhere in this circuit—through the high-voltage source and milliammeter (not shown) and along the wires connecting them—and equal to the current between the electrodes.

So much for what happens when the cathode is relatively negative. The other half of the time, when the cathode is positively charged (Fig. 8–4C), the space charge is simply pulled closer to it, and there is no flow of current. (No electrons are thermionically emitted by the anode, which should be much too cool for that to occur.)

When the voltage applied across a diode happens to be in the *forward* direction, with the anode positive, the tube conducts current easily, and acts almost like a piece of wire with not much resistance. With the voltage in the *reverse* direction, the diode acts (nearly) like an open switch, a (nearly) infinite resistance. Current that would otherwise like to be AC can thus flow in only one direction through the diode, and only half the time (Fig. 8–4D).

A device whose *raison d'être* is to allow the flow of current in only one direction is called a *rectifier*. (An x-ray tube, too, will rectify AC current, but that is not its primary job.) The symbol in Figure 8–5A is standard for a rectifier, such as a vacuum tube diode or a solid-state diode. The arrow points in the direction of flow of conventional current, opposite that of the flow of electrons.

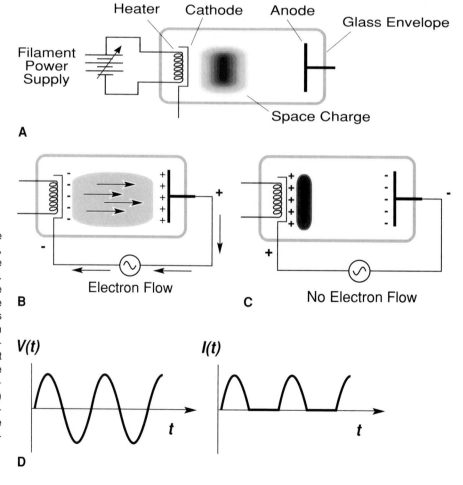

Figure 8–4. Operation of a vacuum tube diode. **A.** The temperature of the cathode, hence the size of the cloud of space charge, are determined by the filament (heater) current. **B.** Application of a positive voltage to the anode alters the space charge equilibrium, causing the flow of electrons from cathode to anode. This flow is the tube current, to be distinguished from the filament current. **C.** When the anode is negative relative to the cathode, tube current ceases. Thus, a diode acts as a one-way valve for electrical current. **D.** The instantaneous voltage $V(t)$ from the source and the current $I(t)$ through the diode are monitored with a voltmeter and an ammeter. $I(t)$ assumes only positive values; that is, current flows in only one direction.

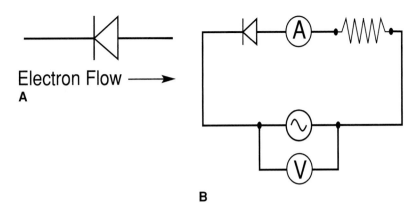

Electron Flow ⟶

A

B

Figure 8–5.   Rectification by a diode. **A.** Standard symbol for a diode. For unfortunate historical reasons, the arrowhead points in the direction of "conventional" current, which is opposite that of the real flow of electrons. **B.** AC voltage applied across a diode and load resistor; current flows only half of every cycle. The ammeter (A) normally reads average current. You have to determine whether the voltmeter (V) reads peak or average (rms) voltage.

The transformation of AC into current that flows in only one direction and for only half a cycle (see Fig. 8–4D) is called *half-wave rectification*. In the circuit of Figure 8–5B, half-wave rectified current is driven through a resistor.

4. THE SIMPLEST X-RAY TUBE CIRCUIT

X-ray photons (and much heat) are produced when high-velocity electrons collide with a metal target. To create an x-ray beam in a controlled fashion, one needs an x-ray tube and its housing, a source of variable low voltage to heat the tube's filament (which doubles as the cathode), a source of adjustable high voltage (preferably DC) to accelerate the electrons through the tube, an exposure timer, and a switch (Fig. 8–6). The voltmeter and ammeter keep track of the voltage directly across the tube and the current through it.

A transformer, diode, timer, and switch combination serves as a rudimentary *generator* or power supply of constant-polarity voltage. When forward biased, the diode is of very low effective resistance (much less than that of the x-ray tube), and practically all the voltage from the transformer is applied across the x-ray tube. When biased in the reverse direction, the

diode is like an open switch, and no voltage appears across the tube. Thus, the voltage supplied to the anode of the x-ray tube is never negative.

It might seem that the diode is not needed, as the x-ray tube itself can rectify the AC. There is a danger, however, that the x-ray tube anode could overheat, and create some unwanted space charge of its own. Without the power supply diode, electrons from the anode would then accelerate in the wrong direction through the tube during the reverse polarity phase of the applied voltage. These electrons could slam into the wire cathode/filament with high kinetic energy, quickly burning it out.

The *peak kilovoltage (kVp)* across the tube, hence the peak energy of the x-rays, can be varied by altering the number of turns that are included in the secondary coil of the transformer (Equation 8–2). The intensity of the beam depends both on the kVp and on the current through the tube. *Tube current*, in turn, is determined by the amount of space charge above the cathode, hence by the temperature of the heater (as established by the filament current). Average tube current, in milliamperes, is measured by the milliammeter.

Our power supply provides half-wave rectified AC, in

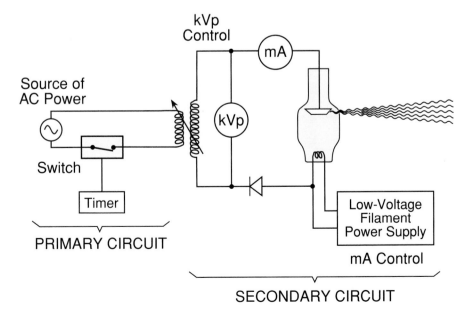

Figure 8–6.   A very simple x-ray tube circuit. The peak voltage applied across the tube is adjusted by changing, in effect, the number of turns in the secondary of the step-up transformer. The average *tube* current is controlled by the cathode temperature (that is, by the *filament* current) and by the peak kilovoltage.

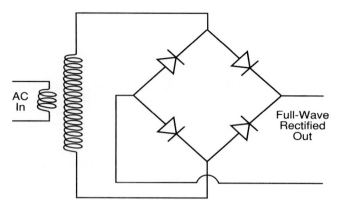

Figure 8–7. Full-wave rectifier circuit.

which the voltage applied to the x-ray tube varies widely. This is less than optimal for two reasons: First, positive voltage is produced (and can drive current through the x-ray tube) during only half of each AC cycle. Second, the applied voltage is near its peak value for only a small fraction of the time, so fewer highest-energy x-ray photons are produced than would be the case if the applied voltage were constant. (Why is *that* relevant?)

We can improve the situation considerably in two ways.

5. FULL-WAVE RECTIFICATION

The first is to replace our single diode, half-wave rectifier with a *full-wave rectification* circuit (Fig. 8–7). Voltage is now produced (and can drive current through the x-ray tube) during both halves of the AC cycle. The left and right sides of Figure 8–8A show the flow of electrons when the upper terminal of the AC source is negative and positive, respectively. The resultant full-wave rectified voltage (Fig. 8–8B) is closer to true DC than is the output of a half-wave rectifier. The next level of im-

provement of this type involves the use of *three-phase power*, as will be discussed in the next chapter.

6. SMOOTHING THE RECTIFIED VOLTAGE WITH A CAPACITIVE FILTER; PERCENTAGE RIPPLE

The second way to improve our voltage supply is to smooth out the rectified voltage with a capacitive filter.

Capacitors, along with resistors, inductors (coils), transformers, and vacuum tubes and transistors, are basic building blocks of electrical circuits. A *capacitor*, represented in circuit diagrams as ⊣⊢, consists typically of a pair of parallel metal foil sheets separated by a thin layer of insulating *dielectric* material. The function of a capacitor is to accept and store charge. When a capacitor is attached to a V-volt battery, some amount q of electron charge will be drawn from one sheet, and the same quantity of negative charge will be pushed onto the second plate (Fig. 8–9). The amount q (coulombs) of charge stored is linear in V (volts):

$$q = C \cdot V \qquad (8.4)$$

The constant of proportionality, C, known as the "capacitance," is measured in SI units in farads, where 1 farad = 1 C/V. C is proportional to the area of the metal sheets (which, for compactness, may be rolled up like a cigar) and inversely proportional to their separation. It also depends on the nature of the dielectric insulating material between them.

> Dielectric substances are made up of highly "polar" molecules (Fig. 8–10A). Each molecule is electrically neutral, but the distribution of electrons on it is nonuniform, with the consequence that its opposite ends seem oppositely charged. When the metal sheets of a capacitor are charged up and produce an electric field within the dielectric material, each such molecule might be rotated somewhat (Fig. 8–10B), so that its charged ends tend, in effect, to neutralize some of the charge stored on the metallic sheets. This allows the capacitor to accept more charge from the battery (i.e., the amount q

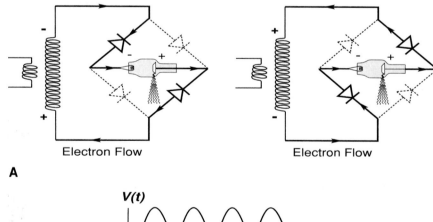

Electron Flow   Electron Flow

A

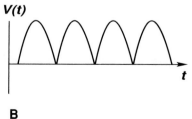

B

Figure 8–8. Full-wave rectification ensures that the voltage applied to the x-ray tube is of the correct polarity at all times. A. The two paths of electron flow, with the two voltage polarities of the source. B. The waveform of full-wave rectified voltage.

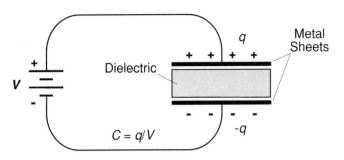

Figure 8–9. A capacitor consists of a pair of metal sheets with dielectric material sandwiched inbetween. Charge of magnitude q is drawn onto each sheet when voltage V is applied. The capacitance is defined as $C = q/V$.

in Equation 8.4 increases) with no change in V. The presence of dielectric material between the plates of a capacitor can increase its capacitance C (and the stored charge) a hundred-fold or so in this fashion.

One of the several important roles of capacitors is in filtering, or smoothing, rectified time-varying voltages. Consider, first, a circuit consisting only of a capacitor attached to a source of AC voltage (such as the secondary of a transformer) plus a voltmeter (Fig. 8–11A). As the upper pole of the transformer grows more positive, electrons are drawn away from the upper plate of the capacitor, leaving it positively charged, too. This continues until the transformer reaches its peak voltage. Thereafter, as the upper pole of the transformer becomes less positive and eventually negative, electrons flow back *to* the upper plate of the capacitor. The graph follows the voltage drop across the capacitor over time.

Now add a single diode to the circuit (Fig. 8–11B). The capacitor again charges up as the upper pole of the transformer goes positive. But after the peak voltage is reached, the diode prevents electrons from flowing back to the upper plate of the capacitor. The plate remains fully charged, and the voltage across the capacitor stays at the peak voltage achieved by the transformer secondary. We have produced our desired constant-voltage power supply.

If there happens to be a resistor (or x-ray tube) of resistance R attached across our filtered power supply (Fig. 8–11C), the capacitor will be able to discharge through it. The *time constant* of this resistor–capacitor (RC) combination, that is, the length of time it takes an appreciable amount of charge to leave the capacitor, is proportional to the magnitudes of both the resistance and capacitance:

$$\text{time constant} = R \cdot C \qquad (8.5)$$

If the time constant is long relative to 1/60 second, then not much charge will leak off before the capacitor is recharged through the diode (Fig. 8–11D), and the voltage will still be fairly (although no longer completely) smooth. The output of a filtered full-wave rectifier power supply is smoother yet (Fig. 8–12).

Voltages from most power supplies are not perfectly smooth, however. The *percentage ripple* is defined as the ratio of the ripple voltage amplitude V_{rip} to the peak voltage:

$$\text{percentage ripple} \simeq 100 \cdot V_{rip}/V_p \qquad (8.6)$$

The percentage ripple for the filtered half-wave and full-wave rectified waveforms in Figure 8–12 are about 20% and 9%, respectively. (Without filtration, the ripple would be 100% for both.) Three-phase voltage supplies can achieve ripple of only a few percent, even without filtration. And modern *constant-potential* generators can supply voltages that are, for all intents and purposes, ripple-free.

It is often not necessary to add a capacitive filter to an x-ray tube circuit. The high-tension cable linking the generator to an x-ray tube behaves, to some extent, like a capacitor, an automatically built-in voltage filter. The potential across the tube may not be perfectly steady, but it will be a lot smoother than it would be without the cable capacitance.

7. TIMING THE EXPOSURE

The last two components of our basic x-ray tube and power supply circuit are the exposure timer and the exposure switch.

Radiographic exposures can be timed in several different

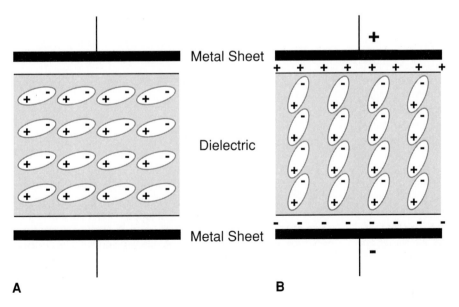

Figure 8–10. Inclusion of dielectric material between the plates of a capacitor increases the capacitance. **A.** One kind of dielectric material consists of polar molecules. **B.** When a voltage is applied, charge accumulates on the metal sheets. The dielectric molecules rotate in such a fashion as to neutralize some of the charge on the plates, allowing more to flow onto them.

A   **B**

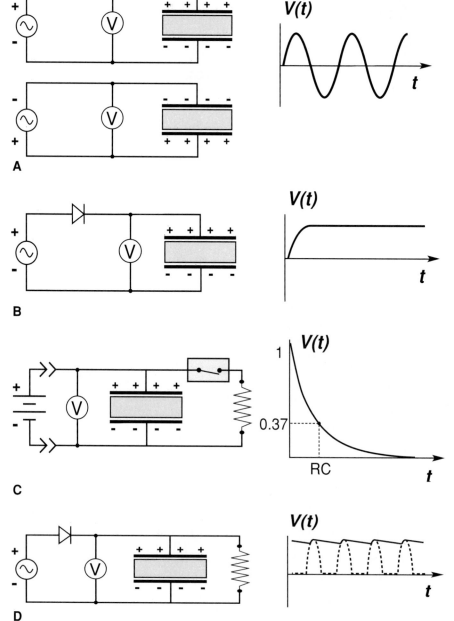

Figure 8–11. Creation of a capacitive filter. **A.** When AC is applied across a capacitor, the charge on it and the voltage across it vary accordingly. **B.** With the addition of a diode, however, charge cannot leave the plates of the capacitor when the polarity of the source voltage is reversed. The voltage across the capacitor rises to the peak value and stays there. **C.** A source of DC voltage is applied across the capacitor, charging it up, and then disconnected. With a resistor in the circuit, however, charge can leak off the capacitor. The time constant (the time required for the quantity of stored charge to fall to 0.37 of its original value) is of magnitude $R \cdot C$. **D.** A source of filtered, half-wave rectified power, applied to a resistor "load."

ways. Some electronic *timers* are based on a resistor–capacitor circuit, similar to a capacitive filter. The timer holds the high-voltage switch closed over the time required to charge or discharge the timer capacitor to a preset voltage; and that time is proportional to the resistance (which may be varied) through which the charge must pass.

More modern, digital timers use a source of fixed, high-frequency pulses. A counting circuit holds the switch closed for the period required to count a predetermined number of pulses.

Alternatively, with *automatic exposure control*, or *phototiming*, a radiation detector continuously monitors the radiation that reaches the radiographic film cassette during an exposure, and shuts off the tube current after the appropriate amount of

photon energy has been delivered (see Fig. 23–6). Chapter 23 will have more to say about phototiming.

8. SWITCHING THE X-RAY BEAM ON AND OFF

The x-ray tube will produce a beam only on the brief (for radiography) occasions that the *exposure switch* is closed. So a way is needed whereby a small control voltage from the timer is capable of switching the high voltage across the tube, and the current through it, rapidly on and off. A "valve" is required whereby, as with a water spigot, one can control a large effect with a relatively small effort.

The simplest solution is to include a solenoid-driven *elec-*

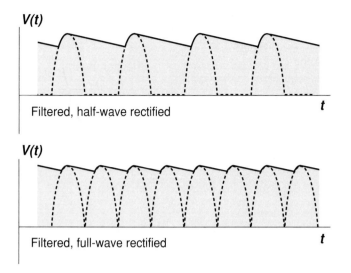

Figure 8–12. With the same amount of filtration, full-wave rectified voltage is much smoother than half-wave rectified voltage.

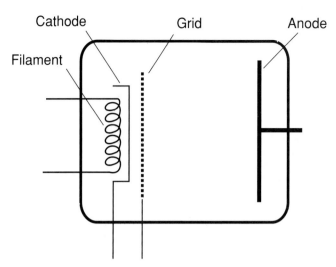

Figure 8–13. Simplified schematic of a vacuum tube triode. Because the grid is close to the cathode, the voltage on the grid has great influence on tube current. As with a water valve, a small effort can control a large effect.

tromechanical switch on the primary side of the transformer. Unfortunately these are slow, erratic, and difficult to maintain, and are seldom used any more.

Another possibility would be to include a vacuum tube diode in series with the x-ray tube, and switch it by controlling its filament temperature: With low filament current, it would act like an open switch; with full filament current, it would function like a closed switch. The response time would be hundreds of times too slow for many applications, however, and the x-ray exposures would not be adequately reproducible.

9. TRIODE VALVES, AND MORE ABOUT SWITCHING

Modern switches are made of *triode* vacuum tubes or their solid-state equivalents. A triode is a diode with a third electrode, a wire-mesh *grid* inserted between the cathode and anode (Fig. 8–13). Exercise 5–5 suggests that the electric field between two flat conductors is proportional to the voltage applied to them and inversely proportional to their separation. As the grid is close to the cathode, even a small voltage between the two can create a large electric field. (The grid also acts by affecting the shape of the cloud of space charge.) Thus, a relatively small negative voltage on the grid can outweigh the effect of a large positive voltage on the anode, and small variations in grid voltage can cause large changes in tube current. Exactly this kind of valve action, incidentally, can be exploited to provide *amplification* of weak audio or radio electric signals, as well.

The tubes that have been developed for switching purposes are highly specialized, gas-filled triodes known as *thyratrons*. These are large and expensive devices that produce much heat, and they have been largely replaced by their solid-state equivalents, known as *silicon-controlled rectifier* (SCR) switches, or *thyristors*. The circuit symbol for a thyristor is the same as that for a diode, except that it indicates a third wire, which brings in the current-controlling *gate* (comparable to the

triode's grid) signal. We shall have more to say about solid-state devices at the end of this chapter.

With a single-phase generator, such as that in Figure 8–6, the timing of the switching must be precisely synchronized with the phase of the 60-Hz line voltage. Opening a switch in an AC circuit causes an abrupt change in the current through it, unless the switching happens to occur when the instantaneous value of the current is practically zero. That leads to a rapid collapse of the magnetic field within any transformer in the circuit, which, in turn, can induce a brief but strong voltage spike. The resultant "arcing" that may occur between the contacts of the switch can be destructive to it and to other circuit elements. This problem has a simple solution for a single-phase generator: Arrange for the exposure switch to be opened and closed only when the value of the current through it is at or near zero (which occurs 120 times a second). The disadvantage of such *synchronous switching* is that one may have to wait as much as 1/120th of a second (8 milliseconds) before closing or opening the switch. And 8 milliseconds is too long an "interrogation time" for some purposes.

An important advantage of three-phase generators, to be discussed in the next chapter, is that techniques (such as "SCR pulsed commutation" and "forced extinction") have been devised that allow for *nonsynchronous switching* (i.e., the timing is totally independent of the phasing of the AC power) on the secondary (high-voltage) side of the step-up transformer. Such methods provide for submillisecond interrogation times.

Another approach, used with some cinefluorography systems, is made possible by a specially designed *grid-controlled x-ray tube* which itself can act as a triode switch. A third electrode (the "focusing cup") within the x-ray tube plays the role of a grid. When the focusing cup is at the same potential as the cathode, the x-ray tube conducts. But if the cup is driven several hundred volts negative relative to the cathode, electrons are prevented from escaping from the space cloud toward the anode, and no x-rays are produced. Rapid switching of x-ray

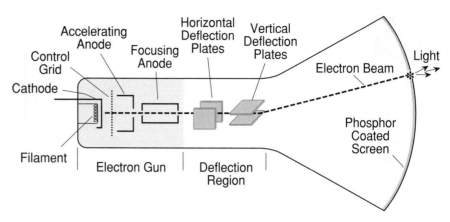

Figure 8–14. The cathode ray tube (CRT) is the heart of the oscilloscope, the computer monitor, and the TV tube. With an oscilloscope, electrons from the cathode are accelerated through and beyond the cylindrical anode and focused into a narrow stream. Voltages applied to two pairs of parallel plates cause the horizontal and vertical deflection of the stream. Where the stream strikes the phosphor at the flat end (screen) of the tube, fluorescent light appears.

output is thus achieved by switching the potential on the focusing cup.

10. THE CATHODE RAY TUBE (ANOTHER TRIODE) IS THE HEART OF THE OSCILLOSCOPE AND OF THE TELEVISION MONITOR

While we're on the subject of triodes . . .

Imaging devices employ electrical signals that vary in time, both to control processes and to convey information. The oscilloscope is an instrument designed to reveal the time dependence of such varying signals. The operation of the television monitors employed to display computerized tomography, magnetic resonance imaging, fluoroscopy, and nuclear medicine images is similar. The heart of an oscilloscope or a TV monitor is a *cathode ray tube*, or *CRT* (Fig. 8–14), which is, in essence, a highly specialized triode.

The anode, rather than being a solid plate as in an x-ray tube, is typically a hollow metal tube. When the grid allows, electrons released from the cathode accelerate through several thousand volts toward the anode, but then coast through and beyond it. Having been *focused* into a narrow beam, the elec-

trons eventually strike the far glass wall, which is coated with a fluorescent material. There they produce a transient spot of light. The number of electrons that reach the phosphor each second and the intensity of the resulting spot of light are determined by the voltage, V_{grid}, on the *control grid*.

An oscilloscope contains two independent pairs of parallel *deflection plates*. A voltage V_y applied to the vertical deflection plates will direct the electron beam (and move the spot of light) up or down by an amount proportional to the sign and magnitude of V_y. Likewise, a voltage V_x applied to the horizontal deflection plates will shift the light spot left and right. The position and brightness of the spot of light on the face of the CRT at any moment thus reflect the instantaneous values of $V_{grid}(t)$, $V_x(t)$, and $V_y(t)$.

Oscilloscopes have been used in imaging in several somewhat different ways. In nuclear medicine, the output of a gamma camera can be fed directly into a CRT (Fig. 8–15). The grid voltage of the oscilloscope is kept far negative, so that no spot of light appears, except when the camera detects a gamma ray. When a gamma ray does interact with the sodium iodide scintillation crystal, the camera's electronics produce voltage pulses V_x and V_y of magnitudes determined by the x and y coordinates of the interaction event, respectively. These are applied to the CRT's deflection plates. Simultaneously, V_{grid} briefly drives the control grid positive, so that the tube con-

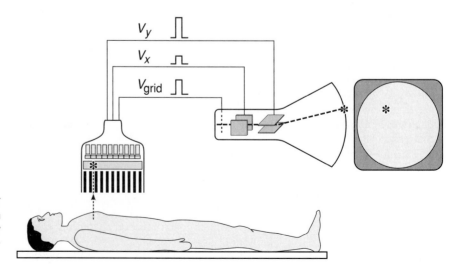

Figure 8–15. One of the ways in which a CRT can be used. In nuclear medicine, a scintillation event in the gamma camera can be recorded by turning the electron stream on, briefly, to produce a pulse of light on the CRT screen.

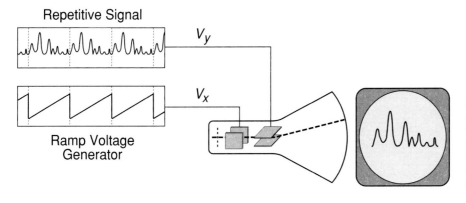

Figure 8–16. Here, a periodic signal voltage is being applied to the vertical deflection plates of an oscilloscope CRT. The beam is swept repetitively left to right in synchrony with the input signal, and left on continuously (except when being snapped back to the left after completion of a sweep). The result is a fixed pattern on the screen.

ducts. A short-lived spot of light is created at the corresponding position on the screen of the CRT, from which it can be recorded on film. (Modern nuclear medicine systems first store the image information in a computer and display the finished product, after computer enhancement, by means of a television monitor or laser camera.)

An oscilloscope may also be used to follow, instead, the time dependence of a single, continuous voltage. The signal of interest is applied to the vertical-deflection plates as $V_y(t)$. Meanwhile, a "ramp generator" produces a horizontal-sweep voltage, $V_x(t)$, that increases linearly with time (Fig. 8–16). The ramp voltage sweeps the electron beam and the light spot from left to right at a constant rate, and thereby defines a time axis. The combined action of the signal voltage and the ramp voltage causes the point of light to trace out a curve with the shape $V_y(t)$. With a "storage oscilloscope," the light trail from a single such sweep may be frozen on the display screen. Alternatively, if the voltage of interest happens to be repetitive and periodic, the electron beam can be snapped back to its starting point at the end of its sweep, like a typewriter carriage return, and a new sweep begun; with proper synchronization, the same pattern is traced out at each pass, again displaying the signal.

A television monitor works in yet a third fashion. The beam is caused to trace the same two-dimensional raster again and again (Fig. 8–17). With each such frame, the grid voltage is made to vary with time in such a manner that the resulting pattern of light intensity on the screen creates a meaningful image. With a TV monitor, incidentally, the beam is deflected by means of magnetic fields from "deflection coils," rather than by electric fields between deflection plates.

11. SEMICONDUCTOR DIODES AND TRANSISTORS

Although older DC power supplies used vacuum tube diodes for rectification, modern equipment employs *solid-state diodes* made of selenium or, more commonly now, *silicon (Si)*.

Recall from Chapter 7, Section 3 that a semiconductor has a nearly full valence band and a nearly empty conduction band, separated by a narrow *forbidden energy band gap* (see Fig. 7–7). In pure silicon (Si), the 1.1-eV gap is sufficiently wide that only a few electrons are thermally excited from the valence into the conduction band at room temperature, and so the electrical resistance is high. Things are quite different, however, when chemical impurities are present.

Each silicon atom has four valence electrons, which it shares with (and thereby attaches itself to) four other Si atoms (Fig. 8–18A). Suppose that a pentavalent atom, such as phosphorus, arsenic, or antimony, replaces an Si atom at some lattice site. Four of its valence electrons will forge tight covalent bonds with adjacent Si atoms; but the fifth will have no place special to go, and will be held only loosely (Fig. 8–18B). Only a slight amount of thermal energy is needed to elevate the fifth electron into the conduction band and, because it gives up that electron so readily, it is said to be a *donor impurity* atom. A semiconductor containing donor impurities is said to be *n-type*, because of the availability of the additional electrons (negative charge carriers).

Boron, aluminum, gallium, and indium atoms, by contrast, are trivalent *acceptor* impurities. As a free atom, an acceptor has only three valence electrons by which it can attach to

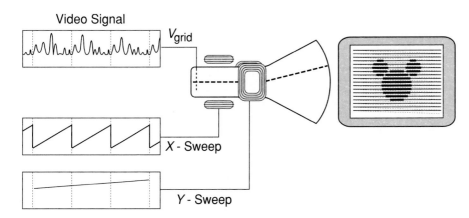

Figure 8–17. The electron beam of a television monitor is swept rapidly from left to right, and slowly downward, in a raster pattern. The video signal is applied to the grid of the CRT, and controls the beam intensity, hence the instantaneous brightness of the point of light on the screen. TV monitors use magnetic, rather than electric, fields to deflect the beam.

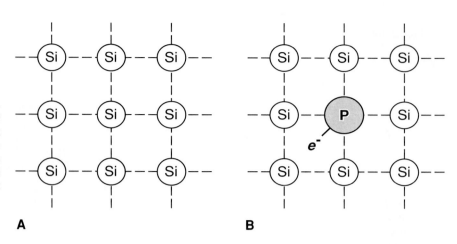

Figure 8–18. Effects of impurities on semiconductors. **A.** Two-dimensional representation of the crystal structure of pure silicon. **B.** When a pentavalent phosphorus atom replaces a tetravalent silicon atom, one of its five electrons is left to dangle loosely, and can easily be pulled away by an applied electric field. Equivalently, it enters the crystal's conduction band.

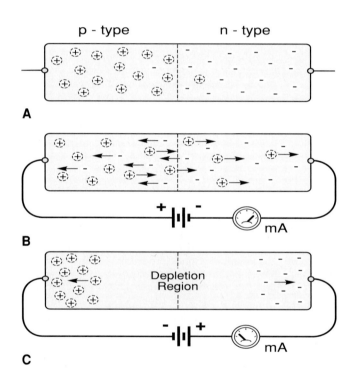

Figure 8–19. Operation of the solid-state diode. A dash indicates the loosely bound, fifth electron of a pentavalent impurity, and a plus sign inside a circle is a hole associated with a trivalent impurity. **A.** Suppose one brings an electrically neutral piece of n-type material into contact with an electrically neutral piece of p-type material, and no potential is applied. Initially, some electrons diffuse into the p-type region. This quickly leaves the n-type material with a slight net excess positive charge, and the other half of the diode with an excess negative charge. This discourages the further net flow of electrons. (There is a similar flow of holes in the other direction, with the same effect.) **B.** With a voltage applied in the "forward" direction, electrons exiting the diode via the p-type material contact are replaced by electrons pumped in through the other side. So, too, with holes. **C.** A "reverse" voltage, however, prevents the flow of current. Hence the diode action. A transistor operates in a similar, but more complex, fashion.

other atoms. But it has an affinity for electrons and, when embedded in a silicon matrix, it tends to pull a fourth one away from a nearby silicon atom. That newly ionized Si atom can, in turn, then steal an electron from *its* neighbor, and so on. In this fashion a *hole*, or localized region of absent electron, can migrate (or be drawn by an electric field) through the semiconductor. Because an electron is a carrier of negative charge, a hole, in effect, transports positive charge. Semiconductor material doped with acceptor atoms is said to be *p-type*.

A diode can be produced by doping one half of a small piece of pure semiconductor with donor impurities and the other half with acceptors. Some electrons from the n-region will tend to diffuse naturally into the p-region (Fig. 8–19A), and holes will diffuse into the n-type material. Suppose that the n-type side is now attached, by way of a *contact*, to the negative pole of a battery, and the p-type to the positive pole (Fig. 8–19B). This establishes an electric field within the material. The electrons that diffused into the p-region will be swept by the field toward and out the positive contact; electrons injected by the battery into the n-type material will replace and follow them. (Likewise, holes will move in the opposite direction.) A considerable current flows even with a low *forward bias*, and the diode displays low resistance in the forward direction.

With *reverse bias*, however (Fig. 8–19C), the nearly free electrons in the n-region will be pulled back from, rather than toward, the p-region. The region inbetween becomes a *depletion layer*, devoid of mobile charge carriers (conduction electrons or holes), and there will be almost no current. Thus, like the vacuum tube diode, the solid-state diode conducts in one direction only.

A triode vacuum tube contains a third (grid) element by means of which a small signal can give rise to large variations in voltage or current. So also a *transistor* consists of three (typically) regions of doped semiconductor arranged in such a fashion that a small control signal input to one of them can regulate the flow of a large current between the others. It would take us a bit too far afield to describe how transistors work. Suffice it to say that diodes and transistors can perform nearly all the kinds of jobs carried out by their vacuum tube counterparts, but are usually thousands of times smaller and more compact, are cheaper, more reliable, and easier to manufacture in large numbers, require no high voltages, and create much less heat (which, otherwise, must somehow be removed).

_____ *Chapter 9* _____

The Nuts and Bolts of Generators

1. **Producing the High-Voltage Alternating Current with an Autotransformer and a Step-up Transformer in Series**
2. **Rectifying the High-Voltage Alternating Current**
3. **Most Modern Generators Are Three-Phase**
4. **Medium-Frequency Generators**
5. **Battery-Powered and Capacitor-Discharge Generators for Mobile X-ray Units**
6. **Constant-Potential Generators**
7. **Falling-Load Generators and Microprocessor Control**
8. **Making the Current (mA) Through an X-ray Tube Independent of the Potential (kVp) Applied Across It**
9. **The Kilowatt Rating of a Generator**

The preceding chapter described, in general terms, the components of a rudimentary circuit capable of powering an x-ray tube. Here we shall develop some of those ideas a bit further, and then employ them in exploring the workings of the various kinds of generators found in the clinic.

In all cases, the objective is to provide nearly constant high voltages across, and precisely determined currents through, an x-ray tube, for exactly controlled periods of time. A number of approaches have been developed to achieve this.

1. PRODUCING THE HIGH-VOLTAGE ALTERNATING CURRENT WITH AN AUTOTRANSFORMER AND A STEP-UP TRANSFORMER IN SERIES

As indicated in Equation 8.2, a transformer can either "step up" or "step down" the voltage from an alternating current (AC) source. Transformers are used in x-ray generators for both purposes.

The simple generator in Figure 9–1 produces a range of high AC voltages (for subsequent rectification and application across the x-ray tube) by means of two transformers in series. The first is a *variable* step-*down* transformer, the setting of which determines the input voltage to the second. It is the second, a step-*up* transformer with a fixed N_2/N_1 ratio, that actually achieves the high voltage.

The first transformer, by means of which the peak kilovoltage (kVp) is chosen, is an adjustable *autotransformer*. A coil of wire serves as the primary, and some (but not necessarily all) of the loops of the same coil act as the secondary as well. If a source of 220 V rms is attached across the primary, for example, the secondary voltage goes from 0 to 220 V rms as the *kVp control* or *selection* switch increases the number of loops that constitute the secondary coil. Thus, when the kVp control is switched, it is actually a relatively low voltage that is being changed. This is much easier on the equipment than would be adjusting high AC voltages directly.

The AC from the secondary of the autotransformer goes to the *step-up transformer*, in which the voltage is increased by a fixed factor of 500 or so. If the peak voltage at each terminal of the secondary is kV$_P$ relative to ground (and the peak drop across the entire secondary is $2 \cdot$ kV$_P$), the peak voltage applied across the x-ray tube, after full-wave rectification, will also be kV$_P$. But because the center of the step-up transformer secondary is grounded, the anode will be kV$_P$/2 *positive relative to ground* potential, at most, and the cathode will be *below ground* by the same amount. As the tube housing and the rest of the world are at ground potential, this approach reduces the likelihood of electrical "arcing" or discharge between points of high voltage and ground. It also usually helps to immerse the wire coils of the transformer in a bath of electrically insulating oil.

_____ **EXERCISE 9–1.** _____

The kVp selection switch is set so that the secondary voltage of the autotransformer is one-third that of the primary. The step-up transformer has a turns ratio of 500:1. What is the kVp, if the input to the generator is 220 V rms?

SOLUTION: The output of the autotransformer is (1/3)(220 V) = 73 V rms. By Equation 8.2, the output of the step-up transformer is (73 V)(500) = 37 kV rms. This corresponds to a peak voltage of 52 kVp.

The filament of an x-ray tube requires about 10 V to achieve thermionic emission temperatures. Its power supply

79

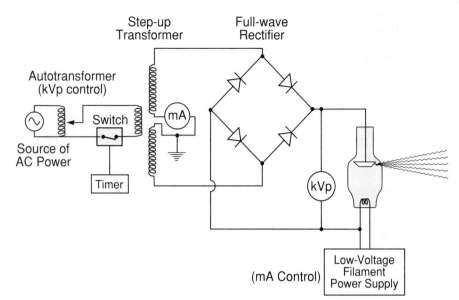

Figure 9–1. Simple x-ray tube circuit. The applied potential (kVp) is determined by adjusting the number of turns picked off in the secondary of the autotransformer. The tube current (mA) is controlled by the filament current (hence, temperature) and by the applied kVp.

therefore contains a step-down transformer and a circuit to stabilize and fine-tune the filament voltage and current.

2. RECTIFYING THE HIGH-VOLTAGE ALTERNATING CURRENT

The high voltage is full-wave rectified before being applied to an x-ray tube. Older generators use vacuum tube rectifiers, but most now employ banks of solid-state diodes. A single silicon diode is intrinsically capable of withstanding a reverse voltage of only about 500 V, independent of its size or construction. But if a 120,000-V source, say, is attached to 300 separate silicon diodes connected in series, the drop across any one of them will be a safe 400 V.

After the tube voltage is full-wave rectified, it is smoothed by the inherent capacitance of the high-tension cables, and sometimes also by added electrical filter.

A significant degree of ripple in the high voltage applied to the x-ray tube is undesirable for several reasons:

- It leads to an imaging beam of inferior quality. As the x-ray tube voltage and current pulsate, the power of penetration and the intensity of the beam will vary, as well; the voltage is therefore near the value that yields best image contrast only a part of each cycle. Also, because the beam is of less than maximum intensity or power of penetration much of the time, the tube must be left on longer to achieve an adequate level of film darkening; hence a loss of resolution through motion of the patient.
- It thermally stresses the tube. As will be seen in Chapter 11, the efficiency of bremsstrahlung production increases with the kinetic energy of the electrons striking the anode. Thus, x-rays will be generated part of each cycle with less than maximum efficiency (i.e., too much heat produced per unit of x-ray beam) if there is significant ripple. Also, 120-Hz thermal cycling is more damaging to the x-ray tube's anode sur-

face than would be the same average power input at a constant rate.
- It leads to unnecessary excess dose to the patient, because the beam is not penetrating enough and has to be left on too long. Proper beam filtration eliminates some of this problem.

3. MOST MODERN GENERATORS ARE THREE-PHASE

Power in which the voltage on a single "hot" wire oscillates about that on the "neutral" (Fig. 9–2), is said to be *single-phase*. So, too, is a generator that makes use of such power.

Full-wave rectified single-phase power contains a significant amount of voltage ripple. For this reason, and also to facil-

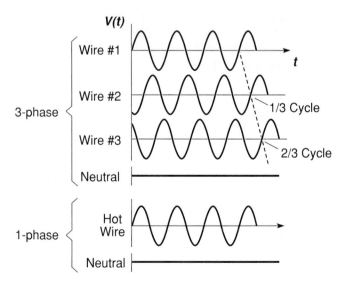

Figure 9–2. Single-phase AC power is delivered on one "hot" wire and one "neutral" wire. Three-phase power arrives on three equally hot wires and one neutral wire. The potentials on the three hot wires are 120 degrees (one-third cycle) out of phase from one another.

itate high-voltage switching and allow short exposure times (less than 1/120 second), most modern x-ray generators are three-phase.

Three-phase power comes into a department on four wires (Fig. 9–2), one of which is "neutral." The time dependencies of the voltages on the three "hot" wires relative to the neutral are identical, but shifted from one another by 120 degrees (i.e., a third of a cycle). All power is carried in the three hot wires, and there is virtually no current in the neutral. The peak voltage difference between any two hot wires is typically between 200 and 500 V, depending on the local power supply and needs.

Transforming three-phase power to high voltage is considerably more complicated than with single-phase, and involves special transformers and circuits. The three hot power lines are attached to three primaries that are arranged in a configuration like an uppercase Greek delta, Δ (Fig. 9–3), and the secondaries are attached in a "Y" or "star" formation. To make things even more confusing, all the primaries and secondaries are wound on the same metal core.

Depending on the details of how these windings and the appropriate rectifiers are connected, the output pulses either six or twelve times per original AC cycle. The percentage voltage ripple factors for single-phase, **six-pulse three-phase,** and **twelve-pulse three-phase** power (full-wave rectified, but before filtration) are 100%, about 13%, and about 4%, respectively (Fig. 9–4).

4. MEDIUM-FREQUENCY GENERATORS

The efficiency of a transformer improves with the AC frequency. This advantage is exploited in a **medium-frequency** *generator,* for which the step-up transformer can be smaller, lighter, and cheaper.

A medium-frequency generator operates somewhat like an old-fashioned automobile ignition system. It starts off with standard single- or three-phase AC power, which it full-wave rectifies and smooths. It chops the resulting, moderately smooth low voltage typically 5000 or 6000 times per second (Fig. 9–5), by means of an *inverter,* a switch that opens and closes automatically and repeatedly. The voltage of this 5- or 6-kHz chopped power can be stabilized easily, so that the peak

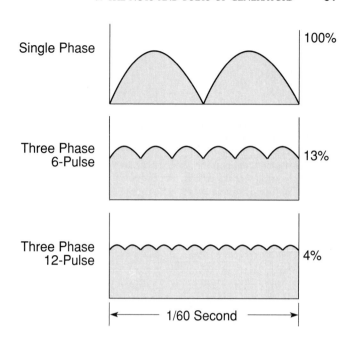

Figure 9–4. Comparison of the ripple for unfiltered full-wave rectified single-phase, six-pulse three-phase, and twelve-pulse three-phase voltage.

voltage it induces in the secondary of the (efficient, small) step-up transformer is constant and independent of variations in the line voltage. This medium-frequency, high-voltage power can be full-wave rectified, smoothed, and applied across the x-ray tube, and the residual ripple is negligible.

5. BATTERY-POWERED AND CAPACITOR-DISCHARGE GENERATORS FOR MOBILE X-RAY UNITS

Some *mobile x-ray units* use single-phase generators that attach to the locally available 110- or 220-V AC. But many hospitals and clinics cannot provide, away from the radiography department, the high levels of AC power required. Also, mobile units

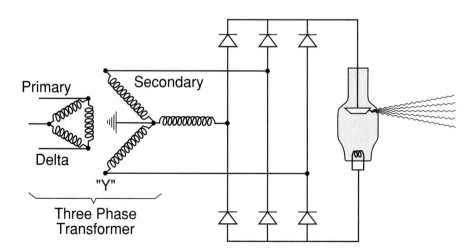

Figure 9–3. Transformers for three-phase power make use of the three hot wires; the neutral wire (unlike the case for single-phase) plays no active role. This circuit produces six-pulse rectified voltage; the circuit for twelve-pulse is more complex.

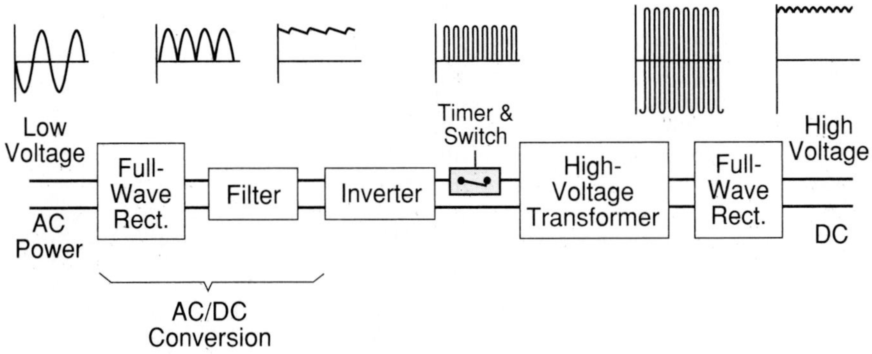

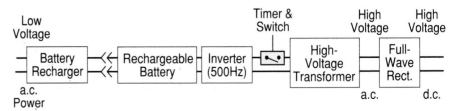

Figure 9–5. The inverter, the heart of the medium-frequency generator, chops DC power several thousand times per second. The resulting relatively high frequency AC voltage can be stepped up with a smaller, cheaper transformer than can a 60-Hz voltage.

may have to operate when electrical power fails or in locations where there is no power.

Use of a rechargeable (such as nickel–cadmium) battery as the source of energy eliminates the dependence on local AC. The battery connects to the primary of the high-voltage transformer by way of an inverter, which closes and opens perhaps 500 times per second (Fig. 9–6). The resulting 500-Hz AC induces high-voltage AC of the same frequency in the transformer's secondary, which can be full-wave rectified, smoothed, and applied across the x-ray tube.

With a **capacitor-discharge generator**, the voltage from the secondary of the high-voltage transformer is rectified and applied across a large capacitor, or bank of capacitors, rather than directly across the x-ray tube. Charge builds up on the plates of the capacitive energy storage system relatively slowly. When the exposure switch is subsequently closed, the accumulated capacitor charge is driven through the x-ray tube. The voltage across the tube drops rapidly from its initial value, when the capacitor is fully charged, but remains high enough long enough to make a radiograph, if the mA-s does not have to be too great.

6. CONSTANT-POTENTIAL GENERATORS

With a **constant-potential generator**, the output voltage is stabilized by means of a "grid bias control" feedback circuit (Fig. 9–7). This circuit continuously monitors the value of the voltage drop across the x-ray tube, and produces a feedback control signal that is proportional to the difference between the actual instantaneous x-ray tube voltage and the desired constant voltage. The feedback signal, in turn, corrects the grid voltages of two triodes that regulate the voltage applied to the x-ray tube; hence the voltage applied across the x-ray tube remains virtually constant.

An additional "switch control voltage" applied to the two

triode grids can turn the voltage applied to the x-ray tube on or off in a fraction of a millisecond. Because it occurs on the high-voltage side of the step-up transformer, this is known as (one form of) *secondary switching*. (As noted in the last chapter, a **grid-controlled x-ray tube** and its specially tailored generator may be employed when rapid switching is required, as in cinefluoroscopy.)

7. FALLING-LOAD GENERATORS AND MICROPROCESSOR CONTROL

During an exposure, the amount of heat accumulated where the electron stream strikes the target of an x-ray tube (along the focal track) increases with time. And the rate at which the anode can safely absorb yet more heat, during the exposure, therefore diminishes. A simple way to deal with this problem is to select the maximum constant value of the x-ray tube current (mA) that the tube can tolerate for the desired kVp and exposure time. But there are better approaches.

A **falling-load** *generator* is designed to minimize exposure times by explicitly accounting for, at any moment during an exposure, the remaining heat tolerance of the anode of the tube. Rather than holding constant, the tube current starts off relatively high, but is caused to fall off with time according to some preprogrammed formula (Fig. 9–8). A falling-current exposure, for some desired mA-s, can be of shorter duration than is possible with a constant-current source. The electronic circuitry that achieves this is now built around a microprocessor.

The integration of microprocessors into generators also provides for the automatic selection of near-optimal technique factors for various anatomic studies. The technologist enters the name of the study ("chest") and perhaps some other relevant information (patient size), and the microprocessor and automatic exposure circuitry do the rest. At present such sys-

Figure 9–6. A high-voltage supply for a mobile x-ray unit makes use of rechargeable storage batteries (such as nickel–cadmium) and operates like a medium-frequency generator. The battery pack is used also for the motor that moves the unit from place to place within the clinic.

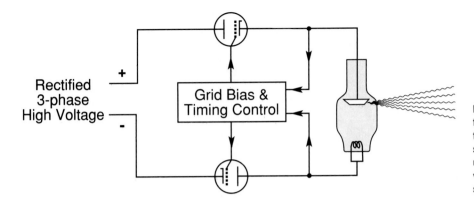

**Rectified
3-phase
High Voltage**

+

−

Grid Bias &
Timing Control

Figure 9–7. The voltage from a constant-potential generator is determined by the current through a pair of triodes. The output voltage is sampled and, by means of a feedback circuit, used to control the triodes so as to stabilize that voltage. The triodes are also used for rapid switching of the x-ray tube.

tems are designed only to mimic the decisions of experienced clinical personnel, however, and cannot improve on the skill of a well-trained technologist. But when combined with a good phototiming system (see Chapter 8, Section 7), this approach results in almost perfect exposure control for all patients and all body parts.

8. MAKING THE CURRENT (mA) THROUGH AN X-RAY TUBE INDEPENDENT OF THE POTENTIAL (kVp) APPLIED ACROSS IT

As indicated in Ohm's law (Equation 7–1), the current through a resistor is linearly proportional to the voltage applied across it (Fig. 9–9). For this reason, a resistor is said to be a *linear* device.

The current through an x-ray tube, by contrast, is *not* simply proportional to the voltage between cathode and anode. With any fixed value of filament current (hence cathode temperature), tube current rises rapidly with increasing tube potential until most of the electrons thermally emitted from the cathode are streaming to the anode (Fig. 9–10A). Higher volt-

ages, then, can do little to increase the flow, and the current-vs.-voltage curve flattens out—the current is said to have *saturated*. A higher cathode temperature, however, will enhance the filament's thermionic emission and increase the tube saturation current.

The primary determinant of tube current is thus the cathode temperature, which is adjusted (by means of the *tube current (mA) control*) by varying the filament current (Fig. 9–10B). But tube current (mA) also depends somewhat on the applied potential, an inconvenience for clinical operation. In any modern generator, tube current is therefore made essentially independent of the selection of high voltage by means of a *space charge compensation circuit*: When the kVp setting is changed, the filament current is automatically adjusted to maintain the tube current unchanged.

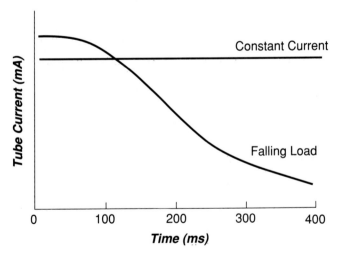

Figure 9–8. The current from a falling-load generator is not held constant during an exposure. Rather, it is made to drop off in such a fashion as to minimize exposure time, taking into account the heat tolerance characteristics of the x-ray tube.

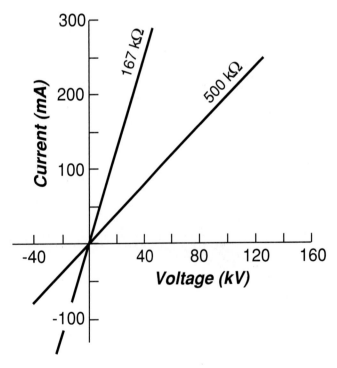

Figure 9–9. A resistor is a linear device. As described by Ohm's law, the current through it, *I*, is proportional to the voltage, *V*, across it: *I = V/R*. This relationship is shown for two different resistances.

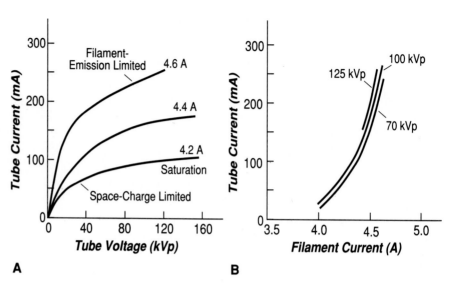

Figure 9–10. X-ray tubes are nonlinear devices. **A.** The current through a typical x-ray tube (mA) increases with applied voltage until it saturates, but there is no strict proportionality. The tube current for any kVp is strongly dependent on cathode temperature, as indicated by the curves for three different filament currents. **B.** Tube current varies rapidly with filament current. Its sensitivity to kVp can be eliminated by means of a "charge compensation" circuit.

9. THE KILOWATT RATING OF A GENERATOR

The *kilowatt rating* of a generator is a measure of its ability to supply power to an x-ray tube. The kilowatt rating is defined as the maximum output capacity under specific operating conditions. In Europe and Japan, the kilowatt rating of a three-phase or constant-potential generator is defined as 100 kVp times the maximum tube current that can be sustained at 100 kVp for 0.1 second:

kilowatt rating
= (100 kVp)(max mA at 100 kVp for 0.1 second)   (9.1)

In the United States, the generator kilowatt rating has traditionally been defined at 80 kVp, but there appears to be a move on to adopt the 100-kVp convention.

The power rating is *not*, in particular, the product of the maximum kVp and the maximum current that the generator can achieve separately. It may be a fairly good indicator, however, of the system's maximum power output.

A generator's power rating should be matched to the requirements of the tube employed. Too large a generator is an unnecessary cost, and one that is too small will underuse the tube.

_____ **EXERCISE 9–2.** _____

A three-phase generator can draw a maximum of 500 mA at 100 kVp for 100 milliseconds. What is the kilowatt rating?

SOLUTION: With SI units, to avoid any confusion with the kilo-'s and the milli-'s: (100,000 V)(0.5 A) = 50,000 W = 50 kW.

X-ray Tubes

In an x-ray tube, the fundamental trade-off is among the needs for high x-ray beam output and a small focal spot (both for good resolution) and adequate heat dissipation (to avoid thermal damage to the tube).

Two partial solutions to this problem are line focusing and rotation of the anode. Heat thereby ends up deposited along the long, circumferential focal track cut by the focal line. The heat radiates and is conducted away, which prevents the instantaneous local temperature from exceeding the melting points of the target and anode materials. Heat radiated from the anode is largely absorbed by the cooling/insulating oil surrounding the tube and, from there, passed by convection to the ambient air.

It is the beam of bremsstrahlung and characteristic x-ray energy, originating at the focal spot, hardened by filters, and shaped by beam restrictors, that is of clinical interest.

1. ANATOMY OF A STATIONARY ANODE TUBE

Slice a stationary anode diagnostic tube longitudinally down the middle, and you will find something like Figure 10–1.

The borosilicate glass *envelope* is evacuated, and must maintain a pressure of less than 10^{-5} mm Hg. (Standard atmospheric pressure is equivalent to what would be found at the bottom of a column of the liquid metal mercury [Hg] 760 mm high, or under 10 m of water.) More air than that in a tube would impede the free acceleration of electrons from cathode to anode. Also, if the tube develops a slow leak (becomes "gassy"), the filament will oxidize away. The wires and other metal elements that pass through the glass envelope have coefficients of thermal expansion different from that of the glass; special alloy seals must therefore be used to ensure the maintenance of the vacuum as the tube repeatedly heats and cools. The envelope may contain a *window*, a small area of diminished glass thickness where the x-ray beam exits the tube.

The **cathode assembly** consists of one or several *filaments*, only one of which is used at a time, and the **focusing cup** for

each (Fig. 10–2). A filament is a helical coil of tungsten wire, similar to the filament of a light bulb; the wire is typically 0.2 mm in diameter, and the helix is 1 to 2 cm long and 2 to 5 mm in diameter. When carrying a current of 3.5 to 5 A, the filament becomes hot enough to emit electrons thermionically. These electrons form a cloud of space charge which, when swept to the anode, gives rise to the tube current.

If a filament is maintained continuously at the temperature required for a radiographic exposure, about 2200°C, the tungsten can evaporate and deposit on the interior surfaces of the tube, over time leading eventually to its failure. When an exposure is not being taken, the filament current is therefore reduced to a much lower **standby** level. The **filament-boosting circuit** then requires a second or so to raise the filament to its exposure temperature, hence the brief delay after the exposure button is pressed. (With a rotating anode tube, the anode must be brought up to speed, as well.) With a two-button system, if the *exposure* button is pressed immediately after the *prep* ("rotor start") button, an interlock circuit prevents the exposure from occurring before the filament and rotor are ready.

Because of the repulsive electric force among electrons, there is a tendency for the electron stream from cathode to anode to spread out, giving rise to too large a focal spot. The *focusing cup* is a block of nickel, held at the same potential as the filament, whose role is to overcome that effect. It is shaped so as to produce an electric field between itself and the anode that compresses the stream of electrons into the required small size and shape at the target.

A *stationary anode* consists of a thin plate of tungsten, 1 cm or so on a side, inset into a large copper block. Tungsten has two physical attributes that make it the target material of choice (except for mammography). First, the efficiency of bremsstrahlung production increases with the atomic number of the target, and that of tungsten, $Z = 74$, is high. Second, it has a high melting point (3380°C) and low vapor pressure (i.e., relatively few tungsten atoms evaporate from the anode at normal anode operating temperatures). It can therefore withstand the high local temperatures produced by direct electron bom-

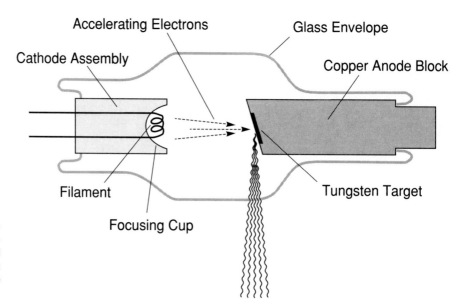

Figure 10–1. Stationary anode diagnostic x-ray tube. Heat is conducted away from the target area into the massive copper block, and from there to the surrounding coolant oil. Such tubes have been replaced by rotating anode tubes for most applications.

bardment relatively well. An alloy of tungsten (90%) and rhenium (10%) is even more resistant to the cracking and crazing that can be caused by thermal cycling, and usually is used instead of pure tungsten.

The role of the copper block of a stationary anode is to conduct heat rapidly away from the tungsten plate and into the oil bath that surrounds the tube. The thermal conductivity and thickness of the tungsten target plate must be such as to protect the copper (melting point = 1083°C) at their interface.

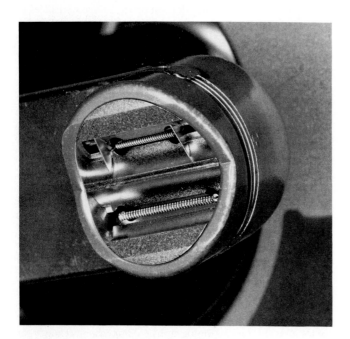

Figure 10–2. Cathode assembly (filaments and focusing cups) of a dual-focus tube. The small filament is used for high-resolution imaging. The larger filament, selected when higher intensities are needed, spreads the heat out over a larger focal region on the anode. *(Courtesy of Varian Power Grid & X-ray Tube Products.)*

Most modern diagnostic tubes have *rotating anodes*, the advantage of which will be described shortly.

2. TARGET ANGLE

The anode surface of a diagnostic x-ray tube and the stream of electrons from the cathode are not perpendicular to one another. The anode surface is canted, rather, by an amount known as the **target** or **anode angle.** The target angle is typically 10 to 20 degrees; that is, the anode is tilted 10 to 20 degrees away from facing the stream of electrons head-on.

When high-velocity electrons are incident on such a canted target, the useful bremsstrahlung x-rays are emitted predominantly in the direction perpendicular to the electron flow and out of the target. (X-ray photons starting off in the opposite direction are fully absorbed by the anode.) Figure 10–3 indicates, for 90-keV monoenergetic electrons entering from the left and striking an anode with a 16-degree target angle, the relative intensity of the x-ray beam produced at any angle.

This angular dependence of bremsstrahlung production is an important factor in the design of the anode. A thick target aligned perpendicularly to the electron flow would absorb most of the photons created in it. With a target that is overly canted, on the other hand, the focal spot would be too large. The target angle should be close to that which gives rise to the greatest usable x-ray beam intensity. But other factors, such as the desired apparent size of the focal spot, are of equal importance.

3. FOCAL SPOT SIZE: RESOLUTION VERSUS HEAT TOLERANCE

The *focal spot* is the region on the anode where the stream of high-velocity electrons collides with tungsten atoms, and from which x-rays are emitted. As will become apparent in Chapter 22, for high resolution (which is often, but not always, of clini-

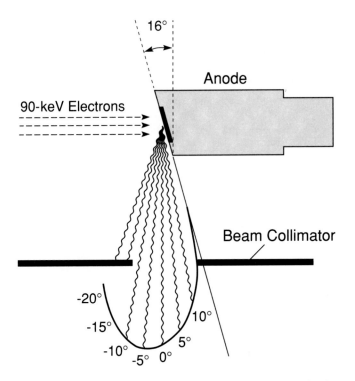

Figure 10–3. Polar diagram of x-ray intensity as a function of emission angle, where the 0-degree direction is perpendicular to the incident electron stream. For any angle the distance from the origin (at the focal spot) to the curve is proportional to the intensity; for this target and electron energy, maximum intensity is emitted at about –5 degrees. The target angle is 16 degrees. (*Adapted from Johns HE, Cunningham JR: The Physics of Radiology, 4th ed. Springfield, IL: Charles C Thomas, 1983 [Fig. 2–16]*).

perature attained by any small region of the anode is determined by its specific heat and mass [Equation 5.5] and by the rates at which heat is entering and leaving it.) The need to prevent such localized overheating limits the possible tube current and, therefore, the intensity of the bremsstrahlung beam.

Thus, during tube selection or design, an optimal balance must be struck, with respect to target angle and focal spot size, between the conflicting needs for resolution, intensity, and anode surface heat tolerance.

4. LINE FOCUSING: LOW TARGET HEAT CONCENTRATION, BUT A SMALL APPARENT SIZE OF THE FOCAL SPOT

Suppose that the electrons from the cathode all landed within a square drawn on the anode. If one looked directly into the beam, through the tube's window, this focal spot would appear to be rectangular (Fig. 10–4A). (Likewise, a coin seems elliptical when not seen face on.) But by focusing the electron stream so as to land along a vertical line (Fig. 10–4B), a more nearly square apparent focal spot can be obtained. With a target angle of 12 degrees, for example, high-energy electrons emitted by the filament might bombard an area on the anode 1 mm wide and about five times that in length, giving rise to a 1×1-mm^2 projected *apparent* focal spot.

The image of the apparent focal spot of a real tube, produced by means of a pinhole camera (Fig. 10–5A), is reproduced in Figure 10–5B. It is not perfectly square, but rather displays a characteristic, nearly rectangular "double banana" shape.

The smaller the anode angle, the longer the line can be. Thus, with line focusing, the area of anode subject to electron bombardment can be increased considerably (and the concentration of heat at any particular point reduced) with no increase in the apparent size of the focal spot. Note that this apparent "foreshortening" of the focal spot occurs in only one direction.

Many x-ray tubes contain two filaments, one larger than the other and made of thicker wire (Fig. 10–2). The larger filament is employed when a greater tube current is required, but

cal importance), one wants as small a focal spot as is achievable.

But if the stream of high-velocity electrons strikes the anode over too small an area, causing intermittent, exceedingly high local temperatures, the resulting thermal stresses and strains can cause the tungsten surface to pit or even crack. (The tem-

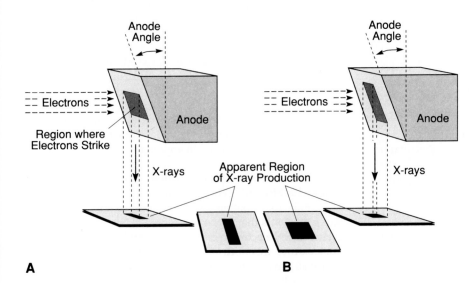

Figure 10–4. Line focusing. **A.** If the electron stream evenly covers a square region on the anode surface, then that region will *appear* to be short and wide when viewed from outside the x-ray tube window. **B.** To produce a focal spot that *appears* square from outside the tube, the electrons must land within an area of target that is tall and narrow. The smaller the anode angle, the longer and/or narrower the focal region (actually bombarded by electrons) must be to produce a square apparent focal spot.

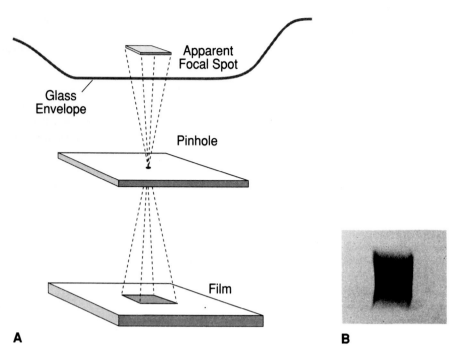

Figure 10–5. The apparent shape of the focal spot should be approximately square. **A.** Obtaining an image of the focal spot for an x-ray tube by means of a pinhole camera. **B.** Pinhole camera image of a focal spot. *(Courtesy of Nuclear Associates.)*

A   **B**

at the cost of a reduction in resolution; for adequate heat dissipation, the electron stream is focused onto a larger area of the anode surface.

Even with a single filament, the dimensions of the focal spot may increase significantly at high tube currents. This phenomenon, known as **blooming,** can diminish image resolution. An increase in focal spot size may also result from a reduction in peak kilovoltage.

Another source of image degradation is the **off-focus radiation** produced by stray electrons that bombard the anode away from the focal spot. The relative amount of x-rays produced off-focus is relatively independent of tube current, but can constitute as much as 25% of the tube's output. Such radiation is usually produced so far off-focus that it does not enlarge the effective size of the focal spot (thereby reducing resolution); but it can diminish the overall image contrast, rather, like the Compton scatter radiation created within the patient.

5. SPREADING OUT THE HEAT ON A ROTATING ANODE

The twin requirements of a small focal spot (to optimize system resolution) and high tube current (for an exposure of brief duration, to eliminate motion blurring) sorely test the ability of an anode to dissipate heat. A significant advance in this struggle came in the 1930s with the development of the rotating anode, which is now to be found in nearly all diagnostic tubes. (Many dental x-ray tubes, which are subject to less punishment, are of the less expensive stationary anode design.)

A standard rotating anode tube appears in Figure 10–6. The anode consists typically of a disk made of molybdenum, graphite, or both, 50 to 125 mm (2 to 5 in.) in diameter, surfaced with a tungsten/rhenium alloy target. It is directly attached, by means of a narrow molybdenum axle, to the "rotor" (also inside the tube) of an *induction motor.* The "stator" of the motor,

outside the tube, consists of coils of wire. The magnetic fields produced by AC current driven through the stator induce currents in the rotor coils, and the interplay of these fields and currents causes the rotor and anode to turn.

An anode usually rotates at about 3000 rpm (i.e., once every 20 milliseconds) and goes around several times during a typical exposure. Thus, with the nearly constant tube current produced by a three-phase generator, each part of the **focal track** will be bombarded by electrons for a few microseconds, and then have 20 milliseconds to radiate away heat before coming around again for another dose of electron bombardment. (In some situations, such as in cineangiography, the anode can be rotated at a higher speed, up to 10,000 rpm. The greater total area of anode surface swept by the electron beam during a 1- to 8-millisecond cine exposure allows use of a higher tube current.)

The advantage of the rotating anode can be illustrated with a simple calculation. Suppose a stream of electrons bombards a stationary anode along a line 6 mm high and 1.5 mm wide (see Fig. 10–4). It covers a region of target (6 mm)(1.5 mm) = 9 mm² in area. What if, instead, the electrons strike the beveled edge of a rotating anode 50 mm from its center? They will cut a swath 6 mm high and (2π)(50 mm) = 314 mm long (Fig. 10–7), which is a region (6 mm)(314 mm) = 1900 mm² in area. The same line of electrons thus irradiates an area 1900 mm²/9 mm² = 200 times greater on a rotating anode than on a stationary anode, with no increase in apparent focal spot size. (If the anode rotates more than once during an exposure, why is it legitimate, in this rough calculation, to ignore the multiple heating of each portion of the focal track?)

Unlike the situation with the stationary anode, with a rotating anode there is no large copper block to absorb the heat and conduct it away to the outside world. Some heat is conducted from the focal track into the rest of the anode, but nearly all leaves the target/anode assembly through the radiation of relatively low energy infrared photons (Fig. 10–8). For-

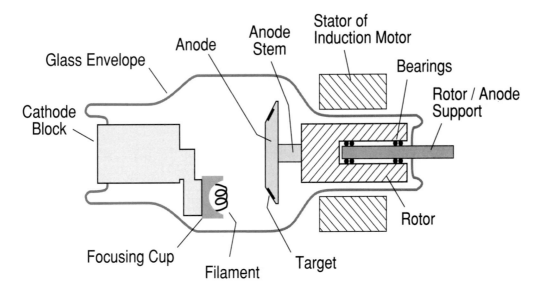

Figure 10–6. Rotating anode diagnostic x-ray tube. All that's needed is a way to mechanically support a rapidly rotating, blisteringly hot anode in a vacuum while applying a high voltage.

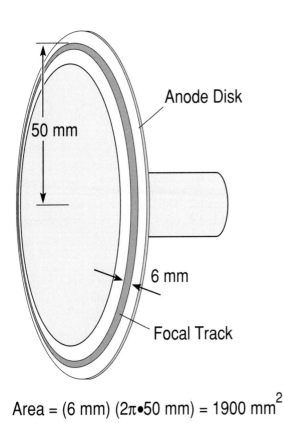

$$\text{Area} = (6 \text{ mm}) \ (2\pi \bullet 50 \text{ mm}) = 1900 \text{ mm}^2$$

Figure 10–7. Comparison of the area of the target region that is directly heated by the electron stream, for stationary and rotating anode tubes. Suppose that for a stationary tube, such as that in Fig. 10–4B, the bombarded region is 6 × 1.5 mm = 9 mm² in area. With a rotating anode tube, the electron stream has the same shape, but it cuts out a 1900-mm² area with each rotation of the anode.

tunately, the higher the target and anode temperatures become, the more rapidly the heat energy is radiated away (Equation 5–6).

Most of the infrared energy radiated from the target and anode is absorbed by a bath of oil surrounding the tube. The oil acts as a thermal conductor between the tube and its housing (and also as an electrical insulator). Transfer of heat from the tube housing to room air takes place by convection, and may be assisted by a fan. A bellows assembly provides for the thermal expansion of the oil, and may be attached to an interlock switch to help prevent overheating.

Molybdenum has a high melting point (2600°C) and is a poor conductor of heat. An axle of this material thermally isolates the rotor bearings and metallic silver lubricant from the anode. (Oils and graphite are unsuitable for use as lubricants at high temperatures in a vacuum.) After each exposure, the rotor is made to slow down, to reduce wear on the bearings. A second or so is therefore required, before an exposure, to bring the anode back up to speed.

Damage to rotor bearings is an infrequent cause of tube failure. Most commonly, the tube becomes gassy, which leads to electrical arcing or a burned out filament. Another source of failure is pitting, cracking, or buckling of the anode surface, which can result in a reduction in the intensity of the usable x-ray beam; it can also cause the electric fields near the anode surface to become distorted, degrading the focal spot.

6. THERMAL RATINGS OF AN X-RAY TUBE: WATT'S A HU?

As an electron from the cathode is brought to an abrupt halt within the target, all of its kinetic energy is converted into other energy forms. Only 1% or less of the kinetic energy of the electron stream becomes bremsstrahlung or characteristic x-ray radiation; the rest is converted into heat. The incident electrons are charged, and expend most of their energy in pushing aside

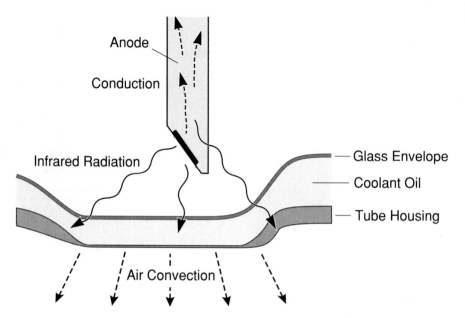

Figure 10–8. In a rotating anode tube, some heat flows from the focal track region of the target to the rest of the anode via thermal conduction. The target and the anode *radiate* infrared photons, which are absorbed by the coolant/insulation oil. The oil conducts heat to the tube's outer housing. From there, it enters the ambient environment by means of air convection, commonly with the assistance of a fan.

electrons belonging to atoms of the target material. Frictionlike forces among them generate heat, just as with electrons driven through a resistive metal wire by a battery. If heat cannot escape from the tube quickly enough, it can cause irreparable damage in seconds.

When the potential across an x-ray tube is (nearly) constant and of magnitude kVp, and the tube current is mA, then by Equation 5.4, heat (plus a relatively very small amount of bremsstrahlung and characteristic x-ray energy) is produced in the anode at a rate of

$$\text{power (W)} = \text{kVp} \cdot \text{mA} \quad \text{(constant potential)} \quad (10.1)$$

The kilo- and milli- cancel one another, leaving the power in the standard SI unit, the watt.

_____ **EXERCISE 10–1.** _____

A diagnostic film is shot at a constant potential of 100 kVp, and with 100 mA, for a time of 0.1 second. At what rate is the tube transforming electric energy into heat and x-rays? What is the total amount of energy so transformed?

SOLUTION: By Equation 10.1, (100 kVp) · (100 mA) = 10,000 W = 10 kW of power is being deposited in the anode during the exposure. That is enough to boil a pot of coffee in a few seconds. The total energy transformed (more than 99% into heat) in 0.1 second is 1000 J = 1 kJ.

For a single-phase generator with 100% ripple, the kVp in Equation 10.1 must be replaced with the effective (rms) value, which is a factor of $1/\sqrt{2} = 0.707$ less:

$$\text{power (W)} = (0.707 \text{ kVp}) \cdot (\text{mA}) \quad \text{(single-phase)} \quad (10.2)$$

With smoothing, the coefficient will be larger than 0.707, but no more than 1.0. Note that while kVp is the peak kilovoltage, mA is the average current.

Heat in x-ray tubes is commonly quantified in terms of a measure that came into standard use when generators were all single-phase. The *heat unit (HU)* is defined as the amount of heat that would be produced in a tube by an unfiltered single-phase generator operating with peak kilovoltage of 1 kVp, an average current of 1 mA, and for a time of 1 second. Hence

$$\text{heat (HU)} = \text{kVp} \cdot \text{mA} \cdot \text{s} \quad \text{(single-phase)} \quad (10.3)$$

Comparison with Equation 10.2 indicates that

$$1 \text{ HU} = 0.707 \text{ W–s} = 0.707 \text{ J} \quad (10.4)$$

independent of the kind (single- vs. three-phase) of generator.

The heating of a tube by a constant-potential generator is about $1/0.707 = 1.41$ times greater than that for a single-phase generator with the same peak kilovoltage, tube current, and duration, and is described either by Equation 10.1 or by

$$\text{heat (HU)} = 1.41 \text{ kVp} \cdot \text{mA} \cdot \text{s} \quad \text{(constant potential)} \quad (10.5)$$

This expression also applies, approximately, for a three-phase, twelve-pulse generator. With three-phase, six-pulse equipment, the factor of 1.41 in Equation 10.5 is commonly replaced by 1.35.

_____ **EXERCISE 10–2.** _____

For the exposure in Exercise 10–1, what is the heat generated in HU?

SOLUTION: By Equation 10.5, heat = 1.41 (100 kVp) · (100 mA) · (0.1s) = 1410 HU.

If a tube is operated improperly, the anode or filament can overheat in a matter of seconds. The conditions of acceptable exposure can be estimated from information supplied by the manufacturer in the form of *rating charts*. The curves in Figure 10–9 reveal the possible combinations of peak kilovoltage, average tube current, and exposure time that a hypothetical tube can just tolerate. Point A, for instance, indicates that with a three-phase generator, the large focal spot, and the standard 3400-rpm anode rotation rate, it is unwise to operate the tube at

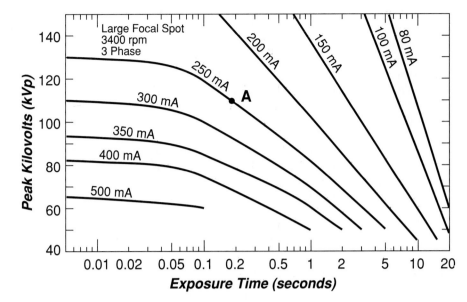

Figure 10–9. Rating chart for a typical x-ray tube, plotting the extreme combinations of peak kilovoltage and exposure time that the tube can tolerate for different values of tube current, with three-phase voltage, large focal spot, and low anode rotation speed. The point marked A indicates, for example, that 110 kVp, 250 mA, and 200 milliseconds constitute one such limiting set of technique factors—none of them can be increased without risking damage to the tube. Similar charts exist for all combinations of filament, anode rotation speed, voltage phase, focal spot size, and sometimes other parameters as well.

110 kVp and 250 mA for more than 0.2 second. Separate curves are provided for every important combination of power source waveform (single- vs. three-phase), focal spot size (small vs. large), and anode rotation rate. (Some tube rating charts show tube current, rather than potential, along the ordinate, and plot curves of constant peak kilovoltage.) As a general rule, you *cannot* apply the rating information on one tube from one manufacturer to another tube design or manufacturer.

The heat accumulated in the anode during a number of exposures, or during a single long fluoroscopic exposure, is determined by the rate of power input, the rate at which heat is radiated or conducted away, and the physical characteristics of the anode (its mass and materials of construction). The capacity of the anode to store heat, however, is limited. It is possible to determine whether the *anode heat-storage capacity* is being exceeded by means of an **anode thermal characteristics** chart which relates, for different rates of anode heating and exposure durations, the heat content. The anode thermal characteristics chart for our tube, which has a heat capacity of 100,000 HU, is

shown in Figure 10–10. Suppose, for example, that during fluoroscopy (with single-phase power), heat is deposited in the anode at the rate of (100 kVp)(4 mA) = 400 HU/s. As indicated by the point marked B, the heat tolerance of the anode will be exceeded after about $8\frac{1}{2}$ minutes of operation.

A **cooling curve** reveals the rate at which a hot anode radiates away heat. (The value of the curve at time $t = 0$ is set equal to the anode heat-storage capacity.) The curve can be used to determine the time required for an anode that has already absorbed a certain quantity of heat to lose any specified amount of it. Separate charts also exist for the tube housing, with and without forced-air cooling.

EXERCISE 10–3.

A certain procedure calls for a 110-kVp exposure at 250 mA for 0.4 second. Is this possible with the tube in Figures 10–9 and 10–10? If not, what is to be done?

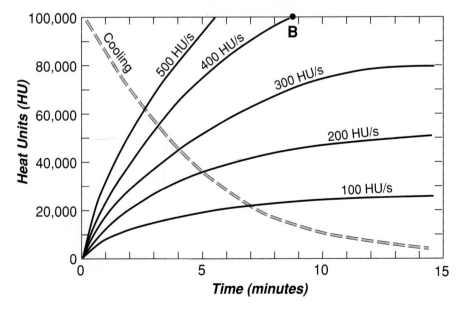

Figure 10–10. Anode thermal characteristics chart for the tube in Figure 10–9, indicating the heat accumulated over time with various rates of anode heating. Also shown is a cooling curve that relates the retained heat as a function of cooling time. The value of the cooling curve at $t = 0$ gives the heat tolerance of the tube. The point marked B reveals that with a heat input to the anode of 400 HU per second, for example, the tube can operate continuously for about $8\frac{1}{2}$ minutes. Cooling curves are also available separately for the tube housing.

SOLUTION: The maximum exposure time that can be tolerated at 110 kVp and 250 mA is about 0.2 second (point A), so the prescribed set of technique factors cannot be used. At a given peak kilovoltage, however, film darkening depends only on the product of exposure current and duration. The prescribed technique factors call for 100 mA-s. A 110-kVp, 200-mA, 0.5-second exposure, also of 100 mA-s, would provide the needed exposure of film and could be handled by the tube.

_____ **EXERCISE 10–4.** _____

How much energy is deposited in the anode of the tube in a $5\frac{1}{2}$-minute-long rapid series of radiographs in which the rate of its delivery averages 400 HU/s? How long must the tube be left to cool for the heat in the anode to fall to half its capacity? Assume a three-phase generator.

SOLUTION: Following the 400 HU/s curve out to $5\frac{1}{2}$ minutes indicates that 80,000 HU will have accumulated in the anode. The cooling curve drops from 80,000 to 50,000 HU in $(3\frac{1}{2} - 1) = 2\frac{1}{2}$ minutes.

_____ **EXERCISE 10–5.** _____

Same as Exercise 10–4, but with a single-phase generator.

SOLUTION: The answers are the same. The anode thermal characteristics chart (unlike the tube rating chart) is concerned with the heat in the anode, not with the fine details of the way it was deposited there.

7. TUBE SHIELDING, FILTERS, AND BEAM RESTRICTORS

The tube *housing* (Fig. 10–11) provides mechanical support for the tube and a container for the oil that surrounds it. It also contains a lead sheath that prevents the escape of x-rays in any direction except through the window. National Council on Radiation Protection and Measurement (NCRP) Report No. 49 stipulates that such **leakage** radiation, when measured at a distance 1 m from the source, "shall not exceed 100 mR (milliroentgens) in 1 hour when the tube is operated at its maximum continuous rated current for the maximum rated tube potential." This has nothing to do, of course, with radiation beam that passes through the housing's exit window, as intended, and then perhaps scatters from the patient, table, and so on.

After emerging through the exit window of the x-ray tube's housing (Fig. 10–12), a beam must pass through one or several kinds of **filters.** The purpose of a filter is usually to remove the lower-energy bremsstrahlung photons, which are diagnostically useless but contribute to patient dose, as will be discussed in the next chapter. The minimum amounts of total (inherent plus added) aluminum filtration that should be employed under various operating conditions for a tungsten target tube are listed in Table 10–1. (The requirements for a mam-

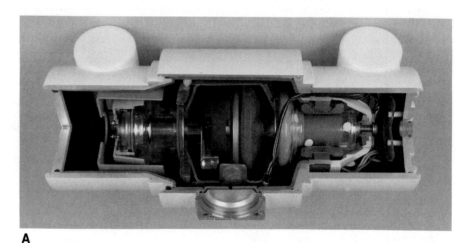

A

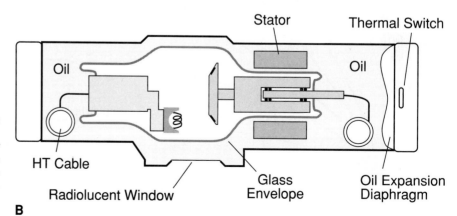

B

Figure 10–11. An x-ray tube and its housing: **A.** The tube itself is diagrammed in Figure 10–6. *(Photo courtesy of Varian Power Grid & X-ray Tube Products.)* **B.** The oil bath serves both to conduct heat away from the tube and to insulate it electrically from the outside world. HT, high-tension.

Stator

Thermal Switch

Oil

Oil

HT Cable

Radiolucent Window

Glass Envelope

Oil Expansion Diaphragm

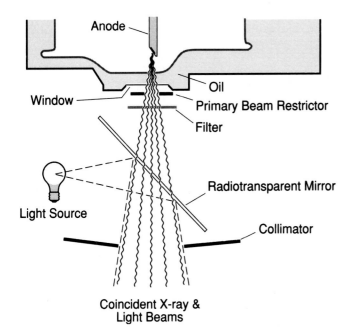

Anode

Oil

Window

Primary Beam Restrictor

Filter

Light Source

Radiotransparent Mirror

Collimator

Coincident X-ray &
Light Beams

Figure 10–12. Filter and collimator structure. The objective is to produce a beam that is of proper "quality" and the desired dimensions and is positioned correctly on the patient. Filtration hardens the beam, removing nonpenetrating but dose-depositing low-energy photons. The collimator shutters determine the beam field dimensions. (These should be made as small as possible, for any particular patient and procedure, to minimize both patient exposure and the amount of image degradation from scatter radiation.) The light field, designed to coincide with the radiation beam, aids in patient positioning.

mography tube with a molybdenum target are different.) There are further conditions on the characteristics of the filtered beam itself (expressed in terms of the half-value layer in aluminum), as will be discussed in Chapter 29.

A modern x-ray system comes equipped with a *primary*

TABLE 10–1. MINIMUM TOTAL BEAM FILTRATION FOR VARIOUS kVp SETTINGS

Tube potential (kVp)	Minimum filtration (mm Al)
Under 50	0.5
50–70	1.5
Above 70	2.5

From National Council on Radiation Protection and Measurement (NCRP): Medical X-ray, Electron Beam, and Gamma-Ray Protection for Energies up to 50 MeV (Equipment Design, Performance, and Use), Report No. 102. Bethesda, MD: NCRP, 1989 (Table 3.1).

beam restrictor and a set of **collimators.** The primary restrictor, with a circular beam port of fixed size, is located close to the tube. Beyond that are the collimators, which can be adjusted so that the beam covers only the region of interest. A bulb and an angled mirror (nearly transparent to x-rays) within the collimator assembly produce a light beam that emerges from the tube housing coincident with the x-ray beam. The light field aids in the positioning of the patient and the setting of the collimator aperture size.

Beam restriction is important for two reasons. First, radiation scattered from the patient's body degrades image quality significantly. And the amount of scatter produced depends strongly (especially for small fields) on beam area.

Second, although there is no direct evidence on the incidence of radiogenic cancers produced at low (i.e., diagnostic) doses, it is prudent to assume that the small risks of radiation-induced carcinogenesis may increase with the volume of tissue irradiated. A fundamental and quite reasonable working hypothesis of radiation safety is that unnecessary exposures should be kept *as low as reasonably achievable* (*ALARA*). And tight collimation is a simple and effective ALARA measure.

Older machines achieved the same effect as collimation, albeit with less convenience and flexibility, by means of attachable *aperture diaphragms* or *cones.*

Chapter 11

The X-ray Beam

The spectrum of an x-ray beam is determined largely by the peak kilovoltage of the tube, the target material, and the amount and kinds of beam filtration.

The most energetic x-ray photons produced (and there are relatively very few of them) have the same energy as the electrons bombarding the anode. Many of the photons created at the low-energy end of the spectrum are preferentially absorbed in photoelectric events in the anode itself or in the glass wall of the tube. An aluminum filter outside it further hardens the beam, reducing even more the component of nonpenetrating, hence diagnostically useless (but nonetheless hazardous), low-energy photons.

Characteristic x-rays are produced if the electrons' kinetic energy exceeds the binding energy of inner-orbital electrons of the target material atoms.

The intensity of the beam generated is proportional to the tube current, and increases (very roughly) with the square of the tube potential. The intensity falls off with the inverse square of the distance from the focal spot. The ability of the beam to penetrate tissues, and to interact differently with different detector materials, depends on the peak kilovoltage, the shape of the voltage waveform, and on the amount and type of filtration.

1. MEASURES OF X-RAY BEAM STRENGTH: PHOTON FLUENCE, ENERGY FLUENCE, INTENSITY, AND EXPOSURE

Over the years, radiology has accumulated a plethora of measures of radiation. Some of these are defined in terms of the _energy deposited_ when radiation enters matter. The gray (Gy) or

rad of **dose** (Table 11–1) refers to ionizing energy imparted per unit mass. The sievert (Sv) or rem of **dose equivalent** even takes into account the biologic effects of the radiation on humans.

It is advantageous to invent other measures of radiation that refer directly to properties of a _radiation beam itself_, rather than to what it does to matter in general (gray) or to people in particular (sievert).

The number of photons n that pass through space per unit of area A (taken at right angles to the beam) is known as the _photon fluence_. If the photon fluence is the same everywhere of interest, this may be written simply as n/A. More generally, the photon fluence varies from place to place, and must be expressed locally as $\Delta n/\Delta A$ (Fig. 11–1A), where a small number Δn of photons pass through a particular small area ΔA.

Photon fluence takes no account of the energies of the photons involved. The photon fluence is the same for 100 x-ray photons/cm² as for 100 infrared photons/cm². Hence the need for the _photon energy fluence_ (Fig. 11–1B), which explicitly incorporates the photon energy: $\Delta n \cdot hf/\Delta A$.

As it stands, this is useful only for a beam of photons that are all of the same energy. With a polychromatic beam, the total energy ΔE passing through ΔA is obtained by summing the energy fluence over all photon energies. Energy fluence can then be defined simply as $\Delta E/\Delta A$, where no mention need be made of the photon nature of the radiation.

In many situations it is necessary to describe the _rate_ at which photon energy flows through space. The energy fluence rate, or **intensity**, I, is the amount of energy fluence per unit time (Fig. 11–1C). For a monochromatic photon beam, this is just

Quantity	SI Unit	Conventional Unit	Relationship
Dose	gray (Gy)	rad	1 Gy = 100 rad
Dose equivalent	sievert (Sv)	rem	1 Sv = 100 rem
Exposure	C/kg	roentgen (R)	1 R = 2.58×10^{-4} C/kg
Air kerma	gray (Gy)	centigray (cGy)	1 cGy = 0.01 Gy

$$I(hf) = (\Delta n \cdot hf / \Delta A) / \Delta t \qquad (11.1)$$

With a polychromatic photon beam, the function $I(E) \cdot \Delta E$ is meant to refer to the intensity of photons with energies that lie in the narrow band from E to $E + \Delta E$. Bremsstrahlung spectra, for example, are commonly presented as $I(E)$ curves. Beware that the term "intensity" sometimes refers to the *integrated intensity*, including photons of all energies.

EXERCISE 11–1.

3×10^{18} photons, of 2.1-eV average energy, pass through a 1-m² area over a 10-second period. What is the intensity in W/cm²?

SOLUTION: $I = (3 \times 10^{18})(2.1 \text{ eV})(1.6 \times 10^{-19} \text{ J/eV})/(10^4 \text{ cm}^2)/(10 \text{ s}) = 10^{-5}$ W/cm², by Equation 11.1. Compare this with Exercise 6–2.

The meaning of intensity is straightforward, but it is not a simple matter to measure x-ray intensity directly in the clinic.

It is much easier (and just as useful) to work with an indirect measure of beam intensity, namely, the exposure or the air kerma.

2. EXPOSURE AND AIR KERMA

Air, which is about 80% nitrogen and 20% oxygen, is the simplest medium that plays a dosimetric role in radiology. As the active ingredient in an **air ionization chamber**, it is also one of the most important.

An idealized ion chamber system is shown in Figure 11–2. Two electrodes suspended in air are attached to a battery via an *electrometer*, a device sensitive to extremely small flows of charge. The battery has pulled some electrons away from the anode and pushed others onto the cathode, creating an electric field between them. As air molecules are uncharged, and unaffected by this field, the region between the electrodes normally acts like an open switch, and no current flows in the circuit. When the air experiencing the electric field is exposed to ionizing radiation, however, the resultant highly mobile electrons

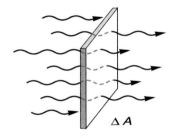

Photon Fluence = $\dfrac{\Delta n}{\Delta A}$

A

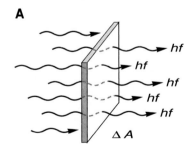

Photon Energy Fluence = $\dfrac{\Delta n \cdot hf}{\Delta A}$

B

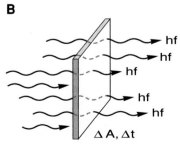

Photon Intensity: $I(hf) = \dfrac{\Delta n \cdot hf}{\Delta A} / \Delta t$

C

Figure 11–1. Measures of x-ray beam quantity. **A.** The photon fluence is the number Δn of photons per unit area ΔA passing through an imaginary surface facing the beam. **B.** The photon energy fluence for a monochromatic beam accounts also for the energy hf per photon. **C.** The intensity I refers to the rate of flow of energy per unit area per unit of time.

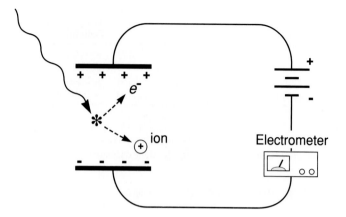

Figure 11–2. The simplest ionization chamber consists of a volume of air located between parallel metal electrodes, and a voltage source plus electrometer combination for creating and measuring a flow of charge. An incident photon interacts with an air molecule, liberating a fast photoelectron or Compton electron, which may, in turn, ionize many other air molecules. The resulting ions and electrons are drawn to the electrodes, and a current registers.

and ions rush to the anode and cathode (perhaps ionizing other molecules along the way), and neutralize some of the charge on them. To reestablish the equilibrium level of charge on the electrodes, the battery pulls new electrons from the anode, through the electrometer, and onto the cathode. It is this flow that the electrometer measures. Clinical ion chambers are compact and small, but they operate essentially the same way.

The electrometer reading depends on the intensity and duration of the irradiation, and on the extent to which the beam interacts with (and deposits energy in) the mass of air within the chamber. The entity actually monitored, namely the amount of ionization charge liberated per unit mass of air irradiated, is known as the *exposure*. Exposure is measured in a unit called the *roentgen* (R), where one roentgen is the amount of ionizing radiation that gives rise to the liberation of exactly 2.58×10^{-4} C of charge (of either sign) through irradiation of a

TABLE 11–2. APPROXIMATE RELATIONSHIP BETWEEN UNITS OF EXPOSURE (ROENTGEN) AND AIR KERMA (GRAY)^a

	Approximately:	
1 R (exposure)	⟵————⟶	1 cGy (air kerma)

^{a}More precisely, 1 R of exposure corresponds to 0.873 cGy of air kerma.

kilogram of air (Fig. 11–3A): $1 R \Leftrightarrow 2.58 \times 10^{-4}$ C/kg. (The SI unit for exposure is the coulomb per kilogram of air; 1 R is smaller than 1 C/kg by a factor of 2.58×10^{-4}.)

Because it is highly reproducible and easily measured, exposure has long been the standard measure of x-ray tube output. One side effect of the change to SI units, however, has been a move to replace exposure with a closely related construct, the *air kerma*, as a measure of x-ray beam strength. At diagnostic energies, air kerma is practically the same thing as *dose to air*, and both are expressed (in SI units) in terms of the gray (1 Gy = 1 J/kg = 100 rad) (Fig. 11–3B). Dose to air, in turn, is tightly linked to exposure; the two, in fact, are proportional to one another: The more ionizing energy you pump into a kilogram of air, the more of it you'll ionize. We shall defer until Chapter 30 a more complete description of air kerma. For the time being, suffice it to say that a 1-R beam corresponds to 0.873 cGy (1 cGy = 0.01 J/kg = 1 rad) of air kerma, and vice versa: 1 R ⟺ 0.873 cGy. Because of their numerical closeness, the roentgen of exposure and the centigray of air kerma are frequently used interchangeably (Table 11–2). In fact, a strong motivation for turning to the cGy of air kerma as the SI unit of beam strength (rather than to the C/kg of exposure) is that the centigray and the (very familiar) roentgen are numerically close. The symbol K_{air} (or K alone) is commonly employed to denote kerma to air, and X stands for exposure.

In this book we shall, in general, use *air kerma* or *exposure* in describing the output of an x-ray tube or the input to an image receptor such as a screen–film system or an image intensifier. We shall keep track of the *intensity*, however, when following the attenuation of a beam passing through matter. The

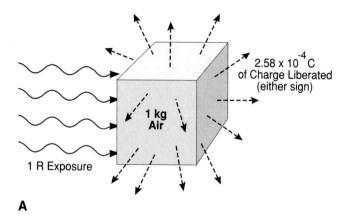

A

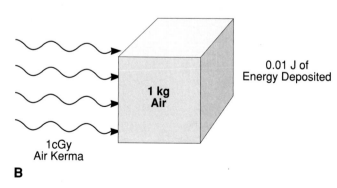

B

Figure 11–3. Measures of x-ray beam strength. **A.** The traditional measure of x-ray beam strength is the roentgen (R). A 1-R exposure will result in the liberation of 2.58×10^{-4} C of charge (of either sign) per kilogram of exposed air. The SI equivalent of the roentgen is the coulomb per kilogram (C/kg). **B.** For diagnostic x-ray beams, air kerma is practically the same thing as the dose to air. The commonly used unit of air kerma is the centigray (cGy). Fortuitously, 1 cGy of air kerma is numerically nearly equivalent to 1 R of exposure.

dose or *dose equivalent* will be appropriate when considering the deposition of ionizing radiation in a patient's body.

As will be shown in Chapter 30, it is easy (and sometimes necessary) to relate energy fluence, exposure, kerma in air, and dose in matter to one another.

3. THE KINETIC ENERGY OF THE ELECTRONS ACCELERATED ACROSS AN X-RAY TUBE IS DETERMINED ENTIRELY BY THE APPLIED VOLTAGE

The central topic of this chapter is the beam of high-energy photons produced by an x-ray tube. Let us back up a step first, however, and begin with the electrons being accelerated from the tube's cathode to its anode.

A modern three-phase or constant-potential generator creates a voltage that is almost constant over time. The amplitude of ripple is of the order of a few percent. Electrons that are thermionically emitted from the cathode and drawn to the anode therefore all acquire about the same kinetic energy. The spectrum of the terminal kinetic energies of electrons accelerated through a potential difference of 100 kV, for example, is a single narrow spike (see Fig. 5–3). The preimpact kinetic energy of the electrons, in electron volts, is numerically equal to the x-ray tube's applied potential, in volts.

> The unfiltered output of a full-wave rectified, single-phase generator, by contrast, varies between 0 kV and the peak voltage 120 times a second. The electrons emitted from the cathode at any particular instant reach the anode in under a microsecond, and their terminal kinetic energy is determined by the value of the tube potential at that instant. For normal radiographic exposures, typically lasting several or several tens of milliseconds, the spectrum of energies of all the electrons that reach the anode will reflect the time dependence of the applied voltage. So, too, will the resultant spectrum of x-rays.

4. BREMSSTRAHLUNG: DIRECT TRANSFORMATION OF ELECTRON KINETIC ENERGY INTO X-RAY PHOTON ENERGY

As discussed in Chapter 4, Section 6, if a moving electron undergoes a rapid change of speed or direction, a portion or all of its kinetic energy will be radiated off in the form of electromagnetic radiation. Such is the case with a *bremsstrahlung* event (Fig. 11–4). An electron with tens or hundreds of kilo-electron volts of kinetic energy penetrates the cloud of orbital electrons of a tungsten atom in an anode, say, and interacts briefly but violently (by means of the electromagnetic interaction) with the nucleus. The more energetic the incident electron, and the more wrenching the change of its velocity, the greater the amount of kinetic energy that is transformed directly into x-ray photon energy.

The bremsstrahlung x-rays produced at an anode (unlike the electrons incident on it) do not all have the same energy. The relative number of photons created is a decreasing function of their energy, rather, and reaches zero at the energy of the incident electrons. A few electrons transform most or all of

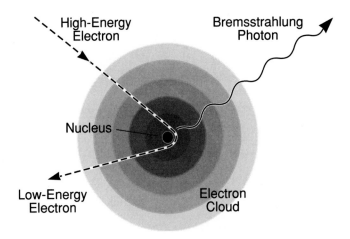

Figure 11–4. A high-velocity electron may penetrate far enough into an atom to be strongly deflected by means of an electric interaction with its nucleus. The electron may then lose some or all of its kinetic energy through the creation of a bremsstrahlung photon.

their kinetic energy into bremsstrahlung radiation, but the vast majority generate lower-frequency photons and waste most of their energy in heating the anode. The results, on balance, are bremsstrahlung production curves of the type shown in Figure 11–5 for 50- and 100-keV electrons.

> The following is a simple, heuristic, non-rigorous explanation of the shape of the bremsstrahlung spectrum. It consists of four steps, and begins by considering the spectrum produced with a very thin foil target.
>
> 1. Imagine that a cross-sectional slice of the region around a nucleus is partitioned into imaginary con-

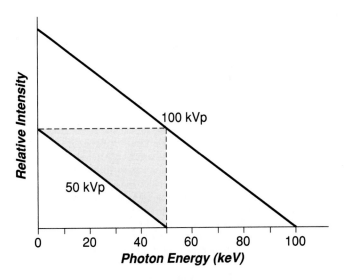

Figure 11–5. Thick target bremsstrahlung spectra produced by 50- and 100-keV electrons, with no beam hardening (by external filters or even by the anode itself) and no creation of characteristic x-rays. The dashed lines indicate that the area under the 100-kVp spectrum is four times that under the 50-kVp curve, suggesting that the integrated intensity (over all photon energies) increases roughly with the square of the tube potential.

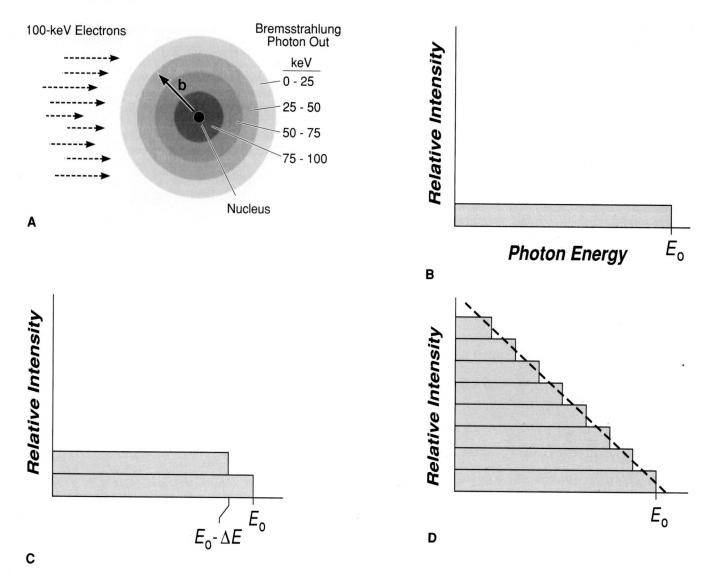

Figure 11–6.   A heuristic explanation of the shapes of bremsstrahlung spectra for both thin-foil and thick targets is given in the text.

centric rings of equal small width, Δb, as with a shooter's target (Fig. 11–6A). The area of a narrow ring is proportional to its radius; that is, the area of the annulus of radius b is $2\pi b \cdot \Delta b$. Suppose that a uniform, monoenergetic stream of electrons of energy E_0 is incident on the region surrounding the nucleus. The number of electrons passing through any ring will be proportional to its area, hence to its radius. Therefore so, too, will be the *number* of photons produced by those electrons: $\Delta n \sim b$. Figure 11–6A shows this for 100-keV incident electrons, and for four ranges of produced bremsstrahlung photons.

2. The electrons passing closest to the nucleus experience the strongest attractive forces, and transform the largest fraction (up to 100%) of their kinetic energy into photon energy. Assume that the *energy* of the typical bremsstrahlung photon created by an electron passing through the ring of radius b is proportional to $1/b$ (which increases as b becomes smaller): $hf \sim 1/b$.

3. Now combine the arguments of steps 1 and 2. The

intensity of the set of photons generated within a ring is determined by the product of the *number* of photons produced (which is proportional to b) and by their *energy* (which is proportional to $1/b$). The intensity of bremsstrahlung photons created within a ring is thus proportional to $\Delta n \cdot hf \sim b \cdot (1/b) = 1$; that is, the intensity of the photons produced by electrons passing through an annulus is (unlike the number of photons or the average photon energy) independent of b. The bremsstrahlung spectrum for a thin foil is therefore constant, up to the energy of the incident electrons, where it drops to zero (Fig. 11–6B).

4. Now for a more realistic, thick target. In passing through a thin foil, the average electron loses ΔE of kinetic energy through weak collisions with the foil material. If our electron stream enters a second thin foil, the bremsstrahlung spectrum will be like the first, but with a peak energy of $E_0 - \Delta E$. The compound spectrum from the first two foils is shown in Figure 11–6C. A thick target may be thought of as being made up of many superimposed foils, and the argument continues along the same line (Fig.

11–6D). The thick target bremsstrahlung spectra for incident monochromatic electrons of two energies were presented in Figure 11–5.

5. EFFECTS OF BEAM FILTRATION AND CHARACTERISTIC X-RAY PRODUCTION ON THE ENERGY SPECTRUM OF THE X-RAY BEAM

The spectrum of a usable diagnostic beam does not look exactly like Figure 11–5, for two reasons. The first has to do with the hardening of the beam as it leaves the tube, and the second with the production of characteristic x-rays. First, beam hardening.

Only a small fraction of the x-rays produced at the anode reach the patient. About half of them start off heading into the anode itself, and are absorbed immediately. Most of the rest are stopped by the lead shielding around the tube.

But even those that are initially moving toward the patient do not necessarily get far. They must survive passage through the tube's glass envelope, the coolant/insulation oil that surrounds the tube, and finally a beam **filter,** such as a 1- to 3-mm-thick sheet of aluminum. The anode, glass window, oil, and added filter *harden* the beam, preferentially absorbing low-energy x-rays (primarily through photoelectric interactions) and thereby increasing the average energy of the remaining photons. The combined filtering action of the anode, window, oil, and *added filtration* is usually expressed in terms of the *equivalent total filtration* that would be caused by some thickness of aluminum alone and is reported in the shorthand units "mm Al."

Because of filtration, relatively few low-energy photons reach the patient, which is generally desirable; low-energy photons penetrate tissue poorly, and thus are diagnostically useless, but they do contribute to patient dose. The amount of beam hardening increases with the amount of filtration, but only up to a point; after most of the low-energy photons have been removed, more filtration mainly lowers the overall intensity of the beam.

_____ **EXERCISE 11–2.** _____

At a constant operating voltage of 80 kVp, the anode and window of an x-ray tube have a combined filtering effect equivalent to 0.5 mm Al. How much added filter is needed to achieve a total effective filtration of 2.5 mm Al?

SOLUTION: A 2-mm-thick aluminum filter is required.

Characteristic x-rays are produced (at energies characteristic of the target material) when the tube potential (in kVp) exceeds the ionization energies (in keV) of inner-orbital electrons of the target atoms. With a tungsten target, characteristic K x-rays are produced with tube potentials above 69.5 kVp (see Table 6–3), and constitute some 30% of total diagnostic beam energy at 120 kVp.

For mammography, the tube is operated at about 25 to 30 kVp, and it is actually the K characteristic x-ray photons of the molybdenum target, occurring at 16 and 19 keV, rather than the bremsstrahlung x-rays, that are principally used for imaging. But for ordinary radiography and fluoroscopy, filtered bremsstrahlung radiation plays the dominant role.

The general shape of the spectrum of a diagnostic beam is distinctive of the bremsstrahlung process, and largely independent of the tube's construction and operating parameters. But the energy of the most energetic photons, the energy of peak photon intensity, and the relative amplitude of the characteristic x-ray lines are determined by the kilovoltage setting. And the shape of the low-energy end of the curve depends on the amount of intentional filtration and other forms of beam hardening.

The spectra of beams obtained at 100 kVp, with a tungsten target and various amounts of filtration, are shown in Figure 11–7. Curve A is the unhardened, purely bremsstrahlung spectrum. Curve B includes the tungsten characteristic x-ray peaks and the effects of beam hardening by the anode itself. Addition of a normal amount of aluminum beam filtration gives rise to curve C.

6. THE LOW EFFICIENCY OF X-RAY PRODUCTION: LESS THAN 1% OF THE ELECTRONS' ENERGY IS TRANSFORMED INTO X-RAY BEAM ENERGY

When electrons from the cathode of an x-ray tube collide with the anode, their kinetic energy is transformed into other forms of energy. With a nearly constant potential (kVp) and a tube

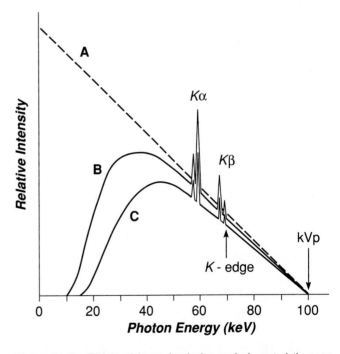

Figure 11–7. Effects of beam hardening and characteristic x-ray production on the spectrum. Curve A is a hypothetical, pure bremsstrahlung spectrum. Curve B is the spectrum of photons coming from a real tungsten target, which itself hardens the beam. Curve C results when the total amount of filtration (inherent plus added) is equivalent to that from 2.5 mm Al. Strong tungsten characteristic x-ray lines may be seen in curves B and C.

current (mA), this energy conversion process occurs, by Equation 10.1, at the rate

$$\text{power (W)} = \text{kVp} \cdot \text{mA} \qquad (11.2)$$

But typically 99% or more of the kinetic energy of the stream of electrons is wasted in heating the anode. The efficiency of bremsstrahlung production is therefore critically important.

As the strength of the electromagnetic interaction of a fast electron with a nucleus is proportional to the charge on the nucleus, the efficiency of the bremsstrahlung process in an x-ray tube is proportional to the atomic number Z of the anode material. This is one important reason why targets of most x-ray tubes are made of tungsten ($Z = 74$) or a tungsten–rhenium alloy.

It also explains why photoelectrons and Compton electrons in a patient's tissues (liberated, for example, by x-rays from a diagnostic tube) radiate away little energy in the form of bremsstrahlung x-rays, even though they may have tens of kilo-electron volts of kinetic energy: They collide with hydrogen, carbon, nitrogen, and oxygen nuclei, all with low bremsstrahlung production efficiency.

This phenomenon can be put to good use. A sample of beta-emitting radionuclide is usually contained directly within a *plastic* (low-Z) vessel with walls thick enough to bring all beta particles to a standstill. In a higher-Z metal container, they would produce more bremsstrahlung photons, which are more difficult to shield against.

The efficiency of the bremsstrahlung process is found empirically (and can be calculated by quantum mechanics) to be approximately

$$\text{efficiency} = 10^{-6} Z \cdot \text{kVp} \qquad (11.3)$$

Equation 11.3 supports our claim that with a tungsten target and normal diagnostic operating voltages, typically $\frac{1}{2}\%$ to 1% of the power pumped into a tube is converted into bremsstrahlung and characteristic x-ray energy. (And of that, only a small fraction exits the tube in the direction of the patient.)

_____ **EXERCISE 11–3.** _____

What is the efficiency of an x-ray tube with a tungsten target operating at 90 kVp?

SOLUTION: By Equation 11.3, efficiency = $(10^{-6})(74)(90)$ = 0.7%.

_____ **EXERCISE 11–4.** _____

A constant-potential tube operates at 100 kVp and 200 mA for 1/20 second, and 5% of the x-ray radiation generated exits through the window as useful beam. How much usable x-ray power is produced?

SOLUTION: Instantaneous power to the anode is (100 kVp)(200 mA) = 20,000 W. About 1% of this is transformed into x-rays and, of that, only 5%, or (20,000 W)(0.01)(0.05) = 10 W, exits through the tube window. Thus, only about (10 W)/(20,000 W) = 0.05% of the power expended in the tube is transformed into useful beam.

7. THE OUTPUT OF AN X-RAY TUBE

The output of an x-ray tube is directly proportional to the number of electrons that undergo bremsstrahlung interactions and, therefore, is linear in the average tube current. It also decreases with the square of the distance r from the focal spot, for the reason discussed in the next section. The dependence on kilovoltage and filtration is more complex, as suggested by Figure 11–8.

The air kerma in centigrays (cGy) at a point r cm from the focal spot may be described roughly (to within 10% or so) by the empirical relationship

$$K_{\text{air}} \text{ (cGy)} = 11 \cdot (2.5/\text{Al})(\text{kVp}/100)^2 \cdot (\text{A-s})/(r/100)^2$$
$$\text{(three-phase or fluoro)} \qquad (11.4)$$

kVp is the applied tube potential, in kilovolts, for a three-phase or constant-potential generator; with a single-phase generator, the output is found to be only about 0.6 as great as that for three-phase. The tube current is expressed in ampere-seconds (A-s, not mA-s). "Al" refers to the total (inherent plus added) equivalent beam filtration, in millimeters of aluminum, and the factor of (2.5/Al) allows you to account approximately for values of total filtration other than 2.5 mm Al.

The exposure in roentgens is numerically greater than the air kerma in centigrays by a factor of 1/0.873.

Figure 11–9 underscores the point that although the intensity of a filtered beam is proportional to tube current for a fixed peak kilovoltage, both the intensity and the peak energy of the photon spectrum increase with peak kilovoltage for fixed tube current.

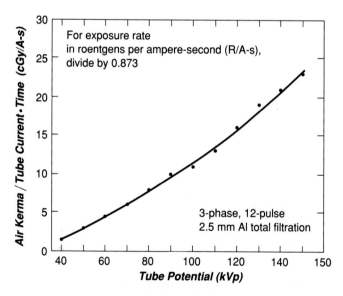

Figure 11–8. Output of a typical diagnostic x-ray tube, with three-phase, twelve-pulse applied voltage and 2.5 mm Al equivalent total filtration. The curve relates, as a function of tube potential, the air kerma rate, in centigrays per ampere-second (cGy/A-s), at a point 100 cm from the focal spot. Equation 11.4 provides the same information. *(After National Council on Radiation Protection and Measurements (NCRP): Medical X-ray Electron Beam and Gamma-ray Protection for Energies up to 50 MeV (Equipment Design, Performance, and Use), Report No. 102. Bethesda, MD: NRCP, 1989 (Table B.3).*

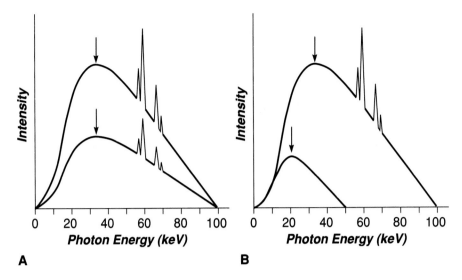

Figure 11–9. Effects of tube current and applied potential on the spectrum and output for a diagnostic tube. **A.** Doubling the tube current doubles the intensity at any photon energy, and the total intensity (integrated over all photon energies) as well. **B.** The effect of doubling the tube potential, from 50 to 100 kVp, is more subtle. The energy of the most energetic photons is doubled, the intensity peak is shifted to higher energy, and characteristic x-ray photons are now produced. The integrated beam intensity is roughly quadrupled (see also Fig. 11–5).

A   **B**

_____ **EXERCISE 11–5.** _____

A 90-kVp, 80-mA, 0.1-second exposure is made with a three-phase generator and a tube with 2.5 mm Al total filtration. What is the exposure 40 inches away?

SOLUTION: Forty inches is approximately 100 cm. By Equation 11.4, the beam strength that far from the source is 11(2.5/2.5 mm)(90 kVp/100)^2(0.08 A)(0.1 s)/(100 cm/100)^2 = 0.07 cGy of air kerma. This corresponds to an exposure of 80 mR.

Fluoroscopy is a special case. Modern radiographic/fluoroscopic systems are usually powered by a three-phase generator. When operating in the fluoroscopy mode, however, the three-phase capability is not (with some systems) employed. Power is tapped off from only one of the three high-voltage lines, rather, and full-wave rectified. But the tube current is very low (several milliamperes, as opposed to several hundred milliamperes for radiography), and the cable between the generator and the x-ray tube provides enough capacitance to smooth the tube voltage very effectively. So even though the applied voltage may be single-phase, here it acts like that from a nearly constant voltage source, and Equation 11.4 therefore describes its exposure rate.

8. THE INVERSE SQUARE EFFECT IS PURE GEOMETRY

For radiation coming from a point source, such as (approximately) the focal spot of an x-ray tube, the intensity or air kerma of the radiation falls off with the square of the distance r from the source. As with Exercise 6–2, this is a purely geometric effect.

Suppose a uniform beam of photons of energy hf are emanating at the rate $\Delta n/\Delta t$ from a point source. At a distance of 1 m, moreover, the area of the beam is 1 m^2. The Δn photons crossing the 1-m^2 area per Δt give rise to 1 unit of intensity. At a distance of 2 m, the area is 4 m^2; so the same number of pho-

tons produced per second produces an intensity of $\frac{1}{4}$ unit of intensity (Fig. 11–10). Generalizing this argument, the intensity falls off with the inverse of the square of the distance r:

$$I(r) \sim 1/r^2 \qquad (11.5)$$

A similar argument applies to the inverse square dependence of air kerma or exposure, as in Equation 11.4.

_____ **EXERCISE 11–6.** _____

The output of an x-ray tube (rate of air kerma) is measured to be 7.3 cGy/min at a distance of 40 cm from the focal spot. What would it be at 65 cm?

SOLUTION: By Equation 11.5, the air kerma rate at 65 cm is reduced from that at 40 cm by a factor of (40 cm/65 cm)^2 = 0.38.

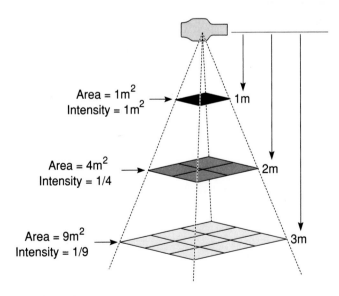

Figure 11–10. The inverse square dependence of x-ray beam intensity on distance from the point source is purely a matter of geometry. The area that the beam intersects increases with the square of the distance, so the number of photons per unit area decreases by the same amount.

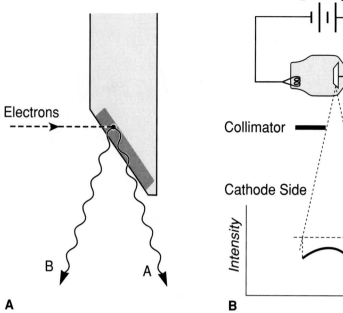

Figure 11-11. The heel effect. **A.** Incident electrons penetrate a good distance into the anode. The set of bremsstrahlung photons emerging in the A direction have to travel farther through metal before reaching the anode surface than do the B photons, and are more attenuated. (They also experience more hardening.) **B.** The shape of the beam intensity-vs.-emission angle curve is a result of the angular dependencies of bremsstrahlung production and self-absorption within the anode and, to a lesser extent, of the inverse square effect.

At 65 cm, the air kerma rate is $(40/65)^2(7.3 \text{ cGy/min}) = 2.8$ cGy/min.

9. THE HEEL EFFECT CAUSES BEAM NONUNIFORMITY

The beam of bremsstrahlung x-rays emerging through the window of an x-ray tube is not of uniform intensity. Indeed, as indicated in Figure 11-11, the part of the beam coming off in the more forward direction (along the line from cathode to anode), commonly called the *anode side* of the beam, is of significantly lower intensity.

At diagnostic energies, as noted in Chapter 10, Section 2, many x-ray photons are emitted in directions nearly perpendicular to that of the stream of incoming electrons. About half of the x-ray photons produced are heading into the anode, where they are absorbed. Of the photons starting off in the general direction of the exit window of the x-ray tube, those head-

ing in a more forward direction have to travel a greater distance through the target material, on average, before escaping it—so that fewer manage to get out. As a consequence, the anode side of the beam can be as much as 30% less intense than the cathode side. This is known as the **heel effect.**

The heel effect is of greater clinical significance for large exposure fields and for small source-to-skin distances, such as in angiography.

Although it is possible to design wedge-shaped beam filters to compensate for the heel effect, this is seldom done. To the contrary, the effect is sometimes put to advantage, by placing thinner parts of the body toward the anode side of the tube, where the beam is less intense. For an anteroposterior (AP) examination of the thoracic spine, for example, it is standard practice to align the patient so that the thinner, upper part of the body is toward the anode side of the tube. The beam is somewhat more hardened and penetrating on the anode side, but the difference in intensity is the dominant effect.

Part 3

Interaction of X-rays with Matter

Chapter 12

X-ray Interaction Mechanisms

1. **Photons of Different Energies Interact with Different Kinds of Matter via Different Mechanisms**
2. **The Case of the Vanishing Photon: The Photoelectric Effect**
3. **In a (Diagnostic Energy) Compton Event, Some X-ray Energy Goes to the Compton Recoil Electron, but Most Goes to the Compton Scatter Photon**
4. **Coherent Scattering, Pair Production, and Other X-ray Interaction Mechanisms**

There are a number of mechanisms by which electromagnetic radiation can interact with matter. The probability that any one of them will come into play depends on the energy of the photons and on the chemical and physical form of the matter with which they might interact.

Diagnostic energy x-ray photons, in particular, interact with matter primarily by means of the photoelectric and Compton (incoherent scattering) mechanisms. In a photoelectric event, all the energy of the incident x-ray photon is transferred to an ejected photoelectron and its atom. In a Compton event, some of the energy of the incident x-ray photon becomes kinetic energy of a Compton electron, and the rest leaves the scene of the collision in the form of a (lower-energy) Compton scatter photon. The coherent scattering mechanism plays only a small role in imaging.

The interaction of x-ray photons with matter was discussed briefly in Chapter 2, Sections 3 through 5.

1. PHOTONS OF DIFFERENT ENERGIES INTERACT WITH DIFFERENT KINDS OF MATTER VIA DIFFERENT MECHANISMS

The portion of the electromagnetic spectrum most familiar to us is the visible, of course, which consists of photons in the energy range 1.8 (red) to 3.1 (violet) eV. When interacting with atoms and molecules, such photons are absorbed in raising outermost-shell electrons to vacant, higher-lying energy states. And photons of these energies are likely to be emitted when the excited atoms and molecules relax to their ground states. (Other, nonradiative, relaxation mechanisms exist, as well. In photosynthesis, for example, relaxation of an optically excited chlorophyll molecule involves many electrochemical steps in which energy is ultimately stored in the high-energy phosphate bonds of ATP.)

Of particular interest to us are the visible light photons emitted by a luminescent material under x-ray excitation. The material must itself be transparent to these photons, so that they can escape and get to the radiographic film, photomultiplier, or whatever form of detector. The energy gap between the filled valence band and the empty conduction band of the pure calcium tungstate in the intensifying screen of a radiographic cassette, for example, is considerably greater than 3 eV. Fluorescence light photons do not carry enough energy to excite valence band electrons into the conduction band and, as a consequence, they pass through the material without being absorbed. The same is true of the sodium iodide crystal at the front end of a gamma camera. So also with the lithium fluoride of a thermoluminescent dosimeter (TLD). In a metal, by contrast, the most energetic electrons in the partially filled conduction band are easily tickled into slightly higher-lying empty states either with the absorption of light photons (which is why metals are not transparent) or by the application of an electric field.

The absorption and emission of light are only a small part of the story of the interaction of electromagnetic radiation with matter. Infrared photons are of lower energies (0.1 to 1.8 eV) than those in the visible range, and are absorbed and emitted principally through changes in the quantized vibrational states of molecules or solids. The energies lie much closer to one another than do electron orbital states, and the energies involved in transitions among them are therefore smaller. As an example, the environmental "greenhouse effect" occurs because visible sunlight easily passes through the atmosphere and heats the Earth's surface. Much of this energy is reemitted in the form of infrared radiation, which is absorbed in the process of exciting transitions among the quantized vibrational states in carbon dioxide, methane, chlorofluorocarbons (CFCs), and certain other atmospheric gases, with a resultant warming of the air.

Similarly, microwave photons (10^{-3} to 10^{-6} eV) induce and are generated in transitions among the vibrational and rotational states of molecules. The radiation in a microwave oven excites such modes in water molecules, resulting in the "frictional" heating and cooking of food.

At the lowest frequencies of interest, electromagnetic interactions are described most simply with classical, rather than quantum, pictures. As the time-varying electric fields of a radiofrequency electromagnetic wave (1 kHz to 100 MHz, corresponding to photon energies of 10^{-12} to 10^{-7} eV) sweep past the wire antenna of a radio receiver, they set its nearly free electrons to oscillating back and forth along it, which induces voltages in it.

On the high-frequency side of the visible portion of the electromagnetic spectrum, an ultraviolet or characteristic x-ray photon is created when an electron falls into a vacancy in an inner atomic orbital (produced earlier when an electron was somehow knocked out of that orbital). X-ray photons, whether produced in this fashion or via bremsstrahlung, will interact with biologic or detector materials almost exclusively, for our purposes, by means of the photoelectric and Compton effects. Other x-ray interaction mechanisms exist, and several will be mentioned later, but the photoelectric and Compton dominate.

2. THE CASE OF THE VANISHING PHOTON: THE PHOTOELECTRIC EFFECT

At the energies used in diagnostic imaging, x-ray photons interact with detector materials (e.g., a fluorescent radiologic screen or the sodium iodide crystal of a gamma camera) and with bone predominantly by means of the photoelectric effect.

The "before" picture of a photoelectric event shows a photon incident on an atom. And "after," there is only an electron rapidly leaving the ionized atom (see Figs. 2–6A and 6–8). Photon in, electron out, and the atom as a whole was given a jolt and ionized. The energy hf_{in} of the absorbed *in*cident photon (of frequency f_{in}) must exceed the ionization energy of the targeted electron. Some of the energy of the incident photon is expended in overcoming the binding of the electron to its atom, and the rest ends up as kinetic energy KE_e of the freed photoelectron:

$$hf_{in} = \text{binding energy} + KE_e \qquad (12.1)$$

The inner-orbital electrons of an atom of high atomic number in a detector material or in bone may be bound tightly (tens of keV of binding energy). Those that constitute the soft tissues (carbon, nitrogen, oxygen) tend to be significantly less. Table 6–4 listed the binding energies of K-shell electrons, (which are the ones most likely to take part in a photoelectric event) for some elements of relevance to imaging.

_____ **EXERCISE 12–1.** _____

What is the kinetic energy of an electron ejected by a 30-keV photon from the K shell of a calcium atom?

SOLUTION: The K-shell electron binding energy is 4.0 keV, so KE_e for the photoelectron is 26.0 keV.

The electric field of an electromagnetic wave is transverse to the direction of its propagation (Fig. 4–6), and it is this field that pulls a photoelectron off its parent atom. An electron ejected by a photon of diagnostic energy is therefore likely to come out nearly perpendicular to the direction of photon propagation.

The important issue in the formation of an x-ray image is the overall probability that a photoelectric interaction will occur—either removing a photon from the x-ray beam or stimulating the image receptor. The likelihood that an x-ray photon will interact with an atom in its path is found to decrease rapidly with its energy, for the most part, and to increase rapidly with the atomic number of the atom. These dependencies may be described quantitatively in terms of attenuation coefficients, and further discussion will be deferred until Chapter 14. For the time being, suffice it to say that in radiography, fewer than half of the x-ray photon interactions that take place in soft tissue do so via the photoelectric effect. (Most occur via the Compton effect.) But nearly all the interactions that occur in bone or in an intensifying screen (both of which have much higher effective atomic numbers) are photoelectric absorption events.

In the collision shown in Figure 2–6A, the struck atom will be left in an ionized state. The atom will soon grab hold of an electron from elsewhere to fill the vacancy left behind. If the photoelectron originated from an inner orbital, a characteristic x-ray photon or perhaps an Auger electron will be emitted as the atom settles back down to its ground state. The energy carried away by the characteristic x-ray (or Auger electron), however, is likely to be reabsorbed by another atom close to the scene of the initiating photoelectric event. Thus, with photoelectric events, virtually all the energy of the incident photon is converted locally into deposited dose. This is not the case with Compton events.

3. IN A (DIAGNOSTIC ENERGY) COMPTON EVENT, SOME X-RAY ENERGY GOES TO THE COMPTON RECOIL ELECTRON, BUT MOST GOES TO THE COMPTON SCATTER PHOTON

At diagnostic energies, the Compton process is the dominant interaction mechanism in soft tissues.

Photoelectric and Compton events both involve the interaction of an incident x-ray with an atom. Either way, an electron is ejected from the atom with some kinetic energy, but there the similarity ends. In a photoelectric event, virtually all the photon's energy is either used to overcome the photoelectron's binding to the atom or imparted to it as kinetic energy. In a Compton collision, by contrast, some of the energy of the incident photon is given to the Compton electron and its atom, but a significant fraction of it leaves the site of the interaction altogether, in the form of a newly created, lower-energy "scatter" photon (Fig. 12–1). The Compton scatter photon and the high-velocity Compton electron both appear at the exact instant of the collision. (This is to be distinguished from the emission of any characteristic x-rays or Auger electrons associated with the subsequent return of a freshly ionized atom to its

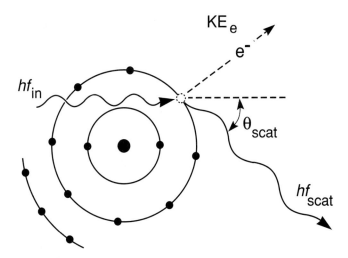

Figure 12–1. With a Compton event, some of the energy of the incident photon is imparted to the Compton recoil electron, and the rest, hf_{scat}, goes to the Compton scatter photon. The scatter photon leaves the scene of the collision at an angle θ_{scat} relative to the path of the incident photon.

nonionized ground state.) Figure 12–2 plots the scatter photon intensity as a function of photon scatter angle, θ_{scat}, for incident x-ray photons of two different energies.

Compton events tend to involve interactions between higher-energy photons and atoms with relatively weakly bound electrons. The binding energy of a struck electron may, therefore, be ignored for most calculations. (When a bowling ball comes barreling down the alley, rubber bands attaching the pins to the floor don't make much difference.) Conservation of energy can then be expressed as

$$hf_{in} = hf_{scat} + KE_e \qquad (12.2)$$

where KE_e is the kinetic energy imparted to the Compton electron, and hf_{in} and hf_{scat} are the energies of the incident and Compton scatter photons.

As discussed in Chapter 5, Section 12, energy and momentum must be simultaneously conserved in a collision of billiard balls. The same is true of a Compton interaction. The geometry of a Compton collision is shown in Figure 12–1. A simple calculation that, in essence, states and combines the conservation of energy and conservation of momentum balance sheets for the incident photon (before the collision) and for the Compton electron and scatter photon (after) reveals that the motions of

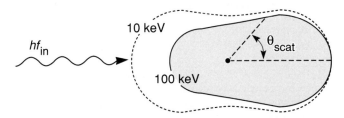

Figure 12–2. Polar diagrams, for two energies of incident photon, of scatter probability as a function of scatter angle. The probability that a scatter photon will come off at an angle near θ_{scat} is indicated by the radial distance from the origin of the diagram to the corresponding point on the curve.

these particles are subject to certain interrelationships. One of these connects the wavelengths of the incident and scatter photons with the photon scatter angle θ_{scat}:

$$\lambda_{scat} - \lambda_{in} = 0.024(1 - \cos \theta_{scat}) \qquad (12.3)$$

where the wavelengths are expressed in Ångstrom (Å). Similar information can be conveyed graphically: Figure 12–3 plots KE_e/hf_{in}, the fraction of the energy of the incident photon that is transferred to the Compton recoil electron, against hf_{in} for several photon scattering angles θ_{scat}.

For a "glancing blow," in which the incident photon barely kisses the atom *en passant* and $\theta_{scat} \approx 0$ degrees, nearly all the energy goes to the scatter photon, $hf_{scat} \approx hf_{in}$, and almost none to the Compton electron, $KE_e/hf_{in} \approx 0$. At the other extreme, maximum possible energy is transferred to the electron for a head-on collision, in which the photon scatters through 180 degrees.

_____ **EXERCISE 12–2.** _____

How is the energy partitioned between scatter photon and Compton electron when a 100-keV incident photon scatters through 60 degrees?

SOLUTION: For the 100-keV photon, about 90 keV of energy goes to the scatter photon, by Figure 12–3, and 10 keV to the Compton electron. For a 5-MeV photon in a radiotherapy beam, the percentages are reversed.

_____ **EXERCISE 12–3.** _____

A 100-keV incident photon scatters through 60 degrees. Use Equation 12.3 to find the energy of the scatter photon.

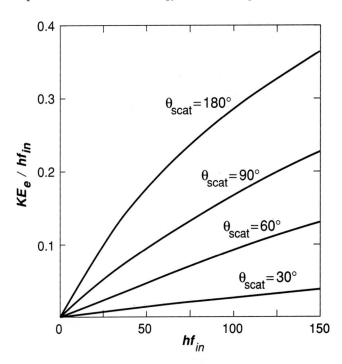

Figure 12–3. Fraction of the energy of an incident photon that is given to the Compton recoil electron, KE_e/hf_{in}, as a function of hf_{in}, for several values of θ_{scat}. You can arrive at this graph easily from Equations 12.2 and 12.3. Try it.

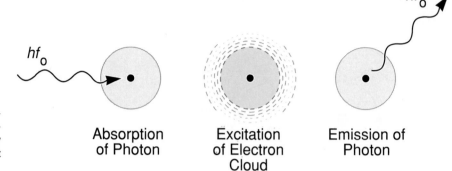

Figure 12–4. With Rayleigh or coherent scattering, a photon is absorbed by the entire electron cloud of an atom. Another is immediately reemitted at a new angle of propagation, but with little or no change of energy.

SOLUTION: By Equation 6.2, $\lambda_{in} = 12.4/100$ keV $= 0.124$ Å. By Equation 12.3, the wavelength of the scatter photon is longer by the amount $0.024(\cos 60°) = 0.012$ Å, regardless of the energy of the incident photon, so that $\lambda_{scat} = 0.136$ Å. From that, $hf_{scat} = 91$ keV.

At any angle, the fraction of the incident photon's energy that is transferred to the Compton electron increases with the energy of the incident photon. It is quite small, however, for photons of under 100 keV. That is, for the relatively low energy photons of diagnostic imaging, $KE_e/hf_{in} \ll 1$ for any scatter angle, and nearly all of the energy is carried off by the scatter photon. This observation will be important when we determine how much dose is deposited in a patient as a result of Compton collisions, and when we consider the degradation of image contrast caused by scatter radiation.

Unlike the photoelectric effect situation, the overall probability of Compton scattering varies only slowly with photon energy or atomic number, as will be seen in Chapter 14.

4. COHERENT SCATTERING, PAIR PRODUCTION, AND OTHER X-RAY INTERACTION MECHANISMS

The photoelectric and Compton effects are the two important (for imaging) mechanisms by which x-rays can interact with matter. It is worth noting, however, that there are others.

In "classical scattering," a photon incident on an atom is scattered with no loss of energy, as with an elastic ball bouncing off a hard floor. The photon merely changes direction of propagation, and the atom is not ionized or even excited. Classical scattering can occur in two different ways.

Several decades before Arthur Compton provided, in 1923, a quantum mechanical explanation for the effect that bears his name, J. J. Thompson had developed a classical theory of "elastic" scattering of radiation by a single atomic electron. Here, a wave of electromagnetic energy does not lose or gain energy, but merely changes direction of propagation. Thompson scattering turns out, in the particular case of long-wavelength incident photons, to be equivalent to Compton scattering. That is, in the limit of very low photon energies, in which scattering occurs with virtually no loss of energy, quantum mechanical Compton scattering reduces to (and may be seen to incorporate) this *Thompson scattering.*

With *Rayleigh* or *coherent scattering*, the electric field of a passing electromagnetic wave expends energy in setting *all* the electrons of an atom into rapid coherent (in-phase) oscillation. The atom's electron cloud immediately thereafter reradiates all this energy as if from a radio antenna (Fig. 12–4). Quantum mechanics would say that the cloud as a whole absorbs a photon, and reemits a photon of the same energy but propagating in a new direction. (To emphasize its fundamental difference in nature from such coherent scattering, Compton scattering is also known as incoherent scattering.)

Coherent scattering events rarely constitute more than 10% of all interactions between diagnostic x-ray photons and electrons, and are usually much less than that. So for simplicity, hereafter we shall include and account for them (even though they are not explicitly mentioned) along with Compton scattering events.

In *pair production* (see Fig. 4–4), the electric field of a high-energy photon interacts with the positive charge of an atomic nucleus in such a way that the photon vanishes, and an electron and a positron materialize in its stead. (This is *not* the way that positrons are produced for use in PET scanning.) The probability of pair production increases with the strength of the nuclear electric field, hence with the atomic number Z of the substance irradiated. By Equation 7.6, $E = mc^2$, the incoming photon must be carrying at least 1022 keV, the energy equivalent of the combined rest masses of the electron and positron. This is an order of magnitude greater than the photon energies one normally encounters in imaging, and we shall not have to consider it further.

Triplet production is similar to pair production, except that the incident high-energy photon is converted into an electron–positron pair in the field of an atomic electron (rather than of the nucleus), and the orbital electron is ejected from its atom in the process. The threshold for this photon absorption process is 2044 keV.

Finally, in a *photonuclear* interaction, the photon is absorbed by a nucleus, which subsequently deexcites by means of whatever processes are available to it. These may include the emission of gamma rays, beta particles, or neutrons. Probabilities for photonuclear events become appreciable only for photons of 10 MeV of energy or more. (In *neutron activation* studies, by contrast, one studies the decay products of the radionuclides produced under *neutron* bombardment.)

Chapter 13

The Linear and Mass Attenuation Coefficients

The preceding chapter explored the two dominant mechanisms of interaction between high–energy photons and matter: the photoelectric effect and Compton scattering. Here we shall pursue that line of study further.

The reason for such interest is that photoelectric and Compton interactions underlie three critically important aspects of x-ray (and gamma ray) image formation:

- High-energy photons are attenuated by the body. In x-ray (transmission) imaging, differential attenuation of the x-ray beam by the various tissues gives rise to the primary x-ray image. In nuclear medicine (emission) imaging, overlying body tissues may attenuate gamma rays emitted by radionuclide distributed within an organ, and that must be taken into account in image interpretation.
- The high-energy photons that constitute the x-ray (or gamma ray) image interact with the detector materials of the image receptor. In radiography, the detector material is the phosphor of an intensifying screen; with some models of computerized tomography (CT), it is the xenon gas of an ion chamber; and in nuclear medicine, it is a scintillating crystal of sodium iodide.
- Photoelectric and Compton events are the first steps by which dose is deposited in the body.

The tendency of high-energy photons to interact either with tissues of the body or with detector materials depends on properties both of the photons and of the irradiated media. This suggests that one can adjust the irradiation conditions so as to maximize the usefulness of the clinical images produced. In carrying out this optimization process, it helps tremendously that aspects of the interactions of an x-ray beam with matter can be quantified. . . . Which brings us to the linear and mass attenuation coefficients.

1. ATTENUATION OF A PHOTON BEAM BY A THIN LAYER OF MATTER

Consider what happens to the number of photons in an x-ray beam, n, as it passes through a very thin layer of attenuating material. "Very thin" in this context means that only a small fraction, at most a percent or so, of the photons are lost from the beam in traversing the layer.

In Figure 13–1, n photons are incident on a thin layer of matter. Of them, a relatively very small number, Δn, are absorbed or scattered in the layer. Δn should be proportional to n; other things being equal, if you double the number of tries, the number of hits will also double: $\Delta n \sim n$.

Similarly, Δn should be proportional (for a thin layer) to the number of atoms in the path of the beam, and hence to the thickness Δx of the layer: $\Delta n \sim \Delta x$.

Combining these two ideas, Δn is linear in both n and Δx:

$$\Delta n = -\mu \cdot n \cdot \Delta x \qquad (13.1a)$$

The constant of proportionality, denoted μ, is called the *linear attenuation coefficient*. The minus sign snuck in because n refers to the photons remaining in the beam, *unaffected* by matter. $\mu \cdot n \cdot \Delta x$ photons are removed from the beam by the layer, so the change Δn in the total number of photons still in it is negative.

_____ **EXERCISE 13–1.** _____

One thousand photons are incident on a thin 0.1-mm thin layer of material. $\mu = 0.5$ cm^{-1}. How many get through?

SOLUTION: By Equation 13.1a, $\Delta n = -(0.5$ cm$^{-1})(1000)(0.01$ cm$) = -5$. Thus, $1000 - 5 = 995$ photons remain in the beam.

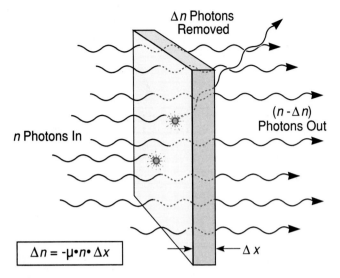

Figure 13–1. "Derivation" of $\Delta n = -\mu \cdot n \cdot \Delta x$. n photons are incident on a slab of material of thickness Δx. The number absorbed or scattered, Δn, will be proportional both to n and to Δx. The number of unaffected photons emerging from the far side, remaining in the "primary beam," is $(n - \Delta n)$

Equation 13.1a is expressed in terms of numbers of photons. Exactly the same argument applies to the beam's energy fluence and to its intensity. Intensity, I, was defined in Equation 11.1 as the rate of energy fluence, or the flow of energy per unit area per second; the change in I in passing through Δx of the material is

$$\Delta I = -\mu \cdot I \cdot \Delta x, \quad \text{small } \Delta x \qquad (13.1b)$$

2. THE LINEAR ATTENUATION COEFFICIENT μ IS THE SPATIAL RATE OF ATTENUATION: $\mu = -\Delta I / I \cdot \Delta x$

Is the linear attenuation coefficient μ anything more than just a simple constant of proportionality?

Absolutely. Its physical meaning may be seen by dividing both sides of Equation 13.1b by $(-I \cdot \Delta x)$:

$$\mu = -\Delta I / I \cdot \Delta x \qquad (13.2)$$

μ is the small fraction $(\Delta I / I)$ of beam intensity that is lost per small amount of thickness Δx of material that the beam traverses. It is thus the *spatial rate*, $-(\Delta I / I)/\Delta x$, at which the intensity diminishes as the beam passes through matter.

Rearranging Equation 13.1a as $\mu = -\Delta n / n \cdot \Delta x$ suggests the equivalent interpretation of μ as the probability $\Delta n/n$ per unit thickness Δx that a photon will undergo a photoelectric or Compton collision. (Appendix 13–1 reviews some useful, elementary ideas about probability.) The greater the value of μ, the more effectively the medium absorbs and scatters photons, and attenuates the beam. The value of μ depends, of course, on both the beam's energy and the physical properties of the irradiated material.

The units of intensity cancel out of the numerator and denominator of Equation 13.2, leaving μ of dimension "per unit of distance." This is consistent with the interpretation of μ as fractional attenuation per unit thickness of matter. One commonly finds μ expressed in *per centimeter*, or cm^{-1}.

From Figure 13–2, it should be apparent that μ is a function of photon energy, material type, and (by comparison of the lung and muscle curves) material density.

EXERCISE 13–2.

It is found that after passing through 2 mm of material, an x-ray beam is only 94% as intense as before. What is μ?

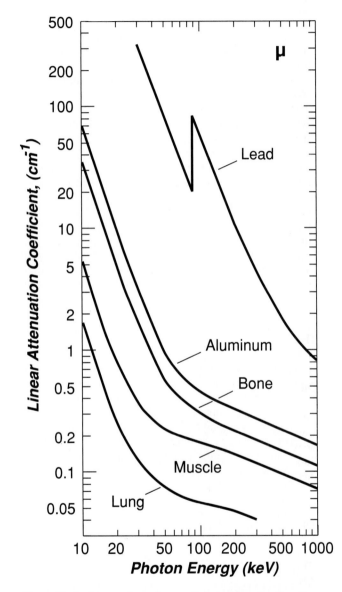

Figure 13–2. Linear attenuation coefficient, μ, as a function of monochromatic photon energy for several materials. Lung and muscle are of nearly identical chemical composition, and the threefold difference in their attenuation coefficients at any energy is attributable to the factor of 3 difference in their densities. At any given energy and density, μ tends to increase with effective atomic number, Z, as will be discussed in the next chapter. At lower energies (below about 30 keV for soft tissue and below about 300 keV for lead), the shape of $\mu(hf)$ is determined by the energy dependence of the probability of occurrence of a photoelectric event. At higher diagnostic energies, the Compton interaction is dominant. (Above 1 MeV, pair production starts becoming important.) (*From Johns HE, Cunningham JR:* The Physics of Radiology, *4th ed. Springfield, IL: Charles C Thomas, 1983 [Appendix A].*)

SOLUTION: $\Delta n/n = 0.06$. By Equation 13.1a, $\mu = (0.06)/(0.2$ cm$) = 0.3$ cm^{-1}.

3. THE LINEAR ATTENUATION COEFFICIENT AS A PROBABILISTIC INTERACTION CROSS SECTION

The linear attenuation coefficient μ is closely related to a parameter that is often used by research scientists to describe photon–atom and similar interactions, the *atomic interaction cross section*.

Photons incident on a thin layer of material see mostly empty space ahead, interspersed with the occasional atom. In this sense, the probability that any photon will undergo a collision in the thin layer is equal to the fraction of the layer's "area," in effect, that is blocked by atoms.

Why bother with two entities, the linear attenuation coefficient of Equation 13.2 and an atomic cross section, when they are similar, and either one alone would do the job? Partly for historical reasons, but also because the two refer to somewhat different perspectives on the same issue. The atomic interaction cross section, as its name indicates, focuses on a characteristic of a single atom. μ, as *its* name implies, refers more to the effect that bulk material (even a "thin" layer can be thousands or millions of atoms thick) has on a photon beam. In any case, "attenuation coefficient" and "interaction cross section" are both commonly used terms that refer to practically the same thing.

4. THE LINEAR ATTENUATION COEFFICIENT IS A FUNCTION $\mu(\rho,Z,hf)$ OF THE DENSITY AND ATOMIC NUMBER OF THE IRRADIATED MEDIUM AND OF THE PHOTON ENERGY

As revealed in Figure 13–2 for several soft tissues, bone, aluminum, and lead, the linear attenuation coefficient is a function of the density, ρ, the (effective) atomic number of the irradiated medium, Z, and the (effective) energy of the photons that constitute the beam, hf:

$$\mu = \mu(\rho,Z,hf) \qquad (13.3)$$

A diagram or table that fully displays the way in which $\mu(\rho,Z,hf)$ depends on these three variables would have to be three-dimensional.

This and the next chapter consider the dependence of $\mu(\rho,Z,hf)$ on the three independent variables. As the functional dependence on *density* is the simplest, we shall begin with it.

5. SEPARATING OUT THE DENSITY DEPENDENCE FROM THE LINEAR ATTENUATION COEFFICIENT μ YIELDS THE MASS ATTENUATION COEFFICIENT $[\mu/\rho]$

It is convenient to separate out the density dependence from the linear attenuation coefficient. This process leaves $\mu(\rho,Z,hf)$ as the product of the density ρ and a new entity, called the

mass attenuation coefficient and denoted $[\mu/\rho](Z,hf)$, which is a function only of the atomic number and the photon energy.

Divide both sides of Equation 13.1b by I, and then multiply and divide the right-hand side by the density ρ:

$$\Delta I \,/\, I = - \,[\mu(\rho,Z, hf)/\rho] \cdot (\rho \cdot \Delta x) \qquad (13.4)$$

It will be important here to keep track of the variables on which μ depends, so they are written out explicitly.

Figure 13–3A displays a thin layer of compressible attenuating material, such as foam rubber or lung, of initial thickness Δx and density ρ. In Figure 13–3B, the layer has been squeezed to half its original thickness, $\Delta x/2$, and consequently to double the density, 2ρ. The product of thickness and density on the right-hand side of Equation 13.4 remains the same, with a constant value of $\rho \cdot \Delta x$. Now, the compression can have no effect on beam attenuation, as the total number of atoms in the beam path is the same; $\Delta I/I$ to the left in Equation 13.4 is therefore also constant. So $\Delta I/I$ and $\rho \cdot \Delta x$ are both independent of the compression. The only other term in the equation, namely, $\mu(\rho,Z,hf)/\rho$, must therefore remain unchanged by the compression as well. $\mu(\rho,Z,hf)/\rho$ is not a function of ρ. Equivalently, $\mu(\rho,Z,hf)$ is proportional to ρ.

This important point, that dividing $\mu(\rho,Z,hf)$ by ρ completely removes the density dependence from it, may be emphasized by expressing the quotient of $\mu(E,Z,\rho)$ and ρ as a new function, denoted "$[\mu/\rho]$," of only the two variables, Z and hf. The function $[\mu/\rho](Z,hf)$ is defined through

$$\mu(\rho,Z,hf) = [\mu/\rho](Z,hf) \cdot \rho \qquad (13.5a)$$

or, equivalently, through

$$[\mu/\rho](Z,hf) = \mu(\rho,Z,hf)/\rho \qquad (13.5b)$$

We could have just as easily designated this new function "Φ" or anything else, but "$[\mu/\rho]$" serves as a useful mnemonic.

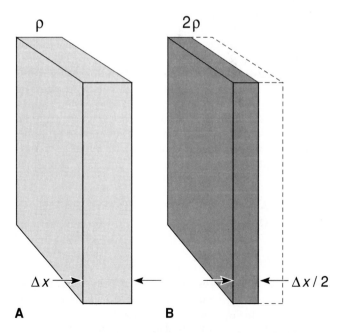

Figure 13–3. If a slice of material such as foam rubber is compressed, the thickness Δx and the density ρ both change, but the product $(\rho \cdot \Delta x)$ remains the same. So, too, does the relative number of photons that interact within the slice, $\Delta I/I$.

$[\mu/\rho](Z,hf)$ is called the *mass attenuation coefficient*, and its units are cm²/g.

___ **EXERCISE 13–3.** ___

Lung tissue, with a normal density of about $\rho = 0.3$ g/cm³ and a linear attenuation coefficient $\mu = 0.15$ cm⁻¹ for some photon energy, is compressed, so that its density is trebled. What happens to the linear attenuation coefficient? What about the mass attenuation coefficient?

SOLUTION: By Equation 13.5a, μ becomes 0.45 cm⁻¹. $[\mu/\rho]$ remains unchanged at 0.5 cm²/g.

___ **EXERCISE 13–4.** ___

The densities of water and of ice are 1.0 and 0.92 g/cm³, respectively. For a certain x-ray beam, μ for water is found to be 0.20 cm⁻¹. What is μ for ice, and how do the mass attenuation coefficients compare?

SOLUTION: $[\mu/\rho]$ is 0.20 cm²/g for water and, therefore, for ice. By Equation 13.5a, μ for ice is 0.18 cm⁻¹.

Equation 13.1b can now be rewritten in the equivalent form

$$\Delta I = -[\mu/\rho] \cdot \rho \cdot I \cdot \Delta x \qquad (13.6)$$

It may seem, at first blush, that replacing μ of Equation 13.1b with the product $[\mu/\rho] \cdot \rho$ of Equation 13.6 makes things more complicated. Actually, it leads to a simplification. The linear attenuation coefficient $\mu(\rho,Z,hf)$ is a function of three variables. $[\mu/\rho](Z,hf) \cdot \rho$ is a function of only two variables (a situation much easier to deal with) multiplied by a third. In other words, a three-dimensional function or table of values for $\mu(\rho,Z,hf)$ is needed for Equations 13.1. The mass attenuation coefficient uses the much more accessible format of a two-dimensional function or table for $[\mu/\rho](Z,hf)$ together with a separate list of the densities of biologic, detector, and shielding materials of interest.

The density of healthy lung, for example, is typically about $\frac{1}{3}$ g/cm³, or roughly a third that of muscle. Its *linear* attenuation coefficient at any given photon energy would also be a third that of muscle. But lung and muscle have virtually the same effective atomic number, and one column listing values of the *mass* attenuation coefficient, $[\mu/\rho]$, for different energies serves them both (Fig. 13–4).

6. THE RADIOLOGIC DEPTH INCORPORATES THE TISSUE DENSITY

___ **EXERCISE 13–5.** ___

Show that $[\mu/\rho](Z,hf)$ may be thought of as the value that the linear attenuation coefficient assumes if a material is compressed or fluffed up to a density of 1 g/cm³.

SOLUTION: Let us do this by way of an example. Imagine a layer Δx thick of tissue of density $\rho = \frac{1}{3}$ and of linear and mass attenuation coefficients μ and $[\mu/\rho]$, respectively. The relative

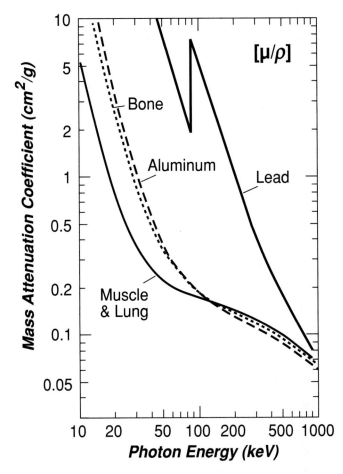

Figure 13–4. Mass attenuation coefficient, $[\mu/\rho]$, as a function of monochromatic photon energy, for the same materials that were considered in Figure 13–2. As they differ only in density, soft tissue and normal lung have the same $[\mu/\rho]$ at any energy. The reason why $[\mu/\rho]$ for bone is greater than that for soft tissue at low energy, but not at high energy, will be discussed in the next chapter. So, too, will the discontinuity in the curve for lead.

attenuation of photons, $\Delta I/I$, will be $-\mu \cdot \Delta x$ and $-[\mu/\rho] \cdot \frac{1}{3} \cdot \Delta x$ with the two approaches. These must be the same, however, indicating that in general, μ does not equal $[\mu/\rho]$.

Now consider the particular situation in which the material is compressed to three times its original density, so that $\rho = 1$, now, and the thickness is $\Delta x/3$. The linear and mass attenuation coefficient pictures yield values for $\Delta I/I$ of $-\mu \cdot (\Delta x/3)$ and $-[\mu/\rho] \cdot 1 \cdot (\Delta x/3)$, respectively. In this case, μ takes on the same numerical value as $[\mu/\rho]$.

> The product $\rho \cdot \Delta x$ appearing in Equation 13.6 is known as the "radiologic depth" or "radiologic thickness," and serves as a useful measure of the amount of material in the path of the beam. It represents the thickness that a layer with the same chemical composition, but of unit density, must have to attenuate as much as a Δx-cm-thick layer of material with density ρ.
>
> This idea remains useful with thick blocks (rather than thin layers) of material. Then, the radiation thickness is obtained simply by multiplying the thickness of the block, x, by the density, radiologic thickness = $\rho \cdot x$, and has the units of g/cm². It is independent of μ and of photon energy.

_____ **EXERCISE 13–6.** _____

The density of cortical bone is about 1650 kg/m³. What is the radiologic thickness of a 2-cm block of such bone?

SOLUTION: The bone density is 1.65 g/cm³, so the radiologic thickness is $\rho \cdot x = (1.65 \text{ g/cm}^3) \cdot (2 \text{ cm}) = 3.3 \text{ g/cm}^2$.

APPENDIX 13–1. Some Useful Ideas About Probability

Iacta Alea Est*

The future is largely unpredictable, but still we must make decisions. These decisions involve estimating, for each action under consideration, both the probability of occurrence of every possible outcome and the significance of its consequences. These estimates must be based, ultimately, on the lessons of past experience. The theories of probability and statistics have been developed largely in the attempt to systematize and optimize the usefulness of this decision-making process, and they have found a variety of important and interesting applications in the radiologic sciences.

People have been trying to settle on a suitable definition of *probability* for hundreds of years. The difficulty arises, in part, because the term is used to describe two very different yet closely related aspects of the same thing.

Probability can refer to the relative frequency with which a certain situation or event is found to occur in a series of repeated observations or measurements. If "heads" comes up half the times that a coin is flipped, then we assume that the probability of obtaining a "heads" on the next toss is 50%. (Many people believe that after a string of six tails with a fair coin, the probability of the next toss yielding a heads will be greater than 50%, but such is not the case.)

Alternatively, probability can reflect an innate property of a system, a characteristic of its inherent state of being. If a coin is exactly the same on both sides, then there should be an equal, 50% chance that either face will come up in a toss.

In practice, one uses an amalgam of these ideas, and doesn't worry too much about the distinction.

You toss 100 fair dice (or one die 100 times), and nearly half land with an even number facing upward; the probability that the next toss will show an even number may be estimated, from this experience, to be about 50%. More generally, if an event is observed $N(\text{total})$ times, and in $N(A)$ of the cases it displays (randomly, and with no form of predetermination or forewarning involved) the characteristic "A", then the experimentally determined probability of A occurring, $P(A)$, is

$$P(A) = N(A)/N(\text{total}) \tag{13.7}$$

One could arrive at this same result without going through the experiment. By the physical symmetry of the situation, the six possible ways a fair die can land are equally likely, and three of them will leave an even number facing up; the a priori probability of a die coming up even is 3 out of 6, or 1/2.

_____ **EXERCISE 13–7.** _____

You search the Weather Bureau's files, and find that the temperature, T, exceeded 32°C (90°F) on 25 of the last 100 Fourth of Julys. What is the probability that $T > 32°$ on next year's Fourth, $P(T > 32°C)$?

SOLUTION: $P(T > 32°C) = 25/100 = 0.25$. But unlike the case of the die, here it is not possible to deduce this result from theory alone (at least not with our current ability to model the weather mathematically). We can only examine the record of Nature's own experiments.

Combining Probabilities

Mutually Exclusive Events. There is no way a die can show a "2" and a "5" simultaneously. Similarly, the maximum temperature in a day cannot be both greater than 32°C and below 21°C. If A and B are two such *mutually exclusive events*, then the probability that one of them will occur is given by

$$P(\text{either A or B}) = P(A) + P(B) \tag{13.8}$$

The probability that one die will show either a "5" *or* a "4" is $1/6 + 1/6 = 1/3$. And the die will come up either "5" or an even number $1/6 + 1/2 = 2/3$ of the time. The *general law of addition for mutually exclusive events* thus provides information on the possible outcomes of a single experiment, such as one day's weather or one toss of the die.

If one of three mutually exclusive events, A, B, and C, definitely must occur, then

$$P(A) + P(B) + P(C) = 1 \tag{13.9}$$

The probability that tomorrow will be above 32°C, or below 21°C, or somewhere between these two limits, for example, is 100%. It is obvious how to generalize this for more than three possible outcomes. Likewise, the probability that the particular event A will *not* occur is $P(\text{not A}) = 1 - P(A)$.

Independent Events. Our study of the Weather Bureau's records has already revealed that $P(T > 32°C) = 0.25$, which implies that $P(T < 32°C) = 1 - 0.25 = 0.75$. Further searching of the Weather Bureau data indicates that no rain fell on 80% of the last 100 July Fourths, $P(\text{dry}) = 0.8$. Then the probability of it being both dry (0.8) and cool (0.75) will be $(0.8)(0.75) = 0.60$. That is, 80% of the 75 cool Fourths were also dry, so that 60% of the last 100 days were both dry and cool. Similarly, the odds that the next Fourth will be wet and hot are $(0.2)(0.25) = 0.05$. The four possibilities and their probabilities of occurrence are summarized in Table 13–1. The probability that the day will fall into one of these four categories, of course, is 100%.

This argument can be formalized as the *general law of multiplication of probabilities for independent events,*

$$P(A \text{ and } B) = P(A) \cdot P(B) \tag{13.10}$$

Equation 13.10 is valid only if the events involved are *independent* of one another. The temperature and humidity must have

---

*"The die is cast." Julius Caesar in 49 BC, upon his decision to cross the Rubicon (a stream that separated Gaul from Italy) illegally with his army, intending to seize power from the Roman Senate. It is an interesting reflection on the complexity of the idea of *probability* that he should choose a fatalistic gaming metaphor for a sequence of events over which he had considerable control.

TABLE 13–1. PROBABILITIES THAT THE FOURTH OF JULY WILL DISPLAY VARIOUS COMBINATIONS OF CHARACTERISTICS

		Wet 0.20	Dry 0.80
Hot	0.25	0.05	0.20
Cool	0.75	0.15	0.60

no bearing on one another. If, by contrast, lower temperatures were likely to *cause* the absence of rain, so that cool days tended automatically to be rain-free, then Equation 13.10 would not work. Much confusion can arise in science, and in the rest of life as well, when people believe that different phenomena are occurring independently (or dependently) when, in fact, they are not.

_____ **EXERCISE 13–8.** _____

You are presented with Q equally difficult radiologic cases. If the probability of making a wrong diagnosis on any of them is q, what are your chances of getting all Q of them right?

SOLUTION: The probability of getting the first one right is $1 - q$, and so also for the second. By the general law of multiplication for independent events, the likelihood of success for both the first and the second is therefore $(1 - q)^2$. Note, especially, that it is not $(1 - q^2)$. By induction, the probability of making no errors in all Q cases is $(1 - q)^Q$.

Chapter 14

Dependence of Attenuation on Atomic Number and Photon Energy

1. **Separating the Total Mass Attenuation Coefficient into Photoelectric and Compton Components**
2. **Dependence of the Photoelectric Mass Attenuation Coefficient on Atomic Number and X-ray Photon Energy**
3. **Photoelectric Contrast Enhancement with Low-Energy X-rays**
4. **A Material Is Relatively Transparent to Its Own Characteristic X-rays**
5. **Dependence of the Compton Mass Attenuation Coefficient on Atomic Number and X-ray Photon Energy**
6. **On the Magnitudes of the Photoelectric and Compton Coefficients**
7. **Why the Photoelectric Mass Attenuation Coefficient Depends So Much More Strongly on Atomic Number and Photon Energy**
   Appendix 14–1. Exponential and Logarithmic Functions

In the preceding chapter, the linear attenuation coefficient for a material, μ, was shown to be a function of its density, ρ, and atomic number, Z, and of the energy of the incident photons, hf. Separating the density out of μ leaves behind the functionally simpler mass attenuation coefficient, $[\mu/\rho](Z,hf)$, which depends on only two variables.

The mass attenuation coefficient can be partitioned into photoelectric and Compton components, $[\tau/\rho]$ and $[\sigma/\rho]$. The two interaction mechanisms differ, and $[\tau/\rho]$ and $[\sigma/\rho]$ are dissimilar functions of atomic number and photon energy. Away from absorption edges, $[\tau/\rho]$ varies with photon energy and the effective atomic number of the medium approximately as $(Z/hf)^3$. At diagnostic energies, $[\sigma/\rho]$ decreases slowly with hf and, with the important exception of hydrogen, is nearly independent of Z.

1. SEPARATING THE TOTAL MASS ATTENUATION COEFFICIENT INTO PHOTOELECTRIC AND COMPTON COMPONENTS

To obtain the best possible image quality and to minimize dose to a patient, it is necessary to operate the x-ray tube at the optimal kilovoltage and to select the most suitable image receptor. Each of these decisions requires an understanding of the dependencies of the photoelectric and Compton interaction probabilities on photon energy and on the properties of the tissues and detector materials irradiated. It simplifies matters to consider the two interaction processes separately.

The *linear attenuation coefficient for the photoelectric effect* is designated τ:

$$\tau = \Delta I/I \cdot \Delta x \quad \text{(photoelectric)} \quad (14.1)$$

Similarly, σ represents the *linear attenuation coefficient for the Compton effect*:

$$\sigma = \Delta I/I \cdot \Delta x \quad \text{(Compton)} \quad (14.2)$$

In nearly all imaging situations, only photoelectric and Compton interactions are of relevance. These mechanisms are independent of one another and "compete" for photons. That is, if an x-ray photon interacts by means of the photoelectric effect, it is no longer available to take part in Compton collisions, and vice versa. (After a Compton event, of course, the new *scatter* photon may well itself undergo a photoelectric or Compton interaction. But for now, we are concerned only with attenuation of the incident primary (unscattered) x-ray photons and creation of the primary x-ray image.) By the general law of addition of probabilities for mutually exclusive events (Equation 13.8), the **total linear attenuation coefficient**, μ, can be expressed simply as the sum of τ and σ:

$$\mu = \tau + \sigma \quad (14.3)$$

τ and σ both are, like the total attenuation coefficient, linear in the density, ρ. $[\mu/\rho]$ is therefore separable as

$$[\mu/\rho] = [\tau/\rho] + [\sigma/\rho] \quad (14.4)$$

The dependence of $[\tau/\rho]$ and $[\sigma/\rho]$ on the effective atomic number of the medium and on the effective photon energy of the x-ray beam are the subject of the rest of this chapter. Through the prescription $[\mu/\rho] \cdot \rho = \mu$ for transforming back and forth between the mass and linear coefficient, and similarly for $[\tau/\rho]$ and $[\sigma/\rho]$, you can easily determine the corresponding properties of μ, τ, and σ.

2. DEPENDENCE OF THE PHOTOELECTRIC MASS ATTENUATION COEFFICIENT ON ATOMIC NUMBER AND X-RAY PHOTON ENERGY

Dependence on Atomic Number, Z

In experiments involving the irradiation of a variety of different materials each composed of a single element, the photoelectric mass attenuation coefficient is seen to increase approximately (but not exactly) with the third power of the atomic number Z of the exposed medium:

$$[\tau/\rho](Z) \sim Z^3 \qquad (14.5)$$

Nearly all materials of medical interest are compounds, and not made up of a single element. One can then replace Z of Equation 14.5 with an *effective atomic number*, Z_{eff}, obtained by averaging the Z's of the various constituent parts of a material in a suitable fashion. A commonly used recipe is

$$Z_{eff} = (a_1 Z_1^n + a_2 Z_2^n + \ldots)^{1/n} \qquad (14.6)$$

where a_i and Z_i represent the relative contribution to the electron density and the atomic number of the ith element in the material, respectively, and the exponent n is typically about 3.5. Hereafter, the unadorned symbol Z will represent the effective atomic number, when appropriate. The effective atomic numbers of some materials of interest are listed in Table 14–1.

Use of Equation 14.6 requires us to know the *electron densities* of materials. The simplest case is atomic *hydrogen*, which consists of a single nucleon (one proton, no neutrons) and one electron. Hydrogen has an atomic weight of 1; that is, the mass of 1 mole (Avogadro's number, 6×10^{23}) of hydrogen atoms is 1 gram. The electron density, in SI units, is thus 6×10^{26} electrons per kilogram of hydrogen atoms.

If atoms contained no neutrons, the electron density would be 6×10^{23} electrons per gram for everything. But the nuclei of the lighter elements *other than hydrogen* consist of roughly equal numbers of protons and neutrons. For biologic materials, in particular, the ratio of atomic number to atomic weight is about one half, $Z/A \approx 0.5$. The nucleus of a normal carbon atom contains six protons and six neutrons, for example, and an ordinary oxygen atom has eight of each. (The Z/A ratio falls below 0.5 at higher Z values, see Fig. 7–11.) There is twice as much mass per electron (i.e., half as many electrons per unit mass) for these materials, compared with hydrogen, and their electron densities are therefore only about 3×10^{26}

electrons per kilogram (Table 14–1). The slightly higher electron densities of water, muscle, fat, and (to a lesser extent) bone reflect on their hydrogen content.

EXERCISE 14–1.

Find the effective atomic number of water.

SOLUTION: The atomic weight of water is 18, so 18 g of it consists of Avogadro's number, N_a (6×10^{23}), of molecules. It contains $2 \cdot N_a$ electrons from hydrogen atoms and $8 \cdot N_a$ electrons from oxygen atoms. Therefore the relative electron densities, the a_i values in Equation 14.6, are 2/10 and 8/10. Then $Z_{eff} = [(2/10)(1)^{3.5} + (8/10)(8)^{3.5}]^{1/3.5} = 7.51$, consistent with the entry in Table 14–1 for water.

Dependence on Photon Energy, hf

It is observed that the probability of occurrence of a photoelectric interaction generally decreases approximately with the third power of photon energy. For any particular material (i.e., with a fixed value of Z),

$$[\tau/\rho](hf) \sim (hf)^{-3} \qquad (14.7)$$

In Figure 14–1, the dashed line marked $[\tau/\rho](hf)$ plots the photoelectric component of the mass attenuation coefficient for soft tissue as a function of energy. As explained in Appendix 14–1, the plot of a "power law" function, such as Equation 14.7, is a straight line on log-log graph paper, and the slope of the curve reveals the exponent (in this case, –3).

EXERCISE 14–2.

Which is more likely to undergo a photoelectric interaction in soft tissue, a 20-keV photon or one of 25-keV energy? How great is the difference?

SOLUTION: From Equation 14.7, the 20-keV photon has an interaction probability that is greater by a factor of $[\tau/\rho](20 \text{ keV})/[\tau/\rho](25 \text{ keV}) = (20 \text{ keV})^{-3}/(25 \text{ keV})^{-3} \sim 2$.

The inverse cube energy dependence of $[\tau/\rho]$ on photon energy is usually valid, but not always so. At photon energies up to a few hundred keV, photon interactions in the element lead are almost exclusively of the photoelectric type. Figure 14–1 shows that $[\tau/\rho](hf)$ for lead jumps discontinuously at 88 keV, where hf equals the electronic K-shell binding energy. Such a break in $[\mu/\rho](hf)$ is known as an **absorption edge.** Photons with energies greater than that of the edge are capable of ejecting photoelectrons from the shell, whereas those of lower energies are not. Hence the interaction probability increases abruptly as the energy of the photon climbs to and reaches that of the edge. Away from the absorption edges, at either higher or lower energies, $[\tau/\rho](hf)$ obeys an inverse-cube rule, Equation 14.7. Figure 14–2 plots $[\tau/\rho](hf)$ for lead on linear paper, for comparison with the log-log plot of Figure 14–1.

To summarize the important characteristics of the photoelectric mass attenuation coefficient: $[\tau/\rho]$ depends on the effective atomic number of the irradiated material and on photon energy, (away from absorption edges) as

$$[\tau/\rho](Z, hf) \sim (Z/hf)^3 \qquad (14.8)$$

TABLE 14–1. PHYSICAL PROPERTIES OF SOME MATERIALS OF RADIOLOGIC INTEREST

Material	Density (kg/m³)	Z_{eff}	Electron Density (electrons/kg)
Hydrogen[a]	0.0899	1	5.97 × 10²⁶
Carbon	2250	6	3.01 × 10²⁶
Air[a]	1.293	7.8	3.01 × 10²⁶
Water	1000	7.5	3.34 × 10²⁶
Muscle	1040	7.6	3.31 × 10²⁶
Fat	916	6.5	3.34 × 10²⁶
Bone	1650	12.3	3.19 × 10²⁶

[a]Standard temperature and pressure (STP).
From Johns HE, Cunningham JR: The Physics of Radiology, 4th ed. Charles C Thomas, 1983 (Table A-3), with permission.

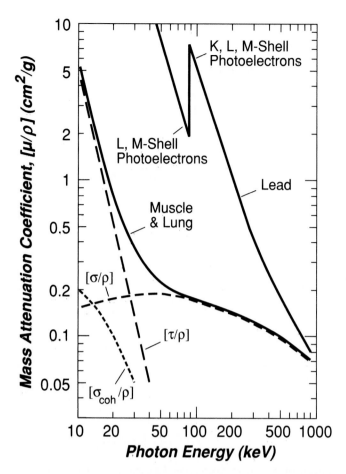

Figure 14–1. Mass attenuation coefficients, $[\mu/\rho]$, for soft tissue and for lead are plotted with the heavy, unbroken lines as functions of energy. *Soft tissue:* $[\mu/\rho](hf)$ is made up predominantly of two components: the photoelectric attenuation coefficient, $[\tau/\rho](hf)$, and the Compton, $[\sigma/\rho](hf)$. The photoelectric component is roughly of the form $[\tau/\rho](hf) \sim (hf)^{-3}$. When plotted on log-log graph paper, such a function lies along a straight line, as explained in Appendix 14–1. The Compton term is nearly constant over the diagnostic range. The coherent or Rayleigh scattering term, $[\sigma_{coh}/\rho](hf)$, is relatively small, and hereafter will be subsumed into the Compton term. *Lead:* In the diagnostic region, attenuation is almost entirely by means of the photoelectric effect. There is a discontinuity in $[\mu/\rho](hf)$, called an *absorption* edge, at each photon energy that equals the binding energy of a shell or subshell of atomic electrons. For lead, the *L*-shell absorption edges occur between 13 and 16 keV, and the *K* edge is at 88 keV. (*Adapted from Johns HE, Cunningham JR: The Physics of Radiology, 4th ed. Springfield, IL: Charles C Thomas, 1983. [Appendix A]; Anderson DW: Absorption of Ionizing Radiation. Baltimore, MD: University Park Press, 1984 [Appendix 9].)*

Things are more complex for photon beams that are not monochromatic, but the general ideas are the same.

3. PHOTOELECTRIC CONTRAST ENHANCEMENT WITH LOW-ENERGY X-RAYS

The fact that $[\tau/\rho]$ depends strongly on Z and hf in this fashion has important implications for radiography. Suppose you are imaging a region of soft tissue, such as a breast. For optimal *contrast* between normal soft tissue and either tumor or

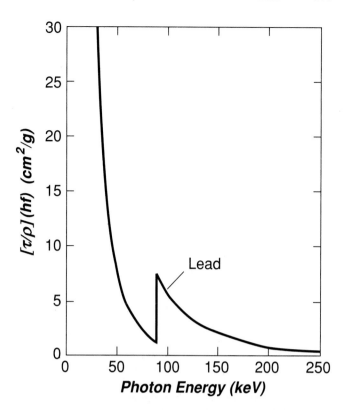

Figure 14–2. $[\tau/\rho](hf)$ for lead, on linear graph paper.

microcalcifications, you attempt to maximize the *differences* in the amounts of attenuation caused in different parts of the x-ray beam by the various tissues. $[\tau/\rho](hf)$ of Equation 14.8 is large for low-energy photons. That is not particularly helpful in its own right; in fact, it reduces the ability of the beam to penetrate the body, which is a distinct disadvantage. But the use of low-energy photons does magnify the *differences* between the attenuation coefficients of tissues with slightly different values of Z, and that can be extremely important. Indeed, it is for this reason that mammography is carried out at very low kVps.

Consider two separate thin pieces of tissue of effective atomic numbers Z_1 and Z_2 and densities ρ_1 and ρ_2, but both of the same thickness Δx. The two will show up on a radiograph as distinct regions if, and only if, the difference in the amounts of attenuation through them, $\Delta I_1 - \Delta I_2 = I \cdot \{[\mu/\rho]_2 \cdot \rho_2 - [\mu/\rho]_1 \cdot \rho_1\} \cdot \Delta x$, is sufficiently large. That is, $\Delta I_1 - \Delta I_2$ will be significant, by Equation 14.8, if

$$\{(Z_1)^3 \cdot \rho_1 - (Z_2)^3 \cdot \rho_2\}/(hf)^3 \qquad (14.9)$$

is large. But as hf appears here in the denominator, $\Delta I_1 - \Delta I_2$ *increases* as the x-ray photon energy *decreases*. It is differences such as $\Delta I_1 - \Delta I_2$ that determine the contrast among tissues in an image, so we conclude that contrast improves with lower peak kilovoltage.

This points to one (but not the only) important consideration in the choice of kVp for an x-ray exposure: Subtle differences in the amounts of photoelectric attenuation occurring in different tissues (because of differences in their densities and effective atomic numbers) may be enhanced, and may give rise to greater contrast in a radiograph, if lower-energy x-ray photons are used. This is readily apparent from Figure 14–3, in which abdominal films were produced at 70 and 100 kVp.

Against this improvement in image quality, however, must be balanced the desirability of the greater overall beam penetration through the body, and of the resulting lower patient dose, that accompany a higher photon energy.

4. A MATERIAL IS RELATIVELY TRANSPARENT TO ITS OWN CHARACTERISTIC X-RAYS

Because of the existence of absorption edges, a material is relatively transparent to its own characteristic x-rays.

The absorption edges of an atomic species lie at energies near, but slightly higher than, those of the atom's characteristic x-rays (Fig. 14–4). A characteristic x-ray photon is emitted when an electron drops from a higher to a lower (bound) orbital. In a photo-electric event, on the other hand, an electron is completely removed from the atom, and that involves a somewhat greater amount of energy. Because the energy of an emission line is a little less than that of the corresponding absorption edge, where μ increases abruptly, a material will attenuate its own characteristic x-rays much less strongly than it does photons of slightly higher energy.

The relative transparency of a material to its own characteristic x-rays has important applications. In a dedicated mammographic system (Chapter 25), the anode of the x-ray tube and the beam filter are both made of molybdenum. The component of the beam of greatest effectiveness for imaging soft tissue differences in breast consists of the relatively low energy (17.4–19.6 keV [Table 6–3]) molybdenum characteristic x-rays. The Mb filter passes these, but strongly attenuates the bremsstrahlung x-rays of energy higher than the *K*-shell absorption edge at 20.0 keV (Table 6–4), which are clinically less useful, for the reason discussed in the last section. It also filters out lower-energy photons, of course, at a rate proportional to $(hf)^{-3}$.

Holmium and other filter materials find similar use in conventional screen–film radiography.

By analogy to electronic circuits that allow passage of lower-frequency signals but block those of higher frequencies, such x-ray filters are sometimes called *low-pass filters*.

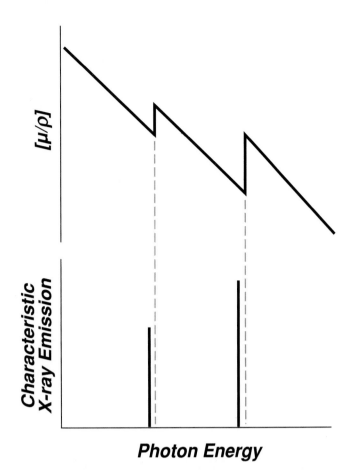

Figure 14–4. An absorption edge for a material and a jump in *attenuation* coefficient occur at an energy slightly higher than the corresponding *emission* lines for the same material. Molybdenum characteristic x-ray photons pass through molybdenum more readily, for example, than do photons of a bit higher energy. A molybdenum filter can therefore be used with a molybdenum-target mammography x-ray tube to pass molybdenum characteristic x-ray photons, while cutting out *higher*-energy bremsstrahlung photons, which would produce lower-contrast images. The filter also removes very low energy bremsstrahlung photons.

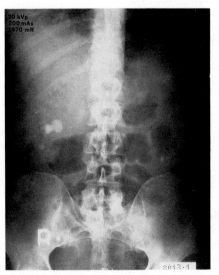
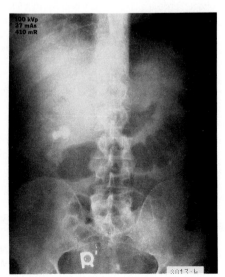

Figure 14–3. Abdominal films obtained at (A) 70 kVp and (B) 100 kVp. The patient has "multiple large and small right renal calculi and a gas-containing abscess in the upper pole of the right kidney. The renal calculi, the renal outlines, the psoas margins, and the trabecular patterns of the bones are best seen on the radiograph made at 70 kVp. . . . At 100 kVp many of the smaller calculi are no longer visible, and even the larger calculi are less distinct. Therefore, in this patient, important diagnostic information is lost as the kVp is increased." (*From the American College of Radiology Learning Files, courtesy of the ACR.*)

A

B

5. DEPENDENCE OF THE COMPTON MASS ATTENUATION COEFFICIENT ON ATOMIC NUMBER AND X-RAY PHOTON ENERGY

In a Compton event, as noted in Chapter 12, Section 3, a high-energy photon collides with a virtually free electron, but imparts only some of its energy to the electron. The rest is transported from the scene of the interaction in the form of a lower-energy scatter photon.

Dependence on Atomic Number, Z

Compton events tend to involve incident photons with energies considerably greater than the binding energies of the affected electrons. Most of the electrons in a material may therefore be thought of as constituting a "gas" of essentially free and independent particles. The physical attribute of a material that would determine its Compton mass attenuation coefficient is therefore the number of electrons per gram. The mass attenuation coefficient depends on Z only to the extent that the effective atomic number influences the electron density (the number of electrons per gram) in this "gas."

As indicated in Table 14–1, all but one (hydrogen) of the elements that make up biologic materials have roughly the same electron density. Biologic tissues, therefore, all have about the same Compton mass attenuation coefficients.

There are, however, subtle differences among the Compton coefficients of biologic materials that arise primarily because of differences in their hydrogen contents. As the electron density of hydrogen is twice as great as for other materials (Table 14–1) the Compton mass attenuation coefficient for bone, for example, is somewhat *less* than that for soft tissue, which contains a greater amount of hydrogen (see Fig. 13–4).

Dependence on Photon Energy, *hf*

A quantum mechanical calculation of the energy dependence of the Compton mass attenuation coefficient leads to a complex expression known as the Klein–Nishina formula. This reveals that $[\sigma/\rho](hf)$ generally decreases with energy. Over the diagnostic range, however, it changes little, and may be viewed as being nearly constant. The dashed curve in Figure 14–1 marked $[\sigma/\rho]$ illustrates this for soft tissue.

To summarize the properties of the Compton mass attenuation coefficient:

$$[\sigma/\rho](hf,Z) \sim \begin{cases} 0.02\ \text{m}^2/\text{kg} = 0.2\ \text{cm}^2/\text{g} & \text{(tissues)} \\ 0.04\ \text{m}^2/\text{kg} = 0.4\ \text{cm}^2/\text{g} & \text{(hydrogen)} \end{cases} \tag{14.10}$$

6. ON THE MAGNITUDES OF THE PHOTOELECTRIC AND COMPTON COEFFICIENTS

Figure 14–1 compared the photoelectric, Compton, coherent (Rayleigh), and total mass attenuation coefficients $[\tau/\rho]$, $[\sigma/\rho]$, $[\sigma_{coh}/\rho]$, and $[\mu/\rho]$ for soft tissue as functions of monochromatic photon energies. Also displayed there is $[\mu/\rho](hf)$ for lead. Figure 14–5A provides similar information in a different format, by showing the *relative* numbers of collisions that occur in the two materials by means of the photoelectric mechanism at any energy. And Figure 14–5B indicates the energy regions in which photoelectric, Compton, and pair production events dominate, as functions of (effective) atomic number.

> With a bremsstrahlung beam, for many purposes (such as finding an "effective" value of $[\mu/\rho]$), one can imagine replacing the real beam with a monochromatic beam of the appropriate "equivalent" photon energy, as will be described in the next chapter. If greater accuracy is required, one must keep track of the relative intensity of the beam (and account for the amounts of different kinds of interactions that occur) at all photon energies.

Figures 14–1 and 14–5 support the claim that at normal diagnostic energies, x-ray and gamma ray photon interactions in soft tissue occur primarily by means of the Compton effect. What does that imply for x-ray imaging? The good side of this is that some of the energy of the incident photons is scattered out of the body and not absorbed locally, resulting in less dose in the tissue. On the other hand, contrast enhancement through kVp reduction works primarily for photoelectric interactions and is less effective where Compton dominates. Also, Compton scattered photons may get to the image receptor and degrade the quality of the image. (Special devices such as radiographic grids and gamma camera collimators help to prevent such scatter photons from ever reaching the detector.)

A photon that makes it through the body without being scattered or absorbed may interact with the *intensifying screen* of a radiographic system, or some other kind of detector. Because the effective atomic numbers of detector materials are relatively high, the interactions occur most probably via the photoelectric process. All the photon energy is absorbed, and little "noise" is introduced by Compton photons emitted and reabsorbed elsewhere within the detector itself.

7. WHY THE PHOTOELECTRIC MASS ATTENUATION COEFFICIENT DEPENDS SO MUCH MORE STRONGLY ON ATOMIC NUMBER AND PHOTON ENERGY

Why should the photoelectric mass attenuation coefficient increase so much more rapidly with atomic number than does the Compton, and fall off so much faster with energy? One partial explanation involves the limitations imposed on the behavior of systems of interacting photons and electrons by the laws of conservation of energy and momentum.

Figure 14–6A illustrates the hypothetical situation in which a photon is absorbed by, and 100% of its energy imparted to, a totally free electron. It is perhaps surprising, but nonetheless true, that Nature does not allow this kind of collision to occur. It is impossible for energy and momentum both to be conserved at the same time for this particular kind of interaction. (This, in turn, has to do with the fact that although a photon carries momentum, it is massless.) As this type of event is forbidden, any interaction between a photon and an electron must involve a third body as well.

> The momentum of a nonrelativistic (i.e., moving much slower than the speed of light) *particle* of mass m and velocity v is $m \cdot v$, (see Chapter 5, Section 12). A judicious mixing of quantum mechanics and the theory of relativity reveals that a *photon* of frequency f carries momentum of magnitude hf/c.

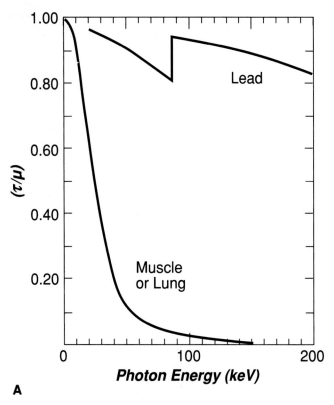

A

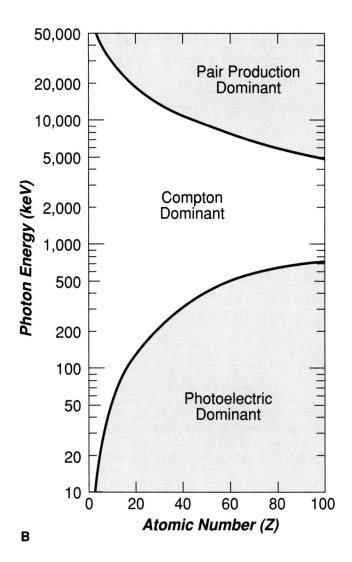

B

Figure 14–5. **A.** Relative fraction of interactions that take place via photoelectric events, $\tau/\mu = [\tau/\rho]/[\mu/\rho]$, for soft tissue and for lead. The curves for most radiation detector materials, such as for the phosphor in a radiographic cassette or for the sodium iodide crystal of a gamma camera, lie somewhere between these two. *(Taken from Fig. 14–1.)* **B.** Another way of demonstrating the energy domains where the photoelectric and Compton interactions dominate, for different materials. For normal radiography (with the exception of mammography), most interactions in soft tissues (low *Z*) take place by way of the Compton process. The average *Z* of bone and most detector materials is much higher, and the photoelectric effect becomes dominant. Pair production does not occur at diagnostic energies.

For the collision in Figure 14–6, the Law of Conservation of Momentum requires

$$hf/c \ (photon, \ before) = m \cdot v \ (electron, \ after)$$

Likewise, by the Law of Conservation of Energy,

$$hf = \tfrac{1}{2}m \cdot v^2$$

These two cannot hold simultaneously, however, as may be seen by dividing one by the other. In other words, the event simply cannot happen. A generalization of the argument holds for all photon energies.

In a real photoelectric event (Fig. 14–6B), a third body is involved in the interaction, namely, the rest of the atom to which the ejected electron had been bound. A three-body collision event can satisfy the two conservation laws at the same time, as small "corrections" in momentum and energy may be imparted to the atom. But for higher-energy photons, or for lower-*Z* materials, the binding of the electron to the atom is relatively very weak and the situation becomes, in effect, like the two-body free-electron scenario of Figure 14–6A. And that is forbidden

from taking place. Thus, with increasing photon energy or decreasing atomic number media, the photoelectric interaction probability simply diminishes. This argument also explains the observation that a photoelectric event is several times more likely to involve a (more tightly bound) *K*-shell atomic electron than an *L*-shell electron, when both are energetically possible.

The Compton effect, by contrast, is an allowed three-body affair (incident photon, struck/ejected Compton electron, and Compton scatter photon) at any energy (Fig. 14–6C), even with totally free electrons. So the preceding constraint does not inhibit such interactions, and $[\sigma/\rho]$ is relatively independent of *hf*.

APPENDIX 14–1. Exponential and Logarithmic Functions

Exponential Functions

Radiology makes much use of exponential functions and logarithms. Because of their importance, it may be worthwhile to review briefly some of their properties.

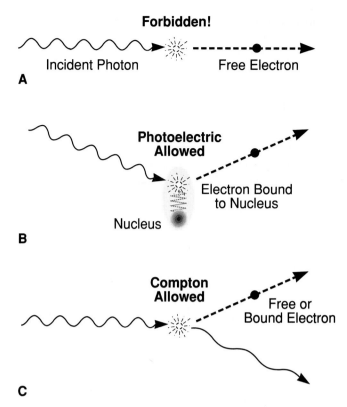

Figure 14–6. Why [τ/ρ] depends relatively strongly on energy. **A.** Total energy and total momentum cannot both be conserved in a photoelectric type of interaction between a photon and a completely free electron, so such an event simply will not take place. **B.** If a small amount of the energy and/or momentum can be imparted to a third body such as a nucleus or an entire atom, however, a photon *can* interact with an electron. But the weaker the binding, the more closely the situation resembles the forbidden free electron scenario, and the lower the probability that the event will take place. **C.** A Compton event, on the other hand, is always a three-body interaction, and it can occur at any energy.

We begin with exponents, and powers of 2 in particular. Two cubed, 2^3, means that the "base" 2 is raised to the "power" or "exponent" 3; that is, it is multiplied by itself three times: $2^3 = 2 \cdot 2 \cdot 2$.

This definition implies a simple rule for the multiplication of two exponentials with the same base: $2^3 \cdot 2^4 = (2 \cdot 2 \cdot 2)(2 \cdot 2 \cdot 2) = 2^7$. When (but only when) the bases are the same, just add the exponents. The multiplication rule and Table 14–2 suggest that exponents of zero and negative numbers also make sense: $2^{-5} = 1/2^5$ and $2^0 = 1$.

_____ **EXERCISE 14–3.** _____

In working with computer-based imaging systems, it is useful to bear in mind that 2^{10} is approximately 1000. Confirm this near equality.

SOLUTION: $2^{10} = 1024.$

The rule for multiplication also indicates the meaning of a noninteger exponent. For example, $2^{0.5} \cdot 2^{0.5} = 2^1$, indicates that the square root of 2, namely, $2^{0.5} = 1.414 \ldots$, is that number which, when appearing twice in a product, yields 2.

TABLE 14–2. SOME POWERS OF 2

⋮		
2^6	=	64
2^5	=	32
2^4	=	16
2^3	=	8
2^2	=	4
2^1	=	2
2^0	=	1
2^{-1}	=	$\frac{1}{2}$
2^{-2}	=	$\frac{1}{4}$
2^{-3}	=	$\frac{1}{8}$
2^{-4}	=	$\frac{1}{16}$
⋮		

The base 2 leads to the "binary" system of Table 14–2, employed by most computers. The number 10 serves as the base for the "decimal" system. (If people had seven fingers on each hand, the common counting system would be based on 14; there is nothing magical about 10.)

The "Naperian" or "Natural" base, which is used throughout the sciences, is designated e and has the value $e = 2.71828183. \ldots$ Just as $\pi = 3.14159 \ldots$ arises in geometry as the ratio of a circle's circumference to its diameter, so also the special constant e occurs naturally in calculus. The meanings of e^b, e^{-b}, e^0, and $e^b \cdot e^c$ follow by analogy to the case of base 2:

$$e^b = e \cdot e \cdot e \cdot \ldots \cdot e, \quad b \text{ times} \tag{14.11a}$$
$$e^{-b} = 1/e^b \tag{14.11b}$$
$$e^0 = 1 \tag{14.11c}$$
$$e^b \cdot e^c = e^{(b+c)} \tag{14.11d}$$

We have been dealing with numbers (in particular, 2, 10, and e) raised to various powers. It is a small step to the definition of an *exponential function*, of the general form $e^{f(x)}$, sometimes written exp $f(x)$. When $f(x)$ itself happens to be linear in x, this assumes a particularly simple form. For $f(x) = bx$ with constant b, for example, $e^{f(x)}$ reduces to

$$y(x) = e^{bx} \tag{14.12}$$

Equation 14.12, commonly referred to rather loosely as *the* "exponential function," is plotted in Figure 14–7 for several positive and negative values of the exponential constant. Any exponential function passes through $y = 1$ for $x = 0$. It is a smoothly increasing (if the exponential constant is positive) or decreasing (when $b < 0$) function of x. In the latter case, the function approaches, but never actually reaches, the abscissa at large values of x.

The exponent must be unitless. The expression $e^{(x \text{ cm})}$, for example, is completely meaningless. If the units of a constant such as μ happen to be cm^{-1}, however, then $e^{-\mu \cdot x}$ is allowed, as the units of μ and x cancel one another, leaving the overall exponent without units.

A point that we shall state (and later use) without proof is $e^{bx} \approx (1 + bx)$ for bx << 1. That is, for values of x near x = 0, an exponential function can be approximated as a linear function. Actually, this reflects a general property of virtually *all* curves: A small enough segment of any sufficiently smooth function looks nearly straight, when magnified.

Many processes occurring in nature display exponential behavior of one sort or another, and all for essentially the same reason: *If the rate of change of a quantity* (dependent variable) with respect to a parameter (independent variable) happens to be always *proportional to the current magnitude of the quantity*, then the quantity must vary exponentially with respect to the parameter (i.e., the dependent variable is an exponential function of the independent variable). As discussed in Chapter 13, for example, the number of x-ray photons (dependent variable) removed from a beam per small thickness (independent variable) of matter traversed is proportional to the number of photons incident on the slice of matter. Exponential attenuation of the beam! But why, then, is Δn linear in Δx (Equation 13.1)? Likewise, in a sample of radioactive material, the number of nuclear decays per unit time is proportional to the total number of radioactive nuclei still present, and the number of remaining nuclei decreases exponentially with time. So also with cell-killing studies: The rate at which cells in a culture are killed per unit of radiation dose is simply proportional, in some situations, to the number of cells still alive, and cell survival is exponential in the dose of radiation deposited. We shall have more to say about these exponential processes, and others, later.

Logarithmic Functions

Now on to logarithms. A logarithm is nothing more than another way of expressing an exponential. The *natural logarithm* of the unitless number w is written $\ln w$ or $\ln_e w$. Then

$$\ln w = z \qquad (14.13a)$$

means nothing more or less than

$$w = e^z \qquad (14.13b)$$

That is, the *logarithm* of w, namely $\ln w$, refers to the *exponent* (z, here) that you must stick on the base e to get w. Equation 14.13a is just the converse of Equation 14.13b, somewhat as $x = y^{1/2}$ is the converse of $y = x^2$.

You may wish to convince yourself of the validity of the following useful relationships involving logarithms:

$$\ln e^z = z \qquad (14.14a)$$
$$\ln 1/a = -\ln a \qquad (14.14b)$$
$$\ln a \cdot b = \ln a + \ln b \qquad (14.14c)$$
$$\ln a^c = c \ln a \qquad (14.14d)$$

___ **EXERCISE 14–4.** ___

Confirm the identity Equation 14.14a.

SOLUTION: ($\ln e^z$) refers to the exponent you must put on the base e to get e^z. That exponent is obviously z.

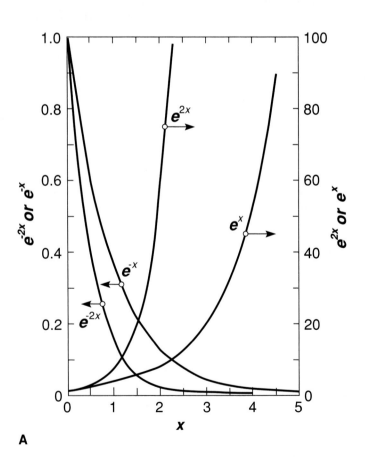

A

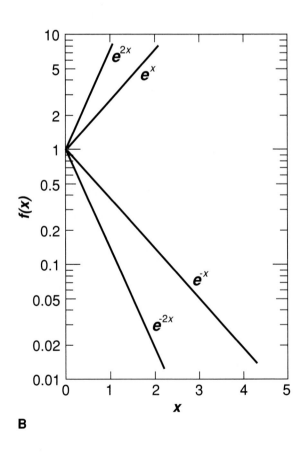

B

Figure 14–7. Examples of exponential functions, with four different values (1, 2, –1, and –2) for the constant in the exponent. **A.** Plotted on linear graph paper. **B.** Exponential functions come out on semilog graph paper as straight lines.

EXERCISE 14–5.

Confirm Equation 14.14b.

SOLUTION: Define some a and y such that $a = e^y$. Then $1/a = e^{-y}$ and, by Equation 14.14a, $\ln 1/a = \ln e^{-y} = -y$. But from $a = e^y$, we also know that $y = \ln a$. Thus $\ln 1/a = -\ln a$.

The *common* logarithm works in the same way as the natural logarithm, written $\log w$ or $\log_{10} w$, but with base 10:

$$z = \log w \tag{14.15a}$$

means exactly the same thing as

$$10^z = w \tag{14.15b}$$

The prescription for taking the common logarithm of a base e exponential is $\log e^q = 0.434q$.

EXERCISE 14–6.

(Challenging). Confirm $\log e^q = 0.434q$.

SOLUTION: Define p through $p = \log_{10} e^q$. Equivalently, $10^p = e^q$. Take the natural log of both sides of this. The left-hand side is now $\ln_e 10^p$, or $p \cdot \ln_e 10$. The right-hand side is $\ln_e e^q$, or q. Therefore $p \cdot \ln_e 10 = q$. As $\ln_e 10 = 2.303$, this becomes $p = 0.434q$. Now, recall the definition of p.

There is a nice approximate expression for a logarithm whose argument is close to unity: $\ln(1 + x) \approx x$, for $x << 1$.

Semilog and Log-Log Graph Paper

Ordinary *linear* graph paper is constructed with vertical lines at $x = n$, where $n = 0, 1, 2, 3, \ldots$, and with equally spaced horizontal lines at integer values of y, as well. Linear functions, of the form $y = m \cdot x + b$, come out as straight lines when plotted on such paper. Other functions, of course, display more complex shapes.

Exponential functions occur so frequently throughout the sciences that a special type of paper has been designed specifically for graphing them. The horizontal lines on *semilog* graph paper are not equally far apart, but rather are spaced in such a fashion that any true exponential will end up lying along a straight line on it. The x axis of semilog paper has a linear scale, but the horizontal, y-coordinate lines occur at distances $\ln n$

TABLE 14–3. FUNCTIONS AND GRAPH PAPER

Function	Example	Plots as Straight Line on this Graph Paper
Linear	$y(x) = m \cdot x + b$	Linear
Exponential	$I(x)/I(0) = e^{-\mu \cdot x}$	Semilog
Power	$[\tau/\rho](hf) \sim (hf)^{-3}$	Log-log

above the origin, where $n = 1, 2, 3, \ldots$. It is because the logarithm is the inverse of the exponential that an exponential function plots out as a straight line on such semilog paper. The curves in Figure 14–7A are replotted on semilog paper in Figure 14–7B. A single kind of semilog graph paper works with any value of the constant b in the exponent in Equation 14.12.

Semilog plots have a variety of applications. If it is suspected that a set of experimental data might be describable in terms of an exponential function, then a graph that turns out to be *straight* on semilog paper provides immediate and unambiguous confirmation. All sorts of functions plotted on ordinary graph paper look as if they might possibly be exponential (if you squint a little), but straight is straight. Also, once it is determined that data do, in fact, lie along a straight line on semilog paper, it is a simple matter to determine the constants of the corresponding exponential function from the graph. Although "least-squares" computer fitting programs can do that more accurately, taking the slope and intercept off a semilog plot is a quick and often adequate first mode of attack. Finally, semilog paper "compresses" the graph of *any* function, thereby increasing the range over which it can be plotted on a single sheet of paper (but, in the processes, distorts its appearance).

Just as an exponential function comes out as a straight line on semilog paper, so also a *power* function, such as x^b, yields a straight line on *log-log* graph paper.

The reason for this may be seen by taking the logarithm of both sides of $y(x) = x^b$, yielding $\ln y = b \cdot (\ln x)$. Plotting this on log-log paper, in which both axes use logarithmic scales, is equivalent to making the transformations $u = \ln y$ and $v = \ln x$. That is, $\ln y = b \cdot (\ln x)$ becomes $u = b \cdot v$, now a straight line.

To summarize, a linear function plots out as a straight line on linear paper, an exponential function yields a straight line on semi-log paper, and a power law function is straight on log-log paper (Table 14–3).

Attenuation of the X-ray Beam in the Patient's Body

As a diagnostic x-ray beam penetrates deeper into the body, energy is removed from it, and so its intensity decreases. Under certain idealized conditions, the intensity, $I(x)$, falls off exponentially with depth, x, according to $I(x)/I(0) = e^{-\mu \cdot x}$, where μ is the linear attenuation coefficient. In practice, attenuation is nearly, but not exactly, exponential.

It is through the process of attenuation of the x-ray beam by a patient's body that radiographic images are formed. It is also how dose is deposited in tissue, either intentionally (in radiotherapy) or as an undesirable yet unavoidable aspect of the radiographic imaging process.

1. THE EXPERIMENTAL STUDY OF PHOTON BEAM ATTENUATION

Attenuation of a type of radiation of interest by a particular material can be studied by means of the experiment shown in Figure 15–1A. Radiation is emitted from a small source (the focal spot of an x-ray tube, for example, or a tiny vial of radionuclide), and a narrow "pencil" beam is produced by means of collimators. A radiation detector, such as an ionization chamber, is placed a large distance from the source, and attached to an electrometer that translates beam intensities into meter readings. A second collimator largely prevents scatter radiation produced within the material under examination from reaching the detector. The study consists of following these readings as various thicknesses of the attenuating material are inserted midway between the source and the detector.

The experimental design of Figure 15–1A is said to be one of *narrow beam* or **good geometry.** The distance between source and detector is large, and the photons that reach the detector are traveling in practically parallel lines. Because of the collimation and because of the large distance between the attenuating medium and the detector, moreover, almost all Compton scatter photons miss the detector. The meter reading is therefore strictly proportional to the number of unscattered photons, those that manage to pass through the medium without undergoing any interactions at all.

With *broad beam geometry*, by contrast, scatter radiation reaches the detector (Fig. 15–1B). This kind of situation, which must be considered in radiation shielding calculations, is generally much more complex than that of good geometry.

The results of a typical study with good geometry, the attenuation by aluminum of the monochromatic (140-keV) gamma rays emitted by a sample of technetium-99*m*, are reproduced in Figures 15–2A and 15–2B on rectilinear and semilog graph paper, respectively. With such a monochromatic source, one finds pure exponential attenuation, for reasons about to be explained. With a bremsstrahlung beam, which has a continuous spectrum, things are a bit more complicated, as will be discussed later.

2. AN X-RAY BEAM LOSES HALF ITS INTENSITY IN PASSING THROUGH A HALF-VALUE LAYER THICKNESS OF MATERIAL

In passing through a thin layer of material Δx thick, the intensity of an x-ray beam, I, is diminished, according to Equation 13.1b, by the small amount $\Delta I = -\mu \cdot I \cdot \Delta x$. The linear attenua-

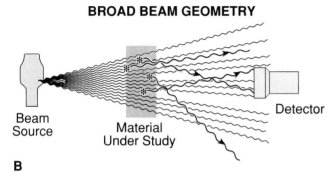

"GOOD" GEOMETRY

Beam Collimator   Detector Collimator

Beam Source   Material Under Study   Detector

A

BROAD BEAM GEOMETRY

Beam Source   Material Under Study   Detector

B

Figure 15–1. Study of the attenuation of photon beams of various spectral compositions by different kinds and amounts of materials. **A.** Under conditions of "good geometry," practically no photons scattered once or several times within the attenuating material will reach the detector. **B.** The "broad beam geometry" scenario must be considered when planning for the shielding of an x-ray imaging room.

tion coefficient, μ, is constant, and the decrease in intensity is linearly proportional to the thickness of the layer.

The more general situation, in which the beam enters a block of the material of arbitrary—rather than very small—thickness, is more subtle. One approach to this more general situation is by way of the **half-value layer (HVL)** thickness. A half-value layer thickness is that amount of a particular material, designated $x_{0.5}$, that will attenuate the intensity of a particular beam to half its initial value (Fig. 15–2), $I(x_{0.5})/I(0) = 0.5$. The actual thickness of the HVL, in centimeters, is determined by the energy spectrum of the photon beam and by the nature of the attenuating medium. In any case, it will be *much* greater than any thin layer Δx. The expression $\Delta I = -\mu \cdot I \cdot \Delta x$ is valid *only* for very thin slices of matter, which attenuate the beam by a few percent, at most.

Under ideal conditions, which is to say with good geometry and monochromatic radiation, the beam is exactly the same after emerging from a HVL of attenuator as when it entered, except that it consists of only half as many photons. If the survivors of this first HVL enter another HVL (which will be of the same thickness as the first), their number will again be reduced by a factor of 2, and so on. Figure 15–3 records the intensity of the beam after passage through various numbers of such HVLs. After transiting N HVLs, the intensity is reduced to 2^{-N} of its original value.

It is useful to be able to express this in terms of the thickness of attenuator, x, rather than the number of HVLs, N. Sup-

pose $x_{0.5}$ is 3 cm. One HVL is 3 cm thick, 2 HVLs will be 6 cm thick, and so forth, and an N-HVL block is $(N \cdot x_{0.5})$ cm thick. Conversely, the number of HVLs in a piece of matter x cm thick is just $N = x/x_{0.5}$. Given an arbitrary thickness of material, x, then all you have to do is determine the number of HVLs, and reduce the beam intensity by a factor of $0.5 = 2^{-1}$ for each:

$$I(x)/I(0) = 2^{-N} = 2^{-x/x_{0.5}}$$
$$N = \text{number of HVLs}, \qquad (15.1)$$
$$x_{0.5} = \text{HVL thickness}$$

The beam intensity thus decreases exponentially with attenuator thickness. The constant $x_{0.5}$ in the exponent of Equation 15.1 is physically meaningful, and its units must be in those of distance, such as centimeters. This leaves the whole exponent, $x/x_{0.5}$, a dimensionless pure number, which it must be for the mathematical expression to make sense. After all, what could possibly be the meaning of $2^{(-3\text{ cm})}$?

_____ **EXERCISE 15–1.** _____

The HVL of a monochromatic beam in a material is 3 cm. What fraction of it remains after passage through 9 cm? What about 10.2 cm?

SOLUTION: $I(9)/I(0) = 2^{-(9\text{ cm}/3\text{ cm})} = 2^{-3} = 0.125$. $I(10.3)/I(0) = 2^{-10.3/3} = 2^{-3.433} = 0.093$.

_____ **EXERCISE 15–2.** _____

Over a time period of one *half-life*, $t_{0.5}$, the activity of a sample of a particular radionuclide falls by a factor of a half. How much of the sample is left after three half-lives? After the arbitrary time t?

SOLUTION: 1/8th; $2^{-t/t_{0.5}}$.

3. THE EXPONENTIAL ATTENUATION OF A MONOCHROMATIC, NONDIVERGENT BEAM WITH GOOD GEOMETRY

We could repeat the preceding argument using tenth-value layers instead of HVLs. The thickness required for the beam intensity to be reduced by a factor of $10^{-1} = 0.1$ would be designated $x_{0.1}$, and the beam would be attenuated by the fraction $10^{-x/x_{0.1}}$ by a thickness x of material.

We might even consider e-value layers. $e = 2.71828183 \ldots$, defined in Appendix 14–1, is a pure number (like 2 and 10) that happens to play an important role in calculus. The beam intensity falls by a factor of $e^{-1} \sim 0.37$ over the *characteristic attenuation thickness* $x_{0.37}$, and in general

$$I(x)/I(0) = e^{-x/x_{0.37}} \qquad (15.2)$$

This notation, with the characteristic e-value layer thickness $x_{0.37}$ in the exponent, is sensible, but it not used in practice. It is customary to define a new entity μ, instead, called the *linear attenuation coefficient*, which is just the *inverse* of the characteristic attenuation thickness $x_{0.37}$:

$$\mu = 1/x_{0.37} \qquad (15.3a)$$

or, equivalently, $1/\mu = x_{0.37}$. Equation 15.2 then becomes

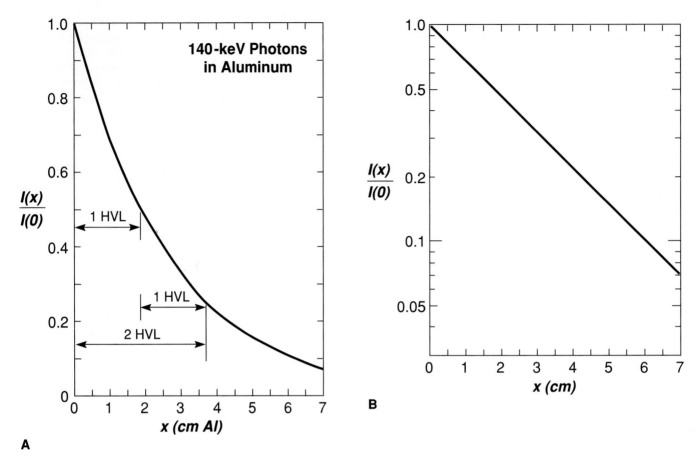

A

B

Figure 15–2. Exponential attenuation of a monochromatic, nondivergent beam under conditions of good geometry. In this case, 140-keV photons are passing through aluminum ($\mu = 0.38$ cm^{-1}). **A.** As plotted on linear graph paper. The intensity falls by the same factor of 0.5 for each half-value layer (HVL) thickness (here, 1.8 cm) of attenuation material in the beam path. **B.** On semilog paper, a purely exponential function plots out as a straight line, as discussed in Chapter 14.

$$I(x)/I(0) = e^{-\mu \cdot x} \qquad (15.3b)$$

This important relationship is known as the Lambert–Beer law, or the *Law of Exponential Attenuation*. The transmission of monochromatic beams through several materials (lung, muscle, and bone at 40 and 80 keV) is demonstrated (on semi-log paper) in Figure 15–4. The value of μ for each curve depends on both the properties of the medium and on the beam energy.

The units of μ are somewhat peculiar. As $x_{0.37}$ is expressed typically in centimeters, μ would be expressed in cm^{-1}, or "per cm."

_____ **EXERCISE 15–3.** _____

The linear attenuation coefficient μ of a particular beam in a given material is 0.231 cm^{-1}. What fraction of the intensity remains after passage through 5 cm?

SOLUTION: $I(5 \text{ cm})/I(0) = e^{-(0.231 \text{ cm}^{-1}) \cdot (5 \text{ cm})} = e^{-1.155} = 0.315$.

_____ **EXERCISE 15–4.** _____

Using Equations 15.3, determine how much the beam is attenuated by an amount of material that happens to equal the characteristic thickness, $x_{0.37}$.

SOLUTION: $I(x_{0.37})/I(0) = I(1/\mu)/I(0) = e^{-\mu(1/\mu)} = e^{-1} = 0.37$.

Equation 15.3b can be expressed in terms of the mass attenuation coefficient as

$$I(x)/I(0) = e^{-[\mu/\rho] \cdot \rho \cdot \mu} \qquad (15.4)$$

by means of the familiar prescription $\mu \leftrightarrow [\mu/\rho] \cdot \rho$. It will be

Figure 15–3. The intensity of a photon beam diminishes by a factor of 0.5 for each half-value layer of attenuating material through which it passes. With exponential attenuation (but *only* with exponential attenuation), the thicknesses of all the half-value layers are the same.

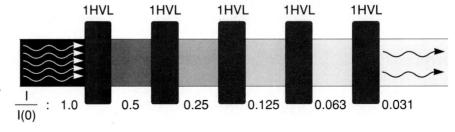

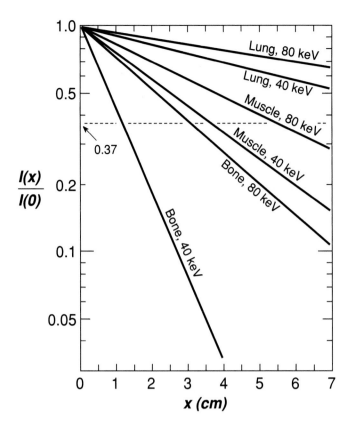

Figure 15–4. Exponential attenuation of 40- and 80-keV monochromatic x-ray beams in lung, muscle, and bone. There are three important messages in this diagram: the spatial rate of attenuation increases with (1) greater density (lung vs. muscle), (2) greater effective atomic number (soft tissue vs. bone), and (3) lower photon energy (80 keV vs. 40 keV). The attenuation coefficient, μ, is the inverse of the characteristic thickness of material, $x_{0.37}$, over which the beam is attenuated by a factor of $1/e = 0.37$.

convenient for the purposes of this chapter, however, to work in terms of the linear attenuation coefficient, instead.

4. THE LINEAR ATTENUATION COEFFICIENT IS THE INVERSE OF THE CHARACTERISTIC ATTENUATION THICKNESS

The magnitude of μ must somehow reflect on the microscopic, local aspects of the photoelectric absorption and Compton scattering of individual x-ray or gamma ray photons by matter. As such, we would expect μ to be a function of photon energy and the chemical properties (i.e., the atomic number) of the attenuating material. It may also be helpful to think of μ simply as the inverse of the characteristic attenuation thickness of material, or distance through it, $x_{0.37}$, over which the intensity of the beam is diminished by a factor of $e^{-1} = 0.37$.

Figure 15–4 illustrates exponential attenuation for several different materials and monochromatic photon energies, hence for different values of μ. The larger the value of μ, the shorter the characteristic thickness $x_{0.37}$, and the more rapidly the beam falls to 0.37 of its preattenuation value. (Making use of Figure 13–2, you may want to convince yourself that in Figure 15–4, $I(x)/I(0)$ does fall to 0.37 for $x = 1/\mu$.) When x-rays are not

readily absorbed or scattered by the atoms in their path, on the other hand, $x_{0.37}$ will be large, μ small, and attenuation of the beam slow.

EXERCISE 15–5.

The characteristic attenuation distance $x_{0.37}$ of a beam in a material is 2 cm. What fraction of it remains after passage through 4 cm? 4.33 cm? 1 cm?

SOLUTION: $\mu = 1/(2 \text{ cm}) = 0.5 \text{ cm}^{-1}$. By Equation 15.3b, $I(4 \text{ cm})/I(0) = e^{-(0.5 \text{ cm}^{-1}) \cdot (4 \text{ cm})} = e^{-2} = 0.135$. Likewise, $I(4.33 \text{ cm})/I(0) = 0.115$; $I(1 \text{ cm})/I(0) = 0.607$.

EXERCISE 15–6.

The characteristic attenuation distance, $1/\mu$, of a beam in a material is 2 cm. What fraction of it remains after passage through 0.01 cm? 0.02 cm? 0.03 cm? Using also the results of Exercise 15–5, plot transmitted intensity as a function of thickness; this shows that for very thin layers (but *only* for very thin layers), the amount of attenuation is proportional to thickness. This observation will be put to use in the next section.

SOLUTION: $I(0.01 \text{ cm})/I(0) = e^{-(0.01 \text{ cm})/(2 \text{ cm})} = 0.9950$. Likewise $I(0.02 \text{ cm})/I(0) = 0.9900$, and so on.

Equations 15.3 and the values of μ (or, completely equivalently, Equations 15.1 and values of $x_{0.5}$) for photon energies and materials of radiologic interest determine, to a large extent, both the ability of an x-ray system to produce useful medical images and the spatial distribution of the dose deposited in the body in the process.

5. LINKING THE RATE OF ATTENUATION (THIN LAYER) AND HALF-VALUE LAYER PICTURES

"But wait a second," you're doubtless thinking right now, "just hold your horses. Somebody has sneakily chosen to give the constant in the exponent of Equations 15.3 the same name and symbol as the constant of proportionality in Equation 13.1, which described attenuation in a thin layer of material. But what reason is there to believe that μ does indeed represent the same thing physically in the two, clearly very different, situations?"

It is easy to connect the general exponential expression to that for the special case of the thin layer and, in so doing, to show that the parameter μ refers to the same physical entity in both.

Assume a particular thin layer of material, of thickness Δx, at a depth of x in a thick block of the material. For monochromatic, previously unscattered photons, the attenuation rate μ of Equation 15.3 is *independent of the depth* of the layer in the material. That fact alone is sufficient information for us to deduce that the shape of $I(x)$ throughout the entire thick block is exponential.

Aside: You may feel that the claim that μ is a constant deserves some support. The interaction of monochromatic x-rays with matter is a random process. The photon collisions occurring within any small volume of material are discrete, relatively few in number, and statistically independent of one another. (Appendix 18–1 will show that photon interaction is an example of a "Poisson" process.) Any still-unscattered photon has no memory, no awareness of how much matter it has already traversed or of what has happened to its identical fellow travelers. The probability that it will undergo a collision over the next millimeter of its travel is therefore independent of its depth in the matter. (Further into the medium there may be fewer photons left and available to undergo collisions, but that's a different issue altogether.) If 1% of the unscattered photons reaching a depth of $x = 2$ cm are removed from the beam in a 1-mm-thick layer, for example, such that $\Delta I/I \cdot \Delta x = 0.01$ per millimeter there, then the *same fraction* will be attenuated in a 1-mm layer buried 20 cm deep. The *absolute numbers* of photons involved will be considerably different in the two situations; that is, many fewer photons reach, and will be lost in, the layer at 20-cm depth. But the fraction, or relative number, attenuated per unit thickness is depth invariant. In other words, $\mu = -\Delta I/I \cdot \Delta x$ is a constant.

Rewrite Equation 13.1 as $\Delta I/\Delta x = -\mu \cdot I(x)$. In Figure 15–5, the rate (at depth x) at which the intensity falls off, $\Delta I/\Delta x$, is seen to be the slope of $I(x)$ at that depth. According to $\Delta I/\Delta x = -\mu \cdot I(x)$, the rate at which photons are removed from the beam at any particular depth is proportional to the number still present in it, $I(x)$. But the intensity diminishes with depth in the block of material. And since $I(x)$ becomes smaller, $\Delta I/\Delta x$ must,

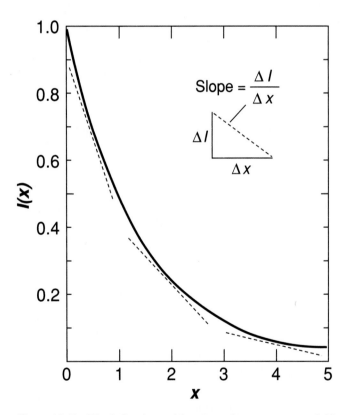

Figure 15–5. Why is the shape of the attenuation curve exponential? The slope of the attenuation curve, $\Delta I/\Delta x$, is the spatial rate of change of intensity. But $\Delta I/\Delta x$ at any depth is proportional to I. As photons are removed from the beam, I becomes smaller, so $\Delta I/\Delta x$ flattens out, in an exponential-like fashion. Pursuing this argument more precisely with the calculus reveals that under idealized conditions, the attenuation is exactly exponential.

too; that is, the graph of $I(x)$ flattens out with greater values of x. This leads to a shape that is at least roughly exponential. When analyzed with elementary calculus, $I(x)$ is seen to be exactly exponential.

Second Aside: A "first-order differential equation" equates the first derivative of a dependent variable to some given function of that variable. In the limit of very small Δ, $\Delta I/\Delta x$ turns into the derivative dI/dx, and $dI/dx = -\mu \cdot I$ is such an equation. The dependent variable is I, its first derivative is dI/dx, and the given function happens to be $I(x)$ itself multiplied by a constant. The objective is to find an explicit form for $I(x)$ that satisfies $dI/dx = -\mu \cdot I(x)$. A standard approach is to take an educated guess at the general form of the unknown $I(x)$, plug it into the differential equation, and see what comes of it. This method confirms that Equation 15.3b is indeed a solution.

It is instructive to make the same point another way: Consider Equation 15.3b for the situation of a small value of x. By Appendix 14–1, when x assumes the very small value Δx, Equation 15.3b reduces to the simpler form

$$I(\Delta x)/I(0) = e^{-\mu \cdot \Delta x} \sim \{1 - \mu \cdot \Delta x\} \qquad (15.5)$$

As $\Delta I = I(0) - I(\Delta x)$, this is equivalent to Equation 13.1b. Thus, the attenuation coefficient of Equations 15.3 is identical to that of Equation 13.1b in the special case in which x happens to be set equal to Δx. But because μ is a constant, totally independent of the magnitude of x, this identity must hold always, for all (not only small) values of x in the exponential expression (Equations 15.3). Equation 15.5 thus provides a strong link between the macroscopic (HVL, thick block of matter) and microscopic (thin slice) views of the x-ray attenuation process.

Exponential attenuation is what one would find for a monochromatic beam under conditions of good geometry. Under less ideal conditions (as with a bremsstrahlung beam that "hardens" as it passes through tissue, or with scatter photons entering the picture), μ will not be depth-independent, and attenuation will not be exactly exponential.

There is an important and useful moral to all of this: Whenever one finds a function (such as the number of photons remaining in a beam, or radionuclei still undecayed in a sample of radiopharmaceutical, or "surviving" cells in a Petri dish undergoing irradiation) whose rate of change with respect to an independent variable (such as depth in matter, or elapsed time, or dose of irradiation) is simply proportional to the magnitude of the function itself, then that function must be an exponential.

The activity, $A(t)$, of a radioactive substance used in a nuclear medicine imaging procedure decays exponentially over time t:

$$A(t) = A(0)\, e^{-\lambda \cdot t} \qquad (15.6)$$

The "transformation constant," λ, is characteristic of the particular radioisotope under examination, and depends on nothing else. See also Exercise 15–2.

The fraction of cells in a culture that survive irradiation, $S(D)$, decreases exponentially, in some situations, with the dose of ionizing radiation deposited, D:

$$S(D) = e^{-D/D_{37}} \qquad (15.7)$$

The constant D_{37} (the commonly seen form for what we would call $D_{0.37}$) depends on the biology of the cells and on the detailed way in which the radiation deposits its ionizing energy within them.

6. THE LINEAR ATTENUATION COEFFICIENT IS SIMPLY RELATED TO THE HALF-VALUE LAYER

The characteristic attenuation distance $x_{0.37} = 1/\mu$ and the HVL thickness $x_{0.5}$ provide different but equally legitimate measures of the rate of beam attenuation. There is a simple and frequently useful relationship between the two.

Consider Equation 15.3b for the particular case in which the attenuator thickness, x, happens to be one HVL: $x = 1$ HVL $= x_{0.5}$. Simply by the definition of $x_{0.5}$, we find $I(x_{0.5})/I(0) = e^{-\mu \cdot x_{0.5}} = 0.5$. Taking the natural logarithm of this leads, with the aid of Equation 14.14a, to

$$\mu \cdot HVL = 0.693 \qquad (15.8)$$

illustrated in Figure 15–6. Remembering this in the equivalent form $1/\mu = x_{0.37} = 1.44 \cdot HVL$ may help provide a feel for the units, magnitude, and physical meaning of μ.

_____ **EXERCISE 15–7.** _____

The HVL of a beam is 3 cm in some medium. What is μ? Find, using Equations 15.1, and 15.3, how much the beam is attenuated in 5 cm.

SOLUTION: $I(5\ \text{cm})/I(0) = 2^{-(5\ \text{cm})/(3\ \text{cm})} = 0.315$. Alternatively, by Equation 15.8, $\mu = 0.693/(3\ \text{cm}) = 0.231\ \text{cm}^{-1}$; then $I(5\ \text{cm})/I(0) = e^{-(0.231\ \text{cm}^{-1}) \cdot (5\ \text{cm})} = 0.315$.

_____ **EXERCISE 15–8.** _____

Which of $1/\mu$ and $x_{0.5}$ is the greater thickness?

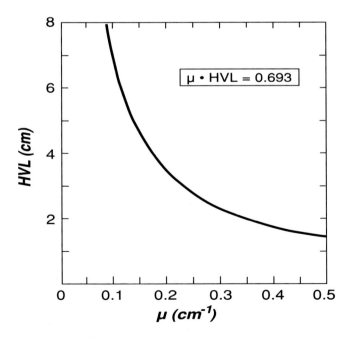

Figure 15–6. The more rapidly a beam is attenuated (i.e., the greater the value of μ), the smaller the amount of material through which it must travel to fall by a factor of 0.5 (i.e., the smaller the HVL).

SOLUTION: $1/\mu$. The beam is reduced to 0.37 of its intensity over a thickness of $1/\mu$ cm, but falls by only a factor of a half over $x_{0.5}$ cm.

7. THE PHOTON MEAN FREE PATH IS EQUAL TO THE CHARACTERISTIC ATTENUATION THICKNESS

The photon *mean free path*, $\langle x \rangle_{\text{photon}}$, is the average distance that a photon travels (or, if you prefer, the distance that the average photon travels) before colliding. The paths of some photons in a very thick block of matter are shown in Figure 15–7A, with interactions indicated by crosses. (For simplicity only photoelectric events are considered here, so that no newly created scatter photons confuse things.) Figure 15–7B indicates the relative number of photons surviving to any depth. From Figure 15–7, we might anticipate that the mean free path length might be somewhere in the range of $x_{0.5}$ or $x_{0.37}$. In fact, the mean free path turns out to be numerically the same as the characteristic attenuation distance, $x_{0.37}$:

$$\langle x \rangle_{\text{photon}} = x_{0.37} = 1/\mu \qquad (15.9)$$

The relative number of x-ray photons surviving at least to the particular depth x is given by Equation 15.3b. The probability that a primary photon at depth x will undergo an interaction event over the next small Δx is $\Delta I/I(x) = -\mu \cdot \Delta x$. By Equation 13.10, the compound probability that a photon will both travel the distance x (give or take a little) and then interact in a slice of thickness Δx is proportional to $(e^{-\mu \cdot x})(\mu \cdot \Delta x)$. The photon mean path length may then be determined from the weighted average of x; that is, $\int x \cdot (e^{-\mu \cdot x}) \cdot (\mu \cdot dx)$. A little integral calculus reveals that the photon mean free path is none other than the reciprocal of μ, (Equation 15.9). The greater the attenuation coefficient, the shorter the path length that the average photon travels before suffering a collision.

This provides yet another interpretation of μ, as the inverse of the photon mean free path.

μ is thus a parameter reflecting three important facets of the physical process of beam attenuation. First, it reveals the macroscopic, global behavior of the beam, through $I(x)/I(0) = e^{-\mu \cdot x}$, where $\mu = 1/x_{0.37}$. Second, it is a measure of the microscopic, local aspects of the photoelectric absorption and Compton scattering of individual x-ray photons by matter, as manifest in the expression $\mu = -\Delta n/n \cdot \Delta x$. Third, $1/\mu$ is the distance traveled by the average photon before interacting with the matter it is passing through. And the third of these interpretations of μ provides a conceptual link between the first two.

8. HARDENING AND SOFTENING A BREMSSTRAHLUNG BEAM ALTER ITS ENERGY SPECTRUM (AND μ)

Under conditions of good geometry, the energy spectrum for monochromatic radiation is unchanged in passage through matter. After traveling through two HVLs of water, for example, the intensity of a beam of 140-keV technetium-99m gamma ray photons is reduced by a factor of 4, but the relative number

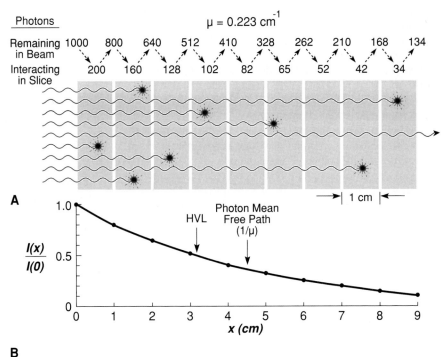

Figure 15–7. The distance that the average photon in a beam travels (= the average distance that a photon travels) before undergoing a collision is called the mean free path. **A.** The number of photons remaining in the beam at any depth, for our example, and the number interacting at that depth. Here, 1000 photons are incident on a thick block of material (partitioned into 1-cm layers for our convenience). With $\mu = 0.223$ cm^{-1}, for example, $n(1\ \text{cm}) = 1000 \cdot e^{-(0.223\ \text{cm}^{-1}) \cdot (1\ \text{cm})} = 800$ remain after passage through the first centimeter, and 200 are removed from the beam. An additional 160 are removed in the second, leaving 640, and so on. Note that the thin-layer approximation suggests (incorrectly) the removal of $\mu \cdot n \cdot \Delta x = (0.223\ \text{cm}^{-1})(1000)(1\ \text{cm}) = 223$ photons in the first 1 cm. (The problem is that here, a 1 cm slice is not thin enough.) **B.** By keeping track, in this fashion, of the numbers of photons interacting at different depths, one can calculate the average interaction depth. With exponential attenuation of a beam, the mean free path is $1/\mu$, (= 4.5 cm, here). The HVL is $0.693/\mu = 3.1$ cm.

of photons at each energy (i.e., the shape of the spectrum) is unaffected. The value of μ is therefore unchanged, as is evident also from the absence of curvature in Figure 15–2B.

For a 100-kVp bremsstrahlung beam passing through a patient, the situation is somewhat different. As Chapter 14 showed, lower-energy photons are almost always removed from a beam much more readily than are those of higher energies. (Indeed, the job of the filter at the exit window of an x-ray tube is to remove useless, but dose-depositing, low-energy photons.) The remaining photons will be of higher average energy, and the beam is said to have been *hardened*. Its photons will be scattered or absorbed at a lower rate, and it will grow more penetrating the deeper it goes. The degree of beam hardening that will occur within a patient decreases rapidly as the amount of initial beam filtration is increased.

With beam hardening, μ is *not* constant, but rather tends to increase somewhat with depth within the medium. As purely exponential attenuation is characterized by a constant value of μ, by definition, beam hardening leads to attenuation that is not perfectly exponential (Fig. 15–8).

_____ **EXERCISE 15–9.** _____

One common measure of the spectral characteristics of a beam is the ratio of the second HVL to the first HVL, as the beam passes through a reference material, such as aluminum or water. For the beam in water in Figure 15–8, what is this ratio?

SOLUTION: The second and first HVLs are 2 and 1.5 cm, respectively, so the ratio is 1.33. The beam hardens considerably in the first few centimeters.

Another process that causes μ to change is the *softening* that arises when lower-energy Compton scatter photons end

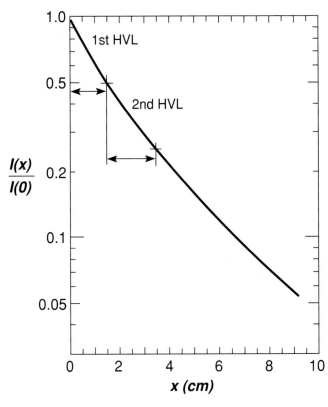

Figure 15–8. For a nonmonochromatic beam, or when scatter radiation reaches the detector, the attenuation is not purely exponential. One measure of beam quality is the ratio of the second and the first half-value layer thicknesses.

up within the beam, when the condition of good geometry does not prevail. Scatter photons are largely removed from a diagnostic beam, before they reach the screen/film cassette, by an antiscatter grid. But scatter, and beam softening, must be taken into account in the calculation of dose within a patient and in planning the shielding requirements for a radiology suite.

To summarize a complicated situation in simple terms: A diagnostic bremsstrahlung beam is normally attenuated nearly, but not exactly, exponentially by the tissues of the patient. And the beam may harden somewhat in the process.

9. EQUIVALENT (EFFECTIVE) ENERGY IS A USEFUL MEASURE OF BEAM QUALITY

Because of hardening (and, to a lesser extent, softening) effects, the bremsstrahlung energy spectrum changes as a beam passes through matter. It is therefore not possible to come up with a single parameter that completely accounts for the energy dependence of the beam's behavior. Still, it is necessary to be able to describe the overall *quality* of the beam at least approximately.

The kVp and HVL in a standard reference material (usually aluminum) together provide a characterization of the beam from an x-ray tube. Although partial, this characterization is adequate for most purposes. It is less reliable for a beam at depth in attenuating material, however, as the distribution of photon energies shifts away from that of simple filtered bremsstrahlung.

The *equivalent (effective) energy* of a polychromatic beam is another approximate but useful measure of beam quality. The equivalent energy is the energy of the photons in a monochromatic beam that would be attenuated at the same rate in some reference material (typically aluminum) as the beam of interest (Fig. 15–9).

Figure 15–10, obtained from Figure 13–2, presents the HVL of a monochromatic beam in aluminum as a function of

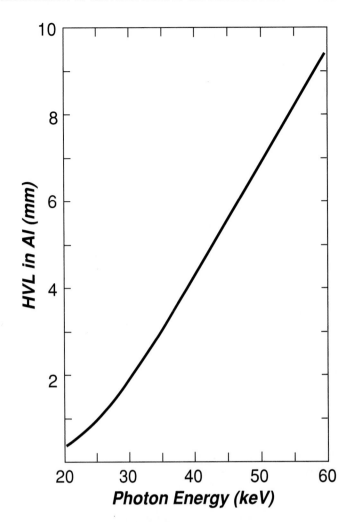

Figure 15–10. HVL thickness (= 0.693/μ) in aluminum as a function of monochromatic photon energy. This chart, together with Table 15–1, allows a rough estimate of the equivalent energies of bremsstrahlung beams for various combinations of potential (kVp) and total filtration.

photon energy. This and Table 15–1 together provide for a rough but quick determination of the effective energy of a bremsstrahlung beam. Table 15–1 displays measured values of HVL in aluminum, in millimeters, as a function of tube potential (kVp) and total (inherent plus added) filtration (millimeters of aluminum, not to be confused with the HVL in aluminum). Once the HVL in aluminum is known, the equivalent monochromatic photon energy can be learned from Figure 15–10.

_____ **EXERCISE 15–10.** _____

What is the quality of the 80-kVp beam produced by a three-phase generator, with 2.5-mm Al total filtration? What is the equivalent energy? What is the HVL in muscle?

SOLUTION: From Table 15–1, the quality is 2.7 mm HVL in Al. From Figure 15–10, the monochromatic energy corresponding to this HVL in Al is 33 keV. μ for a 33-keV beam in muscle is 0.34 cm⁻¹, (Fig. 13–2), so the HVL in muscle is 0.693/0.34 = 2.0 cm.

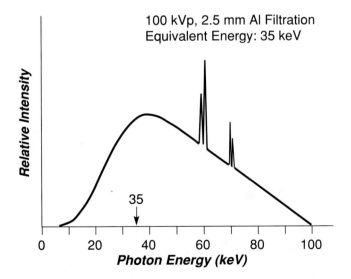

100 kVp, 2.5 mm Al Filtration
Equivalent Energy: 35 keV

35

Figure 15–9. A 100-kVp beam with 2.5 mm Al total (inherent plus added) filtration is attenuated in aluminum at about the same rate as a monochromatic 35-keV beam.

TABLE 15–1. BEAM QUALITY, EXPRESSED AS HALF-VALUE LAYER THICKNESS IN ALUMINUM, FOR VARIOUS COMBINATIONS OF TUBE POTENTIAL AND BEAM FILTRATION[a]

Total Beam Filtration (mm Al)	Tube Potential (kVp)			
	60	80	100	120
1.5	(1.4)	[b]	[b]	[b]
2.5	2.2	2.7	3.3	4.0
	(2.0)	(2.4)	(2.8)	(3.3)
3.5	2.6	3.2	3.9	4.6
	(2.3)	(2.9)	(3.4)	(4.0)

[a]Values are HVL thicknesses in Al (mm), three-phase generator. Values for a one-phase generator are in parentheses.
[b]Minimum of 2.5 mm Al total filtration required for operating potential > 70 kVp.
From National Council on Radiation Protection and Measurements (NCRP): Medical X-ray, Electron Beam, and Gamma-ray Protection for Energies up to 50 MeV (Equipment Design, Performance, and Use), Report No. 102. Bethesda, MD: NCRP, 1989 (Table B.2), with permission.

The effective energy is a construct of limited usefulness. The fact that a beam hardens as it passes through tissue means that its effective energy is only a coarse measure of its overall ability to penetrate a body. Also, clinical situations require fields of finite dimensions; the attenuation coefficient, on the other hand, is defined for the case of good geometry, and measured with very small fields, so that almost no scatter reaches the detector. An accurate description of the interaction of a beam with matter must take both of these factors into account. Still, the effective energy is handy for back-of-the-envelope calculations, and generally gives results that are not too unreasonable. We shall make use of it on several occasions.

10. THE (NEARLY) EXPONENTIAL DEPTH–DOSE CURVE

It should be apparent from past chapters that x-ray energy is *deposited* in matter in a two-step process:

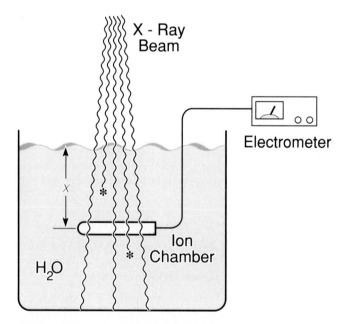

Figure 15–11. Experimental setup for determining percent depth dose (PDD) in water. The important parameters are beam quality (i.e., spectrum, or effective energy), field size at the water surface, and source-to-surface distance (SSD).

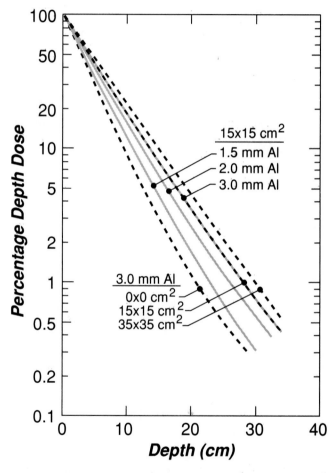

Figure 15–12. PDD curves for three 15 × 15-cm[2] beams of different qualities (expressed in HVL in aluminum; see Fig. 15–10), and dashed curves for three beams of the same quality (3 mm Al) but different field sizes. The lower the equivalent energy, the less penetrating the beam, and the more rapidly the intensity and dose diminish with depth. The larger the field, the more scatter radiation reaches the detector, and the more slowly dose drops off. (*From National Council on Radiation Protection and Measurements (NCRP): Medical X-ray, Electron Beam, and Gamma-ray Protection for Energies up to 50 MeV (Equipment, Design, Performance, and Use), Report No. 102. Bethesda, MD: NCRP, 1989 (Table B.8), with permission.*)

- X-ray photons interact with the matter by means of the photoelectric and Compton mechanisms.
- Then the high-velocity electrons thus liberated expend their kinetic energy in exciting and ionizing other atoms and molecules that they pass near.

The energy per unit mass actually deposited in the matter in this fashion is called the **dose** (see Chapter 5, Section 11).

The relationship between the intensity of a beam at some point in a medium and the dose deposited there will be explored in Chapter 30. But it should come as no surprise that as the intensity of the beam diminishes with depth in the material, so also does the locally deposited dose. And because the intensity falls off nearly exponentially, the dose does as well.

Dose anywhere in a medium may be expressed relative to its value at some reference point. At diagnostic energies, the reference point is commonly taken to be the center of the beam at its point of entry at the surface of the medium. The dose $D(x)$ at depth x on the beam's *central axis* is recorded as a fraction of the dose $D(0)$ at the surface,

$$PDD(x) = 100 \cdot D(x) / D(0) \qquad (15.10)$$

and is called the **percent depth dose.** $PDD(x)$ is a function of the effective energy of the beam (or some other measure of beam quality); its area at the surface, A; and the source to the surface of the medium (or to the skin of the patient) distance, or SSD.

Tables of $PDD(x,A,SSD,hf)$ for water may be obtained by means of the experimental procedure shown in Figure 15–11. The readings from an ionization chamber or diode detector are monitored as it is moved vertically (under computer control) in a tank of water, and the results plotted as a PDD or *depth–dose* curve, as in Figure 15–12. The rapidity with which this curve falls off with depth depends strongly on the energy of the photon beam. In contradistinction to the case of good geometry, here one finds a significant inverse square effect (indeed, the source–detector separation is intentionally being varied) and photon multiple scattering, in addition to simple exponential attenuation of the photon fluence. These three processes (attenuation, inverse square effect, and scatter radiation) combine to determine the shape of the PDD curve. $PDD(x)$ may not be strictly exponential but, perhaps somewhat surprisingly, it is not too far wide of the mark.

Chapter 16

Detecting Ionizing Radiation

1. Ionization
2. The Ionization of Air: Air Kerma and Exposure, Again
3. A Semiconductor Behaves (Somewhat) Like a Solid Gas
4. Materials that Glow
5. The Mechanisms of Fluorescence and Phosphorescence
6. The Scintillation Detector: A Fluorescent Crystal Watched by a Photomultiplier Tube

Energy is transferred from an x-ray photon to matter in a two-step process. First, the x-ray undergoes either a photoelectric or a Compton collision with an atom, resulting in the ejection of a photoelectron or Compton electron. That electron then moves rapidly through the medium, expending its considerable energy (typically several KeV or tens of KeV when first liberated) in exciting and ionizing hundreds or thousands of additional ions. What happens next depends on the nature of the irradiated medium. Of especial interest to us are the effects of ionizing radiation on air, on luminescent materials, and on biologic tissues.

If two electrodes are attached to an adequate voltage, a current will flow when the air between them is ionized. This serves as the basis for the ion chamber radiation detector and for the definition of the conventional unit of exposure, the roentgen (R). In ways, a semiconductor diode behaves like an ion chamber.

A luminescent material responds to ionizing radiation by emitting light. This phenomenon is put to direct use in the display surface of a cathode ray tube, in the screens of a radiographic cassette, in the output screen of an image intensifier tube, and in the scintillation detectors used in computerized tomography (CT), nuclear medicine, and radiation safety.

The exposure of film to x-irradiation is deferred to the next chapter.

The effects of ionizing radiation on tissues will be considered in Chapters 30 through 33.

1. IONIZATION

An x-ray photon transfers energy to a medium in a two-stage process. First, the photon ionizes an atom of the medium by means of a photoelectric or Compton collision. In the second stage, the resultant high-velocity photoelectron or Compton electron subsequently interacts, by means of the Coulombic (electrostatic) force, with atomic electrons along its path; it thereby dissipates its kinetic energy in exciting and ionizing hundreds or thousands of atoms and molecules, leaving be-

hind cations and additional free electrons which, too, dissipate their energy in causing even more excitations and ionizations.

In radiography, it is by means of the first stage alone, photon–electron interactions occurring in the body of the patient, that photons are removed from an x-ray beam by different tissues at different rates. The actual deposition of dose in *tissue*, although of importance for reasons of radiation safety, is not relevant to the formation of the primary x-ray shadow image. For photons striking a radiation detector, however, the situation is very different. There, both the initial photon–electron interaction and the subsequent ionization of the detector material are critically important to the operation of the device. This is all laid out schematically in Table 16–1.

2. THE IONIZATION OF AIR: AIR KERMA AND EXPOSURE, AGAIN

The ionization of air and the concepts of *air kerma* and *exposure* were discussed briefly in Chapter 11, Section 2. Exposure is measured in *roentgens* (R), where one roentgen is the amount of ionizing radiation that liberates 2.58×10^{-4} coulombs of charge (of either sign) per kilogram of air (see Fig. 11–3). Exposure is largely being supplanted by a closely related construct, **air kerma**. Air kerma is, in effect, the dose (deposited ionizing energy per unit mass) to air, and it is commonly expressed in centigrays (cGy).

Exposure and air kerma have two virtues that, together, make them extremely useful constructs. First, they are very easy to quantify through direct measurement. Clinical dosime-

TABLE 16–1. THE TWO STAGES OF PHOTON ENERGY TRANSFER, IN A PATIENT AND IN A RADIATION DETECTOR, AND SOME RELEVANT CONSIDERATIONS

	Patient's Body	Image Receptor
Stage 1: photon–electron interaction	Image formation	Photon detection
Stage 2: ionizations by fast electron	Dose/risk	Detector response

try is of central importance both in the formation of optimal radiographic images and in the minimization of radiation hazards to patients and medical staff. Measurements of exposure or air kerma by means of air-filled ion chambers (Fig. 11–2), form the basis of much of routine dosimetry. Small ion chambers find use in the clinic for checking the outputs of diagnostic and radiotherapy machines, for assessing quantities of radiopharmaceuticals, for performing radiation protection surveys, and as personal dosimeters.

Second, knowledge of the exposure or air kerma at a point in space allows the rapid calculation of dose to adjacent or surrounding tissues or other materials. As will be seen in Chapter 30, if the exposure is determined (by means of an ion chamber) to be X roentgens, then the corresponding dose D in rads is given by

$$D = f_{\text{med}} \cdot X \qquad (16.1)$$

(A similar expression relates dose to air kerma.) The values of the f factor (also called the *exposure-to-dose conversion factor*), f_{med}, depend on the nature of the material being irradiated and on the energy of the beam. For most tissues and energies, f_{med} happens to be numerically near unity. Thus, the exposure (in roentgens), the air kerma (in cGy), and the dose to tissue (also in cGy) at a point are numerically close to one another. As a result, roentgens and centigrays (rads) are often used interchangeably, even though they quantify somewhat different entities.

3. A SEMICONDUCTOR BEHAVES (SOMEWHAT) LIKE A SOLID GAS

In its simplest form, a piece of semiconductor material such as silicon behaves somewhat like an ionization chamber. Imagine that the two sides of a piece of pure silicon or germanium are attached to the poles of a battery, by way of an electrometer (Fig. 16–1A). Normally the valence band of the semiconducting material is almost entirely filled, and the conduction band practically empty. But ionizing radiation excites electrons from the valence into the conduction band, and the magnitude of the resulting current is proportional to the exposure rate.

Clinical detectors are normally not made of pure semiconductor. In part because of problems arising at the metal–semiconductor contacts where wires are attached, the leakage or *dark current* (i.e., the flow through the device even in the absence of radiation) is unacceptably high. The semiconductor diode (see Chapter 8, Section 11) provides a solution to this difficulty.

If a diode is reverse-biased by a few volts (Fig. 16–1B), it normally will conduct only a very slight dark current, of the order of 10^{-13} A. But a significant current will flow while electrons are being liberated within it by radiation. An incoming x-ray or gamma ray (or beta or alpha particle) may expend all its energy in exciting valence band electrons into the conduction band; as a consequence, the diode conducts an amount of charge roughly proportional to the energy of the incident photon or charged particle (Fig. 16–1C). Solid state *photodetectors* operate in a similar fashion, but with electron–hole pairs produced by light, rather than ionizing radiation.

Semiconductor radiation detectors exhibit some significant advantages over ion chambers. Electrons and holes, once produced in a semiconductor, are very mobile, and can be swept to the contacts in a small fraction of a microsecond. That

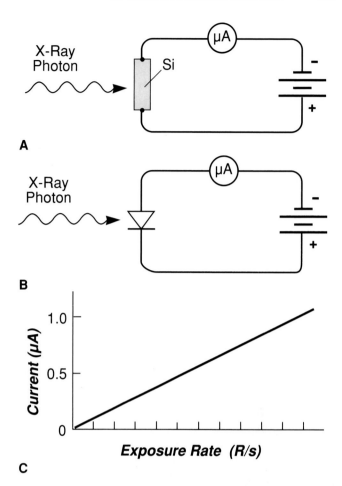

Figure 16–1. Semiconductor radiation detector. **A.** A piece of pure silicon normally conducts only slightly when attached to a source of a few volts. Conduction increases significantly, however, when ionizing radiation excites valence band electrons into the conduction band. **B.** A diode biased in the reverse direction performs even better, because the "dark" current is lower. **C.** The current (in microamperes) through the reverse-biased diode is proportional to the rate of its exposure to ionizing radiation.

fast response allows the detector to follow precisely the subtle variations in output of an x-ray tube as a function of time, as a quality assurance test.

Also, because of its high density ($\rho = 2.3$ g/cm^3 for Si) and the small amount of energy required to produce an ion pair (3 to 4 eV), a diode can be thousands of times more sensitive than an air-filled ion chamber of the same size. As a consequence, it can be built small. A mosaic of independent, microscopic diodes on a single chip, for example, can be used directly for x-ray or optical imaging purposes.

Finally, a diode detector is able to determine the energy spectrum of the ionizing radiation. When an initial x-ray or gamma-ray interaction is a photoelectric event, virtually all the energy of the incident photon is transferred to the photoelectron and eventually expended in the semiconductor material. The number of electrons elevated into the conduction band, and the size of the associated current pulse, is therefore proportional to the photon's energy. (The pulses arising with

Compton events, in which less than the full photon energy is imparted to the Compton electron, would tend to be correspondingly smaller). This provides a way of obtaining the energy spectrum of a radiation beam. Alternatively, an *energy discriminator* circuit can be employed to respond only to those photons of energies within a specified *energy window*. Compton scatter photons of lower energy can be excluded, for example, and thereby prevented from degrading the quality of an image.

4. MATERIALS THAT GLOW

In some radiographic procedures, film is exposed directly to x-rays. Much more commonly, however, the x-rays interact with a luminescent intensifying screen, and it is light from the screen that initiates physicochemical changes in the film. Similarly, the image intensifier and TV monitor of a fluoroscopy system contain luminescent materials. And the front end of a nuclear medicine gamma camera is a luminescent crystal, as is a thermoluminescence dosimeter (TLD) employed for staff or patient personal dosimetry.

Luminescence refers to the emission of visible light by a substance exposed to irradiation or certain other stimuli. If the emission is immediate (i.e., within 10^{-8} seconds), then the process is called *fluorescence*. If there is a delay, then the material is *phosphorescent*. The distinction reflects the different physical mechanisms involved in each, and determines the possible applications. Finally, a *thermoluminescent* material emits light following irradiation, but only upon heating.

Luminescent materials typically are insulator salts that have been highly purified and then, when in molten form, doped with precise amounts of special impurities. The impurities create discrete quantum states, somewhat like the orbitals of free atoms, with energies lying in the forbidden band or band gap between the (nearly filled) valance band and the (practically empty) conduction band of the host material (see Chapter 7, Section 3). Such a state, called an *electron trap*, is capable of holding one electron.

For some kinds of dopant, an impurity atom binds one of its electrons rather loosely. This "trapped" electron will then be almost free, with the trap state lying just below the conduction band (Fig. 16–2). *Phonons*, which are quanta of thermal (vibrational) energy in the solid, will from time to time ele-

vate electrons out of their traps and into the conduction band. Alternatively, a phonon may provide the activation energy needed to dislodge an electron from a trap, after which it drops into a hole in the valence band. The likelihood that a trap is normally filled or empty is determined by the distance (in energy) of the state below the bottom of the conduction band and by the temperature of the medium, which controls the number and energies of the phonons present.

5. THE MECHANISMS OF FLUORESCENCE AND PHOSPHORESCENCE

Whether a *luminescent* material displays *fluorescence, phosphorescence,* or *thermoluminescence* is determined by the dynamics of the traps and electrons.

With one form of *fluorescence*, the traps are normally filled with electrons (Fig. 16–3A). A photoelectron or Compton electron (produced by an x-ray photon) will elevate other electrons out of the valence band into the conduction band (Fig. 16–3B). Electrons that until now were contentedly inhabiting their traps drop immediately into the newly available, lower-energy hole states (Fig. 16–3C), with the emission of visible light photons. Finally (Fig. 16–3D), electrons in the conduction band repopulate the recently vacated trap states.

The individual impurity atoms that serve as electron traps have similar, but not identical, local surroundings. The traps therefore lie nearly, but not exactly, the same distance below the conduction band. The fluorescence photons thus give rise to a band of visible light (Fig. 16–3E), rather than a sharp line spectrum. The wavelengths of these photons do not depend on the energy of the incident x-rays that initiated the process (just as the energies of the characteristic x-rays emitted by an isolated atom after a photoelectric event do not depend on the energy of the instigating x-ray). The total number of holes produced in the valence band, on the other hand, and the *intensity* of the flash of light emitted when they are filled are proportional to the energy of the original x-ray. This makes possible energy discrimination, like that just described for semiconductors.

The electron traps in a typical *phosphor* are normally empty. When a photoelectron or Compton electron lifts electrons into the conduction band, some will drop rapidly into the empty traps. If, for quantum mechanical reasons, a direct transition from a trap to a hole in the valence band is not allowed, then the system must return to its ground state by a more circuitous, and slower, route: phonons of sufficient energy will, from time to time, elevate an electron from a trap back into the conduction band, from which it can fall into a hole, emitting visible light.

Thermoluminescence is similar to phosphorescence, with the difference that the traps lie substantially lower in energy (i.e., further below the bottom of the conduction band). As a consequence, few of the electrons that drop into these traps will be excited back to the conduction band by room temperature phonons. When the sample is heated, however, there will be more and higher-energy phonons capable of doing the job. If the temperature of a sample is raised at a constant rate, then the *glow curve* will be of the form Figure 16–4A. The area under this curve is proportional to the dose imparted to the material. This is the basis for the operation of TLDs (Fig. 16–4B).

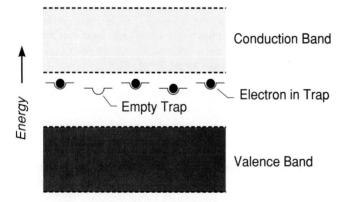

Figure 16–2. Because of the presence of foreign atoms or other imperfections, an insulator may have electron "trap" states with energies lying within the forbidden band gap.

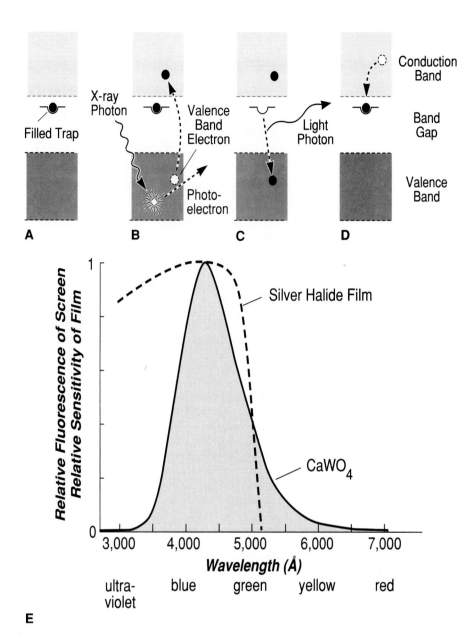

A   **B**   **C**   **D**

E

Figure 16–3. A common mechanism of fluorescence in an insulator involves the filling and emptying of electron traps that lie a few electron volts above the valence band. **A.** Normally, a trap contains an electron. **B.** The fluorescence process is initiated by an x-ray or gamma ray photon. The resulting photoelectron or Compton electron is excited into the insulator's conduction band, and excites other electrons into it as well, leaving behind "holes" in the valence band. **C.** The electron in the trap can drop into a valence band hole, and in the process emits a photon of visible light. **D.** An electron in the conduction band drops into the trap, and the system is ready to go through it all again. **E.** Because of small differences in local physical environments of the individual traps, their distances (in energy) above the top of the valence band are not all the same. For this and other reasons, the visible light emission spectrum is not a sharp peak, but rather a band. The emission band for calcium tungstate (until recently, the standard fluorescent material in radiographic cassettes), shown here, peaks in the blue region of the spectrum. $CaWO_4$ screens are normally used with ordinary silver halide film, which is highly sensitive to blue light, as indicated by the dashed line. Some rare earth screens emit predominantly green light and require films that respond to lower-energy light photons.

6. THE SCINTILLATION DETECTOR: A FLUORESCENT CRYSTAL WATCHED BY A PHOTOMULTIPLIER TUBE

One important application of fluorescent materials, as radiographic intensification screens, has already been mentioned. Another, which finds extensive use in CT, nuclear medicine, radiation safety, and elsewhere, is at the front end of a *scintillation detector*.

A scintillation detector consists of a single crystal of fluorescent material and a *photomultiplier tube* (PMT) (Fig. 16–5). When excited by an x-ray or gamma ray photon, the crystal produces a burst of light. The PMT detects that light and generates a corresponding electrical signal.

A fluorescent material that has found widespread use in medical scintillation detectors is sodium iodide doped about 0.1% by weight with thallium, NaI[Tl]. Because of its relatively high density (3.7 g/cm³) and effective atomic number ($Z_{eff} = 45$), the *intrinsic efficiency* for capturing diagnostic energy x-rays and gamma rays by means of the photoelectric effect is high. The thallium increases the crystal's *conversion efficiency* tenfold, so that as much as 25% of the gamma ray energy imparted may be reemitted from NaI[Tl] as light photons. With the absorption of an x-ray or gamma ray photon, the intensity of the resultant pulse of scintillation light (of mean wavelength 4200 Å) rises for about 30 nanoseconds, and then decays exponentially with a characteristic time of 0.25 microsecond. Sodium iodide is hygroscopic (extracts water out of the air), and the crystal must be protected from moisture. A single crystal is normally employed so that light will not be lost through scattering or absorption at the boundaries of compacted polycrystalline material.

A photomultiplier tube is a vacuum tube that, when exposed to a very faint flash of visible light, generates a pulse of charge. The process begins when a light photon ejects an electron from the bialkali (K_2CsSb) *photocathode* by means of the photoelectric effect. The photoelectron is accelerated through 200 or 300 V toward the first, "tea cup"-shaped *dynode*. On

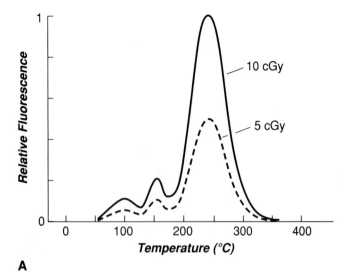

A

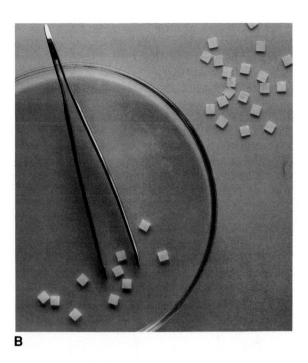

B

Figure 16–4. Thermoluminescent dosimetry. **A.** The glow curves of a thermoluminescent dosimeter (TLD) that was exposed to 5 cGy, read (dashed line), annealed for reuse, exposed to 10 cGy, and read anew (solid line). **B.** The radiation-sensitive component of a TLD badge is a thin chip, a few millimeters across, of thermoluminescent material such as specially doped lithium fluoride (LiF). *(Photo courtesy of Victoreen, Inc., Cleveland, OH.)*

striking it, the first electron dislodges several new ones, each of which is accelerated toward the second dynode, and so on. Typically there are 10 dynodes, each held 100 V more positive than the one before. For every photoelectron originally ejected from the photocathode by a flash of scintillation light, a million or so electrons eventually reach the final dynode, giving rise to a significant voltage pulse. As with the fluorescent screen and film of radiography, it is critical that the spectral response of the PMT be matched to the emission spectrum of the scintillating crystal.

As with the semiconductor detector, an important characteristic of a scintillator/PMT detector is its ability to determine the energy of an incident x-ray or gamma ray. The number of visible light photons produced in the fluorescent crystal with the absorption of a high-energy photon is nearly linear in its energy. But the number of photoelectrons kicked off the photocathode of the PMT is proportional to the number of photons in the light burst. And the same number of electrons reach the final dynode for each of these ejected photoelectrons. The size of the voltage pulse coming out of the detector system thus

Figure 16–5. A scintillation detector consists of a scintillating crystal, such as thallium-doped sodium iodide NaI[Tl], attached to a photomultiplier tube (PMT). The scintillation crystal produces a burst of light of intensity proportional to the energy of the initiating x-ray photon. The light ejects from the photocathode of the PMT a number of electrons proportional to the intensity of the light burst. Every photoelectron is accelerated to the first dynode, where it ejects several secondary electrons. Each of these, in turn, heads for the second dynode, where the process repeats itself. The end result is the arrival of a bunch of electrons at the anode and an output voltage pulse of size proportional to the original x-ray photon energy.

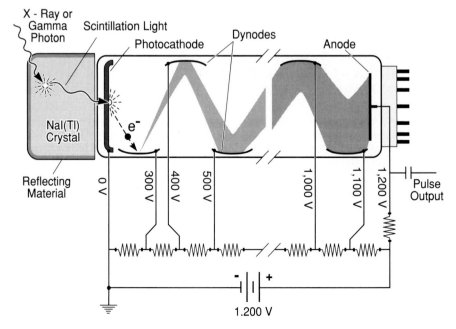

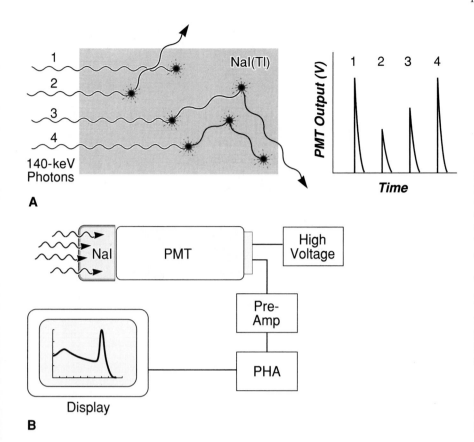

Figure 16–6. A scintillation detector can be used to determine the energies of high-energy photons. But even a monochromatic source produces a complex (rather than a single peak) spectrum. **A.** Four 140-keV photons strike a scintillation detector in sequence. Photons 1 and 4 deposit all their energy within the NaI[Tl] crystal. Some of the energy of photons 2 and 3 escapes as Compton scatter, however, and the PMT output pulses are of correspondingly lower voltage. **B.** The amplitudes of the voltage pulses are assessed by a pulse height analyzer (PHA). The PHA keeps track of the numbers of pulses that arrive with the various voltages, and displays this information as a histogram. The pulse height spectrum for technetium-99*m* is not a single sharp peak at the voltage corresponding to 140 keV. The full width at half-maximum (FWHM) of the 140-keV photopeak is 15 to 20 keV, rather, and there is lower-energy structure in the spectrum attributable to Compton scatter in the NaI[Tl] crystal and to other causes.

provides a direct measure of the energy of the photon that triggered it.

Figure 16–6 illustrates the way this all works, with a sample of technetium-99*m*. Every interacting gamma ray gives rise to an electrical pulse at the output of the PMT, of amplitude proportional to the amount of gamma ray energy actually deposited in the scintillation crystal (Fig. 16–6A). The voltage of each pulse is determined by means of a *pulse height analyzer* (*PHA*) circuit (Fig. 16–6B); and the relative number of pulses as a function of pulse voltage, that is, the *pulse height spectrum* or *distribution*, is displayed as a histogram. The *photopeak* corresponds to the complete absorption of a 140-keV photon; lower-

energy structures in the pulse height spectrum correspond to Compton events in the crystal and a variety of instrumental effects.

As noted earlier, pulse height discrimination makes *energy windowing* possible. A *discriminator* can be set, for example, to accept only those pulses belonging to the photopeak of one radionuclide. That greatly reduces the effects of scatter radiation or, when several radionuclides are simultaneously present, allows the system to respond to the gamma rays from only one of them. Such energy windowing is used in the formation of nuclear medicine images by gamma cameras.

Chapter 17

Mapping Exposure on Film

1. **The Active Ingredient of Film: Microcrystals of Silver Iodobromide**
2. **The Exposure and Development of Film**
3. **The Optical Density of Developed Film**
4. **The Optical Density of Film Is Proportional to the Concentration of Metallic Silver (Ag)**
5. **The Characteristic (H&D) Curve**
6. **The Copying of Radiographs**
7. **Review of the Energy Transformation Processes Occurring in Radiography**

Photographic film has been the principal medium for the formation, storage, and transmission of radiographic images for nearly a century. Although over the next decade computer-based systems may largely supplant it, in some situations film will remain the most convenient and cost-effective way to go.

This chapter describes the composition of radiographic film, the radiation-induced formation of latent images in its silver halide microcrystals, and the development process that transforms some of those microcrystals into flecks of pure silver.

The opacity to light of a region of developed film, as parameterized by the optical density (OD), is directly proportional to the local concentration of metallic silver flecks. The concentration of this silver at a point, in turn, depends on the amount of radiation exposure that the screen–film system experienced there. The response of a screen–film system to irradiation is revealed in the characteristic curve, which relates OD to radiation exposure.

The capture of an x-ray image on film was discussed briefly in Chapter 2, Section 6.

1. THE ACTIVE INGREDIENT OF FILM: MICROCRYSTALS OF SILVER IODOBROMIDE

Radiographic film (Fig. 17–1) is a specialized form of photographic film. An *emulsion* of microscopic silver halide crystals suspended in gelatin forms coatings on both sides (usually) of a *base* of polyester. Antiabrasive *supercoats* on both sides protect the emulsion from wear and tear. Developed film must be nearly transparent where unexposed (although it is usually tinted slightly blue, to reduce eye strain) and possess some obvious mechanical properties: it must be strong but flexible, stable against any aging effects, and fire-resistant. And the emulsion and supercoat must be insoluble, but sufficiently permeable for the developer and fixer chemicals to diffuse in.

The active ingredient in film is the silver iodobromide microcrystals. The halide component consists typically of 90% to

99% bromide ions, and the rest are iodide. The silver halide is usually manufactured so as to form flat triangular microcrystals roughly 1 μm in greatest dimension (Fig. 17–2). Nearly all the silver and halide ions are situated at the sites of a highly regular crystalline lattice: Any ion of either sign is located in the middle of a cube, with ions of the opposite charge at the centers of the cube's six faces.

The crystal structure is not perfect, however, as bromide and iodide ions, which vie for anion sites, have different ionic radii. Because of the resultant mechanical strains within the crystal, a small number of silver ions find it energetically favorable to leave their normal lattice-site homes and settle into random, *interstitial* positions (Fig. 17–3). These interstitial silver ions are not held tightly in place and, with sufficient energy incentive, will wander throughout the crystal. The conditions of preparation of the emulsion (temperature, relative amount

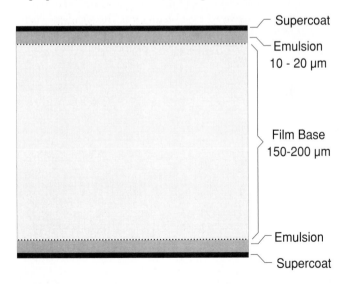

Figure 17–1. Radiographic film consists of a base, an emulsion that contains microscopic crystals of silver iodobromide, and protective coatings.

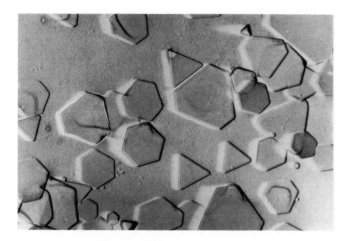

Figure 17–2. Microphotograph of flat, tabular grains of silver halide in film emulsion, with the flat side parallel to the base of the film. *(Courtesy of Arthur G. Haus and the Eastman Kodak Company.)*

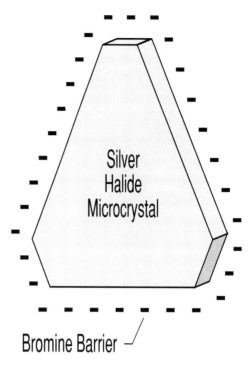

Figure 17–4. A silver iodobromide microcrystal is surfaced predominantly with bromide ions, which erect a negatively charged "bromine barrier" about the crystal. Excess (interstitial) silver ions within the crystal serve to maintain its overall charge neutrality.

of iodide, acidity, etc.) determine the average size of the crystals and the numbers and types of their structural imperfections. These, in turn, strongly affect the photographic properties of the film.

Although each crystal is electrically neutral on the whole, its surface tends to consist predominantly of negatively charged bromide anions (Fig. 17–4), with compensating silver cations at interstitial sites within. This *bromine barrier* strongly repels from the crystal surface any negatively charged ions (in particular, molecules of the developer) diffusing through the gelatin of the film, a fact that is of profound importance when the film is being developed.

2. EXPOSURE AND DEVELOPMENT OF FILM

Exposure of Film

Radiographic film is normally exposed to light emitted (on x-ray stimulation) from a fluoroscopic intensifying screen of a cassette. Collision of one x-ray photon with an intensifying screen results in the release of thousands or tens of thousands of visible light photons. To be transformed (during development) into a fleck of silver, any individual microcrystal of silver iodobromide in the film must have absorbed tens of those light photons.

The photographic process begins for a typical silver halide microcrystal when one light photon from the fluorescent screen liberates an electron (Fig. 17–5A) from one of its Br⁻ anions:

$$Br^- \rightarrow Br + e^- \qquad (17.1)$$

The neutral bromine atom, bearing no charge, is no longer held tightly in place in the ionic lattice, and diffuses out of the crystal, into the film's gelatin, and eventually out of the film altogether.

The electron that is freed from the bromine ion enjoys a more glorious fate. A trace amount of a sulfur-containing agent such as allylthiourea was added to the gelatin during manufacture of the film, and this reacted with the silver iodobromide microcrystals to deposit small *sensitivity specks* of silver sulfide on their surfaces. A sensitivity speck can act something like an electron trap, and is capable of capturing the newly liberated electron.

Having trapped an electron, the sensitivity speck is now negatively charged (Fig. 17–5B). It therefore attracts positively

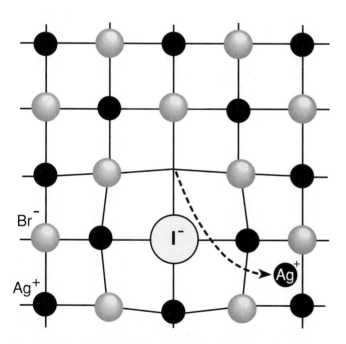

Figure 17–3. The radii of bromide and the iodide ions are different. As a result, small amounts of added iodide give rise to local stresses and strains in a silver bromide crystal. This causes some silver ions to move out of their normal crystal lattice positions and into interstitial locations, from which they can easily be dislodged.

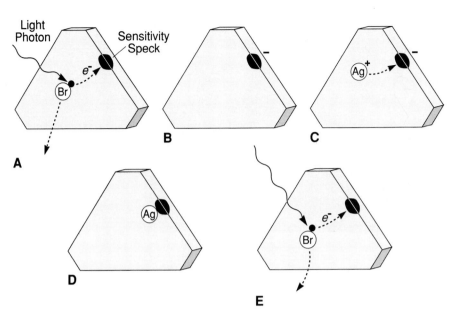

Figure 17–5. Process by which light creates a latent image center at a sensitivity speck in a silver iodobromide crystal. **A.** A light photon removes the outermost electron from a bromide anion. The bromine atom (now uncharged) diffuses out of the crystal. The liberated *electron* wanders through the crystal and is trapped at the sensitivity speck. **B.** The speck is now negatively charged. **C.** It draws an interstitial silver cation to itself. **D.** The electron on the sensitivity speck neutralizes the charge of the silver ion, and the resulting silver atom is deposited there. **E.** Another light photon causes the process to repeat. The deposition of 10 or so silver atoms at the sensitivity speck transforms it into a latent image center. A crystal with a latent image center will be transformed into a fleck of pure silver during the development process.

charged, mobile interstitial silver ions to it (Fig. 17–5C). On reaching the sensitivity speck, a silver ion is neutralized,

$$Ag^+ + e^- \rightarrow Ag \qquad (17.2)$$

and laid permanently to rest within the speck (Fig. 17–5D). The speck is electrically neutral again, and can trap another electron. The process is ready to repeat itself (Fig. 17–5E).

If 10 or so silver atoms are deposited in this fashion, the sensitivity speck becomes a **latent image center** that can trigger the transformation (during the development process) of the entire silver halide crystal into a grain of silver. A "latent image" is not an image in the conventional sense of the word, but refers, rather, to the pattern of silver halide microcrystals that have been activated by light or x-ray photons.

Development of Film

Those silver halide crystals that possess latent image centers are transformed into specks of metallic silver during **development,** and the others are left totally unaffected. This is an all-or-nothing event, in which a crystal either undergoes a complete metamorphosis or remains unaltered.

Developer consists of an alkali to raise the pH to an optimal level, a preservative, a restrainer that reduces fogging, and *developing agents* (Fig. 17–6). A **developer** is a reducing agent, a

donor of electrons to silver cations. The latent image center serves as an essential catalyst for the process. For although the electrons from the developer molecules are repelled by most of the crystal's negatively charged surface, the neutral silver atoms deposited at the sensitivity speck produce a break in the bromine barrier (Fig. 17–7A). At this place the developer can donate its electrons, which enter the crystal and proceed to reduce the remainder of the silver ions (Figs. 17–7B and 17–7C). A silver halide crystal with no latent image center, on the other hand, can successfully ward off the advances of the developer molecules, and thereby remain intact.

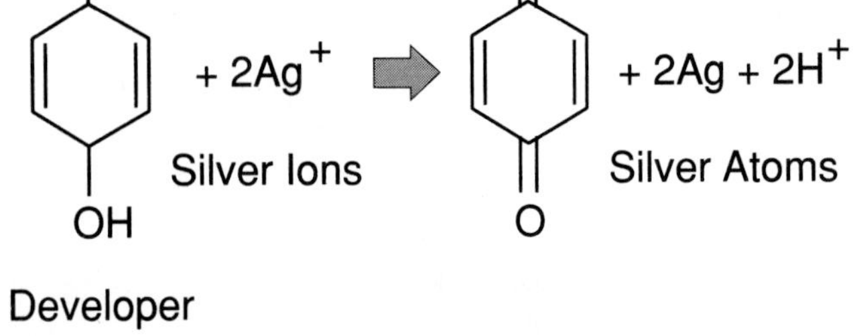

Development converts those silver halide crystals with latent image centers into flecks of silver, but leaves the others unscathed. Over time, however, any undeveloped silver halide crystals still present will spontaneously reduce to silver. It is therefore necessary to remove them from the gelatin soon after development, through the process of *fixation*. **Fixer** contains sodium or ammonium thiosulfate, commonly known as **hypo.** The thiosulfate binds tightly with the remaining silver ions to form a water-soluble complex

$$AgBr + S_2O_3^{2-} \rightarrow Br^- + \text{silver thiosulfate complex} \qquad (17.3)$$

that readily washes out of the gelatin.

To summarize, the postdevelopment concentration of metallic silver, [Ag], in film increases (but not linearly) with the amount of x-ray exposure. And the more silver in the film, the less easily can light get through it.

The situation is somewhat simpler for film exposed directly to the x-ray beam with no cassette. As a single photoelectron or Compton electron can immediately and directly liberate tens or hundreds of electrons and interstitial silver ions in a microcrystal, only one x-ray photon is required to create a latent image center. In the absence of an intensifying screen, the average concentration [Ag] of metallic silver flecks in developed film will then be proportional to the number of high-energy photons originally incident on the undeveloped film, hence to the exposure or air kerma, K_{air}:

$$[Ag] \sim K_{air} \quad \text{(no cassette)} \qquad (17.4)$$

Figure 17–6. The developer hydroquinone is a reducing agent that can give up electrons to two silver ions, transforming them into neutral silver atoms.

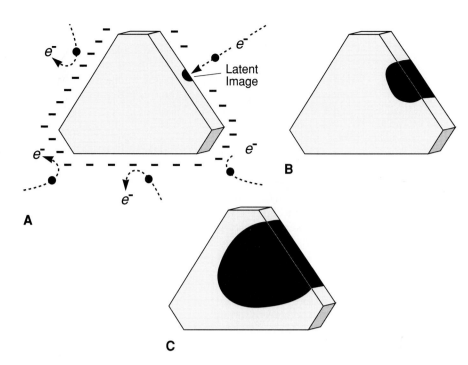

Figure 17-7. During development, silver halide microcrystals with latent image centers (and *only* those) are transformed into microcrystals of pure silver. **A.** A latent image center provides a passageway for electrons, supplied by the developer, through the bromine barrier. **B.** Silver ions are directly transformed into silver atoms by these developer-born electrons. Bromine ions and atoms escape into the emulsion. **C.** Eventually the entire microcrystal consists only of silver atoms.

The process of exposure of film by the light from a fluorescent screen is more complicated than with x-rays alone. So when a cassette is used, the relationship between the density of silver metal in developed film and the x-ray exposure is correspondingly more complex than Equation 17.4.

3. THE OPTICAL DENSITY OF DEVELOPED FILM

The amount of light transmitted through a region of developed film clipped onto a view box depends on the numbers and sizes of the microscopic specks of metallic silver in it. Two useful measures of film opacity are the optical transmissivity and the optical density.

Suppose that a certain x-ray exposure (either with or without a cassette) and subsequent development give rise to film that absorbs 75% of the visible light photons incident on it. That is, visible light of intensity L_0 is incident on the film, and the amount L_t passing through is only a quarter as great, so that the **optical transmissivity**, L_t/L_0, is 0.25. It is just as meaningful to express the transmission as a power of 10, that is, $L_t/L_0 = 0.25 = 10^{-0.602}$, and this, in fact, is the method commonly used in practice. The number in the exponent is called the **optical density (OD)** of the film, and in general

$$L_t/L_0 = 10^{-OD} \tag{17.5a}$$

The optical density may be defined equivalently in terms of the "common" logarithm (i.e., to the base 10) (Equation 14.15), of the fractional transmission:

$$OD = -\log_{10}(L_t/L_0) = \log_{10}(L_0/L_t) \tag{17.5b}$$

From this, as from Equation 17.5a, it should be apparent that the smaller the value of L_t/L_0 (i.e., the more opaque the film), the greater the OD (Fig. 17-8).

---- **EXERCISE 17-1.** _____

To what transmission fraction does an OD of 0.3 correspond?

SOLUTION: By Equation 17.5a, $L_t/L_0 = 10^{-0.3}$, which a pocket calculator readily determines to be 0.5.

---- **EXERCISE 17-2.** _____

A measurement with an optical densitometer indicates that a certain film absorbs 50% of the visible light photons incident on it. What is its OD?

SOLUTION: The fraction transmitted, L_t/L_0, is 0.5. By Equation 17.5b, OD = $-\log_{10}(0.5) = 0.3$.

---- **EXERCISE 17-3.** _____

One hundred percent of the light photons falling on a film pass through it. What is the OD? What about when $L_t/L_0 = 10\%$? 0.01? 0.1%? 0.5%?

SOLUTION: For $L_t/L_0 = 1$, OD = $-\log_{10}(1) = 0$. For optical transmittances of 10%, 1%, 0.1%, and 0.5%, the OD is 1, 2, 3, and 2.3, respectively.

A perfectly transparent film has an OD of 0 (Fig. 17-8). Half the light incident on a 0.3 OD film passes through it. And films with ODs of 1 and 2 transmit 10% and 1% of the light, respectively. The range of ODs occurring within diagnostically useful images is typically about 0.3 to 2.0, corresponding to transmission factors of between 0.5 and 0.01. In normal indoor light, one can barely see black pencil writing on a white page through an OD = 1 film.

Optical density measures an important inherent characteristic of the developed film itself, namely, *how much attenuation of light* occurs within it. OD takes no account of the way in

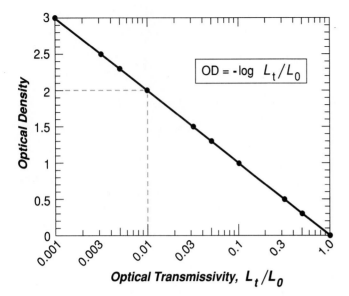

Figure 17–8. Optical transmissivity and optical density (OD). Visible light of intensity L_0 is incident on a film, and the amount L_t passes through it. The optical transmissivity of the film is defined as the fraction, L_t/L_0, that makes it through. At the point indicated, the transmissivity is 0.01, or 1%. The transmissivity can be presented in the fully equivalent form 10^{-OD}, where the number in the exponent is called the optical density (OD). Optical density can also be expressed directly in terms of the transmissivity as $OD = \log_{10}(L_0/L_t)$. An increase in OD by a step of 0.3 or 1 corresponds to a decrease in transmissivity by a factor of 2 or 10, respectively.

which that degree of attenuation was achieved. The amount of x-ray exposure involved, the conditions of developing the film, and other such factors are irrelevant. Only the film's final transmissivity is of importance with respect to the OD.

4. THE OPTICAL DENSITY OF FILM IS PROPORTIONAL TO THE CONCENTRATION OF METALLIC SILVER (Ag)

There exists a simple relationship between the optical density of developed film and the silver concentration or density (i.e., the number of silver grains per square millimeter). This relationship is valid regardless of whether or not a cassette was used in the exposure.

Suppose that a certain concentration of silver metal grains in film results in an optical transmission factor of 10%, hence an OD of 1. What is the effect of doubling the silver concentration in the film? One would get exactly the same net number of grains of silver per square millimeter, hence the same transmission of light, by exposing two separate sheets of film each by the original amount and then superimposing them. One of every 10 light photons passes through the first sheet, and only 10% of those then make it through the second. Thus, only 1 in 100 photons is transmitted through the pair or, equivalently, through a single sheet with twice the silver concentration, and the OD is 2. Similarly, one film with three times the concentration is optically equivalent to a superimposition of three of the original films, with a total OD of 3. Thus, the optical density is linear in the silver concentration,

$$OD \sim [Ag] \qquad (17.6)$$

a relationship valid over the range of clinical exposures. For each equal increment in silver density, the *transmission* is reduced by the same *multiplicative* factor. But because of the way it was defined (Equations 17.5), the optical density increases by the same *additive* amount.

5. THE CHARACTERISTIC (H&D) CURVE

The radiographically important characteristics of a film–screen combination (or of film alone, if exposed directly to x-rays) are recorded in a plot of the optical density against the x-ray exposure or kerma to air. Figures 17–9 and 17–10 provide examples of such *characteristic curves* or *H&D curves* (after F. Hurter and V. C. Driffield who first published one in 1890) plotted on linear or (as is found in practice more commonly) on semilog graph paper. For this particular film–cassette system, an x-ray exposure that gives rise to a kerma to air at the cassette of 1×10^{-3} cGy (corresponding to about 1 mR of exposure) results in a darkening of OD = 1.

The shape of such a characteristic curve depends not only on the properties of the film, but also on the conditions under which it is exposed and developed. We shall reconsider characteristic curves in more detail in Chapter 21.

It is easy to explain the shape of the H&D curve for the particular case of film exposed directly to x-rays, with no intensifying screen present. For direct irradiation of film, the amount of silver laid down is proportional to the exposure or air kerma, $[Ag] \sim K_{air}$ (Equation 17.4). For any film (exposed either with or without a screen), the OD is proportional to the density of deposited silver metal, $OD \sim [Ag]$. Combining these ideas: For direct x-irradiation,

$$OD \sim K_{air} \qquad \text{(no screen)} \qquad (17.7)$$

That is, when there is no screen, the characteristic curve is a straight line on ordinary, linear graph paper.

Above an OD of 2 or so, the silver grains begin overlap-

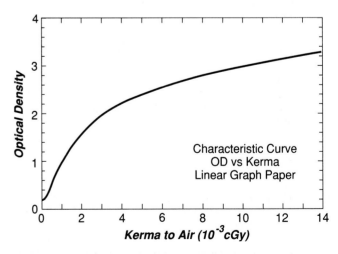

Figure 17–9. The characteristic curve for a film reveals the amount of darkening that will occur with any amount of irradiation. Optical density (after development) may be plotted on linear graph paper against kerma to air in units of 10^{-3} (which is nearly the same thing as exposure in milliroentgens).

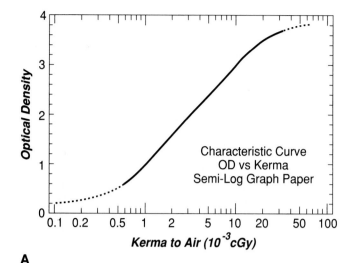

A

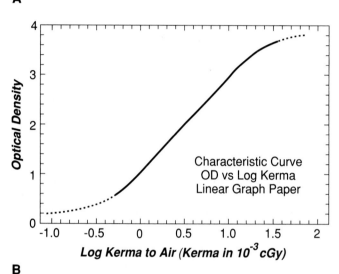

B

Figure 17–10. Characteristic curves commonly make use of a logarithmic exposure scale. **A.** The optical density may be plotted against kerma to air on semilog paper. **B.** Equivalently, the OD could be plotted against the logarithm of the kerma on linear paper.

ping, the OD increases less rapidly with exposure, and Equation 17.7 no longer obtains.

When an intensifying screen is used, the amount of silver deposited in film is not simply proportional to the exposure, and Equation 17.4 does not apply. The characteristic curve is therefore not of the simple form of Equation 17.7.

6. THE COPYING OF RADIOGRAPHS

One can create a copy of a radiograph by producing a contact negative (placing the radiograph over a sheet of unexposed film, shining light on the pair, and developing the fresh sheet) and then making a contact negative of the contact negative. *Radiograph duplicating film* provides a simpler, faster, and generally more accurate way of doing this.

In normal radiography, the optical density of an x-ray film increases with its exposure to x-rays or light. One might expect that with very high exposures, the characteristic curve flattens

out and eventually becomes horizontal (see Fig. 21–2). If every microcrystal has already been given a latent image, more exposure can have no further darkening effect. What actually happens, instead, is that at very high exposures, the characteristic curve eventually dips downward. Above a certain level, where the OD peaks, further exposure causes the film to become *less* opaque, a process known as *solarization*.

> A likely explanation for this peculiar behavior is the *rebromidization hypothesis*. As discussed in Section 2, accompanying the formation of latent images in a microcrystal of silver iodobromide is the release of bromine into the gelatin. Some of this bromine can react with silver atoms of the latent images already established, but normally this effect is of little significance. With a very large exposure and very high resultant bromine concentration in the gelatin, however, bromine can combine with enough silver at the surfaces of some latent images to inactivate them. The rate at which latent images are inactivated with further exposure (and further release of bromine into the gelatin) may become comparable to, and even surpass, the rate at which they are formed. The number of viable latent images then decreases with more exposure, so that the characteristic curve bends downward. In short, *more* exposure means *less* OD.

Commercial duplicating film is radiographic film that has already been solarized. Then, in a film copying machine, the duplicating film is exposed to ultraviolet light through the radiograph to be copied. Regions of higher OD on the original radiograph transmit less ultraviolet light. The corresponding portion of the duplicating film is less exposed and, therefore, ends up staying more opaque. The result is a positive (rather than a negative) copy of the original.

A benefit of the coming of computers to imaging departments is the reduction in the need for film copying and archiving. Images can be sent electronically to an office or other viewing station immediately on request. And if a hard copy is required, it can be generated by laser printer or by photographing a cathode ray tube screen.

7. REVIEW OF THE ENERGY TRANSFORMATION PROCESSES OCCURRING IN RADIOGRAPHY

We shall end this chapter and part of the book with a sketched review of the principal energy transformation processes that take place in the generation of a simple x-ray film. Figure 17–11 indicates the forms of energy present at different stages along the way, the appropriate energy accounting units, and interactions among the various forms of energy and matter.

Electrical power is rectified, and a nearly constant electric potential is applied between the anode and cathode of an x-ray tube. Driving several amperes of current through the filament causes the cathode to become white hot. Electrons are thermionically emitted from it with a potential energy numerically equal, in keV, to the kVp setting of the generator.

As the electrons accelerate, their potential energy becomes kinetic energy. Eventually they collide with the target, and nearly all of their collective kinetic energy is wasted in heating it. (That heat must be removed rapidly through thermal radiation, conduction, and convection to prevent damage to the

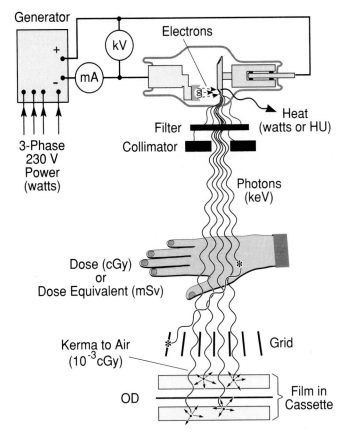

Generator

+

−

kV

mA

Electrons

Filter

Collimator

Heat
(watts or HU)

3-Phase
230 V
Power
(watts)

Photons
(keV)

Dose (cGy)
or
Dose Equivalent (mSv)

Kerma to Air
(10^{-3} cGy)

Grid

OD

Film in
Cassette

Figure 17–11. Some of the energy transformation processes that occur in the creation of a radiograph. Three-phase 230-V AC power fed into the generator is transformed into high voltage DC. Electrons acquire tens of keV in accelerating from the cathode to the anode. Most of the electrons' energy becomes heat and is radiated away. Less than 1% is transformed into x-ray photons. An x-ray beam deposits dose in tissue. For radiation protection purposes, the irradiation is usually expressed, rather, as dose equivalent. With x-ray and gamma ray energy, the dose in centigrays or rads is numerically equal to the dose equivalent in centisieverts or rems. The photons that pass through the tissue and the grid give rise to some kerma in air (in 10^{-3} cGy) or, which is practically the same thing, to exposure (in milliroentgen) at the cassette. Development of the film, which itself involves a number of chemical energy processes, leads to the deposition of silver and the distillation of a medical image.

tube.) But a small fraction (1% or less) of the electron energy is transformed, through the bremsstrahlung process and through the creation of characteristic x-rays, into photons with energies ranging from 0 to kVp keV.

The photon beam emerging from the tube is hardened, as the lower-energy, less penetrating x-rays preferentially undergo photoelectric interactions within the anode itself and with the added filtration. The intensity diminishes with the inverse square of the distance from the focal spot because of beam divergence.

On striking the patient, the beam is attenuated through photon interactions within soft tissue (mostly Compton) and bone (mostly photoelectric), and its intensity falls off roughly exponentially with distance traveled through the body. The intensity of the beam exiting the patient, consisting of both the primary x-ray image and Compton scattered radiation, is a few percent of that which entered. Scatter photons are largely absorbed (photoelectric events) by the lead leaves of a grid.

Most of the x-ray photons that manage to reach the intensifying screens of a cassette interact via the photoelectric (or, to a much lesser extent, the Compton) mechanism. Each photoelectron thereby liberated travels at high velocity for short distances through the screen material, causing it to fluoresce.

The fluorescent light produces latent images in some of the silver halide crystals of the radiographic film. On chemical development of the film, activated silver halide crystals are transformed into microscopic specks of silver metal. And they obscure the light from the light box.

The ability of the beam to penetrate different kinds and thicknesses of tissue, and thus create contrast within the primary x-ray image, is determined largely by the amount of beam filtration and by the kVp applied to the x-ray tube. The overall level of darkness of the film, which depends on both the kVp and the mA-s (tube current times exposure duration), also affects contrast. But kVp and mA-s are the determinants of the amount and distribution of dose within the patient, as well. It is through the selection of the "technique factors" (kVp, mA, and s) that one attempts to achieve a high level of contrast while, at the same time, keeping the patient dose low.

Got it?

III

Analog X-ray Imaging

Part 4

The Formation
of a Radiographic Image

Chapter 18

Contrast, Resolution, and Noise: Determinants of the Diagnostic Utility of an Image

Almost any imaging system acts like a camera. It maps signals transmitted through, or emitted or reflected from, a three-dimensional object onto a two-dimensional surface. The quality of the resultant image is limited by the system's abilities to represent different physical attributes of the object with different shades of gray or color (i.e., to provide adequate contrast) and to capture fine detail, all without permitting unacceptable levels of distortions and interfering signals.

Before considering how the physical characteristics of any particular imaging system determine its capabilities and limitations, it is useful to examine properties of images in general, such as their contrast, resolution, and noise level. Our consideration of noise will include discussion of its statistical nature, and you may wish to review the material in Appendix 18–1, as well as that in Chapter 2, Section 7, before beginning.

1. WHAT DO YOU REALLY WANT FROM A MEDICAL IMAGE?

The Lincoln Monument (Fig. 18–1A), and *Nude Descending a Staircase* (Fig. 18–1B), leave indelible impressions. The Lincoln

Monument is loved for its portrayal of the strength and integrity of the man. *Nude* interprets the essence of the human form by capturing its flow. But does *Lincoln* provide a better image because of its traditional realism? Of course not. The two do quite different things.

One might assume that the quality of a medical image increases with its similarity to the object from which it is taken. But much of the information content of the image is medically irrelevant, and may even distract one's attention away from the diagnostically critical features. What is of importance is not necessarily "realism," but rather the extent to which an image allows the observer to *detect* and *identify* an abnormality and then to *interpret* its meaning so as to determine its cause.

This chapter focuses attention on three especially important measures of the capacity of a medical image to convey clinically useful information, namely, its *contrast, resolution,* and *noise* level. In a particular situation, one or another of these may be of particular significance. But in general all three characteristics are relevant determinants of image quality. Focusing on this standard triad will help in our efforts to assess and describe the diagnostic utility of various kinds of medical images and of the devices that produce them.

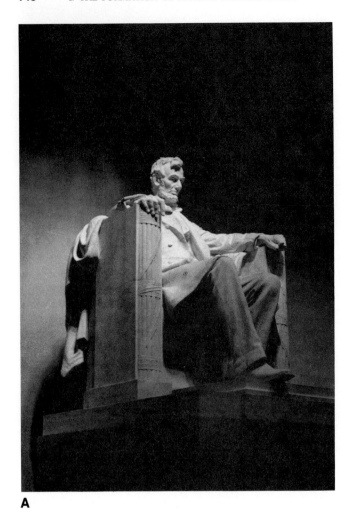

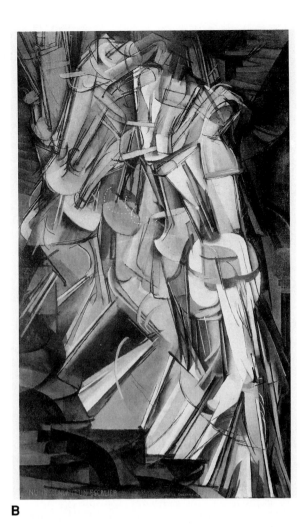

A

B

Figure 18–1. Examples of representations. **A.** The statue within the Lincoln Monument is a *realistic* portrayal of the human form. (*Photo by Gordon Cook.*) **B.** *Nude Descending a Staircase, No. 2,* by Marcel Duchamp (American, born in France, 1887–1968; painted in 1912) captures the essence of *motion. (Courtesy of the Philadelphia Museum of Art: Louise and Walter Arensberg Collection.)*

2. AN IMAGE IS A SPATIAL PATTERN OF INTENSITIES

The word "image" can assume a variety of meanings, depending on the context. In this chapter, an image will usually refer to a pattern of visible light photons. These may be light photons passing through a partially transparent film, or being emitted from the screen of a cathode ray tube, or reflecting from a sheet of paper, or even impinging on the retina. ("Image" can also refer to a pattern of x-ray photons at an earlier point in the radiologic imaging chain, and such situations will be clearly flagged. The pattern of primary [unscattered] x-rays emerging from the body during radiography, for example, is called the *primary x-ray image.*)

Although a pattern of light (or x-rays) could be expressed as a spatial distribution of photon fluence, or energy fluence, or any other determinant or measure of brightness, here we shall talk mainly in terms of *intensities*. Intensity was introduced (Equation 11.1) in the context of an x-ray beam, but the definition is just as valid for light.

Figure 18–2A is a photograph of Nadine Wolbarst that ap-

peared recently in the "Abnormal Behavior" section of one of the racier supermarket tabloids. Figure 18–2B shows how the picture was made. Nadine was bathed in sunlight, some of which was reflected to the camera lens. (Equivalently: Sunlight photons were absorbed by feline atoms, and some were immediately reradiated in all directions, including toward the lens.) Glass **refracts** (bends the path of) light, and a convex lens is a piece of glass precisely sculpted so as to exhibit a remarkable property: The light coming from an object, such as a cat, is focused by the lens in such a fashion that it produces on the *focal plane* an image that is a faithful representation of the source object. The way this happens will be discussed in Chapter 27.

Figure 18–2A is not a bad photograph. There is a fair amount of contrast, nicely picking the various shades of tan in Nadine's coat. The resolution and sharpness are good enough, moreover, for us to make out her whiskers. And there is very little visual noise in the image. You need a magnifying glass to be aware of the grain of the film (or does it arise in the printing of the book?). Most important of all, at least with respect to the transfer of information: the overall image is such that you or I, the final link in the imaging chain, can determine that this is, indeed, a cat. And I, with certain experience that you have not

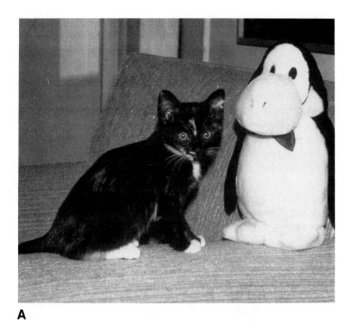

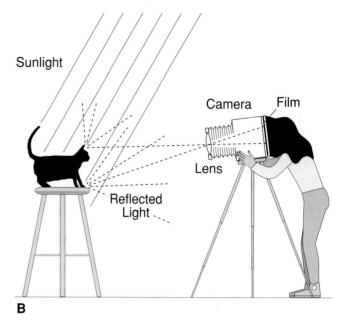

A   **B**

Figure 18–2.   Important qualities of an image. **A.** Nadine Wolbarst and her friend both appear with sharp contrast, high resolution, and little noise. **B.** The making of a photograph: Sunlight, or light from a flash, is absorbed and reemitted by atoms at the surface of the subject. Light photons coming from any point are focused by a lens to a corresponding point on the film.

shared, can even assert with a fair degree of assurance *which* cat she usually is. If the image were blurrier, or in some other sense carried less information or more noise, that would not necessarily be the case.

3. RADIOLOGIC IMAGES ARE USUALLY CONTRAST LIMITED

Once again, three characteristics of an image to a large extent determine (and describe) its usefulness: contrast, resolution, and noise level (Fig. 18–3).

For many radiologic purposes, *contrast* is the issue of greatest concern of the three. Contrast refers to differences in the level of brightness of parts of the image that correspond to anatomically or physiologically different parts of the body. If L_{obj} represents the intensity of light coming from an object or region of interest, and L_{bac} is that from a background or reference region (Fig. 18–4), then a simple measure of contrast might be

$$C = (L_{obj} - L_{bac})/L_{bac} \qquad (18.1)$$

This is just the difference in brightness between the object and the background region, taken relative to the background level.

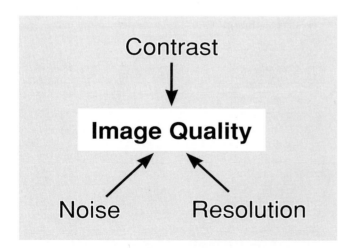

Figure 18–3.   Three important parameters of image quality: the contrast in light intensity (or x-ray fluence, or nuclear magnetic resonance relaxation time, or whatever it is that is being imaged, depending on the modality) corresponding to different parts of the subject; the resolution of fine detail; and the level of interfering noise.

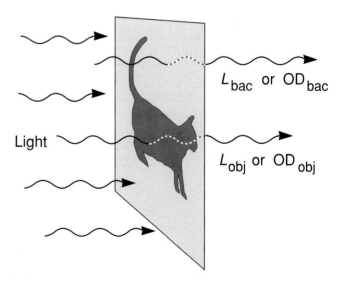

Figure 18–4.   Contrast of an object on film may be defined in terms of the intensities of light coming from it and from the background region (Equation 18.1 or 18.2a) or in terms of optical densities (Equation 18.2b).

In Figure 18–2A, most of Nadine's coat is a medium shade of gray, but the sclera of her eyes are much lighter. Suppose that when the photo is viewed in normal light and at reading distance, $L_{sclera} = 25$ units of light intensity and $L_{coat} = 20$ units. Then the contrast of the white of the eye against the background of fur would be $C = (25 - 20)/20 = 0.25$. A dark-colored object against a light background would yield a contrast numerically quite different, in fact less than zero.

Contrast can be defined equally well in other ways. Instead of the relative difference between the two intensities, for example, one might consider the logarithm of their ratio:

$$C = \log_{10}(L_{obj}/L_{bac}) \qquad (18.2a)$$

Although this may not be as obvious a choice as Equation 18.1, it is every bit as natural and legitimate a measure of the difference between two intensity levels. In the case of our cat's eye, $C = \log_{10}(25/20) = 0.1$. This is comparable to, but not the same as, what we got from Equation 18.1. It is important to spell out clearly how you are calculating C.

The *radiographic image contrast* between two adjacent regions in a film is normally expressed as the difference in their optical densities:

$$C = OD_{bac} - OD_{obj} \qquad (18.2b)$$

This form happens to be fully equivalent to Equation 18.2a. An advantage of defining image contrast as in Equations 18.2 will become apparent in Section 9, when we take into account the physiologic response of the eye to different levels of intensity of light. Note that whether you use Equation 18.1 or Equations 18.2, a value of $C = 0$ means that there is *no* contrast between the regions of interest.

> It is easy to show the equivalence of contrast as defined in Equations 18.2a and 18.2b. If L_0 represents the intensity of light passing through a (nearly transparent) unexposed part of the film, then by the definition of OD (Equations 17.5), $C = OD_{bac} - OD_{obj} = \log_{10}(L_0/L_{bac}) - \log_{10}(L_0/L_{obj}) = \log_{10}(L_{obj}/L_{bac})$, where the last step makes use of Equation 14.14.

_____ EXERCISE 18–1. _____

Seven percent more light is passing through a small area of interest on film than through its surroundings. What is the contrast?

SOLUTION: As the relative amounts of light passing through background and the area of interest are 1 and 1.07, respectively, by Equation 18.1, the contrast would be 7%. With the more common (for film) definition of Equation 18.2a, however, $C = \log_{10}(1.07) = 3\%$. This difference underscores the importance of agreeing on definitions.

Image contrast is determined both by the *subject contrast* produced by the body and by the *receptor contrast* of the image receptor and imaging system. As the next few chapters will show, receptor contrast amplifies the effects of subject contrast. One way that this may (sometimes) be expressed is

image contrast = (subject contrast)(receptor contrast)   (18.3)

With standard radiography, for example, the subject contrast might refer to the contrast in the pattern of x-ray intensities emerging from the patient and passing through the antiscatter grid (i.e., the primary x-ray image plus some scatter photons). It results directly from, and provides information about, non-uniformities in the thicknesses, densities, and chemical composition of the tissues within the body. The receptor contrast of the screen–film system, or *screen–film contrast*, describes its response to different levels of x-ray intensity. It is determined in part by the processes by which the film was manufactured and developed, and on the fluorescence properties of its screens, and can be learned from the characteristic curve. Overall image contrast is affected both by subject contrast and by receptor contrast.

Finally, the perceived image contrast for a film on a light box display depends on the sharpness of the borders between anatomic regions, on their sizes, on the overall level of brightness, on the uniformity of light from the display box, and on the skills of the observer. It is commonly asserted that a contrast on film of a few percent can be picked up visually, but a number of factors affect the threshold of detectability.

4. RESOLUTION, SHARPNESS, AND FINE DETAIL

Resolution is a measure of the quality of detail in a picture. It also refers to the ability of an imaging system to produce that detail. Either way, it may be reported as the minimum separation (in the body) of small objects whose images can just barely be distinguished from one another (in the picture) (Fig. 18–5). If the objects were any closer, their images would blend together. A high contrast between the objects and the background is normally assumed, as are good viewing conditions.

Resolution may be quantified in terms of the ability of an image or system to reproduce detail in a test pattern. The radiographic test pattern in Figure 2–12, for example, consists of narrowing and converging alternating bars of radiopaque and radiolucent material. The images of this device produced with **no intensifying screen,** with a **detail cassette,** and with a **fast cassette** are shown in Figures 18–6A through 18–6C. With *no* screen (Fig. 16–6A), lead stripes 1/24 mm wide (and apart) can

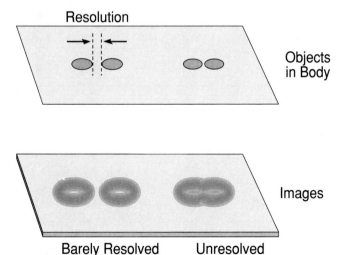

Figure 18–5. When the images of two small objects (lying in a plane parallel to that of the image receptor) in the patient's body can be barely distinguished from one another, their separation defines the resolution of the imaging system.

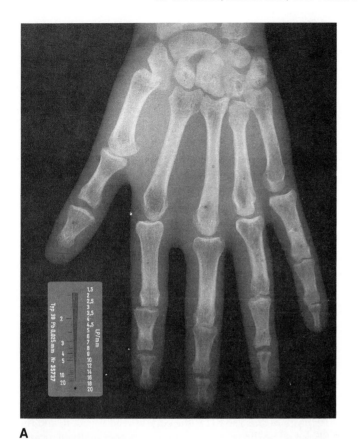

A

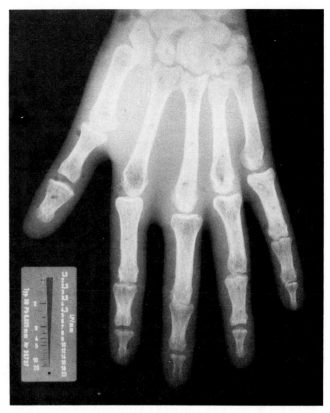

B

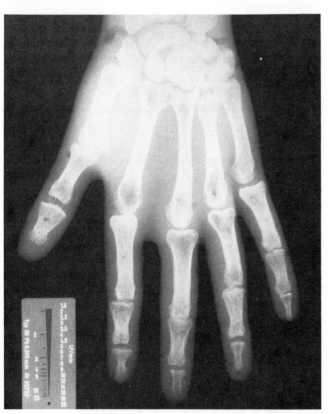

C

Figure 18–6. Quantifying the resolution associated with one component of a radiographic system, the cassette. As the intensifying screens become thicker, the speed increases, but the ability to resolve fine detail is diminished. The resolution test device was seen earlier as Figure 2–12. **A.** When no intensifying screen is used, this film can display better than 12 lp/mm, but it requires a 128-mA-s exposure. **B.** With the same film and a "detail" calcium tungstate screen, only 10 mA-s is required to achieve the same average optical density, and resolution is still better than 7 lp/mm. **C.** The exposure is down to 1.33 mA-s with a "fast" CaWO$_4$ screen, but the resolution is now less than 5 lp/mm. *(From the American College of Radiology Learning File, courtesy of the ACR.)*

just be resolved; in the standard clinical parlance, the resolution is said to be 12 line pairs (lp) per millimeter. The results are almost as good with the detail screen (Fig. 18–6B) (but the radiation dose delivered to the patient is about an order of magnitude lower). With the *fast* screen, however, the resolution is down to 5 lp/mm (Fig. 18–6C). (As will be discussed later, other important determinants of radiographic resolution, in addition to screen speed, are focal spot size and patient motion.)

Another measure of detail is provided by the **point spread function (PSF).** We shall illustrate its meaning with the example of the PSF of a radiographic screen–film combination. An extremely narrow "pencil" x-ray beam is produced by directing an ordinary beam at a metal plate that is fully attenuating except at a pinhole (Fig. 18–7A). The *input* to the screen–film system is this pencil beam of radiation. The output of the system (i.e., the image on film of the point source) will be of somewhat greater dimensions, primarily because of the scattering of x-rays and the diffusion of light *within the fluorescent screen.* After the film is developed, a plot of the *optical density* of the film as a function of distance, *y*, from the center of the image, OD(*y*), is found to be bell-shaped (Fig. 18–7B). Then, knowing the detailed shape of the characteristic curve of the screen–film system, we can estimate the shape of the related bell-shaped curve of the *x-ray photon intensity* that gave rise to the image on film. (This step removes from the analysis the effects of the shape of the characteristic curve, which is not of interest here.) The second bell-shaped curve (of x-ray photon intensity) is the point spread function.

The width of the PSF, and in particular the **full width at half-maximum (FWHM),** halfway to the peak, is a simple numerical measure of the blur introduced into the imaging system by the fluoroscopic screen of the cassette. The greater the FWHM of the PSF, the worse the resolution.

Closely related to the PSF is the *line spread function (LSF),* which measures the system's response to a narrow line (rather than point) x-ray source (Fig. 18–8). Here, the metal plate contains a narrow slit, rather than a pinhole.

Resolution can be reported in terms of any of the preceding parameters. Note that improved resolution will appear as a *decrease* in the separation of resolvable small objects and as a *decrease* in the FWHM of the PSF or LSF, but as an *increase* in the number of line pairs per millimeter.

Sharpness is a different but related measure of image detail, or of the capability of a system to capture it. The image of the outer edge of the bar test pattern is considerably sharper in Figure 18–6A than in 18–6C. The intensities of light from the two images have been measured with a high-resolution optical scanning device and are plotted (Fig. 18–9) as functions of distance from the edge. The dashed line corresponds to the "fast" cassette (or to what one would find with a large focal spot). The *edge spread function* for an imaging system with good resolution (detail screens or no cassette, small focal spot, no motion blurring) falls off faster.

Chapter 24 will describe the *modulation transfer function (MTF),* a different but equivalent measure of a system's ability to capture detail. The MTF, the edge spread function, and the LSF can all be directly related to one another mathematically,

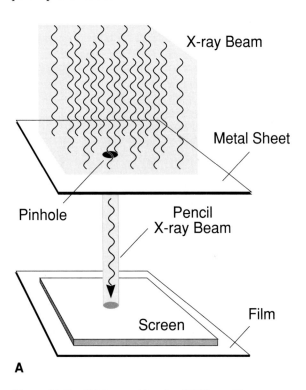

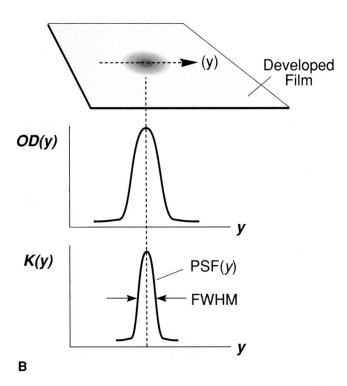

A   B

Figure 18–7. Point spread function (PSF), used here as a measure of the resolution associated with the screen–film component of a radiographic system. **A.** A uniform x-ray beam falls on a metal sheet, and a "pencil" beam of x-rays emerges through the pinhole, to fall on the screen–film combination. **B.** After the film is developed, the dark region created by the pencil beam is scanned with an optical microdensitometer, yielding a plot of the optical density as a function of position, OD(*y*). Making use of the characteristic curve of the screen–film system, a curve of the x-ray beam air kerma or exposure as a function of position, *K*(*y*), is extracted. This is the PSF, and it can be largely parameterized in terms of its full width at half-maximum (FWHM).

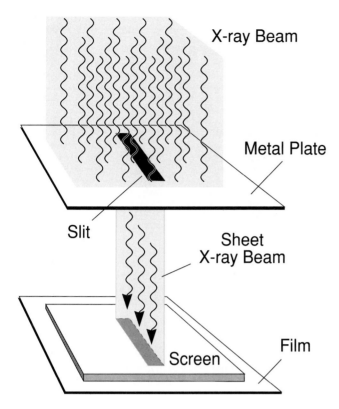

Figure 18–8. After replacing the pinhole in the metal plate with a narrow slit, exactly the same procedure as that described in Figure 18–7 yields the line spread function (LSF).

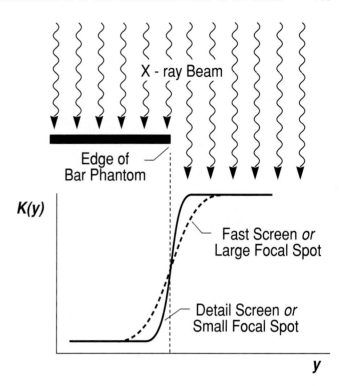

Figure 18–9. The edge spread function is another measure of resolution. X-ray intensity is plotted against position at the outer edge of the bar phantom. The sharper falloff (the solid line) results from use of the smaller focal spot or of a higher-resolution (and slower) cassette.

as is shown in more advanced texts. They also can be derived ab initio for an imaging system through analysis of factors such as focal spot size, intensifier screen thickness, patient motion, and other determinants of image unsharpness.

5. QUANTUM MOTTLE OBEYS POISSON STATISTICS

Seurat's *A Sunday on La Grande Jatte* is composed of many small dabs of paint. From a distance the image seems quite smooth (Fig. 18–10A), but you would have difficulty in making out the finer features. On closer inspection, the size of the individual dabs causes the image to appear blotchy (Fig. 18–10B), and that places an absolute upper limit on possible detail. Sharpness is not what Seurat had in mind, but the objectives of medical imaging are different.

If radiographic film is exposed directly to x-rays, with no cassette, a single grain of silver is likely to be deposited when an x-ray photon interacts with a microcrystal of silver halide (see Chapter 17, Section 2). One cannot make out the individual grains of silver in the developed film without a microscope, and an image will appear smoothly textured. When a cassette is used, however, the grains are deposited in tight, dense clusters. Each cluster is produced by the thousands of visible light photons emitted when a single x-ray photon is absorbed in a fluorescent screen. When such silver grain clusters are too few in number, as with an underexposed radiograph or one taken with too fast a screen, the image does appear dappled or blotchy. This kind of *noise* is known as **quantum mottle.**

It is possible to describe quantum mottle quantitatively. The interactions of x-ray photons with a fluorescent screen occur "stochastically" (randomly), much like the fall of raindrops onto the squares of a sidewalk. In a downpour, where the average number of raindrops is large, the relative differences among squares are not significant. But with a brief sprinkle, only a few drops may land in the average square, and the actual numbers in the individual squares will vary considerably (Fig. 18–11). The relative numbers of squares with 0, 1, 2, 3, 10, or any other integer number of raindrops are given accurately by **Poisson statistics,** discussed in Appendix 18–1.

The average count of drops per square is known as the **mean,** and the **standard deviation** is a direct measure of the width of the distribution of counts about that mean. An important characteristic of the *Poisson* distribution, in particular, is that the standard deviation happens always to be equal to the square root of the mean. If, on average, N raindrops fall per square,

$$\text{mean} = N \qquad (18.4a)$$

then the standard deviation will be

$$\text{standard deviation} = \sqrt{N} \qquad (18.4b)$$

As described by Poisson statistics, the number of raindrops will be less than one standard deviation from the mean, or between $(N - \sqrt{N})$ and $(N + \sqrt{N})$ in about two thirds of the squares. For 95% of the squares, the measurement will lie between $(N - 2\sqrt{N})$ and $(N + 2\sqrt{N})$, and outside that range only 5% of the time. And so on. This important observation is summarized in Table 18–1.

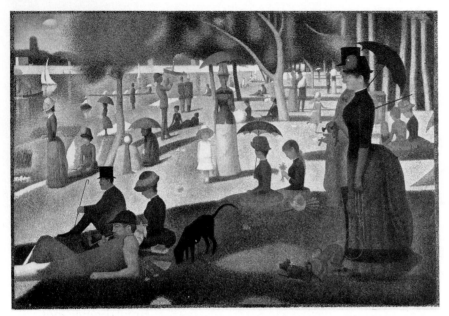

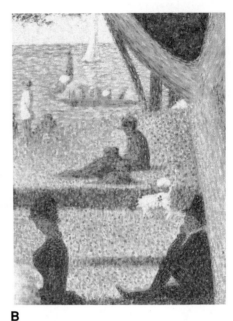

A

B

Figure 18–10. *A Sunday on La Grande Jatte* by George Seurat (French, 1859–1891). **A.** The painting (oil on canvas, 207.6 × 308 cm) seems relatively smooth-textured from normal viewing distance. **B.** Close inspection reveals an image texture similar to that of quantum mottle. *(Courtesy of the Art Institute of Chicago, Helen Birch Bartlett Memorial Collection.)*

Since the standard distribution increases with the square root of the mean, the *relative width* of the distribution, or the *relative variation*, decreases as the mean grows larger:

$$\text{relative variation} = \sqrt{N}/N = 1/\sqrt{N} \qquad (18.4c)$$

The larger the number of counts that occur in the average square, the smaller will be the relative magnitudes of the *fluctuations* in the individual readings about that average, and the more likely it is that the number of counts in any particular square will lie "relatively close" to the mean.

EXERCISE 18–2.

A sidewalk consists of concrete squares, all 1.5 m on a side. After a brief sprinkle of rain, a first-year radiology resident reports that a total of 3270 drops landed on 22 squares. How

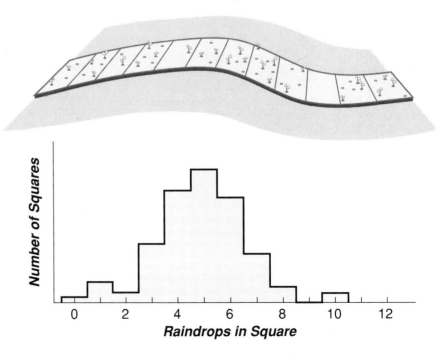

Figure 18–11. When a brief, light shower falls on a sidewalk, the relative number of squares ending up with any particular number of raindrops is given by Poisson statistics.

TABLE 18–1. PROBABILITY OF ANY GIVEN NUMBER OF RAINDROPS LANDING IN A SIDEWALK SQUARE, WHEN THE AVERAGE NUMBER PER SQUARE IS N[a]

	Counts/square				Probability
$(N - \sqrt{N})$	<	actual count	<	$(N + \sqrt{N})$	0.683
$(N - 2\sqrt{N})$	<	actual count	<	$(N + 2\sqrt{N})$	0.950
$(N - 3\sqrt{N})$	<	actual count	<	$(N + 3\sqrt{N})$	0.995

[a]See Table 18–3.

likely is it, roughly, that a typical square, chosen at random, will contain between 120 and 170 drops? More than 170 drops?

SOLUTION: The mean N is $3270/22 = 148.6$ drops and, by Equation 18.4b, the standard deviation is $\sqrt{N} = 12.2$. 120 and 170 are approximately two standard deviations below and above the mean, respectively, so there is about a 95% probability that the number of drops in any square will be between 120 and 170. Five percent of the squares will have counts outside of that range, and in half of those cases (i.e., $2\frac{1}{2}\%$ of the time), the number will exceed 170.

Let's return to x-ray photons falling on a radiation detector, such as a radiographic cassette and film. Suppose that we partition the film, with imaginary lines, into separate squares, as with ordinary graph paper. The squares, or **pixels**, might be, say, 1 mm on a side. We shall now direct a *uniform* x-ray beam at the cassette, and adjust the intensity so that, on average, 100 photons interact per square millimeter of intensifying screen. Each interaction that does occur results in a tiny cluster of silver grains on film. The standard deviation (Equation 18.4b) is 10 clusters. If many 1-mm^2 areas are sampled in different parts of the film, then between 90 and 110 events will be counted in two thirds of the measurements, and the relative variation will be about 0.1, or 10% (Fig. 18–12A). For about 5% of the pixels, the number of clusters will be either less than 80 or greater than 120. One-half percent (0.5%) of the squares will differ from the norm by 30% or more. With this amount of variation from pixel to pixel, the *quantum mottle* in the developed film will be very apparent.

The intensity of the x-ray beam is now increased by a factor of a hundred, and a new film is shot. Ten thousand clusters

are found per pixel, on average. The standard deviation is 100, and the relative variation drops to 1% (Fig. 18–12B). In only 0.5% of the squares will the number of clusters differ from the average by more than 3%. The level of quantum mottle is greatly reduced, and the shading appears much smoother to the eye.

_____ EXERCISE 18–3. _____

Why does film look noisier under a magnifying glass?

SOLUTION: The field of view is smaller, as will be any pixel size selected. The average number of clusters of silver grains in a pixel is less, so that the relative variation is larger.

6. DETECTABILITY REQUIRES SUFFICIENTLY HIGH CONTRAST AND/OR LOW NOISE LEVEL: THE SIGNAL-TO-NOISE RATIO

Section 5 was concerned with the mottle from a uniform x-ray beam, but the implications for imaging are obvious. For a particular anatomic entity to be detected, its impact on an image must be significantly greater than that of the random variations from quantum mottle. In other words, clinical utility requires a high enough signal contrast and/or an adequately low level of noise.

Figure 18–13 illustrates this quantitatively with the example of a 1-mm^2 nodule, embedded in soft tissue, that attenuates an x-ray beam by an extra 2%.

Figure 18–13A shows a hypothetical, idealized case, in which no Poisson statistical variations occur in the number of photons that reach the cassette (i.e., no noise).

Figure 18–13B illustrates the more realistic situation in which 10,000 photons/mm^2 make it through the soft tissue, on average, and the nodule attenuates a further 2% of them; that is, the photon fluence is 200 photons/mm^2 less in the shadow of the nodule than elsewhere. The vertical axis to the right records the number of x-ray photons per square millimeter eventually affecting film, and this is expressed on the left in multiples of the standard deviation, σ. σ is 100/mm^2, so one could say that the nodule is more attenuating than its surroundings by 2σ. But according to Table 18–1, a good 5% of all 1-mm^2

Average: 100 photons/pixel
Standard Deviation: 10
Relative Variation: 10%

101	106	123	98
84	111	107	104
111	91	98	93
108	100	97	102

A

Average: 10,000 photons/pixel
Standard Deviation: 100
Relative Variation: 1%

10,087	10,114	9,900	10,284
9,937	9,986	10,123	10,104
9,841	10,206	10,042	9,881
10,040	9,972	9,906	10,062

B

Figure 18–12. For a Poisson random process, as the average number, $\mu = N$, of photons per pixel increases, so also does the standard deviation in that number, $\sigma = \sqrt{N}$. But the relative deviation, $\sqrt{N}/N = 1/\sqrt{N}$, goes down. The examples shown are for **(A)** 100 photons/pixel and **(B)** 10,000 photons/pixel.

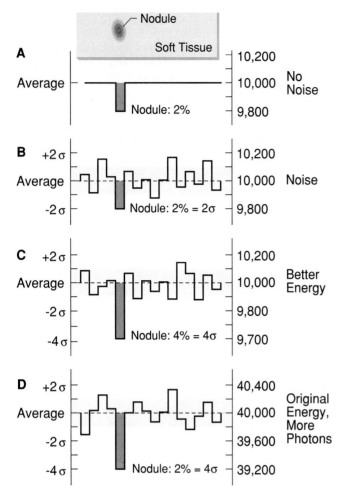

Figure 18–13. Simple illustration of the effect of noise on signal detectability. A nodule, 1 mm in cross-sectional area, attenuates 2% more of a photon beam than does the surrounding soft tissue. Pixels are 1 mm^2 in area. **A.** If there were no random fluctuations in numbers of x-ray photons per millimeter, the nodule would be seen easily. **B.** With 10,000 photons per pixel on average, the standard deviation is $\sigma = \sqrt{10,000} = 100$, and the relative deviation in number of photons, from pixel to pixel, is 100/10,000 = 1%, indicated here by the shaded bar. Roughly one third of all pixels differ (because of naturally occurring, random fluctuations in the numbers of photons) from the average value by at least 1σ, or 100 photons/mm. Five percent of the pixels differ from the average by more than 2σ = 200 photons, i.e., by 2% of the average value. The 2% change caused by the nodule, for which we are looking, can easily become lost in the noise. **C.** Suppose we can improve things, for example, through a change in photon energy or by the addition of nodule-specific contrast material, so that the nodule is much more attenuating. If the nodule now reduces beam intensity 4% more than soft tissue (rather than 2%) but the noise level stays the same, the SNR will have doubled. Fewer than 0.1% of the pixels will differ (because of random processes) from the average by as much as 400 photons = 4σ, and the nodule is likely to be noticed. **D.** Alternatively, one could return to the original energy but improve the statistics by increasing the average number of photons to 40,000/pixel. The standard deviation is now 200/mm^2. The nodule would reduce the number of photons in its pixel by 2% = 800, which now corresponds to 4σ; again, it is visible.

areas differ from background by this amount or more, and the nodule can easily be missed.

If, however, we reduced the photon energy, so that the nodule attenuates 4% excess photons rather than 2% (Fig. 18–13C), but arranged for 10,000 photons/mm^2 still to reach the cassette, the signal stands out clearly, by 4σ, from background.

Likewise, going back to the original energy but increasing the number of photons by a factor of 4, to 40,000, also changes the situation considerably (Fig. 18–13D). The σ is now 200 photon/mm^2. The nodule, which absorbs or scatters an extra 800 photons/mm^2, again differs from background by 4σ.

To summarize the point of Figure 18–13: The greater the number of interaction events per unit area, on average, the smaller the relative amount of random variation that will occur naturally in that number. So if mottle diminishes the utility of an image, as in Figure 2–14, and perhaps obscures an object of interest, a solution to the problem may be to *get better statistics* with more photons. Alternatively, it may be possible to enhance the contrast artificially, as with iodine contrast agent in a blood vessel. Either way, the issue of importance is the magnitude of the clinically significant *signal* relative to the level of background *noise*.

The terminology of electrical engineering is sometimes used in this context. N of Equations 18.4 refers to the average number of photons per unit area required to darken a portion of film to a particular OD. More generally, N is a measure of the average *strength of the signal* in that area. As $\sqrt{N}$ is a corresponding gauge of the level of associated stochastic noise, the inherent **signal-to-noise ratio (SNR)** of the image there is

$$SNR = N/\sqrt{N} = \sqrt{N} \qquad (18.5)$$

The greater the exposure and the average value of N, the smaller will be the *relative* amplitudes of the random fluctuations in N, and the less the *apparent* noisiness. Comparison with Equation 18.4C indicates that the SNR, here, is just the inverse of the relative variation.

Note that in Figures 18–13C and 18–13D, the signal stands out strongly from background noise, and the SNR is much greater than the inherent SNR predicted by Equation 18.5.

7. FORMS OF NOISE OTHER THAN MOTTLE

The preceding definition of the SNR has been concerned with random fluctuation that can be described with Poisson statistics. Quantum mottle is a classic case in point. The natural variations in the number of silver iodobromide grains per unit area of unexposed film, similarly, obeys Poisson statistics, but is rarely discernible in radiography.

A number of imaging modalities make use of detector devices that generate weak electrical signals. These signals may involve the flow of only a few electrons through a circuit, and the number of electrons actually involved at any instant will vary about the average according to Poisson statistics.

Sometimes more noticeable is the noise injected into the sensitive detector electronics by external sources, such as lightning storms, sparking of machinery, and some fluorescent lamps. Poisson noise is thus but one component of this more general category of sources of image degradation, some of which may be of importance. From a broader perspective, "noise" is anything in an image that detracts from its clinical usefulness.

Within the body of the patient, the presence of tissues other than the organ of interest are invariably sources of unwanted signals. With x-ray- or gamma ray-based modalities, Compton scatter photons carry no useful information, but diminish subject contrast. (The problem can be either not enough photons where they should be, leading to mottle, or too many of the wrong kind where they shouldn't be, degrading subject contrast.) Likewise, with magnetic resonance imaging (MRI), any changing magnetic fields present will induce electric currents in the tissues of the patient; these, in turn, will be picked up by the system's radio frequency (rf) detector as a form of noise.

The imaging devices can contribute to the noise in a variety of other ways. Imperfections in computer reconstruction algorithms, for example, may lead to abnormalities in images produced by computed tomography, magnetic resonance imaging, positron emission tomography, and single-photon emission computed tomography. Likewise, cameras and display monitors produce less than perfect images.

It is a major objective of the engineers who design imaging equipment, and of the clinical physicists and engineers who maintain quality assurance on them, to keep all types of noise to an acceptably low level.

8. IN THE EYE OF THE BEHOLDER

Many kinds of medical images are processed and improved with the aid of computers, but few are computer-analyzed or interpreted. Nearly all images, as of the mid 1990s, are still examined and assessed visually for diagnosis by a physician.

The usefulness of an image is thus limited, ultimately, by the ability of the eye to take it in and the brain to make sense of it. The capabilities of the eye and brain thus set the standard in the quest for image quality, and also establish an upper limit on what is really needed. Ideally, the contrast, resolution, and noise of an image should be good enough so that any marginal improvements will be of practically no diagnostic advantage to the observer. Beyond that point, further efforts at improvement may not be cost-effective. In judging image quality, therefore, it is necessary to understand what the eye and brain together can do.

Like a camera, the eye consists of an aperture and lens and a photosensitive surface on which the image is recorded. The photoreceptors of the retina are the *cones* responsible for *photopic* (daylight) vision. (The *rods,* which are involved in scotopic [night] vision, are not of interest here.) Just as the *response* of film to different levels of x-rays or light is revealed in the concentrations of silver grains laid down on development, so also may the *response* of the eye–brain system be described in terms of perceived, or apparent, brightnesses.

It is found experimentally that the apparent brightness of an image is *not* linearly proportional to the intensity of the light coming from it, L. That is, if L increases from 1 to 2, from 2 to 3, from 3 to 4, and so on, the eye–brain system of a person with normal vision will not perceive these changes as equal differences in luminosity.

What kinds of increments in L do, in fact, give rise to equal differences in perceived, apparent brightness? Steps in luminosity *appear* to be equally far apart in brightness only if they

really increase approximately geometrically, as in 1, 2, 4, 8, 16, 32, . . . ; that is, as $L = 2^n$, where $n = 1, 2, 3, ...$ This implies that the physicopsychologic response of the eye is approximately logarithmic in intensity: The apparent brightness is proportional to $\ln L$ or $\log_{10} L$.

> The validity of this claim may be seen by inserting $L = 2^n$ into Apparent Brightness $= \ln L$, and making use of Equation 14.14d. The resulting series, $\ln 2^n = n \cdot \ln 2, n = 1, 2, 3, . . . ,$ increases as $1 \cdot (\ln 2), 2 \cdot (\ln 2), 3 \cdot (\ln 2), . . . ,$ whereas L itself goes as $1, 2, 4, 8, ...$ The geometric progressions $3^n, 10^n$, and so on, would work just as well.

EXERCISE 18–4.

Suppose that the portions of light passing through four adjacent regions of film are of intensities 1/6, 1/18, 1/54, and 1/162 relative to background. Show that to the eye they differ by equal steps of apparent brightness, and that in fact they differ by equal steps of contrast.

SOLUTION: Aside from a factor of $\frac{1}{2}$, the intensities reaching the eye go as 3^{-n}, and will therefore appear to decrease in brightness by equal steps.

Assuming that 100% of incident light passes through unexposed film, the ODs of the four regions are log 6, log 18, log 54, and log 162. With the definition of Equation 18.2b, they differ by equal amounts of contrast.

The eye's ability to distinguish adjacent regions as being separate depends not only on the difference in luminosity from them, but also on their sizes, on the presence or absence of sharp edges between them, and on the level of noise. For x-ray film with *little mottle noise,* and under optimal viewing conditions, one can distinguish large regions with sharp borders that differ in transmission by only a few percent. But with large regions that blend gradually into one another, a difference in intensity of more than 20% may go unnoticed.

So much for *contrast.* What about the eye's *resolution* capability? Under optimal conditions, you can just resolve, at closest focus, a 30 lp/mm black and white optical bar pattern into separate stripes. With the normal viewing distance of about a foot, one can usually make out only about 5 lp/mm in a radiograph on a light box. This limit is to some extent determined by the packing of the cone receptors, which are responsible for acute vision, into the fovea centralis. (Some 35,000 receptors, ranging in diameter from 1 to 3 μm, are fitted into a region about 1.6 mm² in area.) The resolving power of the eye is also affected by various imperfections in the shape of the lens, by eye motion and, to a small extent, even by optical diffraction effects.

9. CONTRAST, RESOLUTION, NOISE, AND THE EYE: IMAGE CONSPICUITY

Contrast, resolution, and mottle noise are three fundamental parameters that describe radiographic image quality. They refer to quite different aspects of an image, and they are affected in different ways by changing the conditions of image formation. But they, and the patient dose, are not necessarily independent of one another, and it is frequently necessary to consider trade-offs that can and should be made among them.

Apparent mottle in an image, for example, is related to the patient dose and resolution. The standard way to reduce quantum mottle in a radiograph is to "improve the statistics" by increasing the number of clusters of silver grains, but with correspondingly less silver darkening from each. One way of achieving this is to use a cassette in which optical dye has been added to the screens' fluorescent material; less light from any scintillation reaches the film, and a smaller, less dense cluster of silver grains is laid down—an approach that also improves resolution. The price, however, is higher patient dose. The great advantage of the relatively new rare earth screens is their ability to provide low-mottle images at relatively low doses.

Similarly, resolution of an image improves, up to a point, with increased contrast and diminished mottle. And, finally, the contrast between regions may vanish with too much mottle. Thus, the separation of image quality into these three parameters is perhaps not so easy as it may have first seemed.

It would be most helpful if we could combine contrast, resolution, mottle, and the capabilities of the eye together in a neat little package, labeled something like "image conspicuity," to serve as an overall figure of clinical utility of images or imaging systems. The fact that each of the three fundamental attributes alone can be analyzed quantitatively suggests that such an integration might be possible. But despite much research activity in the area, and in the closely related field of image analysis by computers, this tantalizing synthesis is yet to be fully achieved.

It complicates matters that different characteristics of images are of primary importance in different diagnostic situations. When looking for hairline fractures, radiographic contrast between bone and soft tissue may already be far more than what is necessary, and only the sharpness of edges is of interest. In a search for soft tissue lesions in the brain with computerized tomography (CT), on the other hand, the contrast is of paramount significance, and the diagnostic utility of the image is limited by the level of mottle and the amount of noise introduced by scatter radiation and by the computer data-reconstruction algorithm. In a lengthy fluoroscopic examination of vessels, in which the contrast may be relatively low despite the introduction of contrast agent, it is important to keep the dose to as low a level as possible, but there must be enough exposure for the required image to be made out through the quantum mottle.

The *contrast-detail* phantom, images of which were shown in Figure 2–14, is useful for studying the ways in which contrast, noise, and resolving capability of an image or an imaging device affect object detectability. Figure 18–14 indicates the levels of contrast required for the detection of objects of different sizes, for the low- and high-noise cases of Figure 2–14. For noise-limited, low-contrast images, the minimum contrast necessary for detection, C_{min}, is related to the area of the object, A, and the signal-to-noise ratio roughly as

$$C_{min} \cdot A^{1/2} \cdot SNR = \text{constant} \qquad (18.6)$$

Thus, as would be expected, less contrast is required for larger objects and when the level of noise is low. A simple explana-

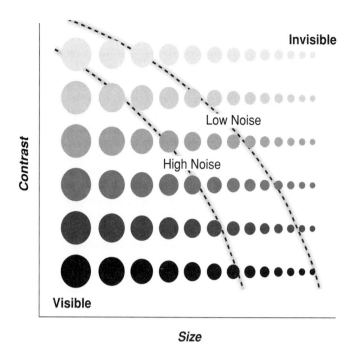

Figure 18–14. Results of tests using the contrast-detail phantom of Figure 2–14 for high-noise and low-noise cases. Each dashed line indicates combinations of size and contrast of objects that are just barely visible above the background noise. This provides one approach to quantifying the overall performance of an imaging system.

tion of this expression will be given later, in connection with the detectability of lesions with gamma cameras.

As noted in the beginning of this chapter, the bottom-line issue is the extent to which images help the physician arrive at correct diagnoses. Fortunately, a wealth of experience acquired over the years provides us with a set of operational ground rules for producing good images. In addition, there exist empirical methods that can help in our attempts to improve on those practical rules. Best known of these is a transplant from electrical engineering known as the *receiver operating characteristic,* or *ROC curve,* method, and it will be described in Chapter 24.

10. THE BENEFIT–RISK TRADE-OFF BETWEEN IMAGE QUALITY AND DOSE

One theme has recurred throughout this chapter: The greater the number of photons used in creating an image, up to a point, the lower the level of quantum mottle and the clearer the picture. But at the same time, for imaging processes that involve ionizing radiation, the radiation hazard to the patient increases as well. It is therefore necessary to settle on some reasonable compromise exposure, for any procedure, that will give adequate pictures but not pose undue risk to the patient.

Let us illustrate this optimization problem with a very simple hypothetical case study. Suppose that a patient presents with symptoms of a disease that is lethal if untreated. There is one reliable radiographic tool that can reveal how to treat it properly. The probability of being able to select the correct treatment increases (up to a point) with diagnostic image quality or signal strength, which is to say, in this case, with exposure, X. The probability of making a correct treatment decision is therefore a sigmoidal function of exposure, $S_{cure}(X)$ (Fig. 18–15). The symbol S is used to emphasize the point that it represents the probability of subsequent patient *survival.*

At the same time, the likelihood that the patient will suffer a lethal radiation-induced cancer from the diagnostic procedure itself also increases with exposure. Equivalently, the probability that the patient will escape the deleterious effects of the diagnostic procedure, $S_{xray}(X)$, decreases from unity slowly with increasing X. It is commonly assumed that, at the exposures encountered in imaging, $S_{xray}(X)$ falls off linearly and very slowly with exposure.

The overall probability of patient well-being, $S_{patient}(X)$, that is, the likelihood that the patient will be cured of the disease and yet not incur a radiogenic cancer during diagnosis, is given by the product of the (independent) probabilities

$$S_{patient}(X) = S_{cure}(X) \cdot S_{xray}(X) \qquad (18.7)$$

according to Equation 13.10. $S_{patient}(X)$ passes through a maximum at some "optimal" exposure, X_{opt}: If the objective is simply to cure the patient and do him or her no irrevocable harm in the process, then X_{opt} is the exposure to use. At lower exposures, the increased risk from the disease would more than compensate for the reduced hazard of the radiation itself, and the converse is true above X_{opt}.

Our little exercise is philosophically interesting, but per-

haps its most important conclusion is that such an analysis need not be used in practice for diagnostic imaging of symptomatic patients. This is true because the radiation risk is extremely small, and $S_{xray}(X)$ changes so very slowly with X. The shape of $S_{patient}(X)$, which is the issue of primary concern, is determined overwhelmingly by that of $S_{cure}(X)$. Figure 18–15 suggests that the approach normally taken by cautious physicians is correct: One should employ sufficient radiation to obtain the necessary diagnostic information, but not follow $S_{cure}(X)$ too far into the region of diminishing returns on additional exposure. And, of course, one should take reasonable radiation safety actions to reduce doses to patients and staff, whenever possible.

But note that although the *individual* radiation risk from a radiologic procedure may be quite small, the collective risk within a *large population* of individuals being examined may be substantial. An approach that works in the emergency room may or may not be suitable in, say, mass screening for breast cancer. In that case, something akin to Equation 18.7 must be reconsidered with greater care.

APPENDIX 18–1. Some Useful Ideas from Statistics

Learning About Populations from Samples: The Mean and the Standard Deviation

Suppose your state's Department of Health is investigating the safety of fluoroscopic examinations. Although it is not feasible to examine the entire *population* of fluoroscopic x-ray machines, it is possible to obtain a meaningful **estimate** of their performance from a sufficiently large and representative **sample.** M machines are chosen at random, and their output rates are measured under identical operating conditions (i.e., same applied high voltage and waveform, tube current, beam filtration, distance from target to measuring device, etc.). We shall denote the output rate of the ith machine x_i.

The simplest parameter for describing the results of the survey is the **sample arithmetic mean** or *average* value of the output rate:

$$\bar{x} = (x_1 + x_2 + \ldots + x_M)/M = (\sum_i^M x_i)/M \qquad (18.8a)$$

This also illustrates the convenience of the short-hand sigma (Σ) notation to denote a sum.

The sample mean in Equation 18.8a was calculated from data taken only from the M machines in the sample, but it should be approximately equal to, and provide a good estimate of, the true **population arithmetic mean** of the entire population* of machines in the state, μ:

$$\bar{x} \sim \mu \qquad (18.8b)$$

More advanced techniques of mathematical statistics allow one to determine the size of a sample needed for estimating a pop-

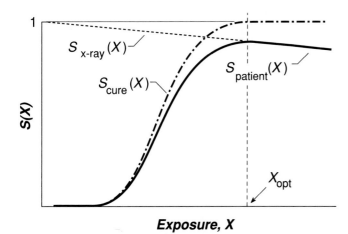

X_{opt}

Exposure, X

Figure 8–15. In a radiographic procedure, optimizing the overall probability of patient survival requires consideration of the needs both to cure the disease and to avoid inducing a cancer with the radiation. The probability of successfully detecting and analyzing the lesion, thereby allowing a cure, $S_{cure}(X)$, is a sigmoidal function of exposure, X. At too low exposures, you won't see much of anything at all, and at high exposures, more radiation won't improve things. (In fact, with too much irradiation, the film will be overexposed, with a decrease in S_{cure}.) The likelihood of the patient surviving the diagnostic procedure itself, that is, of avoiding the induction of a radiogenic cancer, is nearly unity, but decreases very slowly with exposure, $S_{xray}(X)$. The optimal exposure, X_{opt}, is that for which the overall survival probability (Equation 18.7) goes through a maximum.

---

*By convention, the same lower case Greek "mu," μ, is used to represent two completely unrelated entities: the population mean of Equation 18.8b and the linear attenuation coefficient. Similarly, σ can mean either the standard deviation or the Compton coefficient.

ulation parameter, such as the population arithmetic mean, with any desired degree of accuracy and certainty.

The **sample standard deviation**

$$s = [\sum_{i}^{M}(x_i - \bar{x})^2/(M-1)]^{1/2} \qquad (18.9a)$$

serves as a measure of the scatter in the measurements about the mean value. It provides the best estimate of the inherent *population standard deviation*, σ:

$$s \sim \sigma \qquad (18.9b)$$

A related but different issue: Suppose two (and only two) independent factors influence the value of a measurement. The time it takes you to drive to Aunt Ellie's place, for example, depends both on the day of the week (the Bay Bridge is terrible on Saturdays) and on the weather (tends to take longer when it's hot out). Let the uncertainties or variabilities associated with two such independent factors be parameterized by σ_1 and σ_2. Then the overall spread in the measurements may be parameterized by a total standard deviation σ where

$$\sigma^2 = \sigma_1^2 + \sigma_2^2 \qquad (18.9c)$$

Under the Bell-Shaped Curve: The Normal (Gaussian) Distribution

Although a statement of the sample mean and standard deviation may be sufficient for some purposes, more information about the distribution of values of x is provided in the *histogram* of Figure 18–16. For our example of x-ray machines, the total range of possible output rates may be broken into N equal subranges, or "bins" (where N should be selected to be quite a bit smaller than the number of machines, M). The histogram can record either the absolute or the relative number (or fraction) of machines that have an output rate that falls within any particular bin. Equivalently, it records the estimated probability that a machine chosen at random will have an output that falls within the jth bin, P_j. The output rates of some fluoroscopy machines are too low (possibly from a bad x-ray tube) and oth-

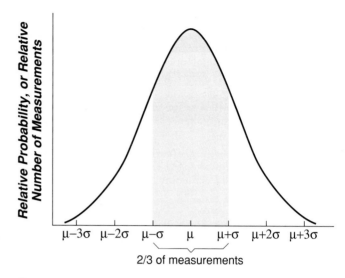

Figure 18–17. It is often possible to approximate a somewhat bell-shaped curve, such as that in Figure 18–16, by means of a Gaussian, or Normal, approximation. The Normal curve of Equation 18.10 is fully parameterized by the average value, μ, and the standard deviation, σ. If some measurable variable is Normally distributed, two thirds of all measurements will lie within the range $\mu - \sigma$ to $\mu + \sigma$. Ninety-five percent of the time, the measured value will lie within 2σ of the mean. See Table 18–2.

ers are unnecessarily high (perhaps indicating a weakness in some other part of the imaging chain, such as the automatic brightness control system), but most of the readings lie fairly close together and nearly centered on the mean value.

As with the results of many other kinds of surveys, Figure 18–16 may be smoothed out and redrawn (Fig. 18–17) in the shape of a bell. A function of the form of Figure 18–17 can be described approximately by the *Gaussian* or **Normal** *distribution*, a continuous function of the form

$$p_{\mu,\sigma}(x) = (2\pi\sigma^2)^{-1/2} \; e^{-1/2 \, (x-\mu)^2/\sigma^2} \qquad (18.10)$$

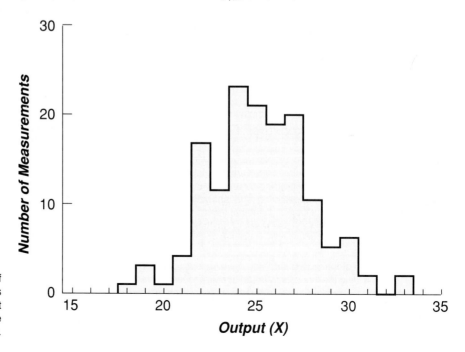

Figure 18–16. Representing the numbers of x-ray machines with different outputs by means of a histogram. The average output, μ, is about 25 units of output, in this example, and the standard deviation, σ, is about 3 units of output.

$p_{\mu,\sigma}(x)$ is symmetric about the population's mean, μ, and its width is characterized by the population's standard deviation, σ. $p_{\mu,\sigma}(x)$ is defined in such a way that $p_{\mu,\sigma}(x') \cdot \Delta x$ relates the probability that (or the relative frequency with which) the independent variable falls within the range from x' to $(x' + \Delta x)$.

If x is Normally distributed, there is a probability of about 2/3 (more precisely, 0.683) that any random measurement of x will fall within one standard deviation of the mean, that is, between $\mu - \sigma$ and $\mu + \sigma$; equivalently, about one third of the time, x will assume a value either greater than $\mu + \sigma$ or below $\mu - \sigma$. Likewise, there is a 95% chance that the measured value of x will lie within $\mu \pm 2\sigma$, and a 99.5% probability that $(\mu - 3\sigma) \leq x \leq (\mu + 3\sigma)$, and so on (Table 18–2).

Rare and Random Events: Poisson Statistics

In 1837, the Frenchman Simeon Poisson derived a distribution function that accounted accurately for the variation, from year to year, in the number of Prussian officers kicked to death by cavalry horses. (No doubt it worked equally well for horses kicked to death by Prussian officers.)

The approach applies to any *Poisson process*, in which discrete, countable, statistically independent events occur relatively rarely, but with a constant probability rate, over a continuous interval of time, distance, or other parameter. When an average of μ events occur in a specified interval (e.g., the mean value, as determined over a decade or so, for the number of Prussians lost *per year*), then the probability $P_\mu(n)$ of seeing exactly n (e.g., 7) of them in any one such interval (year) is given by the *Poisson distribution*:

$$P_\mu(n) = \mu^n \cdot e^{-\mu}/n!, \quad n = 0, 1, 2, \ldots \quad (18.11a)$$

The mean number of events μ in the interval can be any real value, but n must be an integer. (What would 3.3 Prussian officers for the year 1812 mean?) $n!$ is mathematical shorthand for the product of all integers between n and 1; that is, $n! \equiv n \cdot (n-1) \cdot \ldots 3 \cdot 2 \cdot 1$. For the important particular case of $n = 0$, $0!$ is taken to be 1, and Equation 18.11a reduces to $P_\mu(0) = e^{-\mu}$.

Radioactive decay of a radiopharmaceutical provides a perfect example of a Poisson process. The disintegrations of nuclei are discrete, countable (by means of a Geiger counter) events occurring over time, which is continuous. Because of the very short range of nuclear forces, the decay of any one nucleus has absolutely no effect on the subsequent disintegrations of others. The individual decay events are statistically independent, and random. Also, the probability of any given nucleus decaying in a given millisecond is very small. And, finally, the probability of any intact nucleus disintegrating over 1 millisecond is a constant of nature; it will be exactly the same next week as it is today. (Granted, there may be far fewer nu-

clei around next week left undecayed, for a short-lived radionuclide, but that's a totally separate issue.)

Suppose you are measuring the **activity** (number of decays per second) of a sample of a radiopharmaceutical. And suppose further (to simplify things) that the radionuclide has a half-life of several years, so that the activity of your sample will not change appreciably during your study. You count the number of decays that occur in 20 seconds, say, and repeat that measurement a large number of times. The average number of counts per 20 seconds obtained in this fashion can serve as an estimate of μ for use in Equation 18.11a. The Poisson distribution now can reveal the probability that another measurement for 20 seconds will yield exactly n decays, for any particular integer value of n that you choose.

As we shall see, this kind of information can be of great importance in image processing.

___ **EXERCISE 18–5.** _____

Technetium-99m is the workhorse radioisotope of the nuclear medicine department. A day after being injected with a tracer amount of ^{99m}Tc, a patient is examined with a Geiger counter that detects, on average, 3.2 nuclear decays per second. How likely is it that in the next second it will click four times?

SOLUTION: The likelihood of the counter registering four events over the next second (or over any other second in the not too distant future) is given by Equation 18.11a with $\mu = 3.2$ and $n = 4$:

$$P_{3.2}(4) = (3.2)^4 \cdot e^{-3.2}/(4 \cdot 3 \cdot 2 \cdot 1) = 0.18 = 18\%$$

___ **EXERCISE 18–6.** _____

In the first 3 weeks of January, you saw 4.7 ski accident patients per week, on average. How likely is it that in the last week there will be 3? 5? 8? 0?

SOLUTION: Assuming the same ski conditions and comparable populations of vacationers, the probabilities of 3, 5, 8, or 0 patients are given by

$$
\begin{aligned}
P_{4.7}(3) &= 4.7^3 \cdot e^{-4.7} / 3! &= 0.16 &\quad (16\%) \\
P_{4.7}(5) &= 4.7^5 \cdot e^{-4.7} / 5! &= 0.17 &\quad (17\%) \\
P_{4.7}(8) &= 4.7^8 \cdot e^{-4.7} / 8! &= 0.05 &\quad (5\%) \\
P_{4.7}(0) &= e^{-4.7} &= 0.009 &\quad (0.9\%)
\end{aligned}
$$

___ **EXERCISE 18–7.** _____

It is found under a microscope that in a 'uniformly exposed' region of film, 5.4 grains of silver are deposited per square micrometer (μm, or micron). How probable is it that between 4 and 7 grains will be found in a square micron chosen at random in this region?

SOLUTION: This is a Poisson process with $\mu = 5.4$. $P_{5.4}(4) = 0.160$, $P_{5.4}(5) = 0.173$, $P_{5.4}(6) = 0.155$, and $P_{5.4}(7) = 0.120$. The total probability that between 4 and 7 grains will be seen is $P_{5.4}(4) + P_{5.4}(5) + P_{5.4}(6) + P_{5.4}(7) = 0.624$. Why are we allowed to add probabilities like that here?

TABLE 18–2. PROBABILITY THAT A MEASUREMENT OF x FALLS WITHIN A SPECIFIED RANGE FOR VARIABLE x THAT OBEYS A "NORMAL" OR GAUSSIAN DISTRIBUTION, $p_{\mu,\,\sigma}(x)$, PARAMETERIZED BY MEAN μ AND STANDARD DEVIATION σ

Value of x					Probability
$(\mu - \sigma)$	<	x	<	$(\mu + \sigma)$	0.683
$(\mu - 2\sigma)$	<	x	<	$(\mu + 2\sigma)$	0.950
$(\mu - 3\sigma)$	<	x	<	$(\mu + 3\sigma)$	0.995

TABLE 18–3. FOR A POISSON DISTRIBUTION WITH LARGE μ, PROBABILITY THAT A MEASUREMENT OF x WILL FALL WITHIN A SPECIFIED RANGE

Value of x				Probability
$(\mu - \sqrt{\mu})$	<	x	<	$(\mu + \sqrt{\mu})$	0.683
$(\mu - 2\sqrt{\mu})$	<	x	<	$(\mu + 2\sqrt{\mu})$	0.950
$(\mu - 3\sqrt{\mu})$	<	x	<	$(\mu + 3\sqrt{\mu})$	0.995

It is characteristic of the Poisson distribution that the standard deviation, σ, is equal the square root of the mean:

$$\sigma = \sqrt{\mu} \qquad (18.11b)$$

The Poisson distribution can therefore be described *fully* with the single parameter μ. When μ is sufficiently large, moreover, the Poisson function can be approximated by a Gaussian of mean μ and standard deviation $\sigma = \mu^{1/2}$. Then the probabilities of obtaining various counts will be those given by Table 18–3. These are just the probabilities listed in Table 18–2, but rewritten so as to incorporate Equation 18.11b.

The standard deviation increases with the square root of the mean, for the Poisson distribution, but the *relative width* of the distribution, or the **relative variation**, decreases as the mean grows larger:

$$\text{relative variation} = \sigma/\mu = 1/\sqrt{\mu} \qquad (18.11c)$$

This can be expressed also as the *percentage variation* $= 100/\sqrt{\mu}$. According to Equation 18.11c, the larger the average number of counts that occur in an interval of time, for example, the smaller will be the relative magnitudes of the fluctuations in the individual readings about that average value, and the more likely it is that the number of counts in any particular interval will lie "relatively close" to the mean.

___ **EXERCISE 18–8.** ___

There are 100 silver grains per square millimeter, on average, in one uniformly exposed region of developed film. Show that the number of grains differs from this average by less than 10% in two thirds of all such areas.

SOLUTION: $\mu = 100$. As this is a Poisson situation, $\sigma = \sqrt{100} = 10$, which is 10% of μ. The problem amounts to showing that the count is between $\mu - \sigma$ and $\mu + \sigma$ in 67% of the 1-mm^2 areas. We can approximate the Poisson distribution with a Gaussian, of standard deviation $\sigma = 10$. Table 18–3 then shows that there is a two thirds chance that the density of grains will be $\mu \pm \sigma$, or 100 ± 10 grains per square millimeter.

___ **EXERCISE 18–9.** ___

The density of silver grains averages 10,000 per square millimeter in another part of the film. Show that here, in two thirds of such areas, the number of grains differs from the average by less than 1%.

SOLUTION: The same argument used in the previous example reveals that two thirds of all 1-mm^2 areas will contain $10,000 \pm 100$ grains, with a 1% variation rate.

Thus, the larger the average number of events (grains) in an area, the smaller will be the relative magnitudes of the fluctuations in the numbers of these events.

_____ *Chapter 19* _____

Screen–Film Radiography I:
The Primary X-ray Image

1. **Determinants of Image Quality and Dose in Radiography**
2. **The Source of the Beam**
3. **Differential Attenuation and Subject Contrast in the Primary X-ray Image**
4. **An Example—A Thin Bone Embedded in Soft Tissue**
5. **Enhancing Subject Contrast with Contrast Agent or Low kVp**
6. **Tissue Compensation Reduces Some Distracting, Nondiagnostic Contrast**

Chapter 2 sketched the process by which a radiograph is produced. Chapters 8 through 18 expanded on various particulars of the process.

This chapter and the next four retell, once again, the entire story of the creation of a diagnostic x-ray image. This time we shall use concise and rigorous language, as if one imaging professional were describing a novel modality (conventional screen–film radiography) to another, and focus more on the clinical aspects.

Central to all of this will be the themes of image quality (contrast, resolution, and noise) and of the trade-offs between image quality and dose. If you're not ever-vigilant of these issues, you may be getting less than optimal images and exposing the patient or medical staff to unnecessary dose.

1. DETERMINANTS OF IMAGE QUALITY AND DOSE IN RADIOGRAPHY

Standard radiography may be thought of as involving four separate clusters of processes:

1. The generation of a nearly uniform beam of bremsstrahlung and characteristic x-ray photons by means of an x-ray tube and generator. Some aspects of this process (e.g., beam filtration) are generally fixed, whereas others (the technique factors) are adjusted for each procedure and patient.
2. The differential attenuation of this beam (almost entirely through Compton and photoelectric events) by different tissues. The intensity of any portion of the beam transmitted through the body depends on the quality (parameterized, for example, by the effective energy) of the beam, and on the thicknesses, densities, electron densities, and effective atomic numbers of the tissues through which it passes.
3. The detection and recording of the spatial variations in the beam exiting the body. The image receptor nor-

mally consists of a sheet of specialized photographic film sandwiched between the fluorescent screens of a cassette. X-ray photons that have passed through the body are likely to interact with the screen (primarily by means of the photoelectric effect) and cause it to emit fluorescent light, which in turn exposes the film. The greater the transmission of x-rays through some part of the patient, the greater the number of silver halide crystals that will become activated (with the formation of latent images) in the corresponding part of the film, the greater the amount of silver that will be deposited during development, and the greater the developed film's optical density.
4. The viewing and interpretation of the film, and the overall control of the procedure, by the physician.

Table 19–1 indicates the ways in which certain aspects of these four sets of processes directly influence image quality and dose. The size of the tube's focal spot is a primary determinant of image resolution, for example, as will be shown in Chapter 22, but has little effect on contrast for large objects, on noise level, or on patient dose. The tube's kilovoltage setting and amount of beam filtration control the shape of the x-ray photon energy spectrum, which influences the beam's interactions with the various tissues and detector materials; and that, in turn, affects image contrast and patient dose. The bottom row of Table 19–1 is meant to suggest that it is the physician, ultimately, who must ensure that the equipment yields images of maximum utility at low cost in dose to patient and staff. Although physicians will not carry out the necessary quality control program themselves, it is normally their responsibility to make certain that such a program is established and properly followed by suitably qualified technical people.

Table 19–1 does not list all the factors that go into the making of a radiograph, and it does not indicate some secondary relationships. A few designations, moreover, may seem rather arbitrary. The effects of scatter radiation, for example, are noted under "contrast," with "noise" referring to quantum mottle, film

TABLE 19–1. HOW FACTORS OF IMAGE GENERATION INFLUENCE ASPECTS OF IMAGE QUALITY AND DOSE

| | Radiographic Image Quality | | | | | | | |
| | Contrast[a] | | Resolution[a] | | | | | |
	Differential Attenuation	Scatter, etc.	Penumbra	Screen	Movement	Noise[a]	Magnification, Distortion	Patient Dose
Tube/generator								
Focal spot size			X					
Off-focus radiation		x	(x)					x
Beam filtration	x							X
Voltage waveform	(x)				x[b]			x
Technique factors								
kVp	X	x				(x)		X
mA			(x)[c]					
s					X			
mA-s	(x)[d]					X		X
SID[e]			X		x		X	X
Patient								
Thickness	X[f]	X					x	X
Thickness modifiers	All	All						
Compression	x[f]	X						X
Compensation	x[g]	(x)						
Field size		X					(x)	X
Contrast agent	X							
Motion	x[a]				X			
Image receptor								
Scatter rejection		All						All
Grid		X						X
Gap		X					X	X
Screen–film Γ	X[h]							
Screen–film speed					(All)[i]			All
Screen μ					(x)			X
Screen thickness				X	(x)	(x)[a,j]		X
Intrinsic efficiency					(x)	X		X
Screen efficiency				X[k]	(x)	X		X
Film speed					(x)	X		X
Film processing	X[l]	X[l]				X		X[l]
Film granularity						(x)		
Physician/QC	X	X	X	X	X	X	X	X

X, very important connection; **x,** sometimes significant; **(x),** sometimes noticeable; **All,** all items in a subcategory affect image quality or dose.
[a]Contrast, resolution, and mottle influence one another; especially important in the imaging of small objects.
[b]The waveform of the tube potential may affect the exposure time.
[c]Because of blooming.
[d]To the extent that the contrast and the average OD are interrelated.
[e]Source-to-image receptor distance.
[f]The thickness of the portion of the body being imaged influences the choice of kVp.
[g]Without compensation, parts of an image may be over- or underexposed, resulting in reduced gamma and contrast.
[h]Screen–film Γ amplifies subject contrast.
[i]A faster screen–film combination allows shorter exposures.
[j]With a thicker screen, the associated lower sharpness may give the impression of less mottle.
[k]Optical dye in a screen reduces the screen efficiency, but improves the resolution.
[l]Film processing affects Γ, fog, and the average optical density (hence the patient dose).

granularity, and so forth. The reason for this decision should become clear later. And to the extent that contrast, resolution, and noise are interdependent and not fully separable entities, some aspects shown as distinct are, in fact, overlapping.

Still, hopefully, this matrix will help to untangle the most important radiographic processes in a fairly realistic and helpful fashion.

2. THE SOURCE OF THE BEAM

In a typical modern imaging system used primarily for routine radiography, the source of the x-ray beam is a rotating anode tube attached to a constant-potential or three-phase generator capable of putting out a peak voltage of 150 kVp, a maximum average current of 500 mA (when set at voltages considerably lower than the maximum kVp), and a maximum power at 100 kVp (for a 0.1-second exposure) of 50 kW. Most diagnostic films are shot with tube potentials between 50 and 120 kVp, exposure times of 0.01 to 0.1 seconds, and average currents of 50 to 200 mA.

Viewed simply as a generator of heat, like a resistor, the tube expends kVp · mA · s joules of electrical energy during an exposure (Equation 11.2). Practically all of this energy does end up, in fact, as heat in the target. Heat leaves the anode primarily as infrared radiation, much of which is absorbed by a bath of oil surrounding the tube. The oil serves as both a thermal conductor and an electrical insulator between the tube and its housing. Transfer of heat from the housing to room air takes place by convection, and may be assisted by a fan. If a tube is operated improperly, the anode can overheat and become irreparably damaged in a matter of seconds. The conditions and frequency of acceptable exposures may be determined from the rating charts and cooling curves supplied by the manufacturer. Modern systems contain various interlock devices, controlled by temperature sensors and/or microprocessors, to reduce the risk of overheating.

Not *all* the electron kinetic energy, however, is wasted as heat. A small amount is transformed into bremsstrahlung and characteristic x-ray radiation. The efficiency of the bremsstrahlung process ($10^{-6}\ Z \cdot$ kVp) increases with both the atomic number of the target metal and the tube's operating potential (Equation 11.3). With a tungsten/rhenium target and typical diagnostic operating voltages, about 0.5% to 1% of the power pumped into an x-ray tube is converted into x-ray photons.

The general shape of the continuous component of the photon energy spectrum is distinctive of the bremsstrahlung plus beam filtration processes, and independent of the nature of the target material and of all the tube's operating parameters. The peak photon energy, however, is determined by the kilovoltage setting. Characteristic x-ray emission occurs when the generator's kVp setting sufficiently exceeds the energies (in keV) of the target's emission peaks (60–70 keV for tungsten and about 20 keV for molybdenum). Most of the photons at the low-energy end of the continuous spectrum are preferentially absorbed in the anode and glass wall of the tube in photoelectric events. An aluminum filter outside the tube further hardens the beam, reducing even more the component of the lowest-energy, relatively nonpenetrating (but skin dose-imparting) photons. With higher kVp settings, the effective filtration of the anode, glass, and external filter together should be at least equivalent to that of 2.5 mm of aluminum. Additional filtration beyond 2.5 mm of Al has little effect on the shape of the spectrum, except at the highest applied tube potentials, but diminishes beam intensity. Inadequate filtration, on the other hand, can result in patient exposures that are a factor of 2 or more greater than necessary.

Nearly all the x-ray radiation is emitted from the focal spot region of the anode. The integrated intensity of the filtered beam (counting photons of all energies) is linear in tube current and inversely proportional to the square of the distance r from the focal spot. The dependence on kilovoltage and filtration is more complex. The output (in centigrays of air kerma) of a three-phase or constant-potential system, with total filtration equivalent to Al millimeters of aluminum, is shown as a function of applied potential in Figure 11–8, and may be described roughly by the empirical expression

$$K_{air}\ (cGy) = 11 \cdot (2.5/Al) \cdot (kVp/100)^2 \cdot (A\text{-}s)/(r/100)^2$$

$$(19.1)$$

seen earlier as Equation 11.4. Note that current is in amperes, not milliamperes. Output from a tube powered by a single-phase generator is less by a factor of 0.6 to 0.7. Exposure in roentgens may be obtained by dividing the air kerma by 0.873. As a rule of thumb, 1 cGy of air kerma corresponds to about 1 R of exposure and to 1 rem of dose equivalent to tissue.

Because of the angular dependence of the production of bremsstrahlung and the heel effect (see Chapter 11, Section 9), x-ray intensity falls off away from the central axis of the beam, and more rapidly so on the "anode" side of it. This effect is partially offset at depth in tissue, however, by the greater hardening (and, therefore, greater penetrating power) of the beam on the anode side.

Although the *output of an x-ray tube* may be roughly proportional to the square of the applied potential, the *effect on the image receptor* is more complex, for two reasons. First, a higher-kVp beam is more penetrating, so that more of the x-ray energy passes through the patient and reaches the image receptor. Second, the sensitivity of the image receptor may depend on photon energy.

Enough primary photons must transit the patient to produce a suitable average level of darkening of film. Something like 1×10^{-3} cGy of kerma to air (about 1 mR of exposure), give or take a factor of 5, is needed at the radiographic cassette for proper average optical density; the more sensitive rare earth screen–film systems require as little as 0.1 cGy. At the same time, there must be enough contrast among the various tissues of interest to make the image diagnostically useful. Thus the tube should produce an intensity and quality of x-ray energy that leads (after passing through the patient and into the intensifying screen) to a film image that ranges in optical density between about 0.25 and 2.25. Which brings us to the differential attenuation of the beam by the patient.

3. DIFFERENTIAL ATTENUATION AND SUBJECT CONTRAST IN THE PRIMARY X-RAY IMAGE

Chapter 15 explored the attenuation of an x-ray beam by homogeneous blocks of material. Now we shall turn to something closer to a real patient, within whom it is the *variations* in density, atomic number, electron density, and thickness of the tissues that give rise to images, and are of medical interest.

Imagine the beam as consisting of a bundle of separate, slowly diverging *geometric* "rays." The loss in photon fluence or intensity incurred along any one of them in passing through the body is determined, for a given photon spectrum, by the properties of the tissues it traverses. The spatial pattern of unscattered x-ray photon energy emerging from the patient, the composite record of the individual experiences of all of these "rays," is known as the *primary x-ray image*.

The three sources of spatial variation in the primary x-ray image are differences in tissue thickness (Fig. 19–1A), in tissue density (Fig. 19–1B), and in tissue chemical composition (Fig. 19–1C). Each of these contributes to the *subject contrast* defined in Chapter 18, Section 3.

Consider, for example, the effect on a monochromatic beam (for simplicity) of variation in thickness of homogeneous

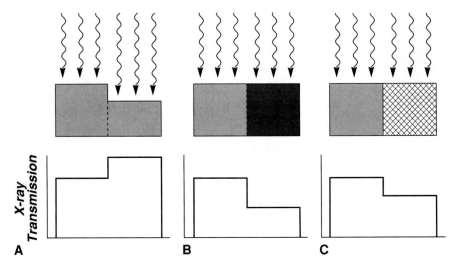

Figure 19–1. The relative amount of x-ray energy that is transmitted through a block of matter depends on the energy of the photons and on certain characteristics of the matter: **A.** Its thickness. **B.** Its density. **C.** Its chemical makeup, in particular the effective atomic number and the electron density.

tissue. We shall define the subject contrast (in the *primary x-ray image*) between two regions of Figure 19–1A in direct analogy to Equation 18.2a, but now in terms of *air kerma:*

$$C_{\text{subject}} = \log_{10}[K_1^{\text{prim}} / K_2^{\text{prim}}] \qquad (19.2)$$

The "air" subscript has been dropped from K, but "prim" (for *primary*) is added to indicate that this kerma contains no scatter radiation. If we ignore the effects of scatter radiation, the contrast depends only on the extent to which photons are removed from the beam in passing through the two regions.

By Equation 15.4, the intensity along a ray is diminished, under conditions of good geometry, by a factor of $e^{-[\mu/\rho] \cdot \rho \cdot x}$ in passage through homogeneous material of thickness x, density ρ, and mass attenuation coefficient $[\mu/\rho]$. From this and Equation 19.2, the contrast in Figure 19–1A is

$$C_{\text{subject}} = \log_{10}(e^{-[\mu/\rho] \cdot \rho \cdot x_1} / e^{-[\mu/\rho] \cdot \rho \cdot x_2}) \qquad (19.3)$$
$$= \log_{10} e^{-\mu \cdot (x_1 - x_2)} = 0.434\mu \cdot (x_2 - x_1)$$

the last step of which made use of $\log_{10} e^q = 0.434q$ (see Exercise 14–6). From the dependence of μ on photon energy, it is clear that the contrast depends on kVp, as was suggested in Chapter 14, Section 3.

EXERCISE 19–1.

Find the subject contrast for the other cases in Figure 19–1 for rays passing through two blocks of the same thickness but different tissues (i.e., different densities or effective atomic numbers).

SOLUTION: $C_{\text{subject}} = 0.434x \cdot (\mu_2 - \mu_1)$, where $\mu = [\mu/\rho] \cdot \rho$.

4. AN EXAMPLE—A THIN BONE EMBEDDED IN SOFT TISSUE

Figure 19–2 follows rays of a 100-kVp beam (three-phase, 2.5 mm Al total filtration) that pass through a 10-cm-thick portion of the body, part of which contains a thin bone. One set of rays traverses 10 cm of unit-density ($\rho = 1$ g/cm³) soft tissue, such as muscle; the other passes through 9.5 cm of soft tissue and 0.5 cm of bone.

The effective photon energies in Table 19–2 were obtained by combining the information in Table 15–1 and Figure 15–10. The equivalent monochromatic photon energy for our beam is 35 keV. The product $[\mu/\rho] \cdot \rho$ for a 35-keV beam in soft tissue is 0.32 cm⁻¹. The ray that transits 10 cm of soft tissue is attenuated by a factor of $e^{-(0.32 \text{ cm}^{-1})(10 \text{ cm})} = 0.041$. The other ray is reduced by $e^{-(0.32 \text{ cm}^{-1})(9.5 \text{ cm})} = 0.048$ in 9.5 cm of soft tissue and by a further factor of $e^{-(0.70 \text{ cm}^2/\text{gm})(1.65 \text{ g/cm}^3)(0.5 \text{ cm})} = 0.56$ in bone, for a total attenuation of $(0.048)(0.56) = (0.027)$. By Equation 19.2, the

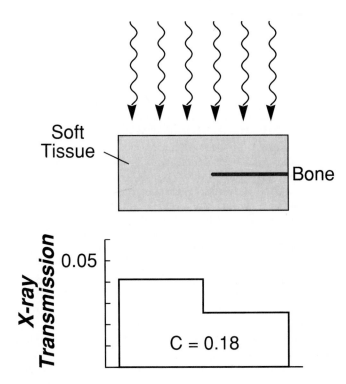

Figure 19–2. This chapter and the next two will explore the example of a 0.5-cm-thick bone embedded in a block (everywhere of 10-cm thickness) soft tissue. An x-ray beam of 35-keV effective energy is directed at our "phantom." The transmissivities through the two regions are 0.041 and 0.027. Only primary (unscattered) photons are considered for now and, by Equation 19.3, the primary image subject contrast is 0.18.

TABLE 19–2. EFFECTIVE ENERGIES, AND CORRESPONDING NARROW-BEAM ATTENUATION COEFFICIENTS[a] IN TISSUES, FOR VARIOUS kVp SETTINGS (THREE-PHASE, 2.5 mm AL EQUIVALENT TOTAL FILTRATION)

Peak Tube Potential (kVp)	HVL in Al (mm)	Effective Energy (keV)	Soft Tissue		Bone	
			$[\mu/\rho]$ (cm^2/g)	HVL (cm)	$[\mu/\rho]$ (cm^2/g)	HVL (cm)
60	2.2	30	0.365	1.9	0.95	0.44
80	2.7	32	0.34	2.0	0.80	0.53
100	3.3	35	0.32	2.2	0.70	0.60
120	4.0	38	0.29	2.4	0.55	0.76
Density (g/cm^3)			1.0		1.65	

[a]Accounting precisely for the shape of the x-ray beam spectrum, for beam hardening in tissue, and for the effects of scatter radiation will yield somewhat different values of $[\mu/\rho]$ and HVL.
See Table 15–1 and Figure 15–10.

subject contrast in the primary x-ray image is $C = \log_{10}(0.041/0.027) = 0.18$.

It is easy to generalize this for application to more realistic situations, where the total attenuation of x-ray photons along a geometric ray is determined by the thicknesses, densities, and attenuation coefficients of all the tissues in its path. Photons traversing material of thickness x_1 and linear attenuation coefficient μ_1 will be attenuated by the amount $e^{-\mu_1 \cdot x_1}$. If the remaining photons then traverse x_2 of linear attenuation coefficient μ_2, their number will be diminished further by a factor of $e^{-\mu_2 \cdot x_2}$. And so on. On emerging from the body, the intensity of the ray is only $(e^{-\mu_1 \cdot x_1}) \cdot (e^{-\mu_2 \cdot x_2}) \cdots$ of its initial value. By Equation 14.11d, this can be rewritten in the more compact form

$$(e^{-\mu_1 \cdot x_1}) \cdot (e^{-\mu_2 \cdot x_2}) \cdots = e^{-\mu_1 \cdot x_1 + \mu_2 \cdot x_2 + \dots)} = e^{-\Sigma \mu_i \cdot x_i} \quad (19.4)$$

and expressed in terms of the mass attenuation coefficients through an obvious generalization. The Σ notation was defined in Equation 18.8a. The sum over the index i may be replaced by an integral when appropriate.

_____ **EXERCISE 19–2.** _____

Assume that a three-phase generator is set for a 100-kVp, 200-mA, 0.02-s exposure, and that the film cassette is 100 cm (40 in.) from the x-ray tube. What is the kerma to air at the cassette in the absence of our thin-bound "patient"? When the patient is present? What is the contrast in the primary x-ray image?

SOLUTION: Equation 19.1 indicates that if there were no patient present, the air kerma at the cassette would be 0.044 cGy = 44×10^{-3} cGy (50 mR).

The part of the beam that traverses 10 cm of soft tissue exits with only 4.1% of that, or 1.8×10^{-3} cGy. A ray that passes through the soft tissue and bone, and is attenuated by a factor of 0.027, leads to an exposure of 1.2×10^{-3} cGy. The contrast in the primary x-ray image is $C = \log(1.8 \times 10^{-3}/1.2 \times 10^{-3}] = 0.18$, as was found above.

Replacing the bremsstrahlung beam with a monochromatic beam, that is, using an effective beam energy, is a fairly crude approximation. The calculation of beam attenuation can

be carried out more accurately by explicitly accounting for the shape of the filtered bremsstrahlung spectrum and for the energy dependence of photon attenuation. That is, one might determine what fraction of the total intensity is in the range 99 to 100 keV and then the attenuation of that (99.5 average keV) component in matter; likewise for the 98- to 99-keV photons; and so on. At the end, by bringing all the components together again, one would have a better estimate of total beam attenuation. A beam of 35-keV effective energy, however, is much easier to use in working through our embedded bone example, to which we shall return in the next two chapters.

5. ENHANCING SUBJECT CONTRAST WITH CONTRAST AGENT OR LOW kVp

The radiographic contrast of 0.18 found above indicates why even a small amount of bone has a very significant effect on the x-ray beam, and partially explains the great success of radiography in bone imaging. The large contrast of bone against its soft tissue background arises because of its relatively high atomic number (i.e., the Z^3 dependence of the photoelectric mass attenuation coefficient) and density.

For some situations in which this kind of differential does not occur naturally, it can be introduced artificially through the use of *contrast agent*. Iodinated media (Z=53 for iodine) allow the imaging of some soft tissue structures such as blood vessels, kidneys, and the ureter. With the discovery of low-toxicity chemical forms, iodine is now used routinely in computerized tomography and digital subtraction angiography as well as in radiography. Similarly, barium (Z=56) or a combination of barium and air ($\rho = 1.2 \times 10^{-3}$ g/cm^3) serves to highlight the alimentary tract.

As discussed in Chapter 14, Section 3, subject contrast also depends on tube potential. Table 19–2 and Figure 13–2 indicate that over the diagnostic x-ray range, μ for bone is always much greater than that for soft tissue. At the lower diagnostic energies, in particular, where the photoelectric effect is important even in soft tissue, μ_{bone} rises $(Z_{bone})^3/(Z_{soft})^3$ times faster with decreasing photon energy than does μ_{soft}. The same phenomenon occurs with fine blood or lymph vessels that contain contrast agent. As a result, one may be able to increase the vessel-to-background subject contrast substantially simply by lowering the tube potential (Fig. 19–3).

Figure 19–3. kVp setting may have a significant effect on the appearance of organs that contain contrast agent. Here, excretory urograms (EXUs) were obtained at **(A)** 70 and **(B)** 110 kVp with an iodinated contrast medium. (The absorption edge for iodine occurs at 33.2 keV.) The renal parenchyma and renal pelvis show up much more clearly on the lower-kVp film. With an iodinated contrast medium, "The best image contrast is usually obtained in the range of 60 to 75 kVp. Radiation exposure to the patient is higher with this technique than with a higher kVp technique, but in view of the increased information content, these lower kVp values are commonly used." *(From the American College of Radiology Learning File, courtesy of the ACR.)*

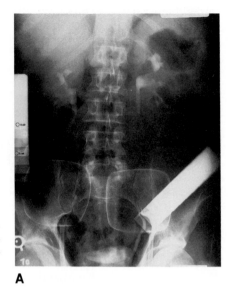

A

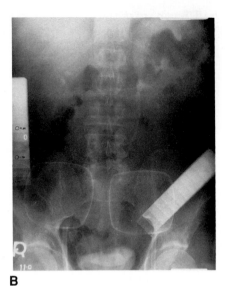

B

Likewise, contrast among soft tissues (e.g., between normal breast tissue and tumor), brought about by differences in density or chemical composition, may be improved by going to lower kVp. (Lower kVp both increases the relative number of interactions that occur via the photoelectric effect and enhances the contrast picked up by those interactions.) The lower-energy beam is less penetrating, however, so one must raise the mA-s to achieve an acceptable overall optical density, with an increased patient dose.

The effect of the overall patient thickness on subject contrast is a little more subtle. Let us, for now, ignore scatter radiation. If the 0.5-cm bone of Section 4 is located within a 14-cm (rather than 10-cm)-thick portion of the patient (Fig. 19–4) the extra 4 cm of soft tissue diminishes both K_1^{prim} and K_2^{prim} in Equation 19.2 by the same factor of $e^{-(0.32\,\text{cm}^{-1}) \cdot (4\,\text{cm})} = 0.28$. This cancels out in the numerator and the denominator, and the subject contrast in the primary x-ray image does not change! Indeed, we can return to the original exposures, and contrast, simply by increasing the mA-s by a factor of $1/0.28$.

When scatter is taken into account, however, as discussed in the next chapter, some of what has just been said will have to be modified. In particular, the contrast degradation resulting from scatter radiation will be seen to increase with overall thickness of the part of the body being imaged. That is a primary reason that the breast is compressed in mammography.

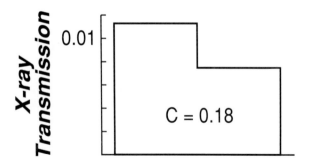

Figure 19–4. An additional 4 cm of soft tissue attenuates both parts of the x-ray beam by the same amount. The subject contrast, as defined by Equation 19.2, does not change. This is no longer true when scatter is taken into account (next chapter).

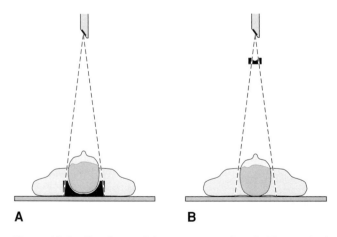

A

B

Figure 19–5. Two forms of tissue compensation: **A.** Wax or plastic compensator. **B.** Wedge filter that attaches to the x-ray tube housing.

6. TISSUE COMPENSATION REDUCES SOME DISTRACTING, NONDIAGNOSTIC CONTRAST

The curvature of a patient's head (and some other anatomic structures) causes rapid changes in optical density that are of no diagnostic utility. Indeed, the spatial variation in exposure of the image receptor may be so great that to achieve a suitable average optical density in the region of interest, other parts of the film will be underexposed, overexposed, or both.

This problem can be largely reduced through *dodging*, or *tissue compensation*. In simplest form, compensation involves the replacement of absent tissue with wax or some other material that is radiologically similar to soft tissue (Fig. 19–5A). Alternatively, the beam can be modified by means of a suitably sculpted metal *wedge filter* or *compensator* that can be attached to the x-ray tube housing (Fig. 19–5B). The level of exposure of the cassette is much more uniform, and the whole film is properly exposed.

With digital radiography, such compensation can be carried out electronically, after the image has been acquired.

Chapter 20

Screen–Film Radiography II: Scatter Radiation and Grids

1. **Scatter Radiation Diminishes Contrast . . .**
2. **. . . But Small Field Size, Tissue Compression, and Low kVp Reduce scatter . . .**
3. **. . . As Do Gaps and Grids**
4. **Grid Parameters**
5. **Grid Cutoff Errors**
6. **Effects of Scatter and a Grid on Contrast: The Embedded Bone Example**

X-ray beam exposure of a patient's body produces not only the primary x-ray image, but also Compton scatter radiation. This scatter, unfortunately, reduces the subject contrast.

The amount of scatter created diminishes with smaller exposure fields and/or lower kVp, and with decreased thickness of the part of the body being imaged (e.g., by means of tissue compression in mammography). The intensity of scatter radiation that eventually reaches the screen–film image receptor can be further reduced through use of a gap or an antiscatter grid.

1. SCATTER RADIATION DIMINISHES CONTRAST . . .

Blue skies and hazy days result from the scattering of light by air molecules and fine droplets of water (or by air pollution). Otherwise, the sun would shine brightly against a star-flecked black backdrop, as would the midday moon. Similarly, the river bottom is lost from view if too much light is scattered from suspended silt.

Just as the stars vanish at sunrise, and the features of the river bottom disappear in its murkiness, so also radiologic images are obscured by Compton scatter photons. The effect of scatter on subject contrast is apparent in Figure 20–1, showing the pelvic region before and after a large fraction of the scatter radiation is removed by means of a grid.

2. . . . BUT SMALL FIELD SIZE, TISSUE COMPRESSION, AND LOW kVp REDUCE SCATTER . . .

What determines the amount of scatter generated in a patient? The most important factors are the cross-sectional area of the beam that strikes the patient, the thickness of the body part being imaged, and the kVp (Fig. 20–2).

The amount of scatter increases rapidly (and subject contrast drops off) with increasing field size, for small fields. Eventually, it levels off for large fields (Fig. 20–3). The reason for this behavior may be seen in Figure 20–4, in which a tank of water is irradiated with beams of different sizes. With a small field of exposure, very few Compton photons arrive at point A on the cassette. (Recall that when studying attenuation of radiation in matter, one usually employs "good geometry," with a very narrow beam, specifically to eliminate the effects of scatter.) That advantage vanishes rapidly as the field grows in size, however, as more tissue is irradiated and produces scatter (Fig. 20–4A). But when a field is already quite large (Fig. 20–4B), not many of the additional scatter photons produced at its edges with further enlargement will reach point A.

A modern radiographic system comes with a *collimator* (Fig. 10–12) that can be adjusted to restrict the field size to the smallest that is clinically necessary for the individual patient. Keeping the field size as small as possible helps to maximize contrast (Fig. 20–5) and also to reduce the radiation dose to patient (and scatter dose to staff, for some procedures).

Tissue thickness is a second factor that strongly influences the amount of scatter generated. Chapter 19, Section 5, showed that subject contrast in the primary x-ray image (not including scatter) is not strongly affected by an increase in the thickness of soft tissue. Unfortunately, of the radiation exiting the patient and heading toward the detector, the primary x-ray image constitutes only a relatively small part; most of it, in fact, may be Compton scatter. The scatter-to-primary ratio increases with overall patient thickness, and the contrast decreases.

In a mammographic examination, the breast is compressed by a radiolucent panel, in part because a reduction of overall tissue thickness leads to less scatter degradation of the image (Fig. 20–6). (Compression also spreads out the breast tissue over a greater area of film, which also improves image quality. It even lowers the average dose to the breast glandular tissues, thereby reducing the [very small] radiation risk.)

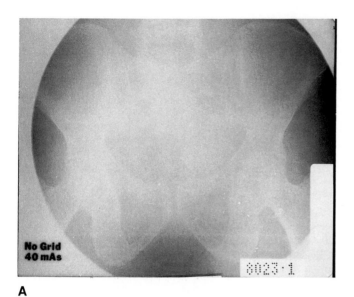

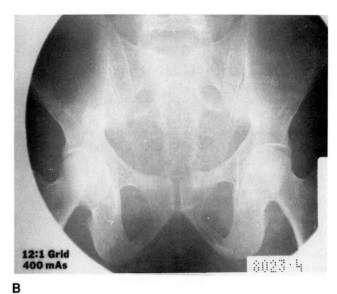

A   **B**

Figure 20–1.   Effect on image quality of removing a large fraction of the scatter radiation. **A.** No grid. **B.** After the addition of a grid of grid ratio 12:1. To maintain the same average optical density, it was necessary to increase the mA-s, and patient dose, by a factor of 10. *(From the American College of Radiology Learning File, courtesy of the ACR.)*

Finally, as discussed in Chapter 19, Section 5, subject contrast usually decreases with increasing kVp. Scatter exacerbates the situation (Fig. 20–7A). Compton photons that escape the patient's body enter the image receptor as misinformation. The relative number of Compton (vs. photoelectric) interactions increases with photon energy. Moreover, there is an increase in the volume of tissue in which are produced scatter photons that have a fair likelihood of escaping the tissue (Fig. 20–7B). Even the probability that a Compton photon will be heading in the "forward" direction (therefore toward the detector) after a single scatter event increases with the energy of the incident x-ray (see Fig. 12–3). All of this argues for a low kVp.

But as will soon be seen, a low kVp is undesirable from a patient dose perspective. This counterbalancing factor is so important, in fact, that one normally takes the kVp as *high* as possible, while maintaining an acceptable degree of contrast. But in some situations, such as with mammography, the need to maximize the contrast is the dominant issue, and one does employ lower energy photons.

In summary, scatter increases with increasing field size,

patient thickness, and kVp. So, to minimize the scatter degradation of contrast:

- Use as small a field as possible.
- Position the patient, compress tissue, or by other possible means minimize the overall thickness.
- Choose a low kVp. But when some contrast can be sacrificed, as is often the case, use a *higher* kVp to lower patient dose. More about that in Chapter 23.

Amount of Scatter
Depends Upon . . . .

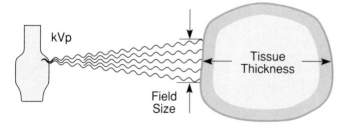

Figure 20–2.   Representation of three important factors that affect the amount of scatter generated in a patient's body: radiation field size, patient thickness, and kVp setting.

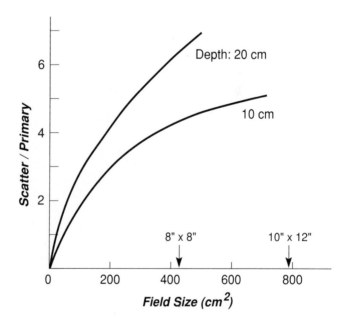

Figure 20–3.   Ratio of scatter radiation intensity to primary beam intensity at a point within the body. The scatter-to-primary ratio depends on the radiation field size, the depth of the point within the body (or, for radiation leaving the body, its thickness), and the energy of the beam.

Figure 20–4. Explanation for the field size dependence of the scatter-to-primary ratio curve of Figure 20–3. **A.** The intensity of *primary* photons arriving at point A is independent of field size, but that is far from the case for *scatter* radiation. When the field is small, even a small increase in its size causes a significant increase in the relative volume of material irradiated, hence in the amount of scatter that is produced and reaches point A. Hence the sharp increase in scatter-to-primary with field size for small fields. **B.** When the field is already large, the law of diminishing returns sets in, and enlarging the field further has little effect at point A.

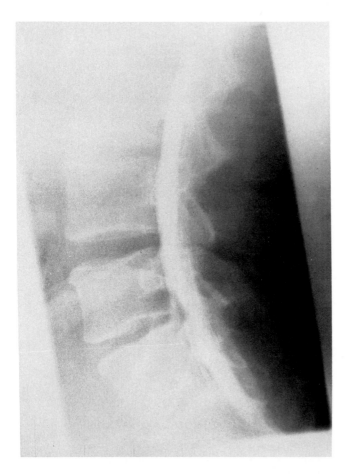
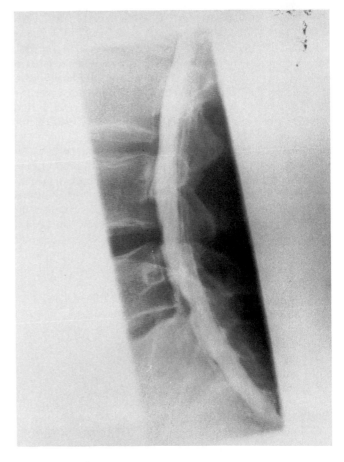

Figure 20–5. Contrast improves with reduced field size, as evident in these lateral myelograms of the lumbar spine. Even though both films used a 10:1 grid, the contrast and visibility of detail increased considerably with tighter field collimation. From a radiation safety perspective, the reduction in irradiated volume compensates for the need to increase the exposure by 50% (as less scatter reaches the image receptor) to achieve the same average optical density. (*From the American College of Radiology Learning File, courtesy of the ACR.*)

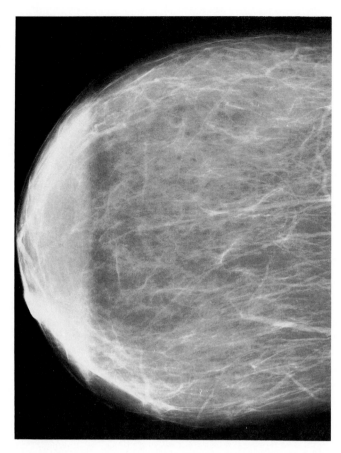

Figure 20–6. Mammographic illustration (cephalocaudal view for 54-year-old woman, normal mammogram) of the effect of tissue thickness on contrast. Only the posterior part of the breast is compressed, because the patient's breast is larger than the compression plate; the higher level of detail there is remarkable. What else contributes to the greater visibility in the posterior part of the breast in this image? *(Courtesy of Thomas G. Langer, MD, University of Virginia Health Sciences Center.)*

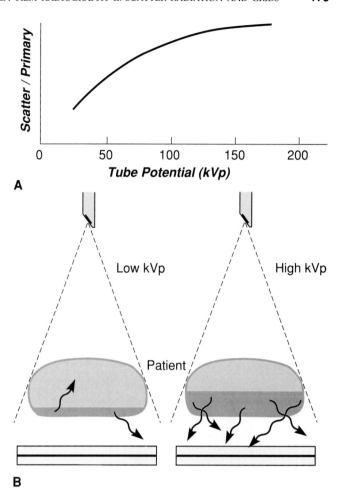

Figure 20–7. Scatter radiation degradation of image contrast tends to increase with photon energy. **A.** Scatter-to-primary ratio as a function of kVp. **B.** Image degrading scatter comes largely from the part of the patient's anatomy that lies closest to the image receptor. As photon energy increases, there is an increase in the volume of tissue in which are produced scatter photons that can escape the body. Also, scatter photons are more likely to come off in a more forward direction, toward the image receptor.

3.   . . . AS DO GAPS AND GRIDS

Figure 20–8 suggests another method of reducing the amount of scatter radiation that reaches the film cassette: Move the patient 10 to 20 cm away from it. The photons that constitute the primary x-ray image continue heading straight toward the cassette. But many of the Compton photons scatter away from the cassette and, with a gap, may miss it altogether. The introduction of a **gap** in this fashion, in some procedures, leads to a magnified image. As the image receptor is moved further from the x-ray source, the tube output must be increased, with a corresponding increase in patient dose.

A more common approach is to employ a *grid*. A grid is somewhat like a Venetian blind, consisting of an array of very thin (0.05 mm or so) sheets of lead foil, separated from one another by weakly attenuating spacers of aluminum or an organic compound. Most of the x-ray photons that make it through the patient's body without interaction will likewise pass along the channels between the lead sheets. Compton scattered photons, on the other hand, enter the grid at skew angles, and nearly all are absorbed by the lead.

The lead sheets in the simplest grids are parallel to one another. There are three standard ways to improve on this. One is to align the planes of lead along the slightly diverging geometric rays of the x-ray beam. The planes of such a **focused grid** are no longer parallel, but rather diverge at the same rate as does the x-ray beam. The grid must be positioned, of course, so that its *convergent* or **focal line** passes through the focal spot of the x-ray tube.

Another grid improvement is to add a second set of lead sheets perpendicular to the first. Such a **crossed** grid can be either parallel or focused. The advantage of a crossed grid is that more of the scatter radiation is filtered out. But with a linear (uncrossed) grid, one can angle the x-ray tube along its length without causing loss of primary radiation from "grid cutoff" (see below); this allows more flexibility in difficult positioning situations.

A third possible improvement is to move the grid continuously during the exposure. A **Bucky** or *Potter–Bucky grid* is shifted in the direction normal (perpendicular) to the planes of

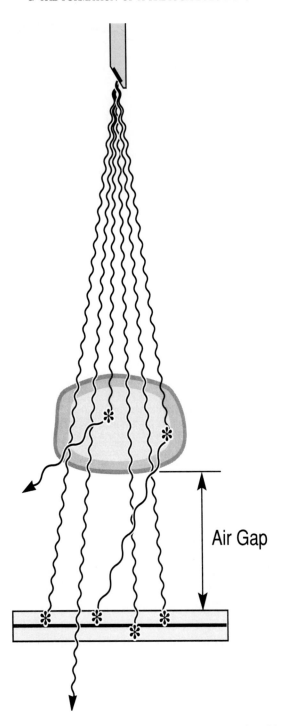

Figure 20–8. With an air gap, much of the scatter produced in the patient will miss the image receptor altogether.

the lead sheets, blurring out their shadows. Several motions can be used: The grid may be moved back and forth in an oscillatory fashion; or shifted fast in one direction and then slowly back; or catapulted rapidly to high velocity and then decelerated exponentially. Some radiologists prefer stationary to Bucky grids—the quality of modern grids is high enough that the shadow lines may not be overly distracting, and stationary systems are cheaper, have no moving parts that break down, and result in less dose to the patient.

With a single-phase generator, the motion of the grid must be carefully controlled. If, over the interval between x-ray pulses, the grid shifts a distance equal to the separation between the sheets of foil (or some multiple thereof), then the shadows of the sheets will overlap at times of high exposure rate, and their image will be pronounced, somewhat as a movie camera may stroboscopically freeze the spokes of a turning wagon wheel.

4. GRID PARAMETERS

The effectiveness of a grid increases with its thickness, T (also called its height or depth), and as the separation, W, of the lead sheets decreases (Fig. 20–9). Put another way, T is the length of the channels through the grid and W is their width; the greater the value of T/W, the more difficult it is for scatter photons to make it all the way through. The **grid ratio,** defined as

$$\text{grid ratio} = T/W \qquad (20.1)$$

is therefore an important determinant of the grid's usefulness. Ratios for most grids lie between 4:1 and 16:1.

_____ **EXERCISE 20–1.** _____

The thickness of the grid is 3 mm, and the lead sheets are separated by 0.25 mm of filler. What is the grid ratio?

SOLUTION: By Equation 20.1, the grid ratio is (3 mm/0.25 mm) = 12, or 12:1.

The thickness of the lead foil itself is ignored in the definition of grid ratio, but is accounted for in the *lead content*. Lead content is expressed in g/cm^2 and determined, in effect, by cutting out a cylinder 1 cm^2 in cross-sectional area through the grid (Fig. 20–10) and weighing the lead obtained. It increases with the thickness of the lead foil, the height of the grid, and the number of sheets per centimeter.

Four parameters are commonly used to describe the performance capabilities (as opposed to construction) of a grid: the Bucky factor, B; the primary transmission, T_p; the selectivity; and the contrast improvement factor.

The **Bucky factor,** sometimes called the grid factor, is the ratio of the total amount of radiation (primary image plus scatter) incident on the grid to that which passes through it (Fig. 20–11):

$$B = \text{incident total/transmitted total} > 1 \qquad (20.2a)$$

Always a number greater than 1, B is also the amount by which the mA-s must be increased to offset the decrease in total amount of radiation reaching the cassette when a grid filters out much of the scatter (and some of the primary image) radiation:

$$B = \frac{\text{exposure with grid}}{\text{exposure without grid}}, \quad \text{for same optical density}$$

$$(20.2b)$$

As with a gap, a price to be paid for enhanced signal-to-noise is greater patient dose.

The Bucky factor depends on the grid ratio and on the photon energy, as indicated in Table 20–1. This reflects the kVp

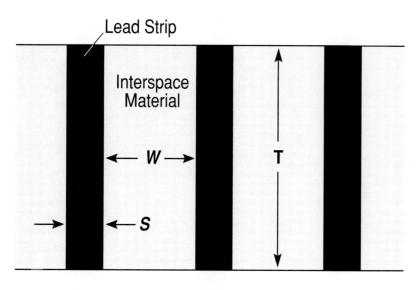

Lead Strip

Interspace Material

W

T

S

Grid Ratio: T/W

Figure 20–9. A grid, seen from end on. The lead sheets are S thick and T tall and separated by distance W. The grid ratio, T/W, is one of the primary determinants of the effectiveness of a grid at removing scatter while leaving an adequate primary photon image.

dependence of the relative numbers of photon interactions that occur in the patient's body by means of the Compton and photoelectric mechanisms and the kVp dependence of the effectiveness of the grid in rejecting scatter photons.

_____ **EXERCISE 20–2.** _____

A 100-kVp, 4-mA-s exposure gives an acceptable average optical density with no grid. By how much must the mA-s be increased if an 8:1 grid is added?

SOLUTION: By Table 20–1, increasing mA-s by a factor of 4 would be about right.

Of the primary (unscattered) radiation incident on a grid, the *primary transmission* is the relative amount that is actually transmitted through it,

T_p = transmitted primary/incident primary < 1   (20.3a)

with values ranging typically from 50% to 75%. One might suspect T_p to be determined by the relative amount of open channel confronting a primary photon approaching the grid,

$$T_p \sim W/(W + S) \qquad (20.3b)$$

where S is the thickness of the lead sheets, and W is the separation between them (see Fig. 20–9). Experimentally measured values of T_p are somewhat less than this.

The *selectivity* of the grid is the ratio of the primary photon transmission to the scatter radiation transmission:

$$\text{selectivity} = \frac{\text{primary transmission}}{\text{scatter transmission}} \qquad (20.4)$$

Lead Content: g/cm^2 of Lead

1-cm^2 Area

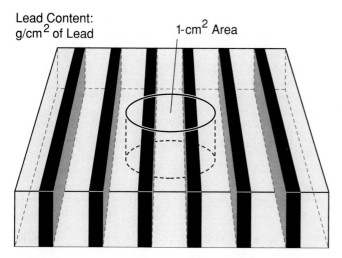

Figure 20–10. If a plug of 1-cm^2 cross-sectional area is drilled out of a grid, the mass of lead removed defines the "lead content" (g/cm^2).

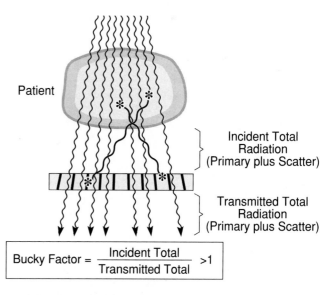

Patient

Incident Total Radiation (Primary plus Scatter)

Transmitted Total Radiation (Primary plus Scatter)

$$\text{Bucky Factor} = \frac{\text{Incident Total}}{\text{Transmitted Total}} > 1$$

Figure 20–11. The inverse of the Bucky factor measures the fraction of radiation (primary plus scatter) that is removed from a beam when a grid is put in place. The Bucky factor itself is therefore the factor by which the output of the x-ray tube must be increased to return the cassette to its pregrid level of exposure.

TABLE 20–1. TYPICAL VALUES OF THE BUCKY FACTOR[a] FOR VARIOUS GRIDS AND kVp SETTINGS

			Grid Ratio			
	No grid	2:1	4:1	8:1	12:1	16:1
			Bucky Factor			
70 kVp	1	1.1	2.7	3.5	4.0	4.5
95 kVp	1	1.1	2.7	3.8	4.3	5.0
120 kVp	1	1.1	2.7	4.0	5.0	6.0

[a]Factor by which output of x-ray tube must be increased to maintain the same air kerma at the cassette when the grid is inserted.
National Council on Radiation Protection and Measurements (NCRP): Medical X-ray, Electron Beam, and Gamma-ray Protection for Energies up to 50 MeV (Equipment Design, Performance, and Use (Report No. 102). Bethesda, MD: NCRP, 1989 (Table B.4).

In general, the more effective a grid is at diminishing scatter, the more primary x-ray image is also lost in the process. The selectivity is a measure of the success with which the grid can remove scatter while passing the primary x-ray image.

A most important measure of the usefulness of a grid is the **contrast improvement factor**, or **relative contrast**:

contrast improvement factor
$$= \text{contrast with grid} / \text{contrast without grid} \qquad (20.5)$$

Typical values of relative contrast are recorded in Table 20–2. It increases most significantly with lead content and grid ratio, but also depends on the Bucky factor, primary transmission, patient thickness, field size, and kVp.

5. GRID CUTOFF ERRORS

There are a number of ways that a grid can be inadvertently misused, and as a group these go by the name of **primary beam cutoff errors**. With each, some problem in the system setup geometry reduces the size or quality of the primary x-ray image reaching the cassette.

In Figure 20–12, for example, a focused grid was put in place with its divergence pointing the wrong way. In Figure 20–13, the orientation is correct, but the grid is too close to (or too far from) the x-ray tube, a situation known as focus–grid distance decentering. And the grid in Figure 20–14 is shifted laterally. It is usually fairly easy to correct any of these problems, or combination of them, once they are detected.

Since any beam is divergent, with a parallel grid the transmission is diminished toward the edges of the field, or cut off, because of the mismatch of geometries. Although not an

"error" in the above sense, this situation may be thought of as a special case of focus–grid distance decentering. The effect can be reduced either by increasing the distance of the grid from the source of the x-ray beam, if the tube can produce more intensity, or by selecting a grid with a lower grid ratio.

6. EFFECTS OF SCATTER AND A GRID ON CONTRAST: THE EMBEDDED BONE EXAMPLE

Let us return to the bone in soft tissue of Chapter 19, Section 4, and consider the effects of scatter created in the patient's body and of a grid placed in front of the image receptor.

The reason for the dependence of contrast on scatter is suggested by Figure 20–15. In the upper graph, the heights of the open blocks correspond to $K_{\text{soft}}^{\text{prim}}$ and $K_{\text{bone}}^{\text{prim}}$, the values of primary beam (no scatter included) kerma in air at the screen–film cassette for x-ray photons transmitted through 10 cm of soft tissue alone and for those passing through 9.5 cm of soft tissue plus the 5 mm of bone. We have defined the *subject contrast in the primary x-ray image* as the logarithm of the ratio of the kermas, exposures, transmitted intensities, and so forth (see Equation 19.2).

When the same amount of scatter radiation, K_{scat}, is added to each part of the beam, the subject contrast changes from $\log_{10}(K_{\text{soft}}^{\text{prim}} / K_{\text{bone}}^{\text{prim}})$ to $\log_{10}(K_{\text{soft}}^{\text{prim}} + K_{\text{scat}}) / (K_{\text{bone}}^{\text{prim}} + K_{\text{scat}})$. It is a simple matter to show that C_{subject} decreases as K_{scat} grows larger. Scatter reduces contrast.

For our example, Exercise 19–2 demonstrated that the air kerma at the cassette is 1.8×10^{-3} cGy for x-ray photons transitting only through soft tissue, but 1.2×10^{-3} cGy for the part of the beam passing through the bone. Suppose that about 3

TABLE 20–2. TYPICAL VALUES OF THE RELATIVE CONTRAST[a] FOR VARIOUS GRIDS AND kVp SETTINGS

			Grid Ratio			
	No grid	2:1	4:1	8:1	12:1	16:1
			Relative Contrast			
70 kVp	1	2.0	3.0	4.8	5.3	5.8
95 kVp	1	1.5	2.0	3.3	3.8	4.0
120 kVp	1	1.3	1.5	2.5	3.0	3.3

[a]Contrast relative to that with no grid, using a 20-cm-thick water phantom and a test pattern.
National Council on Radiation Protection and Measurements (NCRP): Medical X-ray, Electron Beam, and Gamma-ray Protection for Energies up to 50 MeV (Equipment Design, Performance, and Use (Report No. 102). Bethesda, MD: NCRP, 1989 (Table B.4).

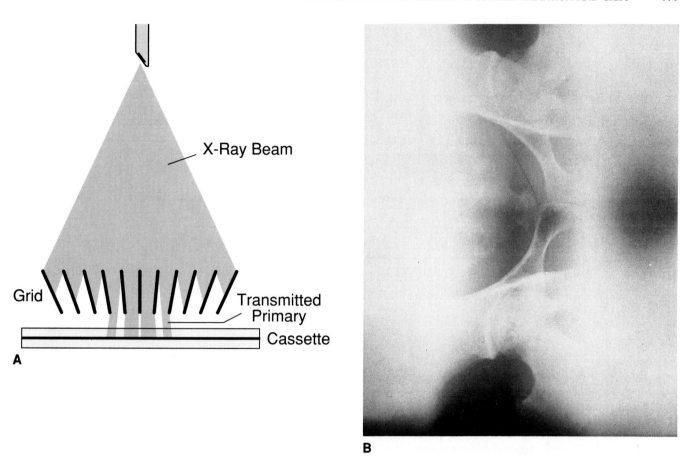

Figure 20–12. Example of a grid cutoff error. **A.** A focused grid faces the wrong way, so that only those x-ray photons near the center of the beam will pass through to expose the cassette. **B.** The result of such a cutoff error. (*From the American College of Radiology Learning File, courtesy of the ACR.*)

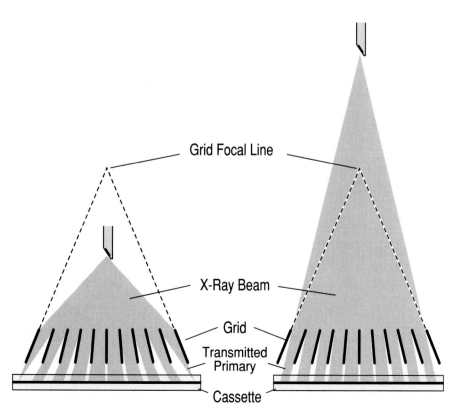

Figure 20–13. Cutoff errors that arise when a focused grid is too close to, or far from, the x-ray tube focal spot.

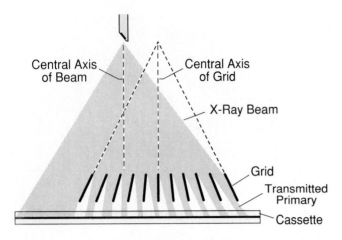

Figure 20–14.   A focused grid not centered relative to the x-ray beam.

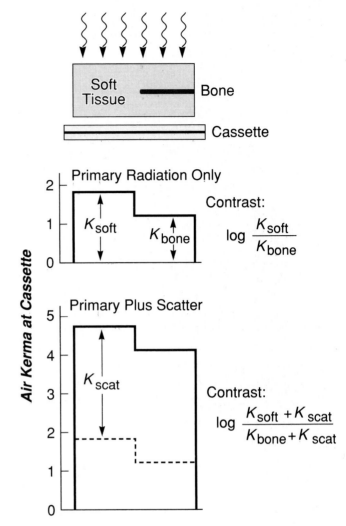

Figure 20–15.   A return to the embedded bone example of Chapter 19, Section 4. The contrast, as defined in Equation 19.2, may be generalized so as to include scatter radiation. The contrast decreases as the relative amount of scatter (scatter-to-primary ratio) at the image receptor increases.

$\times\ 10^{-3}$ cGy of scatter is superimposed on the entire primary x-ray image. The subject contrast is now $C_{subject} = \log_{10}(1.8 + 3)/(1.2 + 3) = 0.060$, considerably less than what is obtained with no scatter.

> How realistic is it to assume that scatter exiting the patient is 2 or 3 times as intense as primary x-ray beam? Figure 20–3 provides a partial answer. Another rough indication can be extracted from Figure 15–12. Consider the three curves labelled 3 mm Al; these correspond to a beam with a 3-mm HVL in aluminum, which should be fairly close to the quality of our beam. The dose imparted by the very narrow beam $(0 \times 0\ \mathrm{cm}^2)$ falls to about 5% of its entry value in passing through 10 cm of water. The scatter contributions of the 15×15 and 35×35-cm^2 beams, on the other hand, raise the dose at 10 cm of depth to 15% to 20% of the surface dose. This would suggest that for the photon beam of our beam quality exiting a 10-cm-thick patient, perhaps a quarter or a third of the intensity consists of primary photons, and the rest is scatter.

A grid can undo some of the loss of contrast brought about by scatter. Table 20–2 indicates that an 8:1 grid improves contrast for a 20-cm-thick phantom by a factor of about 3. For a 10-cm-thick patient such as ours, there will be much less scatter (relative to the primary beam intensity), so the grid will be correspondingly less helpful, the contrast enhancement factor for our situation being closer to 2. Even this, however, will raise the overall contrast from 0.06 to about 0.12.

According to Table 20–1 and Exercise 20–2, use of the grid will reduce the total kerma to air at the cassette (primary plus scatter) by a factor of about 4, so that the average kerma to air at the cassette is roughly 1×10^{-3} cGy (which is what it was before scatter and the grid came in). Is this enough to produce an image on film with a good average optical density? That depends on the screen–film system, as will be seen in the next chapter.

Chapter 21

Screen–Film Radiography III: Films and Screens

1. **The Characteristic Curve of a Screen–Film System Plots Optical Density Against the Logarithm of the Relative Air Kerma or Exposure**
2. **Speed, Latitude, and Gamma**
3. **Film Exposed Directly to X-rays**
4. **Use of a Screen Reduces Patient Dose . . .**
5. **. . . But Diminishes Resolution and Sharpness . . .**
6. **. . . And May Increase Quantum Mottle**
7. **Effects on Mottle and Resolution of Increasing the Screen–Film Speed**
8. **Rare Earth Versus Calcium Tungstate Screens**
9. **Effect of Screen–Film Gamma on Contrast: The Embedded Bone Example**

The primary x-ray image is created in the body of the patient, but transformed into a visual image by means of the image receptor. Although the image receptor in radiography may be film alone, much more commonly it is film sandwiched between the intensifying screens of a cassette.

The basic exposure–response behavior of a screen–film combination (or of a film alone) is contained within the characteristic curve, a plot of optical density against the logarithm of the relative air kerma or exposure. The most important information, however, is summarized in terms of three parameters: speed, latitude, and gamma.

Use of a cassette significantly reduces patient dose and/or exposure duration, but at the cost of some loss of resolution and perhaps some increase in mottle. Rare earth screens, which are largely displacing those made of calcium tungstate, generally offer comparable or better image quality but at lower dose.

1. THE CHARACTERISTIC CURVE OF A SCREEN–FILM SYSTEM PLOTS OPTICAL DENSITY AGAINST THE LOGARITHM OF THE RELATIVE AIR KERMA OR EXPOSURE

As suggested in Chapter 17, Section 5, for a given set of irradiation and film development conditions, the response of a screen–film system (or of a film alone, when no cassette is being used) to different levels of x-ray exposure may be described completely in terms of the *characteristic curve*.

An ordinary plot of optical density against air kerma or exposure at the cassette would be perfectly legitimate, and is sometimes employed, as in Figure 17–9. (Hereafter, both "air kerma" and "exposure" will be used loosely as abbreviations for "air kerma or exposure.") But it is more common practice, instead, to modify the mode of information presentation in two

ways: One (1) uses a *logarithmic scale* for air kerma, as in Figure 17–10, and (2) plots the optical density (OD) against the logarithm of the *relative air kerma* (or, equivalently, one graphs OD against relative air kerma on semilog paper). This approach offers several conveniences.

First, the *relative* air kerma. In the clinic, one rarely knows the exact beam strength at a cassette. The amount (in units of optical density) by which a poor film is over- or underexposed, however, is often fairly obvious. A characteristic curve in which air kerma is expressed (along the *x* axis) relative to some convenient reference value provides all the information needed to remedy the problem.

Suppose that a radiograph is shot with a screen–film combination described by Figure 21–1, which was taken from Figure 17–10. With particular kVp and mA-s settings, the average OD in the anatomic region of interest is found to be 2.8. We may not know the precise value of the absolute air kerma or exposure (in cGy or mR) at the image receptor, but the characteristic curve still reveals the amount by which we must decrease the air kerma to get down to an average OD of 1.3, say, in the repeat film: We have to reduce relative exposure from 40 to 7. We could, most simply, decrease the mA-s by a factor of about 7/40.

A relative scale offers another benefit: The units of beam quantity (cGy or mR) cancel out, and the choice of the measure of beam quantity (air kerma or exposure) becomes totally immaterial.

Plotting the *logarithm* (to the base 10) of the relative air kerma is helpful in three ways. Each increment of 0.3 in the log of the relative air kerma, each additional equal step along the *x* axis by that amount (Fig. 21–1), corresponds to another doubling of the relative air kerma. Second, the clinically relevant portion of the characteristic curve tends to be fairly straight when OD is graphed against the logarithm of relative air kerma; then differences or changes in OD are nearly propor-

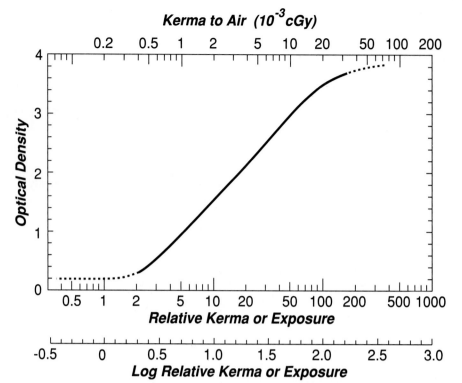

Figure 21–1. Characteristic curve for the screen–film system of Figure 17–10. The upper scale uses air kerma, in units of 10^{-3} cGy, as the independent variable. Bear in mind that 1×10^{-3} cGy of air kerma corresponds approximately to 1 milliroentgen (mR) of exposure. The second scale uses either the air kerma or the exposure, relative to an arbitrary fiducial level (which, in this case, happens to fall at 0.2×10^{-3} cGy, within the fog portion of the curve). The lowest scale presents the *logarithm* of the relative kerma or exposure.

tional to differences or changes in log exposure. Third, as the exposures grow larger, the logarithm increasingly compresses the upper end of the number scale, in a way that allows a wide range of (relative) exposures of interest to be displayed.

The characteristic curve of a screen–film system consists of six distinct parts (Fig. 21–2). At very low doses, the **toe** of the curve emerges out of the **fog** that occurs normally in developed film even without any exposure. Above the toe lies the so-called **linear** part of the curve, in which changes in the OD are approximately proportional to changes in the *logarithm* of the (relative) air kerma. The characteristic curve on semilog paper is nearly straight here. This is the only part of the characteristic curve used in standard radiography. Elsewhere, the dependence of OD on exposure is weaker; that is, the sensitivity of the image receptor to variations in exposure is poorer. The linear portion terminates in a **shoulder**, above which the curve flattens out and **saturation** sets in. Finally, **solarization** (see Chapter 17, Section 6) occurs at exposures much higher than those encountered in the clinic.

2. SPEED, LATITUDE, AND GAMMA

A complete characteristic curve reveals more about a screen–film system than one normally needs to know to make a good film. Much of the important information can be summarized, and presented more simply, in the form of three parameters: the speed, the latitude, and the gamma.

Speed is a measure of the ease with which the middle of the useful OD range is reached. A **fast** film or screen–film combination requires relatively little exposure to achieve that level of darkening. Speed is formally defined as the *inverse* of the air

kerma, K (in cGy), or the exposure (in R) required to achieve an OD of 1 above and beyond fog level:

$$\text{speed} = 1/K \qquad (\text{for OD} = 1 + \text{OD}_{\text{fog}}) \qquad (21.1)$$

The fog level for curve a in Figure 21–3 is OD = 0.2, for example, and the kerma to air required to produce an OD of 1.2, point A, is 1.3×10^{-3} cGy. The speed is thus $1/(1.3 \times 10^{-3}$ cGy$) = 770$ cGy^{-1}. The smaller the amount of radiation needed to reach the reference OD level, the faster the system. In Figure 21–3, the characteristic curves a and b are identical to one another, except that curve b is displaced to the right by a log relative exposure of +0.6 relative to curve a, and requires four times the exposure to reach any particular OD. As will become apparent later in this chapter, the speed of a screen–film system is determined by the choices of screen and film, the kVp, the film processing conditions, and other factors.

_____ **EXERCISE 21–1.** _____

Find the speed of screen–film b of Figure 21–3.

SOLUTION: The OD of fog is 0.2, and the air kerma required to produce an OD of 1.2 is 5×10^{-3} cGy. The speed is therefore $1/(5 \times 10^{-3}$ cGy$) = 200$ cGy^{-1}. As suggested above, this is about four times slower than the film of curve a.

Latitude refers to the range of exposures, or of log relative exposures, over which the film is radiographically useful, such that the characteristic curve is nearly straight and the OD is between about 0.25 (where a bit more than half the incident light photons pass through it) and about 2.25 (0.6% optical transmittance),

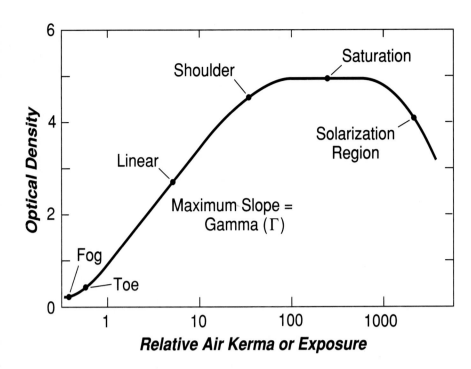

Figure 21–2. A complete characteristic curve, in which optical density is plotted against the relative air kerma or relative exposure (with a logarithmic scale), consists of six parts. Commonly seen are the fog, typically with an OD of 0.1 to 0.2; the toe; the linear region, where nearly all radiographic exposures are made; and the shoulder. The saturation and solarization regions normally are not displayed or used.

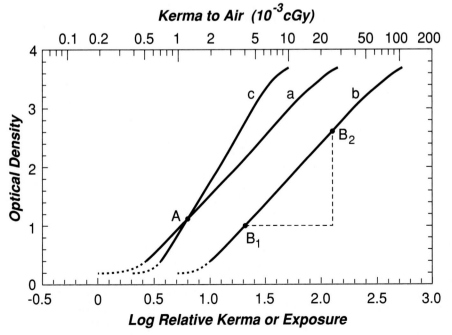

Figure 21–3. The screen–film systems of curves a and c are faster than that of curve b, as less air kerma is required to reach an OD of 1.0 above fog level. The latitude for curve c is less than for a or b, and its gamma is correspondingly greater. The gamma is determined from the differences in optical densities and log relative exposures for two points that lie in the linear portion of a curve. With curve b, for example, the optical densities for points B_2 and B_1 are 2.6 and 1.0, respectively, with a difference of 1.6; the log relative kermas differ by 2.1 − 1.3 = 0.8; therefore, $\Gamma = 1.6/0.8 = 2$.

latitude = K(OD = 0.25) to K(OD = 2.25)   (21.2)

Outside this spread, the film is either *underexposed* or *overexposed*.

Although regions with ODs in the range 0.25 to 2.25 are usable, and even more opaque parts can be explored with a "bright light," the eye is most effective at picking out patterns with ODs between about 1.0 and 1.5.

_____ **EXERCISE 21–2.** _____

Find the latitude for screen–film system a of Figure 21–4.

SOLUTION: Latitude = 0.4×10^{-3} to 4×10^{-3} cGy. Expressed in terms of log relative exposure, the latitude is about $1.4 - 0.3 = 1.2$.

The *gradient* is the rate at which the optical density changes with the logarithm of the exposure or relative exposure, that is, the slope of the characteristic curve, over the exposure range of interest:

$$\text{gradient} = (OD_2 - OD_1)/(\log_{10} K_2 - \log_{10} K_1)$$
$$= (OD_2 - OD_1)/(\log_{10} K_2/K_1) \qquad (21.3a)$$

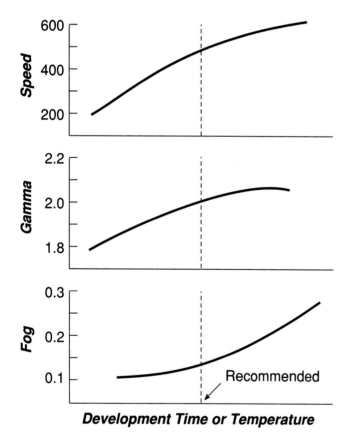

Figure 21–4. The characteristics of developed film depend on the development process itself. Of particular importance are the temperature of the developer fluid and the time that the film spends in it. The optimal conditions suggested by the manufacturer are based largely on consideration of a desirable combination of speed, gamma, and fog levels.

The gradient is greatest, and the screen–film system is most responsive to small variations in exposure, in the linear region, and almost always one attempts to operate there. The slope of the characteristic curve in the linear region is called the **gamma**:

$$\text{gamma} = \Gamma = (OD_2 - OD_1)/(\log_{10} K_2 - \log_{10} K_1)$$
$$= (OD_2 - OD_1)/(\log_{10} K_2/K_1) \quad \text{(linear region)}$$
$$(21.3b)$$

Screen–film systems used in radiology have gammas typically between 2 and 3.5.

_____ **EXERCISE 21–3.** _____

Find the gamma of curve b in Figure 21–3.

SOLUTION: Consider points B_2 and B_1, where $K = 25 \times 10^{-3}$ cGy (OD = 2.6) and $K = 4 \times 10^{-3}$ cGy (OD = 1.0). $OD_2 - OD_1 = 2.6 - 1.0 = 1.6$ and $\log 25 \times 10^{-3} - \log 4 \times 10^{-3} = \log 25/4 = 0.8$. (Equivalently, the log relative kermas at the two points are 2.1 and 1.3, with a difference of 0.8.) By Equation 21.3b, $\Gamma = (1.6)/(0.8) = 2.0$.

As evident from curves a and c of Figure 21–3, the greater the gamma, the smaller will be the latitude. If a high gamma is required to accentuate contrast in one part of a film, the dynamic range may be so limited as to leave other important regions too dark or transparent. That is, a high gamma may be helpful in bringing out subtle contrasts, but it results in the loss of perhaps important information at the two ends of the OD scale. One of the great advantages of a computer-based *digital radiographic system* is that its response can be adjusted (i.e., the *dynamic range* selected) separately for any region of interest of the image.

It is instructive to cast Equation 21.3b in a somewhat different form. The subject contrast between two regions of a patient's body was defined in Equation 19.2 as $C_{subject} = \log_{10}(K_2/K_1)$. The corresponding visual contrast in developed film (see Equations 18.2) is $C = (OD_2 - OD_1)$. Inserting these into Equation 21.3b yields

$$C = \Gamma \cdot C_{subject} \qquad (21.4a)$$

seen earlier as Equations 18.3. There, the gamma was called the receptor or screen–film contrast.

Another way of saying the same thing: By Equation 18.2, radiographic contrast may be expressed in terms of the intensity, L, of transmitted light as $C = (OD_2 - OD_1) = -\log_{10} L_2/L_1$. Inserting this and the definition of $C_{subject}$, Equation 19.2, into Equation 21.4a gives $-\log_{10} L_2/L_1 = \Gamma \cdot (\log_{10} K_2/K_1)$ or, equivalently,

$$L_2/L_1 = (K_2/K_1)^{-\Gamma} \qquad (21.4b)$$

In radiography, the gamma of a film or screen-film system is almost always greater than 1. By either Equation 21.4a or 21.4b, this will enhance subject contrast. Suppose that the gamma happens to be precisely 1. A 2:1 difference in the amount of x-ray energy passing through two regions of the patient's body will result in a 2:1 difference in the transmittance of the corresponding parts of the developed film. With a gamma greater than 1, this differential will be accentuated.

The speed of a screen–film system (or of a film alone, if no screen is used) depends strongly on the details of the process by which the film is manufactured. More film darkening will occur per crystal with larger crystals of silver halide. Larger crystals generally are also more sensitive. For both reasons, larger microcrystals result in a faster film. The speed also varies with the reducing power of the developer, its temperature, and the time and degree of agitation in the development process, as indicated by Figure 21–4. Similar considerations apply to the gamma, latitude, and fog level. An important advantage of an automatic film processor (Fig. 21–5), in addition to its being faster, more convenient, and less labor intensive, is the high uniformity in the quality of developed films.

The above description of the properties of film is of more than academic interest. A complete characteristic curve can be produced rapidly and easily in the clinic by means of a **sensitometer** and **optical densitometer,** as will be discussed in Chapter 29, to check both the film quality and the processor performance.

3. FILM EXPOSED DIRECTLY TO X-RAYS

As shown in Chapter 17, Section 5, for film exposed directly to x-rays (with no screen), the optical density is linear in x-ray exposure, and the characteristic curve is straight on ordinary rectilinear graph paper, up to ODs of 2 or more.

The characteristic curves for nonscreen film exposed at several different values of kVp are shown in Figure 21–6A. The sensitivity of film to direct exposure by x-rays (i.e., the speed) depends on the energy of the photons. Figure 21–6B displays the relative speed of a typical radiologic nonscreen film as a function of x-ray tube voltage. The decrease in the rate of film darkening at higher voltages is a direct consequence of the falling attenuation coefficients for silver and bromine atoms. Perhaps more surprisingly, the film speed

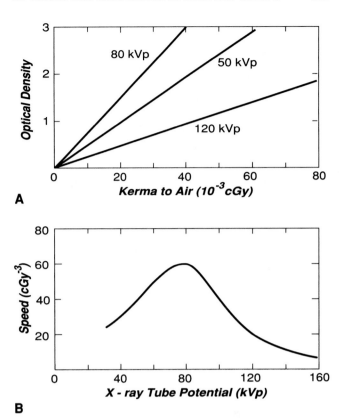

A

B

Figure 21–6. Effect of kVp on film exposed directly to x-ray energy (no screen). **A.** The film is faster with an 80-kVp exposure than with either a higher or a lower potential. **B.** Speed as a function of kVp.

declines also at low energies, above but near the absorption edges of these ions (at 26 and 13 keV, respectively). Here, photoelectric attenuation of the x-ray beam is relatively high, but much of the energy of an incoming photon is expended in overcoming the atomic binding energy, and subsequently lost in the form of characteristic x-ray photons that escape the crystal altogether.

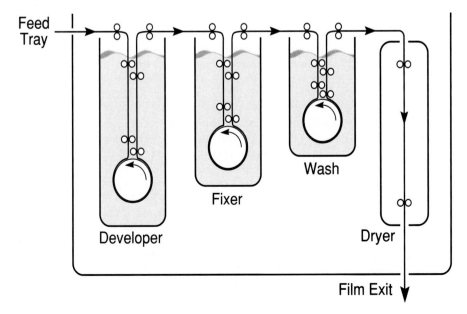

Figure 21–5. A processor, in which film is passed through developer and fixer, and then washed and dried, all automatically. It is important that an automatic film processor be kept at peak performance by means of a comprehensive quality assurance program.

The variation in film speed with photon energy is a relatively small effect, and the relationship of darkening to kVp, for a fixed mA-s,

$$OD \sim K \sim (kVp)^2 \tag{21.5}$$

is determined primarily by the kVp dependence of the x-ray tube output (see Equation 19.1).

4. USE OF A SCREEN REDUCES PATIENT DOSE ...

For some applications where high detail is required and the amount of tissue irradiated is relatively small, such as in dental work or in the search for fine fractures in the bones of the extremities, film is often exposed directly to x-rays. In general, however, radiologic **intensifying screens** are used, and reduce patient exposure by one or even two orders of magnitude, that is, by a factor of 10 or 100. Also, a much lighter mA-s load is placed on the x-ray tube; and with rare earth screens, a less powerful, and less expensive, generator is required.

In a standard radiographic cassette, a sheet of double-emulsion film is sandwiched snugly between two screens made of a polycrystalline fluorescent material embedded in a transparent binder. The crystals of fluorescent material are typically about 10 μm in dimension. The screens are protected by a cleanable transparent plastic coating, and the system is made rigid by means of a metal frame and backing. An x-ray photon passes through the cardboard front of the cassette and interacts with one or the other of the two screens, inducing a scintillation of visible light. This light exposes the emulsion primarily on the adjacent side of the film. The amount of **crossover** exposure of the emulsion on the opposite side of the film (Fig. 21–7) is normally relatively small and, for some new

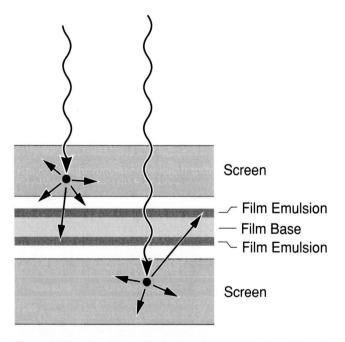

Screen

Film Emulsion
Film Base
Film Emulsion

Screen

Figure 21–7. One source of loss of spatial resolution is crossover, in which light produced by one screen exposes the emulsion adjacent to the opposite screen. (Compare this with Figure 2–7.) Modern radiographic films have largely eliminated this problem.

films, virtually absent. Each screen may be backed with a layer of reflecting material, which reduces the loss of the light that starts out heading in the wrong direction. The back screen may be made thicker, to compensate for the attenuation of the x-ray photon beam that occurred in the front screen; then the same amount of light reaches the emulsion on each side of the film.

Until recently, the fluorescent material in nearly all intensifying screens was calcium tungstate. The spectrum of light from a $CaWO_4$ screen (see Fig. 16–3E) is practically independent of the energy of the x-ray photons producing the emissions. Calcium tungstate screens emit in the region 4000 to 5000 Å (400 to 500 nm) of the electromagnetic spectrum, with a peak at about 4300 Å . The sensitivity of a typical silver halide film as a function of visible and ultraviolet photon energy is also shown in Figure 16–3E. These two spectra largely overlap, and the predominantly blue light emitted by the tungsten screen is well suited for creating latent images in such film.

_____ **EXERCISE 21–4.** _____

What would be the effect on contrast and speed of using single-emulsion film (rather than the standard kind, in which both sides of the film are coated)?

SOLUTION: Contrast and speed both would be halved. Consider the converse problem: Suppose the ODs in two regions of a single sheet of emulsion are 0.6 and 0.8, so that the contrast is 0.2. Superimposing two such planes of emulsion would take the ODs to 1.2 and 1.6, respectively, for a contrast of 0.4. The same kind of argument applies to the film speed.

The *intensification factor* of a screen is defined as the ratio of the air kerma required to produce a given optical density (typically OD = 1) without a screen to that needed with the screen:

$$\frac{\text{intensification}}{\text{factor}} = \frac{K \text{ (film alone)}}{K \text{ (screen plus film)}} \quad \text{for OD} = 1 \tag{21.6}$$

Aside from the fog, this is just the ratio of the speed of the screen–film system to that of the film alone. There are hundreds of possible combinations of commercial screens and films, but most fall into the three general categories commonly referred to as "fast" or "high speed," "par speed," and "detail." Some typical physical characteristics of calcium tungstate screens in these classes are listed in Table 21–1, along with their intensification factors for a tube potential of 100 kVp.

The reason for the relatively high efficiency of screens in converting x-ray energy into film darkening should be clear from the hypothetical example outlined in Table 21–2. Suppose that 1000 photons from an x-ray tube operated at 100 kVp are incident on a film alone, and another 1000 are incident on the same kind of film in a cassette.

With the *directly exposed film*, about 3% of the photons interact with silver bromide crystals. It may be assumed that for each of these 30 events, a latent image is formed.

With a cassette, the thickness, density, and mass attenuation coefficient of the screen are such that perhaps 30% of the x-ray photons, or 300, undergo photoelectric interactions. The *intrinsic efficiency* of a calcium tungstate screen in converting x-ray energy to visible light energy is about 5%. The effective energy of a 100-kVp beam is about 35 keV, by Table 19–2. So

TABLE 21–1. TYPICAL CHARACTERISTICS OF CALCIUM TUNGSTATE INTENSIFYING SCREENS (100 kVp)

Speed	Intensification Factor (100 kVp)	Phosphor Thickness (μm)	Resolving Power (lp/mm)
Fast, high speed	100	150–300	3.5
Par speed	50	100–130	5
Detail	25	50–75	7

5% of the energy of the typical 35-keV photon (i.e., 1750 eV) is reemitted as light. Most of this emitted light is blue, of 3-eV photon energy; (1750 eV/3 eV) = 600 (rounding off) light photons are produced for every x-ray photon absorbed.

Thus, the 1000 initial x-ray photons result in the generation of (300)(600) = 180,000 light photons. With a *screen efficiency* of 50%, half of these visible photons (i.e., 90,000) escape the screen and enter the film. A viable latent image is formed in one silver halide crystal for every 100 light photons, on average, that enter the film. The grand total number of latent images generated by the 1000 x-ray photons incident on the cassette is 900.

The intensification factor of the screen (i.e., the ratio of the numbers of latent images formed per x-ray photon with and without the screen) is therefore 900/30 = 30.

The intensification factor for a screen–film system is a function of peak kilovoltage, because of the dependence of the screen and film attenuation coefficients on x-ray photon energy. (Indeed, we were careful to note that the intensification factors listed in Table 21–1 applied at one particular tube potential.) Figure 21–8 illustrates the intensification factor, as a function of tube kVp, for a typical par speed calcium tungstate screen and film. The speed of the system increases with kVp over much of the diagnostic range. The *K*-absorption edge of tungsten lies at 69.5 keV, which explains the upturn in the intensification curve above 100 kVp. The *K* edges of silver and bromine (of importance for a film used with no cassette) are at 26 and 13 keV, which leads to the decline in intensification factor below 50 kVp. CaWO$_4$ screens are therefore more effective with high-kilovoltage procedures than with low. As we shall soon see, the dependence of rare earth screens on tube potential is different.

The conversion of x-ray energy to light (see Chapter 16, Section 4), depends in part on the thermal excitation of electrons into and out of traps. As a consequence, the intensification factor of a tungsten screen decreases by about 25% with a

10°C increase in cassette temperature. Rare earth screens display a much smaller temperature dependence.

As may have become apparent even from the highly simplified discussion above, the physical processes taking place when a screen is employed are subtle, and preclude a simple derivation of the shape of the H&D curve. Their complexity is further indicated by the *breakdown of the reciprocity law*. For film exposed directly to x-rays, it is found that the OD depends on the magnitude of the exposure, but not on the length of time over which it takes place. This behavior is called **reciprocity**. With film exposed to light, on the other hand, the OD resulting from very long exposure times is lower than what one finds with shorter times, even though the total air kerma delivered and amount of light produced are the same. This occurs because a sensitivity speck in a grain of silver halide must accumulate a "critical mass" of silver atoms to generate a stable latent image. If the exposure rate is too slow, some silver has time to be freed thermally and leak away from the sensitivity speck while others are still being drawn to it, and criticality is not achieved. Reciprocity failure also occurs for screen–film systems with very short exposure times. Fortunately, reciprocity failure is not observed within the range of exposure times normally employed clinically.

5. . . . BUT DIMINISHES RESOLUTION AND SHARPNESS . . .

Use of a cassette reduces patient dose, but it also may worsen resolution. Figure 18–6A, for example, was made without an intensifying screen, and has a resolution of better than 12 line pairs per millimeter. The "detail" screen used in Figure 18–6B still manages to achieve 7 lp/mm, but with a patient dose that is 13 times less. The "fast" screen of Figure 18–6C required only 1% of the nonscreen image exposure, but provides less than 5

TABLE 21–2. SAMPLE CALCULATION OF A SCREEN INTENSIFICATION FACTOR

	Film Alone	Cassette
X-ray photons incident	1000	1000
(fraction absorbed)	(3%)	(30%)
X-ray photons absorbed	30	300
(light photons/X-ray)	—	(600)
Light photons produced	—	180,000
Light photons reaching film	—	90,000
(photons/latent image)	(1 x-ray)	(100 light)
Latent images formed	30	900
Intensification factor		<30>

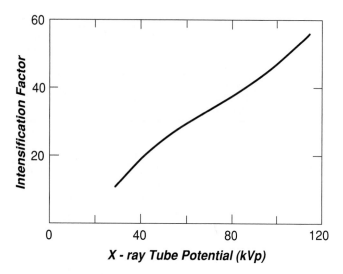

Figure 21–8. Increase in the intensification factor of a par speed calcium tungstate screen with the x-ray tube potential.

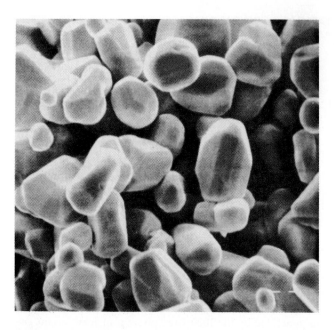

Figure 21–9. Individual crystal grains of the rare earth phosphor YTaO$_4$:Nb, taken at 2500× magnification with a scanning electron microscope. The average crystal is about 6 microns across. *(From L. Brixner et al., SPIE Vol. 555—Medical Imaging and Instrumentation '85, 1985, with permission.)*

lp/mm resolution. Why should the reduction in exposure come at the cost of less information on fine detail?

A burst of visible light is produced when an x-ray photon is absorbed by the screen. Light is emitted in all directions from the point at which the scintillation occurs, and will fall on an area of film significantly greater than the size of a single crystal of silver halide—or of a (much larger) crystal of the screen phosphor, for that matter. Reflection from the screen's reflecting layer, diffusion and scattering (at the boundaries between phosphor crystals [Fig. 21–9]) of light within the screen, poor screen–film contact, and crossover further enlarge the area of film that is illuminated. The intensity of this light diminishes with the distance from the point where the x-ray event occurred, on the other hand, because of the inverse square effect

and because of absorption by the screen itself. On balance, the distribution of the intensity of light that eventually reaches the film from a single scintillation may be described by a bell-shaped curve (Fig. 21–10) typically 0.2 to 0.6 mm across. The width of this curve depends on the type of screen, and also on the distance from the point of x-ray interaction (in the screen) to the film. The resulting dot of film darkening is considerably larger and blurrier than what would be produced by an x-ray

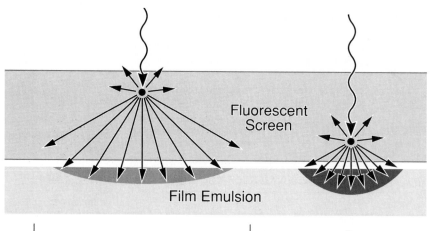

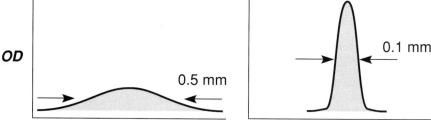

Figure 21–10. An x-ray photon that interacts (in the fluorescent screen) closer to the film results in a more compact cluster of silver microcrystals in it. Hence the potential for better resolution with thinner screens, in which all the light is generated close to the film.

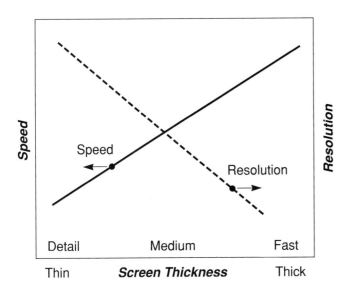

Figure 21–11. Thicker screens are faster, with less patient dose, but provide poorer resolution.

photon interacting directly with a single alkali halide microcrystal in film.

There is a reciprocal relationship for screens between speed and resolution, as affected by screen thickness (Fig. 21–11). It is possible to improve the resolving capability of a screen by reducing the dimensions of the light bursts it generates. The most important way of doing this is to decrease the screen's thickness. The dimensions of a cluster of silver microcrystals produced by a single x-ray photon, that is, the effective width of the bell-shaped curve in Figure 21–10, increases with the distance between the place in the screen where the x-ray photon is absorbed and the film. With a thinner screen, the photoelectric interactions all occur closer to the film, and the bursts of light will have less room within the phosphor to spread out before exposing it. But a thinner screen transforms fewer of the incident x-rays into flashes of light, and more x-ray exposure is therefore required to achieve an acceptable optical density. Resolution is better, but the screen is slower.

Chapter 22 will say more about the effect of screen blur on the overall resolution of a radiographic system.

6. … AND MAY INCREASE QUANTUM MOTTLE

Compton scatter reduces image quality, but is manifest only as a general reduction in image contrast. *Quantum mottle* is a form of noise that is directly visible.

The formation of a radiographic image is a stochastic process; it depends on the random interactions of large numbers of x-ray photons with the body, the detecting system, or both. What determines the apparent level of quantum mottle in a radiograph is the number of x-ray photons that actually give rise to the distinct points of light that produce the image. As indicated earlier in Figure 2–14 and in Chapter 18, Section 5, if the number of x-ray photons interacting with the screen decreases, even if the light from each increases so as to maintain a constant average OD, then eventually the image will start to look blotchy, or mottled. The problem, quite simply, is that not

enough information is being conveyed, relative to the level of noise, to produce an adequate representation of the object being examined. The weak link in the imaging chain is an insufficient number of x-ray photons used in the creation of the primary x-ray image.

There are sources of noise for screen–film systems other than random fluctuations in the number of x-ray photons per unit of area striking the screen (quantum mottle). Stochastic (random) variations occur also in the amount of energy actually absorbed per interacting x-ray; in the physical properties of the screen itself (giving rise to *structural mottle*); and in the number of silver halide crystals per unit area of undeveloped film (*film granularity*). Only the last of these, film granularity, is of any clinical significance, however, and then only for portions of film that are either under- or overdeveloped.

7. EFFECTS ON MOTTLE AND RESOLUTION OF INCREASING THE SCREEN–FILM SPEED

Dose *to the patient* and the intensity of the beam transmitted through the patient *to the cassette* both depend on the output of the x-ray tube. In efforts to reduce patient dose, therefore one also cuts down on the air kerma, K_{s-f} delivered to the screen–film system.

The optical density of developed film increases with both the speed of the screen–film system and the amount of radiation K_{s-f} that reaches it:

$$\text{OD} \sim (K_{s-f})(\text{screen–film speed}) \qquad (21.7)$$

Thus, to decrease patient dose (hence K_{s-f}) with no reduction in average OD, we must increase the speed of the screen–film system.

Let's spell out the meaning of Equation 21.7 explicitly (Fig. 21–12). Suppose we have a fluorescent screen of thickness x and mass attenuation coefficient $[\mu/\rho]$. The OD will depend on the number of x-ray photons that reach the cassette (i.e., on K_{s-f}); on the probability that an x-ray photon incident on the screen will interact with it, $e^{-[\mu/\rho] \cdot \rho \cdot x}$; on the amount of light produced per x-ray interaction (**intrinsic efficiency**); on the fraction of that light that escapes the screen to expose the film (**screen efficiency**); and on the sensitivity of the film. The system speed is determined by all but the first of these:

$$\text{screen–film speed} \sim (e^{-[\mu/\rho] \cdot \rho \cdot x})(\text{intrinsic efficiency})$$
$$\times (\text{screen efficiency})(\text{film speed}) \qquad (21.8)$$

These are just the factors that were considered in Table 21–2.

In their attempts to increase the system speed, primarily to reduce patient dose, manufacturers might vary the screen thickness or x-ray attenuation coefficient, the efficiency of the screen at transforming x-rays into usable light, and the film speed. These different approaches to the problem, however, have different effects on mottle and resolution (Table 21–3).

Relative to a given screen–film combination (Fig. 21–13A), one can improve the speed (reduce the needed number of incident x-ray photons) with no change in either the degree of mottle or the average OD (i.e., with no change in the number of bursts of light produced or in the brightness of each) by increasing the probability that any particular x-ray photon incident on the screen will interact with it. This can be accomplished by making the screen thicker (Fig. 21–13B), which

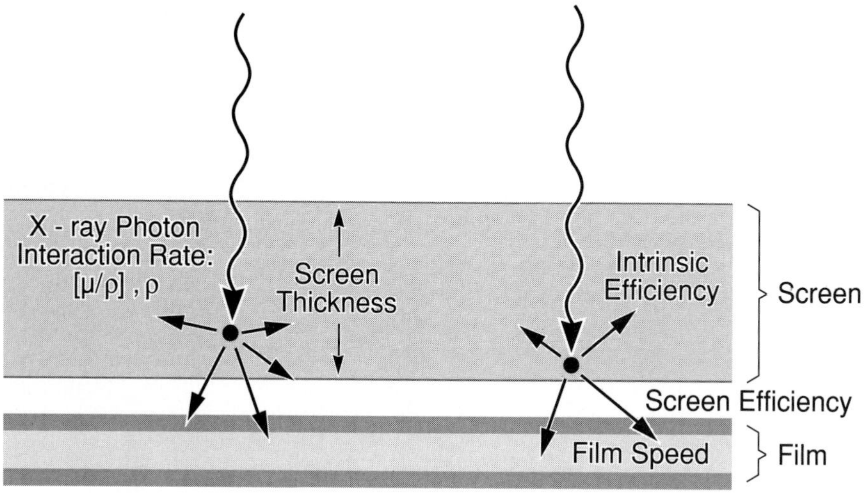

Figure 21-12. Variables that can be manipulated to affect the speed of a screen–film system include the probability that an x-ray photon will be absorbed, which depends on the mass attenuation coefficient (i.e., the chemical composition), the physical density of the screen material, and its thickness; the amount of light that reaches the film, which is a function of both the efficiency with which light is produced and its ability to escape the screen; and the speed of the film itself.

results in a loss of resolving power, or by raising its effective attenuation coefficient, μ (Fig. 21-13C). The latter approach does not diminish resolution, but does require the use of a screen of higher physical density, or electron density, or atomic number, or with a helpful absorption edge. As the number of scintillations ultimately generated remains the same either way, the level of quantum mottle is unaffected.

An alternative method of increasing screen speed is to keep the x-ray interaction probability the same, but increase either the light output from each interaction that does occur (Fig. 21-13D) or the effect of the light that is produced (Fig. 21-13E). That is, one can increase the intrinsic (x-ray-to-light conversion) efficiency of the screen, or the screen efficiency (with a better reflecting back layer or a less absorptive optical dye), or the film speed. Any of these three approaches results in larger but fewer clusters of silver grains in the developed film and a worsened level of quantum mottle. If the screen speed is changed in such a way that only a fourth as many x-ray photons are employed and each produces a dot four times darker, for example, the average OD will be the same but, by Equation 18.5, the signal-to-noise ratio will be $\sqrt{4} = 2$ times worse. In other words, more mottle.

8. RARE EARTH VERSUS CALCIUM TUNGSTATE SCREENS

Until the 1970s, nearly all screens were made of polycrystalline calcium tungstate. Recently, however, **rare earth** screens have come into widespread use. They are substantially faster, as in-

dicated by Table 21-4 and of comparable resolution. The level of quantum mottle, although somewhat worse than for slower screens, is acceptable for most applications. They bring about increases in speed by means of both higher attenuation coefficients and greater energy conversion efficiencies.

The bulk of the phosphor material in these screens consists of oxysulfide, oxybromide, tantalate, or other compounds of gadolinium (Gd), lanthanum (La), or yttrium (Y). Gadolinium and lanthanum are rare earth elements, members of a family with atomic numbers running from $Z = 57$ to $Z = 71$ in the Periodic Table. They are chemically very similar to one another and, as a consequence, notoriously difficult and expensive to obtain in pure and separate form. (Yttrium is not a rare earth, strictly speaking, but it behaves like one.) Efficient fluorescence requires that trace amounts of **terbium** (Tb), **thulium** (Tm), europium (Eu), niobium (Nb), or other *activator* be added to the phosphor. Terbium, thulium, and europium, incidentally, happen to be rare earths themselves.

Some of the fluorescence mechanisms of doped rare earth screens are different from those of $CaWO_4$. An x-ray photon may be absorbed by means of a photoelectric interaction with an atom of the rare earth phosphor matrix material, for example, but with a good part of the energy being immediately transferred to the dopant atoms, which are the actual emitters of much of the light. These impurities behave much like loosely held, nearly free atoms, and their emission spectra consist of relatively sharp lines, a situation reminiscent of that of the hydrogen atom of Chapter 6. Thus, the color of the light from a rare earth phosphor depends largely on the atomic energy levels of the dopant. In thulium-activated lanthanum oxybromide

TABLE 21-3. EFFECTS ON IMAGE QUALITY AND PATIENT DOSE OF VARIOUS METHODS OF INCREASING SCREEN–FILM SPEED

To Increase Speed, Increase . . .	Effect on Image Quality		Patient Dose
	Mottle	*Resolution*	
Screen μ ($[\mu/\rho]$ or ρ)	Same	Same	Less
Screen thickness	Same[a]	Worse	Less
Intrinsic efficiency (x-ray-to-light conversion)	Worse	Same	Less
Screen efficiency (e.g., less dye)	Worse	Worse	Less
Film speed	Worse	Same	Less

[a]Increasing screen thickness may reduce the apparent mottle, because of the increased screen blur.

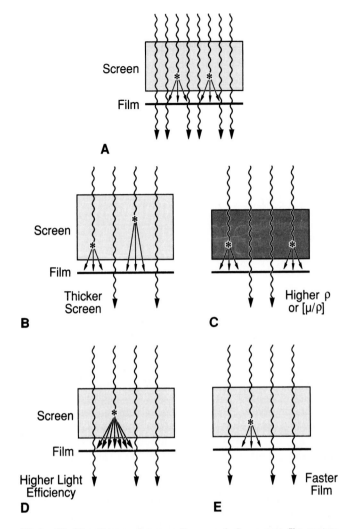

Figure 21–13. One can increase the speed of a screen–film system **(A)** and thereby reduce patient dose, with **(B)** a thicker screen; **(C)** a screen of higher mass attenuation coefficient, [μ/ρ], or physical density, ρ; **(D)** a screen with greater intrinsic efficiency (light emitted per unit of x-ray photon energy absorbed) or screen efficiency (fraction of the light produced that escapes the screen); or **(E)** faster film. The first two of these can be achieved with no worsening of mottle. But use of a thicker screen causes a loss of resolution.

Rare earth screens have higher mass attenuation coefficients than calcium tungstate, for most of the x-ray photons involved in forming the image, and greater intrinsic efficiencies.

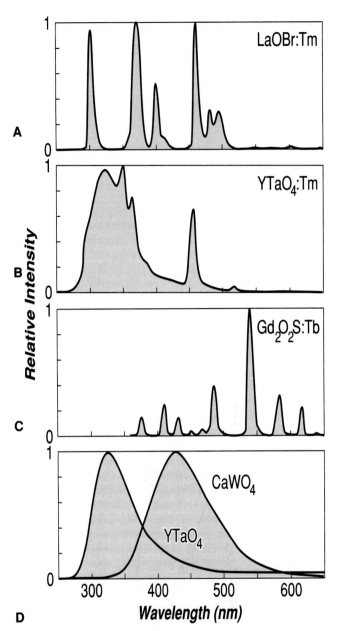

Figure 21–14. The energies of the emission spectral lines of a rare earth phosphor are characteristic primarily of the impurity dopant, but the relative intensities of the lines are affected by the nature of the host material. 1 nm = 10^{-9} m = 10 Å. **A.** LaOBr:Tm. As with calcium tungstate screens, rare earth screens doped with thulium emit primarily in the blue, and allow use of ordinary blue-sensitive radiographic film. **B.** $YTaO_4$:Tm. Comparison with (A) reveals the influence of the host matrix material. **C.** Gd_2O_2S:Tb. Terbium emits largely in the green, and special "ortho" film has been developed to make best use of it. **D.** Undoped $YTaO_4$ and $CaWO_4$. *(Courtesy of Jack Beutel EI: Du Pont de Nemours & Co., Inc.)*

($LaOBr$:Tm), for example, the thulium impurity ion gives rise to strong emission peaks in the blue part of the spectrum (Fig. 21–14A). The peaks occur at the same energies in *thulium*-activated yttrium tantalate ($YTaO_4$:Tm), but the host material affects the relative intensities of the lines (Fig. 21–14B). With terbium-activated gadolinium oxysulfide, by contrast, the dopant emits predominantly in the *green* (Fig. 21–14C). Special **orthochromatic** films, with molecules of green-sensitive dye adsorbed to the surfaces of the silver halide crystals, have been developed for use with such phosphors. The emission spectra of calcium tungstate and undoped yttrium tantalate are shown, for sake of comparison, in Figure 21–14D.

The compositions of some commercial screens, the color of the emitted light, and the speeds of screen–film combinations, are shown in Table 21–5. Speed is taken relative to that of a par speed $CaWO_4$ screen, and matched film, exposed at 70 kVp.

The enhanced speeds of rare earth screens relative to those of $CaWO_4$ screens are partly attributable to the energies at which the relevant phosphor's *K*-absorption edge occurs. Fig-

TABLE 21–4. TYPICAL VALUES OF AIR KERMA, IN 10^{-3} cGy, AT THE FRONT SURFACE OF A SCREEN–FILM SYSTEM USED AT AND ABOVE 70 kVp[a]

Screen[b]	Resolution (lp/mm)	Slow Film[c] (relative speed: 0.5)	Medium Film[c] (1)	Fast Film[c] (2)
Two CaWO$_4$ Screens, Used with Blue-Sensitive Film				
Slow (relative speed: 0.5)	7	4	2	1
Medium (1)	5	2	1[d]	0.5
Fast (2)	3.5	1	0.5	0.025
Two Rare Earth Screens, Used with Green-Sensitive Film				
Slow (relative speed: 1)	8.5	2	1	0.5
Medium (2)	6	1	0.5[e]	0.25
Fast (4)	4.3	0.5	0.25	0.125
Extrafast (6)	3.5	0.33	0.17	0.08

[a]For example, an average air kerma of about 2×10^{-3} cGy, or an exposure of about 2 mR, is required for slow film with a medium-speed calcium tungstate screen (1×10^{-3} cGy of air kerma corresponds to about 1 mR of exposure). Typical values of resolution are also listed.
[b]Screen speeds relative to Du Pont Par speed CaWO$_4$ screens (2 screens).
[c]Film speeds relative to Du Pont Cronex 4 film (double emulsion).
[d]Du Pont Par speed screens with Cronex 4 film.
[e]3M Trimax 4 screens with XD film.
After NCRP Report No. 102, Table B.6.

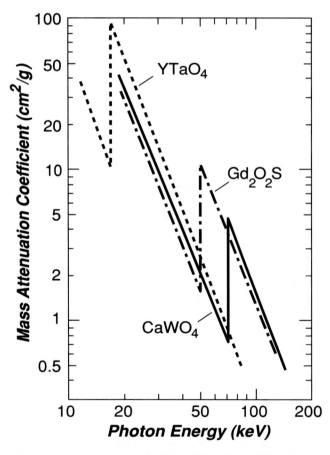

Figure 21–15. Rare earth screens are faster than calcium tungstate in part because they convert x-ray energy to light more efficiently. Also, as indicated here, they more readily intercept x-ray photons in the range of energies important in image formation.

ure 21–15 shows the dependence of the x-ray attenuation coefficients of tungsten, gadolinium, and yttrium on photon energy. Most x-ray photons from a tube operating at diagnostic voltages have energies considerably less than the K-edge of tungsten at 69.5 keV (see Table 6–4). But the absorption edge of gadolinium occurs at 50.2 keV. Gadolinium is therefore able to make better use of photons in the range 50.2 to 69.5 keV, emerging from a patient, than can calcium tungstate. This is even more so for lanthanum (K edge at 39.0 keV) and yttrium (17.0 keV).

Capturing x-ray photons more efficiently is only part of the story. Equally importantly, rare earth screens get more use out of the x-ray photons that do interact. In the example illustrated in Table 21–2, it was noted that the intrinsic efficiency of a calcium tungstate screen is about 5%; on average, 5% of the energy of an x-ray photon absorbed in the phosphor is transformed into light energy. The corresponding fractions for rare earth screens are in the range 10% to 20%.

For both reasons (attenuation coefficient and conversion efficiency), the speed advantage of rare earth screens, relative to CaWO$_4$, is greatest for tube potentials in the range 70 to 90 kVp. And because of this greater sensitivity of rare earth screens to lower-energy photons, it is generally possible to operate at lower x-ray tube voltages. This results in better contrast, leads to the production of less heat in the tube, and requires the services of a less powerful and expensive generator.

_____ **EXERCISE 21–5.** _____

How much faster is a typical rare earth screen than a calcium tungstate screen?

SOLUTION: The difference in attenuation coefficients leads to an improvement by a factor of about 1.3. The ratio of intrinsic efficiencies is of the order of 12%/5% = 2.4. Taking them together, the rare earth screen is faster by a factor of, perhaps, 3.

TABLE 21–5. CHARACTERISTICS OF SOME CALCIUM TUNGSTATE AND RARE EARTH INTENSIFYING SCREENS[a]

Speed Class	Screen (Manufacturer)	Film	Phosphor	Spectral Emission
100	PAR (DU)	Cronex 4	$CaWO_4$	Blue
100	Lanex Fine (K)	T-MAT-G T-MAT-L	Gd_2O_2S: Tb	Green
100	Quanta Detail (DU)	Cronex 10 Cronex 10L Cronex 10T	$YTaO_4$: Tm	UV/blue
100	Ultra-Vision Detail (DU)	UV-G UV-L	$YTaO_4$	UV
250	Hi-Plus (DU)	Cronex 7 Cronex 10	$CaWO_4$	Blue
250	Lanex Medium (K)	T-MAT-G T-MAT-L OC	$Gd_2 O_2S$:Tb	Green
250	Quanta Fast Detail (DU)	Cronex 10 Cronex 10L Cronex 10T	$YTaO_4$: Nb	UV/blue
250	Ultra-Vision Fast Detail (DU)	UV-G UV-L UV-C	$YTaO_4$	UV
400	Lanex Regular (K)	T-MAT-G T-MAT-L OC	Gd_2O_2S: Tb	Green
400	Quanta III (DU)	Cronex 7 Cronex 10 Cronex 10T Cronex 10L	LaOBr: Tm	UV/blue
400	Quanta V (DU)	OTG	80% Gd_2O_2S: Tb 20% LaOBr: Tm	Blue
400	Quanta Rapid (DU)	Cronex 10T Cronex 10L	90% $YTaO_4$: Nb 10% LaOBr: Tm	UV/blue
400	Ultra-Vision Rapid (DU)	UV-G UV-L UV-C	$YTaO_4$	UV
600	Lanex Fast (K)	T-MAT-G T-MAT-L	Gd_2O_2S: Tb	Green
600	Quanta Super Rapid (DU)	Cronex 10 Cronex 10L Cronex 10T	LaOBr: Tm	Blue

[a]Manufacturers: K, Kodak; DU, Du Pont. Speed class relative to 100-speed for PAR $CaWO_4$ screen and Cronex 4 film exposed at 70 kVp.
Courtesy of Jack Beutel EI: Du Pont de Nemours & Company.

The improvement in speed that comes from the increased intrinsic efficiency is accompanied by an increase in quantum mottle. (The component of enhanced speed achieved through the greater effective μ involves no such increase.) This problem is not as severe in very fast screens as one might suspect, however, because their somewhat poorer resolution blurs out the appearance of mottle.

9. EFFECT OF SCREEN–FILM GAMMA ON CONTRAST: THE EMBEDDED BONE EXAMPLE

In Chapter 19, Section 4, we estimated the primary x-ray image contrast for a thin bone embedded in soft tissue. Chapter 20, Section 2, modified this estimate to account for scatter that is created in the patient's body, but partially eliminated by a grid. Here we shall return one last time to this example, and consider the effect of the screen–film gamma on final image contrast. The screen–film system being used has the characteristic curve shown in Figure 21–1.

At the end of Chapter 20, Section 6, it was noted that, in our example, the kerma to air behind 10 cm of soft tissue and a grid was about 1×10^{-3} cGy, and that the *subject contrast* in the x-ray image (primary plus scatter) was about 0.12. By Equation 19.2, this means that behind the bone, the kerma is 0.76×10^{-3} cGy. The corresponding values of OD produced in the film are 0.98 and 0.75, by Figure 21–1. The *total image contrast*, defined as the difference in optical densities, is thus 0.23. The subject contrast has thus been amplified approximately by the amount of the gamma of the screen–film system ($\Gamma = 2$), in accord with Equation 21.4a.

_____ **EXERCISE 21–6.** _____

It is felt that an average OD of 1 for the region of interest is too low. What effect would increasing the mA-s (hence the exposure) by 50% have on the radiographic contrast?

SOLUTION: The new kermas are 1.5×10^{-3} cGy and 1.14×10^{-3} cGy, with corresponding ODs of 1.34 and 1.11; the contrast is 0.23. Thus, if you are in the straight portion of the characteristic curve, changing the exposure of the image receptor does not change the contrast.

As noted in Chapter 19, Section 4, replacing the bremsstrahlung beam with a monochromatic beam is an approximation. Our estimate of the total contrast can be made more precise by explicitly accounting for the shape of the bremsstrahlung spectrum, beam hardening effects, and the energy dependence of the response of the imaging system.

Chapter 22

Screen–Film Radiography IV: Magnification and Resolution

1. **The Image Is Magnified Because the Beam Is Divergent**
2. **Distortion Is Caused by Nonuniform Magnification**
3. **Unsharpness Arising from the Shape of the Object Being Imaged**
4. **Unsharpness Resulting from Motion of the Patient or of the Imaging System**
5. **Geometric (Penumbra) Unsharpness Caused by the Finite Size of the Focal Spot**
6. **Unsharpness Produced by the Image Receptor Itself (Screen Blur)**
7. **A Simple Measure of Combined Motion, Penumbra, and Screen Unsharpness**
8. **Magnification Radiography for Greatest Detail**

In most situations, the clinical utility of a radiograph is limited by its ability to differentiate an object of interest from background. In others, contrast is not a problem, but the accurate representation of fine detail is. The issues are different, and so are the factors that complicate the task at hand.

This chapter provides a largely qualitative discussion of resolution and unsharpness and of the related topics of magnification and distortion. Chapter 24 reconsiders resolution, and image quality in general, in the quantitative terms of the modulation transfer function (MTF).

We begin by examining the simple geometry that determines the size of an image at the film cassette, and which can lead to geometric distortions in it.

1. THE IMAGE IS MAGNIFIED BECAUSE THE BEAM IS DIVERGENT

If you hold your hand in front of a flashlight in a dark room, the size and sharpness of the shadow on the wall will depend on the distances of the hand from the bulb and from the wall. (The unsharpness increases with the diameter of the bulb, as well.) The magnification occurs because of the divergence of the beam of light. You can increase the magnification (and the blur) of the image by moving your hand closer to the light source and/or further from the wall. The same thing happens with radiographs, and for the same reason.

Figure 22–1 is a reminder that the lengths of the bases of similar (same shape) triangles are proportional to their heights. Suppose that a flat object lies a distance SOD (source-to-object distance) from a point source of x-ray (or light) energy, and in a plane parallel to the imaging plane. The cassette itself is SID (source-to-image receptor distance) from the tube. If the object is OB in dimension, then the image size IM will be greater by the amount

$$M = \mathrm{IM}/\mathrm{OB} = \mathrm{SID}/\mathrm{SOD} \qquad (22.1)$$

The factor M is known as the **magnification**, and it depends only on the relative distances of the object and the receptor from the point source of the x-ray (or light) beam.

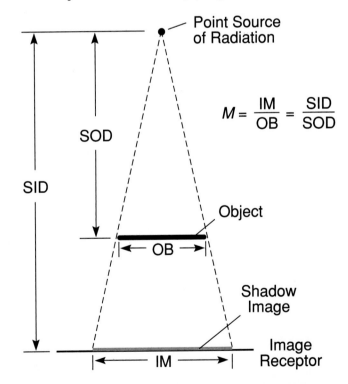

$$M = \frac{\mathrm{IM}}{\mathrm{OB}} = \frac{\mathrm{SID}}{\mathrm{SOD}}$$

Figure 22–1. The lengths of the bases of equivalent triangles are proportional to their heights: IM/OB = SID/SOD. If the geometry is such that an object of size OB produces an image of size IM, the magnification M is defined as $M = \mathrm{IM}/\mathrm{OB}$. SOD and SID refer, respectively, to the source-object distance and the source-image receptor distance.

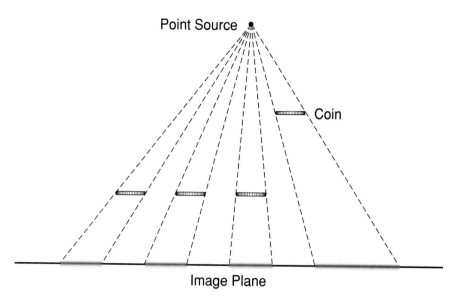

Point Source

Coin

Image Plane

Figure 22–2. Identical circular coins in a plane (the object plane) will produce, in a parallel image plane, images that are circular and all of the same size.

EXERCISE 22–1.

A patient is placed so that a vertebral body and the sternum are 5 and 25 cm from the cassette, respectively. The cassette is 100 cm from the focal spot of the x-ray tube. By how much are the images of the vertebral body and the sternum magnified?

SOLUTION: By Equation 22.1, for the vertebral body, $M = 100/95 = 1.05$. For the sternum, there is 33% magnification.

In clinical imaging the magnification is a number always larger than 1, but it is normally desirable to keep it as close to unity as possible. We shall see why in Section 8.

2. DISTORTION IS CAUSED BY NONUNIFORM MAGNIFICATION

Figure 22–2 shows, perhaps surprisingly, that silver dollars at different locations on a plane that lies parallel to a radiographic cassette will cast shadows that are circular and all of the same

size. When the coins lie in planes at different distances from the cassette, however, their images will be magnified by different amounts, in accord with Equation 22.1.

The different parts of any three dimensional object cannot help but lie in different planes and, as a consequence, the image of the object will be **distorted**: those portions lying farther from the plane of the image receptor will be magnified more. The image of identical balls with centers lying in a plane, for example, will be neither circular nor of the same size (Fig. 22–3). Likewise, the image of a coin tilted relative to the plane of the image receptor will be elliptical in shape, and the nature of the distortion will depend on the position of the coin in the beam.

3. UNSHARPNESS ARISING FROM THE SHAPE OF THE OBJECT BEING IMAGED

There are four common sources of unsharpness of x-ray images (Fig. 22–4): unavoidable blur stemming from the geometric shapes of the structures being imaged; relative motion of

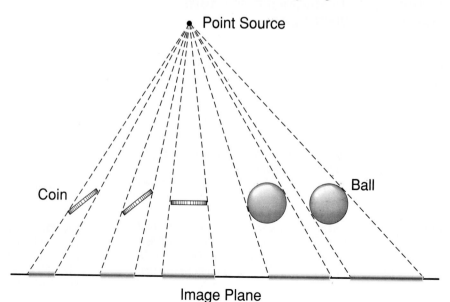

Point Source

Coin

Ball

Image Plane

Figure 22–3. Because of distortion, balls and circular coins not lying parallel to the image plane will produce images that are neither circular nor of the same size, in general, even if their centers are all at the same height above the image plane.

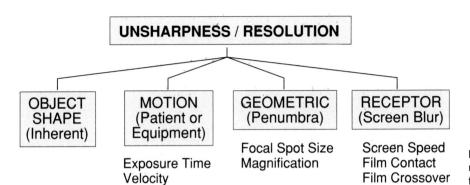

UNSHARPNESS / RESOLUTION

OBJECT SHAPE (Inherent)	MOTION (Patient or Equipment)	GEOMETRIC (Penumbra)	RECEPTOR (Screen Blur)
	Exposure Time Velocity	Focal Spot Size Magnification	Screen Speed Film Contact Film Crossover

Figure 22–4. Principal sources of unsharpness in images, and some clinically controllable factors that affect them.

patient and the equipment; penumbra arising from the finite size of the focal spot; and blur created by the image receptor itself, such as from the diffusion of light within the fluorescent screens of the film cassette. These effects are separable from one another, and will be considered individually.

The first source of image unsharpness is the inherent three-dimensional shape of the object being imaged. Blur will occur at the edge of an object that is partially attenuating (Fig. 22–5), unless the edge happens to be flat, and lying parallel to the diverging rays of the x-ray beam. Occasionally it is possible to reduce this effect somewhat through positioning of the patient.

4. UNSHARPNESS RESULTING FROM MOTION OF THE PATIENT OR OF THE IMAGING SYSTEM

Another possible source of unsharpness is motion of the patient or organ being imaged, or the imaging system (Fig. 22–6). If the object of interest within the patient moves with velocity v during an exposure of duration Δt, for example, then it travels the distance $v \cdot \Delta t$. Because of the magnification by a factor M, the region of unsharpness in the image will be roughly

$$\Delta IM = M \cdot v \cdot \Delta t \qquad (22.2a)$$

in dimension.

Of greater importance than the absolute amount of blur in the image is the degree to which the blur degrades its quality. For a small object in the body, a good measure of relative un-

sharpness is the ratio of the amount of the blur in the image to the overall size of the image of the structure or object of interest (Fig. 22–7). For a structure or object of size OB, the image size is $IM = M \cdot OB$. The relative **motion unsharpness** due to motion, $\Delta IM/IM = M \cdot v \cdot \Delta t / M \cdot OB = v \cdot \Delta t / OB$, depends on the velocity of the motion and on the exposure duration. One perhaps surprising result is that the *relative* unsharpness, $\Delta IM/IM$, is independent of the magnification. As the amount of blur increases with magnification, so also does the size of the object's image, and the two effects cancel. The same is not true for the other kinds of unsharpness.

It is an inconvenience, and of no benefit, that the relative unsharpness depends on the actual size of the object being imaged. We therefore refine the concept a bit, and formally define the **relative unsharpness**, U, as $\Delta IM/IM$ for a 1-mm reference object in the body (OB = 1 mm). Then the motional relative unsharpness reduces to

$$U_{mot} = v \cdot \Delta t / (1 \text{ mm}) \qquad (22.2b)$$

The absence of a dependence of U_{mot} on image magnification is indicated in Figure 22–8 for 10 mm/s motion and a 0.02-second exposure.

In some situations motion is unavoidable. (In conventional tomography, carefully designed motions are introduced intentionally, so as to blur out images of all objects except those in a single thick slice of the tissue of interest.) In most standard radiographic situations, motion is fortunately not a serious problem, because of the short exposure times involved.

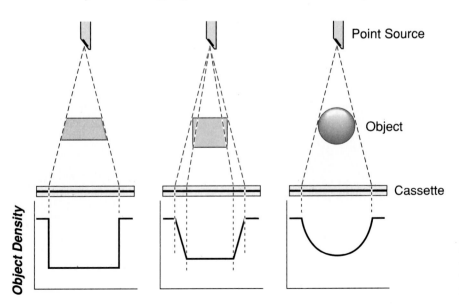

Figure 22–5. Inherent unsharpness. The sharpness of the edge of an image depends on the degree to which the corresponding edge of the object follows the lines of divergence of the x-ray beam.

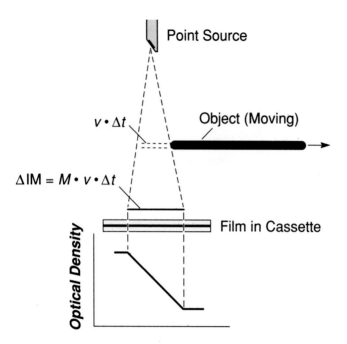

Figure 22–6. Motion unsharpness. Motion-induced blur increases with the distance that the object being imaged moves relative to the imaging equipment (or vice versa) during an exposure.

5. GEOMETRIC (PENUMBRA) UNSHARPNESS CAUSED BY THE FINITE SIZE OF THE FOCAL SPOT

If there were no other sources of blur, a perfect, infinitesimal focal spot would give rise to perfect images. The x-ray shadow of a sharp-edged object in the patient's body would have sharp edges, in particular (Fig. 22–9A), and the image of a tiny speck of highly attenuating material would itself be a tiny speck.

An x-ray tube's focal spot is not infinitesimal, however, but rather typically on the order of 1 mm in effective dimen-

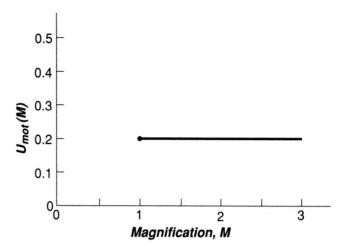

Figure 22–8. The relative unsharpness resulting from motion, U_{mot}, is independent of the amount of magnification, M. Note that M cannot be less than 1.

sions (as would be seen looking into the beam). As a result, the x-ray shadow even of a sharp-edged object will be imperfect: A point at the image receptor directly behind the edge will be exposed by part, but not all, of the source of radiation (Fig. 22–9B); the intensity therefore falls off relatively gradually in this **penumbra** region, rather than abruptly, and the image of the edge is fuzzy. Similarly, a single attenuating speck now produces a blurred spot. This blurring, or loss of resolution, is known as **geometric unsharpness**, and it is the predominant source of unsharpness in normal radiography.

The width ΔIM of the penumbra region of the image at the cassette can be estimated from the image of the edge of an object situated SOD away from the focal spot. If the image receptor is SID from the focal point, and the focal spot is of dimension F, then by similar triangles, $\Delta IM/(SID - SOD) = F/SOD$, or

$$\Delta IM = F \cdot (SID - SOD)/SOD = F \cdot (M - 1) \qquad (22.3a)$$

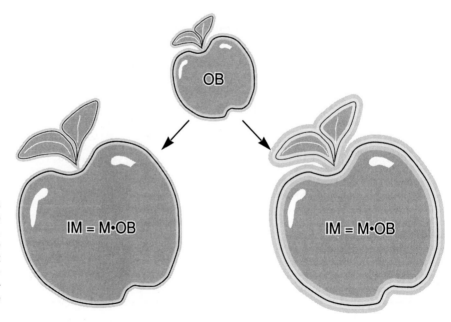

Figure 22–7. The large apple to the right was created simply by doubling the size (and the width of the region of blur) of the smaller image. The large apple on the left contains the same *absolute* amount of blur as the small apple; that is, the image increased in size without a proportionate increase in the amount of blur. The *relative* unsharpness is smaller, and you are more able to resolve fine detail.

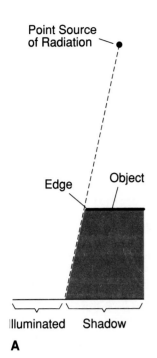

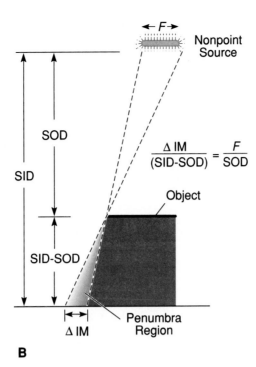

$$\frac{\Delta IM}{(SID-SOD)} = \frac{F}{SOD}$$

A

B

Figure 22–9. Geometric (penumbra) unsharpness. **A.** A point source of radiation will cast a sharp shadow of a sharp-edged object. **B.** There appears a region of blur, or penumbra, at the edge of the shadow image produced with a nonpoint source. The width of the penumbra region, DIM, is proportional to the dimension of the source, F. It also depends on the distances of the object from the source, SOD, and from the image plane, SID–SOD.

The last step followed from Equation 22.1. The amount of geometric unsharpness thus increases with the size of the focal spot and with the amount of magnification (Fig. 22–10). Note that when the object being imaged is against the image receptor, so that M = 1, there is no geometric unsharpness.

The relative unsharpness caused by penumbra, U_{pen} = $\Delta IM/IM$, for a 1-mm object depends on M as

$$U_{pen} = [F/(1 \text{ mm})](1 - 1/M) \qquad (22.3b)$$

Unlike the case of motional blurring, U_{pen} becomes larger with greater amounts of magnification; that is, as an image is magnified, the penumbra increases even faster. If penumbra is the dominant source of unsharpness, then one produces the best pictures by using the least amount of magnification. U_{pen} curves appear in Figure 22–11 as functions of magnification for a 1.0-mm focal spot, and for a 0.1-mm focal spot employed in magnification mammography.

Nearly all x-ray tubes used in general radiography contain two filaments, which give rise to focal spots typically 0.6 and 1.0 mm in dimension. If an adequate exposure can be obtained with a low mA, the smaller filament may be employed. If a thick part of the body is being imaged, however, or if a pulse of very short duration is required, so that a higher current is needed, the heat must be spread out over a larger focal spot on the target surface, as produced by means of the larger filament, with the associated loss of resolution. Higher tube currents

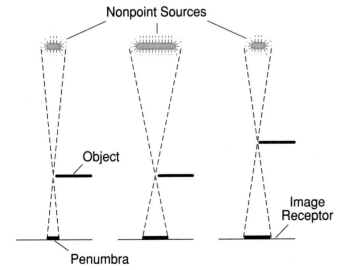

Figure 22–10. The amount of penumbra increases with the size of the source of radiation, and also for an object closer to the source.

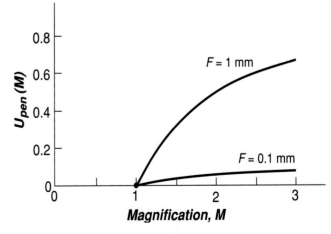

Figure 22–11. The relative geometric unsharpness resulting from penumbra, U_{pen}, increases with focal spot size and with magnification. This component of total relative unsharpness can therefore be kept down by using a small focal spot and little magnification.

lead to blooming, in addition, with an additional increase in U_{pen}.

Finally, as the plane of the focal spot is not parallel to that of the film (Fig. 22–12), penumbra unsharpness is somewhat less pronounced on the anode side of the image. The magnitude of this effect depends on the anode angle.

_____ EXERCISE 22–2. _____

The end of a rib is 30 inches from the 1.2-mm focal spot of an x-ray tube and 10 inches in front of a film cassette. The rib is 1.1 cm across, as seen by the beam. How much magnification is there, and how much geometric unsharpness?

SOLUTION: By Equation 22.1, the magnification is $M = 40/30 = 1.33$. By Equation 22.3a, penumbra introduces about $\Delta IM = (1.2 \text{ mm})(0.33) = 0.40$ mm of unsharpness into the image. The relative unsharpness for an object of unit dimensions (Equation 22.3b) is $(1.2 \text{ mm}/1 \text{ mm})(1 - 1/1.33) = 0.30$.

6. UNSHARPNESS PRODUCED BY THE IMAGE RECEPTOR ITSELF (SCREEN BLUR)

The final important source of image unsharpness in radiography is the diffusion and scatter of light within the intensifying screens of the cassette.

As discussed in Chapter 21, Section 4, a burst of visible light is produced when an x-ray photon is absorbed by the screen. Light is emitted in all directions from the point within

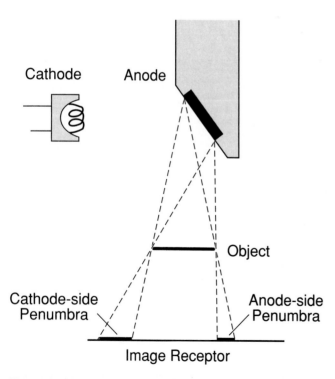

Figure 22–12. For purely geometric reasons, because of the angling of the target, the amount of penumbra unsharpness is greater on the cathode side of an image.

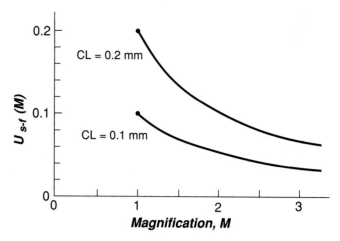

Figure 22–13. Screen–film unsharpness. The amount of blur introduced by a screen is totally independent of the image size, so magnification decreases the _relative_ unsharpness. The screen–film component of relative unsharpness, $U_{s\text{-}f}$, can therefore be kept down by using a detail screen (in which case the dimension CL of a typical cluster of silver grains appearing in the developed film is small) and high magnification.

the screen at which the scintillation occurs, and will fall on an area of film much larger than the size of a single crystal of silver halide. The result is a round cluster of silver grains, densest at the center and tapering off at the edges. The average dimension of such clusters, CL, depends on the properties of the screen (especially the thickness and the concentration of dye in it), but is typically a fraction of a millimeter. The **image receptor** (_screen–film_) **unsharpness** will be exacerbated by poor physical contact between film and screen, or by crossover.

The amount of unsharpness introduced into an image by the screen–film system itself is independent of magnification:

$$\Delta IM = CL \text{ (constant)} \qquad (22.4a)$$

The relative unsharpness decreases with magnification, however:

$$U_{s\text{-}f} = CL/(1 \text{ mm}) \cdot M \qquad (22.4b)$$

The larger the image, the less conspicuous will be a blemish of fixed size. $U_{s\text{-}f}$ is plotted against M in Figure 22–13 for two values of image receptor unsharpness, CL = 0.1 and 0.2 mm.

Table 22–1 lists typical values of the effective **blur** for several categories of screen. Comparison with the results of Exer-

TABLE 22–1. TYPICAL AMOUNTS OF BLUR FOUND IN VARIOUS SCREEN–FILM SYSTEMS

Screen–Film Speed	Blur (mm)
Mammographic	0.15–0.2
Detail	0.2 –0.35
Par speed	0.5 –0.6
High speed	0.6 –0.7

After Sprawls P. Jr: Physical Principles of Medical Imaging, Rockville, MD: Aspen, 1987, p. 271.

cise 22–2 suggests that a detail screen introduces less unsharpness into an image than does the penumbra resulting from focal spot size.

> When image receptor blur is a problem, one can select a thinner screen or one containing more optical dye. Either way, the size of a typical cluster of silver grains will diminish (and mottle will improve). But as a consequence, the mA-s will have to be increased. Thus there is a fundamental trade-off for screens between resolution and speed, noted in Chapter 21, Section 5, in connection with screen thickness. The cost for better resolution is greater patient dose.

7. A SIMPLE MEASURE OF COMBINED MOTION, PENUMBRA, AND SCREEN UNSHARPNESS

In the clinic, all three factors (motion, penumbra, and image receptor unsharpness) may combine to limit resolution. To obtain a measure of overall relative unsharpness, one might consider simply adding the terms in Equations 22.2b, 22.3b, and 22.4b. That, however, would tend to produce an overestimate (why?), and a judicious blend of the Pythagorean Theorem and some relevant statistics suggests that a better approach is to add the three relative unsharpnesses in quadrature, as with Equation 18.9c:

$$U_{\text{total}} = \sqrt{(U_{\text{mot}}^2 + U_{\text{pen}}^2 + U_{\text{s-f}}^2)} \qquad (22.5)$$

A similar expression holds for absolute values of the unsharpness, ΔIM.

If any one (or two) of the three terms in Equation 22.5 is significantly smaller than the others, then it can be ignored.

___ **EXERCISE 22–3.** _____

In the procedure of Exercise 22–2, in which the relative penumbra unsharpness for a rib was found to be 0.3, the motions of the patient during the short exposure cause motional blurring of the image of less than 0.01 mm. The unsharpness from the screen is about 0.2 mm. What is the total relative unsharpness?

SOLUTION: The relative unsharpness for motion is, by Equation 22.2b, $U_{\text{mot}} = 0.01$ mm/1 mm = 0.01. Likewise, by Equation 22.4b, $U_{\text{s-f}} = (0.2 \text{ mm})/(1 \text{ mm}) \cdot 1.33 = 0.15$. By Equation 22.5, $U_{\text{total}} = (0.01^2 + 0.3^2 + 0.15^2)^{1/2} = 0.34$ mm. The total unsharpness is only a bit more than that of the geometric unsharpness alone, and the motion and blur contributions are relatively unimportant.

Equation 22.5 applies to any imaging system, of course, if $U_{\text{s-f}}$ is replaced with the appropriate image receptor unsharpness. Typical ranges of total unsharpness for some of the standard modalities are indicated in Table 22–2.

8. MAGNIFICATION RADIOGRAPHY FOR GREATEST DETAIL

Because of beam divergence, a radiographic image is always at least a little larger than the patient. But for normal radiography, the patient is placed close to the film cassette and, by Equation 22.1, that means little magnification. If the cassette is moved away from the patient, the output of the x-ray tube must be increased accordingly (to achieve a suitable average optical density), leading to more patient dose. To reduce distortion, moreover, both patient and image receptor are kept as far from the x-ray tube as its capacity to dissipate anode heat will allow. Again, little magnification.

To summarize, the general rules of thumb are:

- Maximize the distance between patient and x-ray tube.
- Minimize the distance between patient and cassette.

Sometimes, however, one may need to image fine structures with high resolution. It then may help to magnify the image, for although the geometric unsharpness increases with the amount of magnification, the screen–film blur does not, and it becomes relatively less important. In some circumstances, you gain more than you lose by magnifying.

Figure 22–14 plots U_{total}, the total relative unsharpness (Equation 22.5) against M for two cases: For one curve, the

TABLE 22–2. TYPICAL VALUES OF BLUR (AND APPROXIMATE SIZE OF THE SMALLEST OBJECT OR DETAIL THAT CAN BE IMAGED)

Modality	Blur (mm)
Radiography	0.1–0.5
Fluoroscopy	0.5–1
Computed tomography	1.0–2
Magnetic resonance imaging	1–3
Ultrasound	2.0–5
Nuclear medicine	3–10

After Sprawls P. Jr: Physical Principles of Medical Imaging, Rockville, MD: Aspen, 1987 (Fig. 1.6).

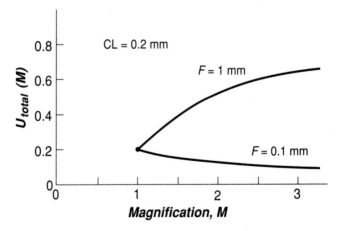

Figure 22–14. Total unsharpness, as defined in Equation 22–5, as a function of magnification, for two quite different clinical situations. With routine radiography, one might choose a large focal spot (e.g., $F = 1.0$ mm) and little magnification. For finest detail, however, a small focal spot (0.1 mm) and some degree of magnification (typically $M = 1.5$) serve better.

focal spot size and screen blur are 1 and 0.2 mm, respectively, and the geometric unsharpness dominates. This is typical of the situation normally found for general radiography. The image is sharpest for little or no magnification.

Magnification radiography makes use of an x-ray tube with an especially small (typically 0.1 mm across) focal spot. For this curve in Figure 22–14, the same screen was used as before. Relative unsharpness seems to improve with increasing *M*. But fo-

cusing the electron stream onto a very small region of the anode can easily damage it, so a low tube current (mA) is employed. A (detail) screen is required for an adequate optical density to be obtained over an acceptably short exposure time (so that motion does not become a problem). The optimal amount of magnification is then determined through a balancing of penumbra, screen blur, patient motion, tube output, and patient dose effects. A value of *M* = 1.5 is commonly adopted.

Screen–Film Radiography V: Optimal Technique Factors

1. **kVp: The Trade-off Between Image Contrast and Patient Dose**
2. **Source-to-Image Receptor Distance (SID): The Trade-off Between X-ray Tube Heating and Patient Dose**
3. **Selection of the Optimal Screen–Film System and Technique Factors**
4. **Some Clinical Examples**
5. **Automatic Exposure Control Takes Out Much of the Guesswork**

For a properly maintained radiographic system, image quality and patient dose are determined largely by the choice of radiographic technique factors. In selecting technique factors for a particular study and patient, it is necessary to optimize the clinical benefit–cost ratio for a number of trade-offs—in the choice of kVp, for example, the trade-off between contrast and patient dose. Fortunately, the solutions to most such optimization problems have been found through trial and error in the clinic, with some assistance and explanations from theory.

1. kVp: THE TRADE-OFF BETWEEN IMAGE CONTRAST AND PATIENT DOSE

Chapter 19, Section 5, and Chapter 20, Section 2, indicated that subject contrast in the primary x-ray image decreases with increasing tube potential, and that the inclusion of scatter enhances that effect. Does this mean that one should always try to optimize contrast by using the *lowest* possible operating voltage? To the contrary! In practice, one normally does the opposite, raising the tube potential to the *highest* value that will still yield an adequate level of contrast. The primary reason for adopting this strategy has to do with dose to the patient.

Figure 23–1 illustrates the distributions of dose deposited by two beams in soft tissue. The high kVp beam readily penetrates the tissue. The other, of lower energy, is much less penetrating. Let us adjust the mA-s for the two situations so as to end up with the same average level of radiation intensity exiting the body and entering the film cassette. (We are ignoring the energy dependence of the sensitivity of the image receptor.) The diagram indicates that a far greater volume of tissue is taken to higher doses with the less penetrating, lower-kVp beam; more radiation must be pumped in on one side to obtain the necessary intensity coming out the other. So in terms of patient dose, a higher tube potential is preferable.

A second, less significant, argument supports this conclusion. A photon with energy less than about 25 keV will most likely interact with soft tissue by means of the photoelectric effect, depositing all of its energy locally as dose. The photoelectric effect is dominant in bone up to about 45 keV.

At higher energies, however, the Compton interaction assumes greater importance in both materials. Then the incident photon imparts only a small portion of its energy to the Compton electron; the rest is transported from the site of the collision, and perhaps out of the patient, in the form of a scatter photon. The Compton collision contributes as fully to the formation of an image as does a photoelectric event (i.e., an x-ray photon is removed from the beam), but at much less cost in patient dose. The use of a grid to remove the Compton scatter radiation, on the other hand, calls for an increase in the exposure by the amount of the Bucky factor (see Equation 20.2b). Finally, the photon energy dependence of the sensitivity of the image receptor must be taken into account.

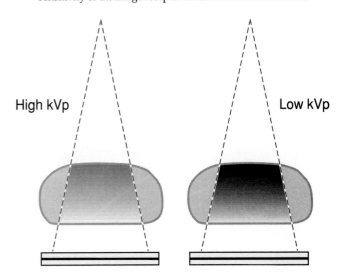

High kVp   **Low kVp**

Figure 23–1. The average dose deposited in the patient depends strongly on the power of penetration of the beam. The amount of energy that must be pumped in, on the beam entrance side, to achieve a specific air kerma at the film cassette, in particular, increases rapidly as the kVp decreases.

Consideration of dose has left us on the horns of a centrally important dilemma. Lower photon energy may lead to better contrast, but it also imparts more dose to the patient. The way out, however, is straightforward. When the subject contrast is strong, as in the imaging of a bone or barium-coated bowel, the best approach is to use a higher tube potential, with reduced patient dose. When the contrast is marginal at high kVp, the need for greater primary x-ray image contrast, and for less scatter degradation, calls for a lower kVp. In mammography, for example, potentials are typically between 25 and 30 kVp, because of the critical need for maximum contrast among masses of soft tissues.

2. SOURCE TO IMAGE RECEPTOR DISTANCE (SID): THE TRADE-OFF BETWEEN X-RAY TUBE HEATING AND PATIENT DOSE

A similar argument suggests the advantage of a large *source-to-image receptor distance* (SID). Figure 23–2 shows two beams, both of the same relatively high energy. The source of the first is far from the patient, and undergoes little divergence within the patient. When the SID is small, however, the entrance dose must be much higher to achieve the same exit dose, purely because of the geometry, that is, the inverse square effect associated with beam divergence. For a given film exposure, then, the average patient dose decreases as the SID increases. (Increasing the SID thereby gives the impression of improving the beam's power of penetration; but this is quite different from increasing the half-value layer [HVL] by raising the kVp.) Also, as noted in the last chapter, increasing the SID reduces the amount of image distortion, again for geometric reasons (less beam divergence).

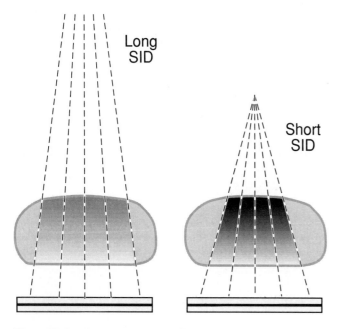

Figure 23–2. A strongly diverging beam, brought about by a short source-to-image receptor distance (SID), has the same effect as a low kVp; the beam is less penetrating, in effect (but now for purely geometric reasons), and more entrance dose is required to achieve the necessary exposure of the image receptor.

Unfortunately, the amount of x-ray radiation that must be produced to obtain the necessary intensity level at the image receptor, and the associated heating (and wear and tear) of the x-ray tube, increase with the square of SID, because of the beam divergence. Image quality is also an issue, to some extent. A higher tube current may cause blooming of the focal spot, with loss of resolution. Likewise, a longer exposure time may lower resolution, because of patient motion. Again, important trade-offs.

The range of SIDs used in clinical practice has been arrived at by balancing these considerations of image quality, patient dose, and x-ray tube longevity. As a general rule, in most situations one should use as large an SID as the equipment can readily tolerate. Dental radiography is one notable exception. And sometimes a relatively small SID (but not less than 40 cm = 15 in.) is employed in mammography.

3. SELECTION OF THE OPTIMAL SCREEN–FILM SYSTEM AND TECHNIQUE FACTORS

Clearly there are numerous variables that one must decide on to obtain even the simplest of useful radiographs. Fortunately, some theory and much practical experience provide guidance in all of this.

A first consideration is the choice of screen–film combination. Although an independent radiologist or small community hospital may stick with only one or two screen–film combinations for all standard radiographic applications, teaching hospitals may well make use of many specialized systems. In the latter case, should one ever have to select a screen–film combination, a reasonable approach for a particular study consists of two steps: First, select as fast a screen as can provide images with the necessary resolution and sufficiently low mottle. Second, pick a film with a spectral response matching the fluorescence emission of the screen. The screen–film gamma should be high, to enhance subject contrast, yet not so great as to restrict latitude excessively.

The various factors that influence contrast and patient dose are indicated in Figure 23–3. The operating kVp (and filtration), in particular, is determined by optimizing the trade-off between contrast and dose for the screen–film combination and for the type of study and particular anatomy (thickness) of the individual patient. In general, thicker body parts call for higher-energy, more penetrating beams. And if contrast is not an issue, one can keep the dose down with a high tube potential, for a patient of any thickness. Use of as large an SID as the x-ray tube can readily accept also helps to minimize patient dose.

Finally, an mA-s is chosen that will lead to a comfortable average optical density over the region of interest. This involves a consideration of kVp, patient thickness, SID, attenuation by the table and grid, and speed of the screen–film system (Fig. 23–4).

With regard to the first of these factors, in particular, the output of an x-ray tube increases (and the required mA-s decreases) roughly as the square of kVp (see Equation 19.1). When film is being exposed without a screen (so that optical density is linearly proportional to exposure), the optical density is roughly proportional to the square of the kVp. When a screen is used, film darkening is found to increase, for fixed

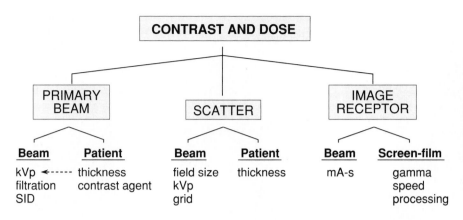

CONTRAST AND DOSE

PRIMARY BEAM — **SCATTER** — **IMAGE RECEPTOR**

Beam	**Patient**	**Beam**	**Patient**	**Beam**	**Screen-film**
kVp ◄-----	thickness	field size	thickness	mA-s	gamma
filtration	contrast agent	kVp			speed
SID		grid			processing

Figure 23–3. Factors that can strongly influence image contrast, patient dose, or both. For example, scatter radiation, which reduces contrast and increases patient dose, is affected by both beam field size and patient thickness. Likewise, the thickness of the patient influences choice of kVp (hence the penetration capability of the primary beam), and kVp is a prime determinant of contrast. Which of these factors affects only contrast or dose alone? (See Table 19–1)

mA-s, approximately as $(kVp)^n$, where the exponent n is typically around 4. In summary,

$$OD \sim \begin{cases} (kVp)^4 & \text{screen} \\ (kVp)^2 & \text{no screen} \end{cases} \quad (23.1)$$

___ **EXERCISE 23–1.** _____

In an attempt to improve contrast, a cassette film shot at 75 kVp is to be retaken at 60 kVp. How should the other technique factors be changed?

SOLUTION: With the same mA-s, the optical density would decrease by a factor of roughly $(60/75)^4 = 0.4$. To maintain the same optical density, the mA-s should be increased by a factor of $1/0.4 = 2.5$.

4. SOME CLINICAL EXAMPLES

In searching for a hairline fracture in a bone of the hand, contrast is not a major issue, nor is dose. The image is sharpness-limited, and what is required is resolution. The resolution is determined primarily by focal spot size and the speed of the screen–film combination. With the small focal spot (operated at low current, to avoid blooming), and a detail rare earth screen and perhaps single-emulsion film, a resolution of 10 lp/mm or more is achievable. Because the required mA-s is relatively low (small tissue thickness), and because the hand can be held immobile, motional unsharpness is not a problem. A tube potential of 50 to 60 kVp might be used to maximize the dose efficiency of the screen.

If a fine vessel containing a small amount of iodine contrast agent is to be imaged, the signal-to-noise ratio would be greatest with near-monochromatic photons of energy just above iodine's K-absorption edge at 33.2 keV. The tube is therefore operated at about 60 to 70 kVp with a 0.1-mm *holmium filter*; with the K edge of holmium at 56 KeV, the filter removes penetrating but inefficiently detected *higher*-energy photons from the beam before they enter the patient. A detail rare earth screen will allow adequate imaging with a relatively low skin dose.

An abdominal series may involve a search for fluid (or air) against a background of soft tissue. Resolution is relatively unimportant, but contrast must be maximized. The amount of contrast required for an abnormality to be detected depends on the difference in its optical density from background, its size, and the sharpness of its edges. For a thin patient, a potential of 70 kVp and a grid might be selected to enhance contrast and

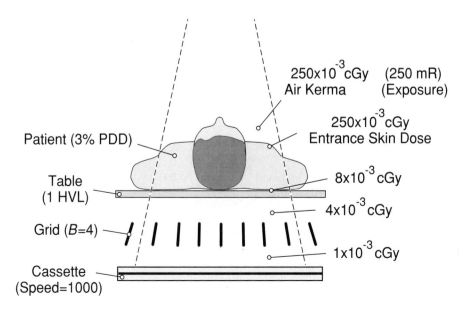

Patient (3% PDD)

Table (1 HVL)

Grid (B=4)

Cassette (Speed=1000)

250×10^{-3} cGy   (250 mR)
Air Kerma   (Exposure)

250×10^{-3} cGy
Entrance Skin Dose

8×10^{-3} cGy

4×10^{-3} cGy

1×10^{-3} cGy

Figure 23–4. Typical values of air kerma in centigrays that one might find at different places along a diagnostic beam. This example assumes a 3% percentage depth dose (PDD), which implies that the beam exiting the patient is about 3% as intense as that entering. (But as both entrance skin dose and, much more so, exit dose contain scatter contributions, this does not mean that the intensity of the exit primary image is 3% that of the entrance intensity.) The patient table attenuates the beam by a factor of a half, here, and the Bucky factor (B) is 4. All the values one would find in a particular situation, except for the desired input to the image receptor, depend strongly on patient thickness; all of them depend on kVp.

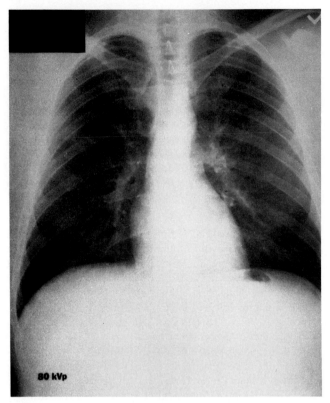

A

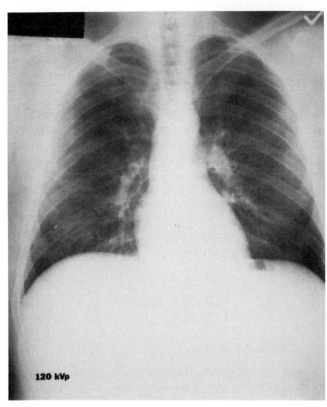

B

Figure 23–5. Routine conventional posteroanterior chest films, taken at relatively **(A)** low and **(B)** high kVp with a 6-foot SID, a 10:1 grid, 2.5 mm Al filtration, and a par speed calcium tungstate screen–film system. "The lower kVp film presents a higher contrast (often referred to as a shorter gray scale) than does the high kVp film. This is seen both in the mediastinum and in the pulmonary markings. . . . On the low kVp film, bones are also better seen, although it is to be emphasized that in the vast majority of cases a chest radiograph is concerned with diseases of the lungs, pleura, mediastinum, and diaphragm rather than of bones. Furthermore, the bones could hide significant pathology of these structures, such as small pulmonary nodules. The high kVp film shows better visualization of the mediastinal structures and has a lower entrance skin exposure. Overall, both films are of diagnostic quality; however, the high kVp film is preferred." This situation is to be compared with those of Figures 14–3 and 19–3. *(From the American College of Radiology Learning File, courtesy of the ACR.)*

reduce scatter degradation. A par speed screen requires more mA-s and (hence patient dose) than would a fast screen, but may be preferable because of the smaller amount of mottle.

In a double-contrast, lower gastrointestinal series examination for polyps or small ulcerations, the colon is coated with barium emulsion and then filled with air. A high degree of contrast is provided by the barium–air interface at the bowel wall. Many films are taken, so it is important to keep the dose low for each, using a tube potential of 120 to 150 kVp.

For a chest film, high contrast among soft tissues (brought about by a low kVp) would be desirable, but a significant price to pay for the contrast would be a significantly reduced effective latitude (Fig. 23–5). Working at 120 kVp is normally preferable, primarily to provide a longer gray scale. It also keeps down the relative number of photoelectric events in bone and hence rib shadowing, and leads to lower overall patient dose.

The above choices of technique factors are typical, but in practice, *technique factors* may vary considerably from patient to patient and from institution to institution. Tables of technique factors should be determined for different individual imaging systems at the time of initial acceptance testing, and confirmed through periodic quality assurance procedures.

5. AUTOMATIC EXPOSURE CONTROL TAKES OUT MUCH OF THE GUESSWORK

Because of variations among patients, x-ray tube aging, and other factors, the setting of the mA-s can be a hit or miss business, very chancy, even with tables of technique factors. **Automatic Exposure Control (AEC)**, or **phototiming**, offers a way around that problem. An AEC system monitors the radiation passing through the patient directly, and cuts off the tube output after a preselected amount of radiation has reached the screen–film.

Several methods of carrying this out are illustrated in Figure 23–6. A large, flat radiation-transparent ionization chamber (or a small fluorescent screen, viewed through an optical fiberoptic *light pipe* by a light-sensitive photomultiplier tube) may be placed between the patient and the film cassette and attached to an electrometer. The electrometer controls the exposure switch of the generator, and terminates the production of x-rays when the appropriate level of exposure is reached. Because it is positioned directly in front of the screen–film system, the AEC leads to the appropriate amount of average film darkening, regardless of patient thickness. A backup timer ter-

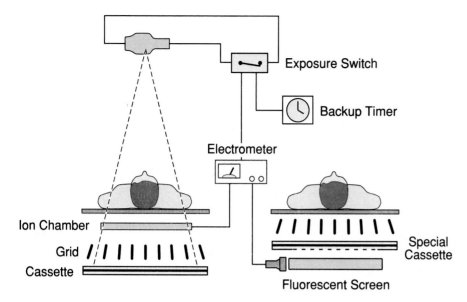

Figure 23–6. Two automatic exposure control (AEC) systems. To the left, an ion chamber that is nearly transparent to the x-ray beam is positioned immediately behind the patient. An electrometer monitors the quantity of radiation delivered and, at a predetermined level, opens the exposure switch. There is also a backup timer, should the AEC fail to operate properly. A second configuration places the exposure monitor (a fluorescent screen observed by a photomultiplier tube, in this case) behind the cassette. The cassette is of special design, with a back cover that is transparent to x-rays, rather than being made of metal.

minates the exposure after a short period, should the phototimer fail.

Alternatively, a special fluorescent screen and photomultiplier tube can be located behind the cassette. The cassette must have a cardboard back, rather than metal. The phototube measures the light output of the AEC screen, which in turn is proportional to the amount of radiation incident on the cassette.

Three or more independent sensors may be positioned at various places in the field of the x-ray beam, allowing control of the tube by exposure to one region of interest or by an average over several.

Some phototimers in current use take tens of milliseconds to measure the x-ray exposure and turn off the x-ray tube. Recommended exposure times for rare earth screens, however, are often an order of magnitude less than that. Phototiming can

then be used only if adequate imaging is obtained when shooting at a lower exposure rate and for a longer time. This incompatibility will be encountered less frequently in the future, as older AEC systems are upgraded or replaced.

At the other extreme of exposure times, an AEC backup timer system is required to terminate an exposure automatically after 600 mA-s above 50 kVp, and after 2000 mA-s at lower potentials. This is intended to protect the patient from excessive exposure in case of AEC malfunctioning.

A final caveat. Automatic exposure control is not really completely automatic. To avoid serious errors, and to ensure optimal choice of kVp and mA-s for the individual patient, the system still requires the services of an alert, skilled radiographer.

The Modulation Transfer Function and Other Measures of Imaging System Capabilities

Several quantitative parameters have been devised that correlate with the abilities of imaging devices to perform clinical tasks. Such parameters can be employed both for intercomparison between systems and for quality control of a particular system over time. One of the most widely used of these is the *modulation transfer function* (*MTF*), a measure of how well a system handles contrast and different levels of fine detail. Before turning to the MTF, however, it is necessary to discuss *representations* of images and the *Fourier representation*, in particular. It's not as painful as it may sound.

Before beginning, you may want to take a glance at the Appendix 24–1, which reviews some properties of periodic functions such as $\sin (k \cdot x)$.

1. DIGITAL REPRESENTATION OF AN IMAGE

The quantitative study of imaging makes use of various **mathematical representations** of images. Perhaps a good place to begin is with a brief discussion of the simplest of these, the **digital representation.**

Let us consider the creation of a digital representation of an ordinary radiograph by means of a computer-controlled, laser-scanning film densitometer (Fig. 24–1A). The radiograph is partitioned by an imaginary *matrix* or grid (like ordinary graph paper) of many thousands of tiny, square **pixels**, or *picture elements,* each with its own value of transmittance or optical density. By means of a computer-controlled mechanical or electro-optical device, a narrow laser beam pointing down from above is stepped from pixel to pixel throughout the film

in a well defined pattern, and a photodetector on the far side of the film monitors the intensity of transmitted laser light at each location. At any instant, the x and y coordinates of the beam define the **address** of a pixel. The voltage from the photodetector measures the **value** of the image at that address, and can be transformed into an ordinary number (digitized) by means of an electronic *analog-to-digital converter* (ADC). The entire image can be stored in computer memory, or transmitted to a colleague, as the set of the many thousands of pixel addresses and corresponding pixel values. An example of this appears in Figure 24–1B.

The set of addresses and values that constitute the digital representation can be changed back into a visible image by reversing the process. With a laser printer, this involves "painting" on photosensitive paper with a laser beam. The address for a point in the image, stored in the computer's memory, directs the laser beam to the corresponding point on the paper. The stored intensity value for that address determines the brightness of the laser light there, hence the darkening of the paper. The reconstructed image is made up of many thousands of separate pixels, each with its own shade of gray, somewhat like a newspaper photo. The smaller the pixels (hence the greater their number), and the greater the number of gray levels of light shading employed, the more closely the displayed image will resemble the original radiograph. But also, the greater the level of computer memory and speed required.

It may seem most natural to represent an image in this way and, in fact, computerized tomography (CT), magnetic resonance imaging (MRI), digital subtraction angiography (DSA), and other computer-based modalities make extensive

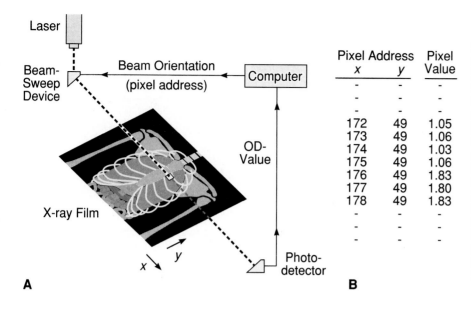

Pixel Address		Pixel
x	y	Value
-	-	-
-	-	-
-	-	-
172	49	1.05
173	49	1.06
174	49	1.03
175	49	1.06
176	49	1.83
177	49	1.80
178	49	1.83
-	-	-
-	-	-

Figure 24–1. System for digitizing a chest radiograph. **A.** Imagine that the film is partitioned into square pixels, perhaps 0.1 mm on a side. Under control of the computer, the narrow laser beam (pointing down into the film from above) is swept in the x direction, from one edge of the film to the other; the beam then steps one pixel in the y direction, and the x sweep is begun anew. This process is repeated until the entire film has been covered. For any pixel address (i.e., laser beam position), a photodetector (below the film) puts out a voltage proportional to the intensity of light transmitted through the film there. This pixel *value* is digitized and entered into the computer. **B.** A small portion of the table of pixel addresses and pixel values that constitutes the digital representation of the x-ray image.

use of the digital representation. But there are other, equally legitimate ways to achieve the same end. The **Fourier representation**, in particular, is of special importance in imaging technology, as we shall see in dealing with CT and MRI. It is also intimately involved with the definition and use of the modulation transfer function.

2. FOURIER REPRESENTATION OF AN IMAGE

In 1815, Jean-Baptiste-Joseph Fourier demonstrated that just about any function or curve, no matter how irregular in shape, can be represented as a combination of sine and cosine functions of the appropriate frequencies and amplitudes (or, equivalently, of sine functions of the correct frequencies, amplitudes, and phases).

Consider, for example, the square wave of Figure 24–2A that repeats itself periodically with some fixed spatial frequency of f_0 copies per meter. This function might correspond to the optical density of film containing a pattern of alternating black and white stripes. The simplest approximation to this square wave is just

$$\tfrac{1}{2} + (2/\pi)\,\sin(2\mu f_0 \cdot x) \qquad (24.1a)$$

(Fig. 24–2B), where the constant $2/\pi$ causes the sine wave (chosen to be also of frequency f_0) to stick up a bit above the flat top of the square wave. The sum

$$\tfrac{1}{2} + (2/\pi)\{\sin(2\pi f_0 \cdot x) + \tfrac{1}{3}\sin(6\pi f_0 \cdot x)\} \qquad (24.1b)$$

(Fig. 24–2C) does a lot better. The second sine term is chosen to have three times the frequency and one-third the amplitude of the first; its crests and troughs fill in the gaps and diminish the peaks of $\sin 2\pi f_0 \cdot x$, resulting in something quite a bit closer to a square wave. Adding a $5f_0$ **component** (Fig. 24–2D), is better yet. And the graph of the infinite series

$$\tfrac{1}{2} + (2/\pi)\{\sin(2\pi f_0 \cdot x) + \tfrac{1}{3}\sin(6\pi f_0 x)$$
$$+ \tfrac{1}{5}\sin(10\pi f_0 \cdot x) + \ldots\} \qquad (24.1c)$$

is indistinguishable from Figure 24–2A. Our square-wave function can thus be expressed as a *Fourier decomposition* into sine functions of judiciously selected frequencies and amplitudes. The lowest frequency in this series, f_0, which is the same as that of the function being represented, is called the **fundamental**, and integer multiples of it are its **harmonics.**

In practice, of course, it is not possible to manipulate all the terms in an infinite series individually. But the higher frequency contributions to the sum become small, in most imaging situations, and one can **truncate** the series at some harmonic, retaining only the lower-frequency terms. The spatial frequency at which the truncation is made, however, determines the amount of fine detail the image can present (just as pixel size places an upper limit on resolution for a digital representation).

As shown in Figure 24–2E, it is possible to summarize the results of a Fourier decomposition by means of a *spectrum*, displaying the amplitude of any sine term component as a function of its frequency. The spectrum here consists of distinct spikes at discrete values of the frequency and is said to be *discrete*. The same terminology was used earlier in connection with certain photon and electron energy spectra.

More generally, nearly any one-dimensional curve (not only a periodic one), or any function of one variable, can be represented as an appropriate combination of sine terms. The Fourier representation of a single rectangular (up and down) step (Fig. 24–3A), for example, contains contributions at *all* frequencies, as indicated by its *continuous* spectrum (Fig. 24–3B). In the mathematics of imaging, it is sometimes helpful to think of a nonperiodic function of interest as being one cycle of an extended, periodic function (Fig. 24–3A). It can then be represented (approximately) by means of a simple series, with a discrete spectrum.

The above arguments can easily be extended to two or more dimensions. The product

$$\{\sin(6\pi f_x \cdot x)\}\{\sin(2\pi f_y \cdot y)\} \qquad (24.2)$$

is itself a pattern periodic in two dimensions, and it should be apparent that *any* two-dimensional image can be represented

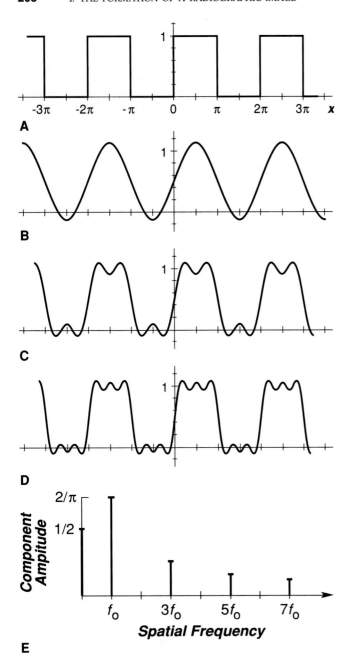

Figure 24–2. Fourier representation of a periodic function, such as a square wave. **A.** The value of the square wave function might represent the optical density one finds in scanning across a pattern of black and white stripes. **B.** The simplest Fourier approximation of the square wave consists of a constant plus a single sine term (Equation 24.1a). **C.** An improvement in the representation (Equation 24.1b). **D.** A further improvement, by adding in the $5f_0$ component. **E.** The spectrum of any periodic function, such as a square wave, is discrete. The complete series continues indefinitely, containing an infinite number of terms. In practice it is necessary to truncate the series at some finite value of the spatial frequency.

as a combination, with the appropriate frequencies and amplitudes, of terms like Equation 24.2. The spectral contents of some objects commonly seen in radiography are shown in Figure 24–4.

There is no need here to describe how a Fourier decomposition is performed (in practice it usually involves a computer-

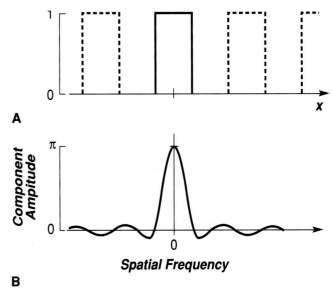

Figure 24–3. Fourier representation of a non-periodic function, such as a single rectangular step. **A.** Mathematically it is often convenient to think of a non-periodic function as a periodic function of very large period; that is, the series for the periodic square wave function is determined, but then the blocks are moved mathematically far apart from one another. **B.** By this (or other) mathematical machination, it is found that the spectrum of a single block is continuous, containing components at *all* spatial frequencies (not just at integer multiples of a fundamental frequency, f_0).

based process known as the *fast Fourier transform*), but suffice it to note that it *can* be done. Such mathematical manipulations are central to the image reconstruction processes that form the heart of CT and MRI.

If it seems that a lot of mathematical machinery is required to perform a Fourier analysis, just bear in mind that the ear and

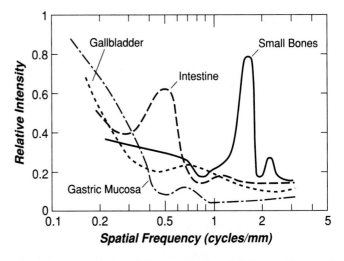

Figure 24–4. Typical spatial frequencies found within x-ray images of several representative organs. The bones of the foot, for example, contain fine structure, and require high resolution (i.e., ability to capture high spatial frequencies) for faithful image representations. (Redrawn from Pfeiler M, et al., Die Intensitäts-verteilung im Strahlenrelief als Eingangsgrösse beim Röntgenfernsehen, in Elektromedizin, Band 12/1967.

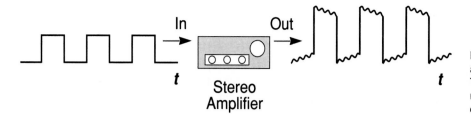

Figure 24–5. Distortions in an audio amplifier arise because the device is not strictly linear. That is, it does not amplify all frequency components by the same amount. (Also, it may introduce phase shifts among them.)

brain together are very effective at doing so. They can often pick out individual instruments or notes in a symphony with ease. The eye, by contrast, cannot do the same. It perceives a super-positioning of blue and yellow light as being green. But a glass prism breaks sunlight into its spectral components—Fourier decomposition!

3. THE MODULATION TRANSFER FUNCTION (MTF)

Images are generated, processed, stored, and transmitted by imperfect systems. Some such systems are more imperfect than others, however, and methods are needed to determine and describe the extent to which a piece of equipment degrades the images created in it or passing through it. The *modulation transfer function* (MTF) provides one such method.

The problem is one sadly familiar to all of you Bach aficionados. Glenn Gould hasn't sounded quite so lively lately, so you compare the output of your audio amplifier with a known input signal. Your worst fears are confirmed. The stereo system affects high- and low-frequency signals differently (Fig. 24–5) and leads to significant tonal distortion.

It is not apparent from Figure 24–5, however, exactly where the difficulties lie. It is much more revealing to examine the response of the system to monochromatic (consisting of only one frequency) sinusoidal input signals systematically (Fig. 24–6). The *frequency response* curve shows how the amplitude of the output signal varies with the *frequency* of the input sine wave (the *amplitude* of the input being held constant), and

it should be flat over the range of audible frequencies. The frequency response actually measured can tell a good deal about how well the amplifier is working.

Since an image can be expressed as a Fourier combination of sine waves of different spatial frequencies, amplitudes, and phases, one can do exactly the same thing with an imaging system or with any of its constituent parts. The MTF of an imaging system is the spatial counterpart to the stereo amplifier's frequency response function.

Before defining the MTF formally, let us briefly revisit the issue of image contrast. Equation 18.1 defined the optical contrast of a single, localized object against a fairly uniform background as $C = (L_{obj} - L_{bac})/L_{bac}$, where L_{obj} and L_{bac} refer to the intensity of light coming from the two regions (Fig. 24–7A). You can view this as the amplitude of the object's *signal above the average background* value, *relative to background*.

If the signal of interest happens to be one that varies sinusoidally within the image (Fig. 24–7B), a corresponding definition of contrast might be $C = L_{amp}/L_{bac}$, where L_{amp} and L_{bac} refer to the amplitude of the light intensity wave and the average background light level, respectively. Now, from Figure 24–7B, it is apparent that the intensity of the light varies between a maximum value of $L_{max} = L_{bac} + L_{amp}$ and a minimum of $L_{min} = L_{bac} - L_{amp}$. We can therefore represent the signal amplitude, L_{amp}, as $\frac{1}{2}(L_{max} - L_{min})$. Likewise for the background, $L_{bac} = \frac{1}{2}(L_{max} + L_{min})$. The contrast then becomes $(L_{max} - L_{min})/(L_{max} + L_{min})$. More generally, the **modulation**, M, of *any* periodic signal, S (not only one of varying light intensity), may be defined as

$$M = (S_{max} - S_{min})/(S_{max} + S_{min}) \qquad (24.3)$$

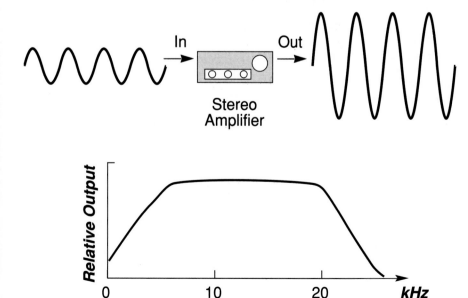

Figure 24–6. One way to check out your stereo. Use monochromatic signals, one at a time and all of the same amplitude, as input, and plot the output amplitude (and phase shift) as a function of frequency.

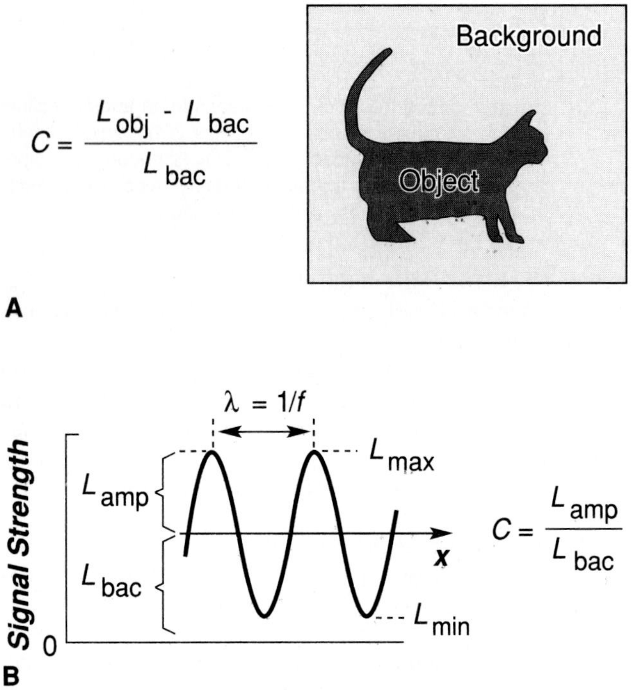

$$C = \frac{L_{obj} - L_{bac}}{L_{bac}}$$

A

$$C = \frac{L_{amp}}{L_{bac}}$$

B

Figure 24–7. The modulation transfer function (MTF) makes use of the idea of contrast, introduced in Equation 18.1. **A.** For a non-periodic image, the contrast may be defined as the relative amount by which an object stands out from background. **B.** For a periodically varying pattern (or for a Fourier component of an image), the same idea can be expressed in terms of the amplitude of the wave relative to background.

That is, the *modulation* refers to the *contrast*, relative to its background or average value, of a *periodically* varying signal. A signal with a modulation of 1 carries maximum possible information, whereas one with $M = 0$ carries none.

Now on to the modulation transfer function. We are interested in the effect that an image processing device has on a signal, in particular, on its modulation. Suppose the *input* to the device is a signal of frequency f and modulation $M^{in}(f)$. In carrying out its appointed image processing task, the device may degrade the image somewhat. The value of the *modulation* of the *output* signal, $M^{out}(f)$, will be smaller (Fig. 24–8) even if its *amplitude* is larger. The extent of the degradation for our signal of frequency f is indicated by the modulation transfer ratio, $M^{out}(f)/M^{in}(f)$. The **modulation transfer function, MTF(f),** is the function that records the modulation transfer ratio for all frequencies:

$$MTF(f) = M^{out}(f)/M^{in}(f) \qquad (24.4a)$$

The MTF is commonly normalized relative to a value of 1 at $f = 0$,

$$MTF(0) = 1 \qquad (24.4b)$$

As with an audio amplifier, an imaging device will invariably be more successful at handling signals of some frequencies than of others. In most cases, the response is best at low spatial frequencies, diminishing with increasing frequency, so that the MTF falls off from a maximum value of unity near $f = 0$.

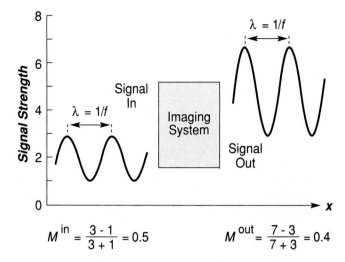

$$M^{in} = \frac{3 - 1}{3 + 1} = 0.5 \qquad M^{out} = \frac{7 - 3}{7 + 3} = 0.4$$

Figure 24–8. An example of the way in which the modulation of a periodic signal, or of a Fourier component thereof, can change in passing through a device. The input signal is 1 in amplitude and the average background is 2, so $M^{in} = 0.5$. This can also be expressed in terms of the maximum (3) and minimum (1) values of the signal, as $M^{in} = (3–1)/(3+1) = 0.5$. The modulation of the output signal is found, in similar fashion, to be $M^{out} = 0.4$, which is less than M^{in}. The device has degraded the image quality.

EXERCISE 24–1.

Three signals, of spatial frequencies 1, 2, and 3 cm^{-1}, enter an imaging device. All are 100% modulated, $M^{in}(f) = 1$ (Fig. 24–9A). What are the modulations of three corresponding output signals? Draw MTF(f).

SOLUTION: The input and output modulations were determined from Equation 24.3 and recorded in Table 24–1, and the MTF at each frequency was determined from Equations 24.4. MTF(f) is shown in Figure 24–9B.

The MTF(f) is thus a measure of the ability of the imaging system to handle contrast as a function of spatial frequency. In a sense, it is also a generalization of the resolution. The greater the MTF(f) of an imaging system at high spatial frequencies, the more adept it is at capturing fine detail. The rolloff region of the MTF(f) curve indicates the image component frequencies for which the system runs into trouble.

It is necessary to conclude this introduction to the MTF with two qualifications. First, the MTF is formally defined only for a device that is *linear*, that is, for which the output is linearly proportional to the input. This is the case with an inten-

TABLE 24–1. VALUES OF M^{in}, M^{out}, AND MTF(f) FOR SEVERAL VALUES OF f FOR THE SYSTEM OF EXERCISE 24–1

f (cycles/cm)	M^{in}	M^{out}	MTF (f)
1	1	(4 – 0) / (4 + 0) = 1	1
2	1	(3 – 1) / (3 + 1) = 0.5	0.5
3	1	(2 – 1) / (2 + 1) = 0.33	0.33

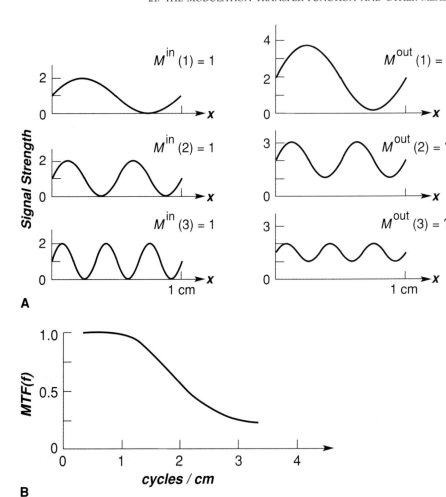

Figure 24–9. Input and output signals for Exercise 24–1. **A.** All three input signals, of spatial frequencies 1, 2, and 3 cycles per centimeter, are of unity modulation, $M^{in}(f) = 1$. The output modulations, however, are frequency dependent. One cannot simply subtract away the same amount of background from all three output signals as a quick fix, as the amount of background in the output is frequency dependent. **B.** A plot of MTF$(f) = M^{out}(f)/M^{in}(f)$.

sifying screen, for example, but is not so for film, in general; as is evident from a characteristic curve, neither the transmittance nor the optical density is strictly linear in exposure. Still, the errors introduced by assuming linearity for film are relatively small.

Second, an imaging device may not only reduce the modulation of a signal, it may also introduce *phase shifts* into it. Phase shifts are critically important in some imaging situations, and must be taken into account, but for simplicity we shall not consider them further here.

4. THE MODULATION TRANSFER FUNCTION OF A FLUORESCENT SCREEN

Let us illustrate the meaning of the MTF with the example of the fluorescent screen of a particular radiographic cassette. In Figure 24–10 the cassette is being irradiated with a spatially modulated x-ray beam, in which the intensity varies sinusoidally with a spatial frequency of f cycles/mm across its face. The source of such a pattern might be a uniform x-ray beam that passes through a carefully sculpted piece of attenuating material whose thickness varies appropriately in space. The input to the cassette is a *signal* of frequency f and amplitude X_{amp}, superimposed on a uniform background of intensity X_{bac}. The input modulation is at this frequency $M^{in} = X_{amp}/X_{bac}$ $= (X_{max} - X_{min})/(X_{max} + X_{min})$.

In a similar fashion, the output (the pattern of light intensity emitted from the screen) corresponding to this input is experimentally determined to be of amplitude L_{amp}, superimposed on a background of average value L_{bac}. The output modulation is thus $M^{out} = L_{amp}/L_{bac} = (L_{max} - L_{min})/(L_{max} + L_{min})$. The modulation transfer function is the modulation transfer ratio M^{out}/M^{in} displayed as a function of spatial frequency f.

In practice, one would more likely use a pattern of closely spaced slits cut in a sheet of lead of uniform thickness, giving rise to a "square-wave" pattern of x-ray intensities as input signal, and then perform some fancy mathematical back-peddling to arrive at MTF(f).

Alternatively, instead of a sinusoidal or square-wave pattern of x-ray energy, one could use as input a very narrow pencil beam (see Chapter 18, Section 4). The resultant image is a blurred point of light. (As light bursts can occur at various depths within the phosphor, the measured point spread function represents an average, in effect, of all their contributions [Fig. 24–11].) As is shown in more advanced texts, MTF(f) can be directly related to the Fourier spectrum of the point spread function (PSF) of that image.

There is a simple explanation for the general shape of the MTF(f) curve for the fluoroscopic screen of a radiographic cassette. As discussed in Chapter 21, Section 5, and Chapter 22, Section 6, a burst of visible light appears, and radiates outward

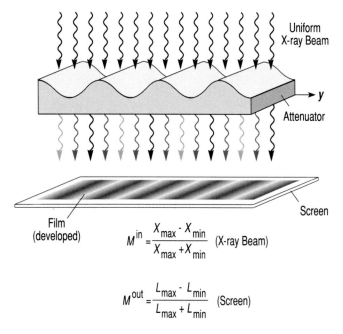

$$M^{in} = \frac{X_{max} - X_{min}}{X_{max} + X_{min}} \quad \text{(X-ray Beam)}$$

$$M^{out} = \frac{L_{max} - L_{min}}{L_{max} + L_{min}} \quad \text{(Screen)}$$

Figure 24–10. A conceptually simple, but technically difficult, way to obtain MTF(f) for a radiographic screen. An x-ray beam that varies sinusoidally in space (the input signal) is created by means of a spatially modulated attenuator, and falls on the screen. The resulting pattern of light is mapped by scanning the screen with a light meter or by exposing film (in which case the shape of the characteristic curve must be taken into account). The MTF at this frequency is the ratio of the output and input modulations. After the MTF for this spatial frequency is obtained, the process is repeated at other frequencies.

in all directions, when an x-ray photon is absorbed by a cassette screen. This results, in the developed film, in the creation of a cluster of silver grains with a bell-shaped point spread function (Fig. 24–11 and Chapter 18, Section 4). It is the shape of this PSF that determines the form of the screen's MTF curve. Consider what happens when a sinusoidally modulated x-ray beam falls on the cassette (Fig. 24–12). If the wavelength of the input pattern is long relative to the full width at half-maximum

(FWHM) of the PSF, then the finite dimension of any single cluster of silver grains has little effect on the output image. When the spatial period of the test pattern is comparable to the FWHM of the PSF, however, the output image on film becomes blurred, and the output modulation diminishes.

The PSFs for several typical screen systems are presented in Figure 24–13, along with the derived MTFs. Since the FWHM of the system PSF increases with greater screen thickness or screen transparency to light, the MTF begins its rolloff at lower frequencies. Also shown, for comparison, is the MTF of a perfect cassette, which is unity for all spatial frequencies.

5. MODULATION TRANSFER FUNCTIONS FOR AN X-RAY TUBE FOCAL SPOT AND FOR PATIENT MOTION

Similar arguments suggest a shape for the MTF(f) of an x-ray tube's focal spot. The effects of the finite dimensions of a real focal spot are not discernible in the image of a low-spatial-frequency pattern. But penumbra-type degradation becomes significant when the period of the image pattern is comparable to the size of the projection of the focal spot. Thus the MTF(f) is unity for signals that vary slowly in space, but falls rapidly above a spatial frequency characteristic of the focal spot size and magnification (Fig. 24–14).

Similar arguments allow the calculation of the MTF associated with patient motion. Larger amplitude and more rapid motions lead to an MTF(f) that falls off faster at lower spatial frequencies.

6. OVERALL IMAGE QUALITY: THE SYSTEM MODULATION TRANSFER FUNCTION

The MTF is useful not only in comparing focal spots, fluorescent screens, and other items, but also in determining how the overall performance of a complete radiologic system is influenced by the behavior of its separate components. Suppose

Figure 24–11. Because of the inverse square effect and the scattering, diffusion, and absorption of light within the screen, the spatial distribution of emerging scintillation light depends on the depth within the screen at which the initiating x-ray interaction takes place. (The points of interaction of four particular x-ray photons are shown on the left-hand side of the figure; light photons are being emitted at one of them.) The overall point spread function (PSF) for the screen is thus an average of the individual x-ray photon PSFs for all depths.

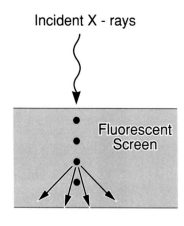

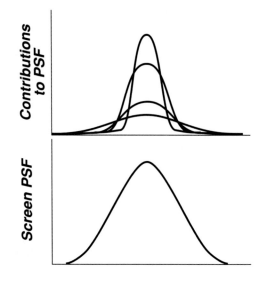

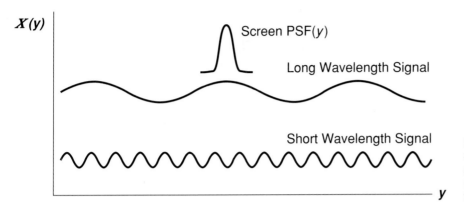

$X(y)$

Screen PSF(y)

Long Wavelength Signal

Short Wavelength Signal

y

Figure 24–12. The dimensions of the clusters of silver grains have a significant effect on a sinusoidal image unless the cluster dimensions happen to be much less than the wavelength of the image pattern.

that an imaging system consists of separable stages in series, where the output of each stage serves as the input to the next. The MTFs at frequency f of the various stages are $MTF_1(f)$, $MTF_2(f)$, $MTF_3(f)$, and so on. The behavior of the whole system at that frequency is described by the product

$$MTF_{sys}(f) = MTF_1(f) \cdot MTF_2(f) \cdot MTF_3(f) \ldots \quad (24.5)$$

Typical MTFs associated with screen blur, focal spot pen-

umbra, and patient movement during the exposure are plotted (on log–log graph paper) in Figure 24–15 along with the composite, total system MTF(f). From Equation 24.5 and Figure 24–15 it should be apparent that even if only one component has a low MTF at some frequency, then the MTF for the entire system will be low there. The imaging chain is truly as strong as its weakest link.

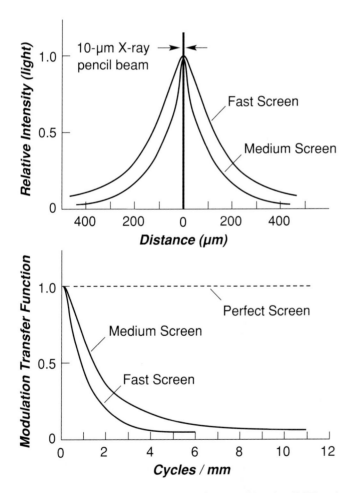

Figure 24–13. Typical shapes of the point spread function (PSF) and the modulation transfer function (MTF) for fast (relatively thick screen) and medium speed calcium tungstate cassettes.

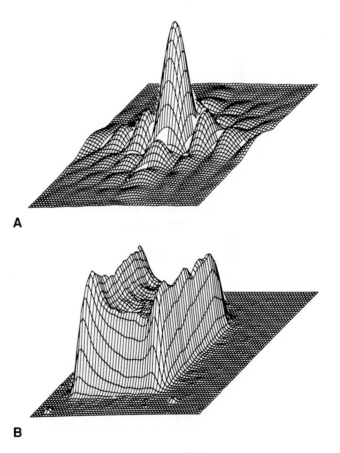

Figure 24–14. **A.** Three-dimensional representation of the modulation transfer function for the focal spot of an x-ray tube. This was derived, through some complex mathematical manipulations, from **(B)** a (two-dimensional) image of the focal spot obtained by means of a pinhole camera. *(From Wagner RF, et al.: Toward a unified view of radiological imaging systems. Part 1. Noiseless images. Med Phys 1974; 1:11–24.)*

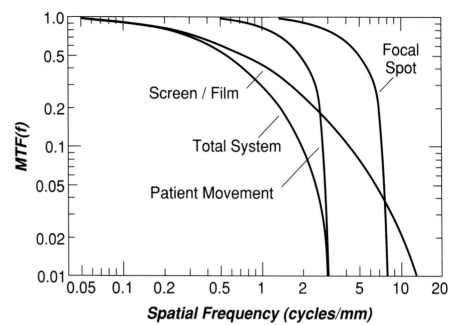

Figure 24–15. The total MTF(f) function for a complete radiographic system (including patient motion) can be constructed out of the MTF(f) functions of its constituent parts through use of Equation 24.5.

_____ **EXERCISE 24–2.** _____

From Figure 24–15 and the component MTFs, find the value of the total MTF(f) at a spatial frequency of 2 cycles/mm.

SOLUTION: At 2 cycles/mm, the component MTFs for focal spot, patient motion, and screen blur are about 0.90, 0.43, and 0.23, respectively. By Equation 24.5 these combine to give MTF_{sys}(2 cycles/mm) = 0.09, in agreement with the "Total System" MTF line in the figure.

This may seem like a lot of work that can be circumvented just by examining a typical exposed film. But the use of MTFs (or of equivalent formalisms) can be invaluable in the study of complex imaging systems. The approach may reveal where losses of information occur, and may suggest methods of correcting or compensating for them.

7. IMPROVING IMAGE QUALITY: FREQUENCY COMPENSATION AND DECONVOLVING WITH THE POINT SPREAD FUNCTION

If MTF analysis indicates that the capabilities of an imaging system fall off too rapidly at high spatial frequencies, say, then _frequency compensation_ can be employed to boost the response where needed.

Suppose that, as a signal is passed through an imperfect system, problems show up, in part, as a loss of high-frequency signal components in the output. One can compensate somewhat for this problem by passing the signal, before or after, through another system that preferentially amplifies at higher frequencies. For imaging, unlike the case of stereo, this generally involves feeding the signal into a computer and employing digital techniques. (Alternatively, one could use a digital filter to diminish the low frequency components.) This frequency **compensation** will cause the final signal to be closer to

the original input than would use of the imperfect system alone. The process will amplify the high frequency components of noise as well, and one must determine whether that is an acceptable price to pay for sharper images. Frequency compensation of this type is relatively easy to implement, and commonly employed in the computer-based digital modalities.

There is another (closely related) method, based on the point spread function, that may be used to compensate for system imperfections. Suppose that the imaging system under study is a screen–film combination. Suppose also that the input is a small x-ray beam that is rectangular in cross section with sharp edges. This input may be thought of as consisting of a set of perfectly abutting, very narrow pencil beams (Fig 24–16A). The output is then created through the superpositioning (overlapping) of the corresponding individual pencil beam PSFs (Fig. 24–16B). The image of the rectangle is degraded in a predictable fashion, with great blurring of its edges (Fig. 24–16C), and the wider the pencil beam PSF, the greater the loss of image fidelity. The mathematical process of forming the output image in this fashion is known as the _convolution_ of the input image with the PSF of the imaging system.

If the PSF for the system is known, one may be able to reverse the process, and _deconvolve_ an output image, to arrive at a better representation of the input. One can, in effect, account systematically for the degradation brought about by the system, and reconstruct aspects of the truer image that was originally put into it.

8. THE WIENER SPECTRUM OF THE NOISE

As anyone knows who has ever had a teenager, or been one, noise comes in a remarkable variety of forms. In any of its guises, however, noise always does essentially the same thing: It obscures messages of interest by interjecting extraneous signals that carry no information, or information that is irrelevant, or (worst of all) information that seems relevant but is wrong.

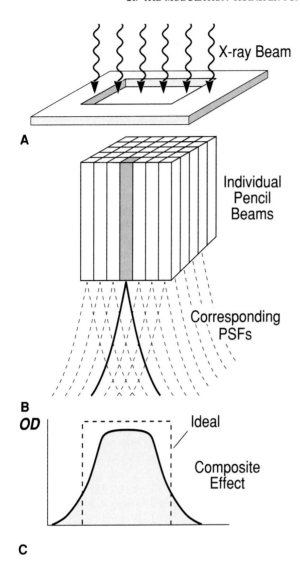

Figure 24–16. Deconvolving with the point spread function (PSF). **A.** Suppose we wish to form the screen–film image of a small rectangular opening in a piece of attenuating metal. The rectangular x-ray beam that passes through the collimator may be thought of as being made up of separate, very narrow "pencil" beams that abut one another perfectly. One of these is highlighted. **B.** Our beam then falls on an intensifying screen, and the "image" of each individual pencil beam defines, in effect, the PSF. **C.** The image of the entire rectangular beam consists of the superpositioning of the individual PSFs corresponding to all the pencil beams. The shape of the PSF will be especially relevant where the image is changing rapidly, in our example, at the interior edges of the collimator

There have been attempts to account, in the MTF formalism, for image degradation resulting from different kinds of noise, and some of these involve the *Wiener spectrum*. Consider, for example, the noise associated with film granularity. When observed through a magnifying lens, a developed sheet of uniformly exposed film is not the same everywhere. The number of silver grains per unit area varies, rather, in accord with the dictates of Poisson statistics. If a microdensitometer is used to scan such a film, its output will be a voltage (corresponding to the optical density) that looks something like Figure 24–17A. This signal may be fed into a computer, and its Fourier spec-

trum determined. This process is repeated a number of times, and the resulting set of Fourier representations averaged together. At each frequency, the value of the average Fourier component (the amplitude of the spectrum) is then squared. This, finally, is the Wiener spectrum (Fig. 24–17B), a measure of noise power as a function of frequency.

Different noise sources, such as film granularity and quantum mottle, yield different Wiener spectra. The exact shape of the curve may suggest ways in which the signal-to-noise can be improved.

9. JUDGING PERFORMANCE WITH RECEIVER OPERATING CHARACTERISTIC (ROC) CURVES

The MTF is useful in indicating some kinds of weak links in an imaging chain. But that is a far cry from assessing the ability of a system to provide images from which a physician can detect and classify tissue irregularities. The receiver operating characteristic (*ROC*) curve is a construct, borrowed from our radio engineering colleagues, by means of which we can quantify the overall success with which an imaging system plus observer together will generate clinically correct diagnoses.

Suppose that some disease causes the liver to enlarge. It is reported in the literature that in a nuclear medicine imaging study of several hundred adults known to have the disease, the apparent sizes (i.e., areas on the display) of the livers obey a bell-shaped, Normal distribution (Fig. 24–18A). For healthy adults, the organ sizes are again Normally distributed, but with a significantly smaller mean value. It is fairly easy to tell the two situations apart, except for livers in the range of sizes where the distributions overlap.

You propose to use apparent liver size for purposes of diagnosis. You pick, somewhat arbitrarily, the size marked C in Figure 24–18A to serve as the diagnostic cutoff level: You will diagnose patients with a liver of apparent size larger than C as having the disease, or *positive*, and the others you will call *healthy*, or *negative*. A positive finding is a *true positive* (TP) if a biopsy reveals unequivocally that your image-based diagnosis was correct. With a *false positive* (FP), on the other hand, your imaging study indicates that there is an abnormality but the results of your study are wrong. So also for the negatives: A negative diagnosis is a *true negative* (TN) only if there really is no abnormality present; and an imaging study that misdiagnoses a diseased liver as being healthy is *false negative* (FN). The four possibilities are laid out in Table 24–2. The populations of false-positive and false negative patients, for example, are indicated in Figure 24–18A with shading and hatching, respectively. An individual patient with an imaged liver size just above C could easily be either true positive or false positive.

Naturally you are interested in learning about and being able to discuss the reliability with which you and the imaging system together will make diagnoses of the true positive, true negative variety. Several simple parameters have been devised for this purpose. Suppose that your study consists of a total of N_{total} cases and that N_{TP} of them turn out to be TP (and so also for the other entries in Table 24–2). The **accuracy** of your method is defined as the fraction of cases that are diagnosed correctly:

$$accuracy = (N_{TP} + N_{TN})/N_{total} \qquad (24.6)$$

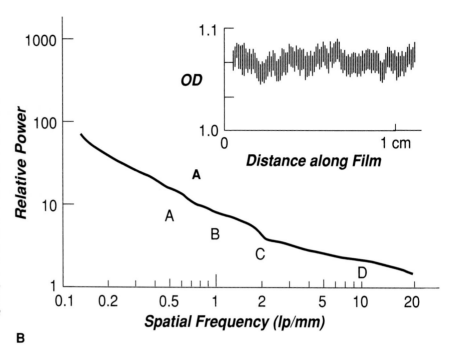

Figure 24–17. Wiener (or noise power) spectrum. **A.** The inset shows the variations in voltage output, or in optical density (OD), as a microdensitometer slowly scans a uniformly exposed and developed piece of film. **B.** This typical radiographic Wiener spectrum displays some characteristic structure: Region A corresponds to large-scale irregularities in screen construction, film development, and so on. Region B is "white noise" caused by quantum mottle. Region C reflects the general rolloff of the imaging system modulation transfer function (MTF) at these spatial frequencies. And region D records another form of white noise, associated with film or screen graininess. *(After Johns HE, Cunningham JR: The Physics of Radiology, 4th ed., Springfield, IL: Charles C Thomas, 1983 [Fig. 16–29].)*

The **sensitivity** (also called "true-positive fraction") is

$$\text{sensitivity} = N_{TP}/(N_{TP} + N_{FN}) \qquad (24.7a)$$

where the term in the denominator is the number of cases in which disease really was present (whether diagnosed correctly or not). **Specificity** (*true-negative fraction*) refers to the relative number of healthy patients diagnosed as such:

$$\text{specificity} = N_{TN}/(N_{TN} + N_{FP}) \qquad (24.7b)$$

These parameters are useful, but they depend on the choice of diagnostic cutoff level. If you moved the cutoff level C in Figure 24–18A far to the left, for example, *everything* would be called positive, and the test would be clinically useless. So where should you place the diagnostic cutoff level? The ROC method helps to resolve this problem.

For our example, the ROC curve plots the true positive rate against the false-positive rate (Fig. 24–18B) for the various possible choices of the cutoff organ size. The areas under the curves of Figure 24–18A indicate that with cutoff level C, to obtain a true-positive rate of about 85%, we must accept about a 15% false-positive rate. This yields point C in Figure 24–18B. If you feel that no more than 5% false positives is tolerable, you can increase the organ cutoff size to point C′ in Figure 24–18A, but you find that the true positive rate falls to 70%. This yields a second point on the ROC curve. Conversely, if you are intent on catching more of the true positives, point C″, the number of false positives that sneak in also increases. By assuming a range of values of the threshold organ size, you can generate the entire ROC curve, the solid curve in Figure 24–18B.

Ideally, your ROC curve would look something like the dashed line in Figure 24–18B, with all true positives and no false positives. But several factors conspire to prevent that. First, the liver may happen to be unusually large within a healthy individual, or small within one who has the disease; you would obviously have no control over the false positive or negative that would result. But also, the image of the liver has

a blurred border, and the apparent size will depend on the strength of the image relative to the background noise level. The percentage of correct diagnoses might therefore increase with the signal-to-noise ratio (Fig. 24–18C), or with the strength of the image signal. Likewise, the abilities of the viewer play a role in all of this. As the image quality and physician skill improve, the ROC curve should come closer to the ideal.

If different imaging systems or techniques (which might lead to different values of the signal-to-noise ratio in Fig. 24–18C) or different viewers yield dissimilar ROC curves, then the one with the curve closest to the ideal will most likely give correct results.

APPENDIX 24–1. Waves in Time and Space: The Sine Function

Many natural phenomena are oscillatory in time or space. The sine and cosine functions of trigonometry are often appropriate for their description.

The value of sin θ for the particular angle θ can be defined as the ratio of the altitude of a right triangle to its hypotenuse:

$$\sin \theta = \text{altitude}/\text{hypotenuse} \qquad (24.8)$$

(Fig. 24–19A). Calculated in this fashion, sin θ is recorded as a function of the independent variable θ in Figure 24–19B. The cosine function, cos θ, is similarly defined as the ratio of the base of the triangle to the hypotenuse.

After the angle θ has run from 0 to 360 degrees, sin θ repeats itself:

$$\sin(\theta + 360°) = \sin \theta \qquad (24.9)$$

Because of this, it is said to be a **periodic** function with a periodicity of 360 degrees.

Angles can be expressed either in degrees or in radians, which are defined in terms of the radius and circumference of

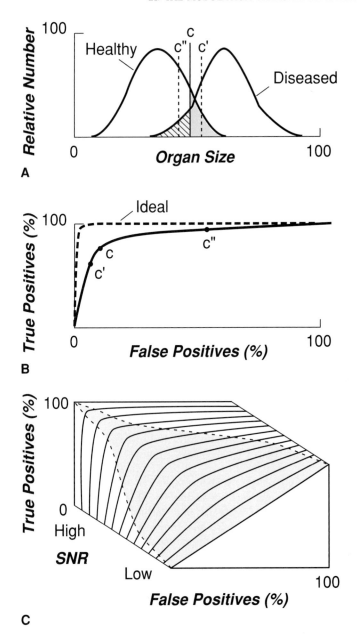

A

B

C

Figure 24–18. Construction of a receiver operating characteristic (ROC) curve for a hypothetical clinical test based on hepatomegaly as detected by imaging. **A.** Distribution of liver sizes for a population of healthy patients and for those with the disease. Somewhat arbitrarily, the organ size marked *C* is chosen initially as the clinical threshold: Larger liver images are assumed to indicate presence of the disease. **B.** Point *C* relates the percentage of false positives (FP) that come along with the true positives (TP) for this choice of clinical threshold liver size. *C'* and *C''* do the same for other threshold organ sizes. A number of points such as these define the ROC curve. The ideal ROC curve is indicated by the dashed line. If several different imaging machines (or clinical techniques, or clinicians, and so on) yield dissimilar ROC curves, the system with the curve closest to the ideal will provide the most reliable diagnostic information. **C.** The ROC curve becomes more like the ideal as the signal-to-noise ratio (SNR) improves.

TABLE 24–2. POSSIBLE COMBINATIONS OF IMAGE-BASED AND CONFIRMED-CORRECT DIAGNOSES

Pathology Report	Image-Based Diagnosis	
	Positive	*Negative*
Positive	TP	FN
Negative	FN	TN

a circle: One **radian** is the *angle* subtended by a segment of the circumference that happens to be exactly one radius, *r*, in length (see Fig. 24–19A). As the entire circumference is 2π radii ($2\pi r$) in length, 360 degrees corresponds to 2π radians:

$$2\pi \text{ radians} \approx 360° \qquad (24.10)$$

Although defined in terms of a geometric angle, θ can take on more abstract meanings. We are concerned here primarily with things that vary periodically in time or space. The vertical motion of a hummingbird's wing, for example, may be described approximately as a sinusoidal function of time, *t*:

$$y(t) = A \cdot \sin(2\pi f \cdot t) \qquad (24.11a)$$

A is the **amplitude** of the sweep of the wing in meters. Its **frequency**, *f*, is expressed in the units cycles per second, or hertz (Hz). That is, over $t = 1$ second, the angle $2\pi f t$ goes through 2π radians or 360 degrees *f* times. The function $y(t)$ is said to have a **period** of $1/f$ second.

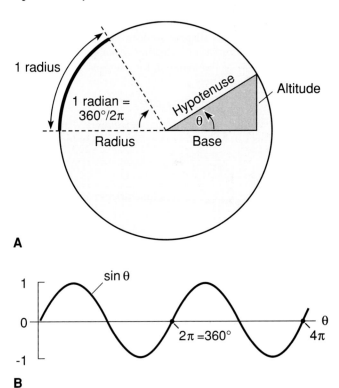

A

B

Figure 24–19. Some definitions from elementary trigonometry. **A.** The sine, cosine, and other trigonometric functions can be defined in terms of ratios of the base, altitude, and hypotenuse of a triangle. The radian is the angle subtended when a line of length equal to the radius of a circle is laid out along its circumference: 2π radians correspond to 360 degrees. **B.** The sine function, $\sin \theta$, is periodic, and begins repeating itself at $\theta = 360$ degrees $= 2\pi$ radians.

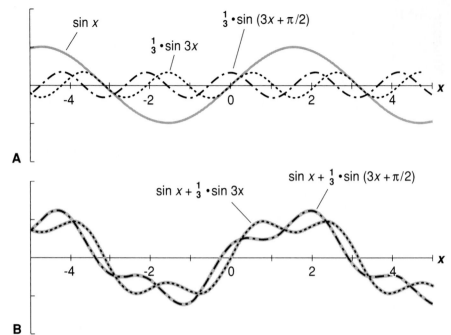

Figure 24–20. Significance of phase. **A.** Three simple functions—$\sin x$, $\frac{1}{3} \cdot \sin 3x$, and $\frac{1}{3} \cdot \sin (3x + \pi/2)$, where the last two differ only by a 90-degree phase shift. **B.** Phase *is* important: $\{\sin x + \frac{1}{3} \cdot \sin 3x\}$ vs. $\{\sin x + \frac{1}{3} \cdot \sin (3x + \pi/2)\}$. If the term in braces were a contribution to a Fourier representation of an image, the phase angle could well have a visible effect.

The **angular frequency**, ω, in radians per second, is defined through $\omega = 2\pi f$. Equation 24.11a can then be expressed in the equivalent form

$$y(t) = A \cdot \sin \omega \cdot t \qquad (24.11b)$$

Some phenomena display smooth periodic behavior in *space*. A photomicrograph of a feather reveals spatial undulations in thickness of the material, for example, nearly of the form

$$y(x) = B \cdot \sin(2\pi f \cdot x) \qquad (24.12a)$$

where f now corresponds to the **spatial frequency**, in *cycles per millimeter*. This can be expressed equivalently in terms of the *spatial period* or *wavelength*, λ, as

$$y(x) = B \cdot \sin(2\pi x/\lambda) \qquad (24.12b)$$

Typical units for λ might be millimeters per cycle. A third,

equivalent form, involving the spatial angular frequency, k (e.g., radians per mm), is

$$y(x) = B \cdot \sin k \cdot x \qquad (24.12c)$$

This is illustrated with the solid and broken curves in Figure 24–20A for the particular cases $k = 1$ and $k = 3$ (radians per unit length).

Sometimes you will find a sine or related function that contains a constant **phase factor.** The phase of a periodic function refers to the angle at some starting or reference time or place. The phase of an isolated function is usually not of much interest, but if there are several such functions, their *relative phases* can be critically important. Figure 24–20B, for example, compares the sum of $\sin x$ and $\frac{1}{3} \sin 3x$, both when the two functions are in phase at $x = 0$ and when they differ in phase at $x = 0$ by 90 degrees $= \pi/2$.

Part 5

Other Analog X-ray Imaging Modalities

Chapter 25

Mammography

1. **Enhancing Soft Tissue and Microcalcification Contrast with a Low kVp and Tissue Compression**
2. **A Dedicated Mammography System Employs a Special X-ray Tube, Compression Device, Grid, and Cassette**
3. **The Xerographic Process: A Photoconducting Selenium Plate as Image Receptor**
4. **Xerography Enhances Edges Around Calcifications**
5. **Mammographic Doses and Risks**
6. **Other Methods of Breast Imaging**

Breast cancer strikes approximately one in eight American women. Fortunately, 5-year survival for stage I patients, in which the lesion is small and limited to breast tissue, is of the order of 90%. Clinical examination and self-examination may allow detection while the disease is still at an early stage, but mammography may indicate its presence before it is palpable.

In 1989, the American College of Radiology (ACR), the American Medical Association (AMA), the National Cancer Institute (NCI), and other major medical organizations recommended, in addition to routine clinical breast examination, a mammogram every 1 or 2 years for women between the ages of 40 and 49 and an annual mammogram after age 50. Women with a family history of the disease or other risk factors may require closer surveillance. A 1990 survey by the NCI found that 64% of American women over 40 have had at least one mammogram, up from 37% in 1987. It is hoped that this situation will continue to improve as insurance companies and other sources pay for more screening mammograms.

Mammography, whether for mass screening or in the testing of a woman who displays symptoms of breast cancer, must be able to reveal not only subtle differences in the density and composition of breast parenchymal tissue, but also the presence of minute calcifications (specks of calcium hydroxyapatite, $Ca_5(PO_4)_3OH$, typically 100 μm in dimension). Thus there is a need not only to maximize the subject contrast, for the detection of soft-tissue lesions, but also to obtain a high degree of resolution and low noise. Latitude must be wide enough to ac-

commodate both the thick tissue near the chest wall and the skin at the edge of the breast, moreover, and the dose must be low. Although each of these objectives may be easy to achieve separately, having to satisfy them all at the same time is no simple task.

1. ENHANCING SOFT TISSUE AND MICROCALCIFICATION CONTRAST WITH A LOW kVp AND TISSUE COMPRESSION

The amount of contrast found among the soft tissues of the breast is determined by both the subject contrast and the receptor contrast (Equations 18.3 and 21.4).

The various tissues of the breast are radiologically similar, but not identical. The fibrous, ductal, and glandular tissues have nearly the same radiological properties as water, with effective atomic number $Z_{eff} = 7.4-7.6$ and density of about $\rho = 1.0 \text{ g/cm}^3$. For fat, $Z_{eff} = 5.9-6.5$ and $\rho = 0.9 \text{ g/cm}^3$.

Subject contrast is enhanced in mammography by imaging with lower-energy photons, where the attenuation coefficients of the soft tissues and the differences among them (which is the important thing) are greatest. The photoelectric effect dominates and, according to Equations 14.8 and 14.9, the linear attenuation coefficients of normal and pathologic tissues, of effective atomic numbers Z_{norm} and Z_{path} and densities ρ_{norm} and ρ_{path}, differ by a factor of

$$\mu_{norm}/\mu_{path} \sim (Z_{norm}/Z_{path})^3 \, (\rho_{norm}/\rho_{path}) \qquad (25.1)$$

It is such differences that must be seen for diagnosis.

Likewise, although contrast is rarely an issue in imaging bones, the search for microcalcifications in the breast is another matter. Enhanced visibility, brought about by low kVp, can increase the likelihood of their detection. Figure 25–1 estimates the contrast for 1 mm³ of glandular tissue, and for a 100-μm calcification, relative to normal breast tissue, as functions of monochromatic x-ray energy (not including the degradation in contrast resulting from scatter).

Compton scatter radiation degrades subject contrast, but the amount of scatter present can be reduced in several ways. The first and foremost of these is physical **compression** of the breast between the image receptor (grid and screen–film cassette) and a parallel, radiotranslucent paddle. Although the process causes varying degrees of discomfort for patients, the results with respect to image quality are striking (Fig. 20–6). (Indeed, being able to see the benefits of compression, on sample films left in the examination room, may provide encouragement to the reluctant patient.) Compression reduces the thickness of tissue that must be traversed by the x-ray beam. As a consequence, the breast exposure needed to achieve an adequate level of radiation at the image receptor is lower. Less scatter is produced, and there is less dose to breast tissue, as

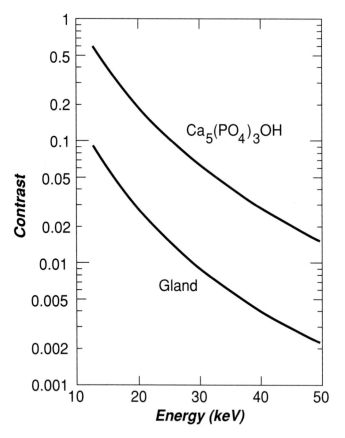

Figure 25–1. Contrast, relative to normal breast tissue, for a 100-μm microcalcification and for 1 mm of glandular tissue, as functions of monochromatic photon energy. This indicates the advantage of creating mammograms with lower-energy photons. *(After Webb S, ed.,* The Physics of Medical Imaging. *Philadelphia: Adam Hilger, 1988 (Fig. 2.7), with permission.)*

well. Compression also causes much of the breast tissue to be spread out and of uniform thickness; as a result, the image contains less overlapping of tissue shadows and is of nearly uniform average optical density. Compression even helps to eliminate motion unsharpness.

Scatter can be reduced further in mammography, as in other forms of x-ray imaging, by means of *tight collimation* of the beam about the region of interest. And a *moving grid* can reduce the scatter-to-primary ratio for a large or dense breast by as much as a factor of 3. When fine detail must be examined, an *air gap* not only leads to magnification and (when used with a microfocus tube) improved resolution, but also reduces scatter. Either a grid or an air gap increases average dose to the breast by a factor of 2 or 3 but, for a properly maintained dedicated mammography system, the doses are so low that the benefits of increased clarity far outweigh any increment in radiation risk, especially for difficult cases.

2. A DEDICATED MAMMOGRAPHY SYSTEM EMPLOYS A SPECIAL X-RAY TUBE, COMPRESSION DEVICE, GRID, AND CASSETTE

Any new radiographic system intended for breast imaging (whether screening or diagnostic) should be **dedicated**, with a specialized mammographic x-ray tube, compression device, grid, and image receptor (Fig. 25–2). Most new systems use a mammographic screen–film cassette as the image receptor.

The x-ray tube in a dedicated screen–film mammographic system should* employ a molybdenum (Mo, $Z = 42$) target and be operated (with a three-phase or constant-potential generator) in the range 25 to 32 kVp. The strong emission of molybdenum K-shell characteristic x-rays, between 17.4 and 19.8 keV, produces a beam that is not highly penetrating, but that provides high contrast in tissue that is not too thick (the typical compressed breast being 3 to 8 cm across). Higher tube potentials yield lower contrast, as a greater fraction of the photon interactions occur by means of the Compton mechanism (for which the radiologic differences among soft tissues are less and scatter is produced). With voltages below 25 kVp, on the other hand, poorer beam penetration leads to greater dose to the breast, with little improvement in image.

The window of a molybdenum-anode tube is a thin sheet of beryllium, as absorption of lower-energy photons by glass could attenuate the beam excessively. Added molybdenum filtration is preferable to aluminum, as a material is relatively transparent to its own characteristic x-rays, (see Chapter 14, Section 4). A molybdenum filter, typically 0.03 mm thick, passes the Mo characteristic x-rays, but removes much of the bremsstrahlung radiation above the 20.0-keV molybdenum K-absorption edge, which is less effective in imaging. Figure 25–3 shows the spectrum of a 30-kVp constant-potential beam with 0.03 mm of added Mo filtration. A filtered 30-kVp beam

---

*These "should's" follow the 1987 recommendations of the Conference of Radiation Control Program Directors (CRCPD) and the Center for Devices and Radiological Health (CDRH) of the Food and Drug Administration (FDA) for *screening* mammograms. Optimal imaging parameters for nonscreening mammography may be somewhat different.

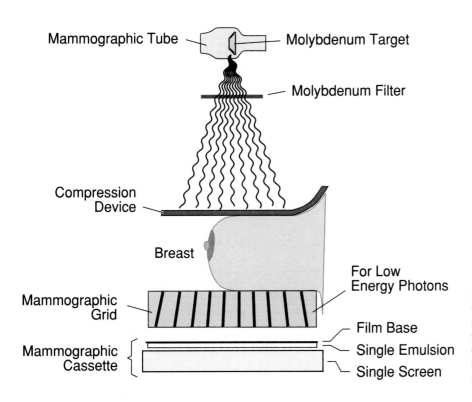

Mammographic Tube — Molybdenum Target

— Molybdenum Filter

Compression Device

Breast

For Low Energy Photons

Mammographic Grid

Film Base
Single Emulsion
Single Screen

Mammographic Cassette

Figure 25–2. A dedicated mammographic system differs from a standard radiographic unit in that it employs an x-ray tube with a molybdenum target and a molybdenum filter; a compression device; a low-photon-energy grid; and a single-screen detail cassette containing single-emulsion film.

should have a half-value layer thickness (HVL) in aluminum of 0.3 to 0.37 mm.

A breast should always be compressed, when possible, both to increase image contrast and to reduce tissue dose. It is becoming routine practice to use a grid for most patients, especially when a breast is difficult to compress and/or contains very dense glandular tissue. Only a special mammographic grid (designed for very low energy x-rays) should be employed.

In the past, mammography was sometimes performed with film and no screen, but modern detail rare earth and calcium tungstate mammographic screens provide adequate res-

olution at a small fraction of the dose. A mammographic cassette, which contains only a single fluorescent screen for better resolution, should be used. Because of the low x-ray energy, a single thin screen can absorb more than 50% of the photons that reach it. The cassette is oriented so that the x-rays pass through the film before entering the screen. That way, light is emitted predominantly from the layer of screen closest to the film, where the x-rays first strike, so that light diffusion and the resultant loss of resolution are lower. The film has emulsion only on the side adjacent to the screen, to reduce crossover. In some mammographic cassettes, film and screen are drawn into close physical contact by means of a vacuum.

Clear visualization of microcalcifications 100 to 200 μm in dimension requires an overall system resolution of 15 lp/mm. The inherent resolution limitation imposed by the screen is a bit less than 20 lp/mm. Working through the geometry outlined in Chapter 22, Sections 5 through 8, suggests that a 0.4-mm effective focal spot is needed. If magnification radiography is to be used (or if the film is to be inspected with a magnifying glass), for a more detailed examination of microcalcifications or certain other masses, then an even smaller focal spot is required. Some mammographic tubes are designed to produce two focal spots, one 0.4 mm or so in dimension for normal mammography (with a grid), and the other about 0.1 mm across for magnification (with no grid) by a factor of 1.5 or 2. Magnification mammography should not be used for screening.

Higher speed and greater contrast can be achieved for some films with "push processing," or the extended processing cycle. Film that has been left in the developer for up to 4 minutes, and is therefore overdeveloped, results in greater average optical density (OD) and enhanced contrast. To obtain the same optimal average optical density (about OD = 1.2) as would result with normal development, a lower exposure is used, with correspondingly less dose to the breast. This re-

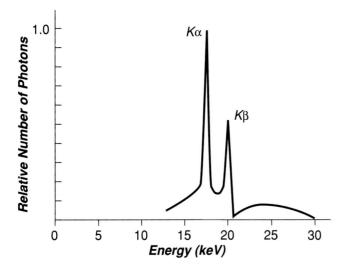

Figure 25–3. The emission spectrum for a molybdenum-target x-ray tube (plus molybdenum beamfilter) is dominated by the molybdenum characteristic x-ray peaks at 17.4 and 19.8 keV. Such a tube is normally operated between 26 and 32 kVp.

quires an initial adjustment of the automatic exposure control (AEC) system, which most dedicated systems employ.

As with other forms of radiography, various possibilities for applying *digital technology* to mammography are being explored actively. Digitization offers a number of advantages, which will be discussed in upcoming chapters. It is generally held, however, that digital systems do not yet provide adequate spatial resolution.

The use of *stereotactic mammography*, for the precise placement of biopsy needles, will be discussed in the next chapter.

3. THE XEROGRAPHIC PROCESS: A PHOTOCONDUCTING SELENIUM PLATE AS IMAGE RECEPTOR

Xerographic mammography is a form of radiography that employs a thin sheet of photoconducting amorphous selenium, rather than a fluorescent screen and film, as the image receptor. No darkroom or solutions are needed, nor are there problems with storing unused or developed film. But a special machine is required to develop the image and fix it on paper. The final product, a blue or black image on white paper, is viewed by reflected (rather than transmitted) light.

Amorphous selenium is a semiconductor with a 2.3-eV energy band gap (see Chapter 7, Section 3). (An "amorphous" material is vitreous, glass-like, with the atoms in random positions; in a crystal, by contrast, the atoms are positioned so as to constitute a three-dimensional, periodic lattice.) It is also a *photoconductor*. In the dark, the resistivity of amorphous selenium is very high. But visible light photons of 2.3 eV (yellow-green) or greater energy can excite electrons from the valence to the conduction band, where they can flow readily in response to an applied electric field. Similarly, when an x-ray photon interacts to produce a high-energy photoelectron or Compton electron, which in turn excites many other electrons into the conduction band, the local conductivity of a small volume of the material can increase by orders of magnitude. When the source of exciting light or x-rays is removed, the material returns immediately to a state of high resistivity.

A xerographic cassette contains a *xerographic plate*, (Fig. 25–4), rather than a fluorescent screen. The plate consists of a thin (150 to 300 μm) layer of amorphous selenium, supported by a 2-mm-thick rigid substrate of aluminum. The selenium and aluminum are separated by a very thin (0.1 μm) layer of aluminum oxide, a good insulator. An overcoating of organic material protects the selenium from abrasion and from chemicals.

The first step in recording an image is to *sensitize* a xerographic plate and insert it into a cassette. A uniform positive charge is deposited on the outer (away from the aluminum substrate) surface of the selenium. The device that causes this to happen, either a "scorotron" or a "corotron," produces a strong electric field in the vicinity of several long, straight wires; the field is sufficiently intense to ionize air molecules, and it drives some of them into the selenium plate. A uniform positive charge is thus laid down on the outer surface of the selenium as the wires sweep across it. To compensate for this positive charge, the same amount of electron charge flows into the aluminum substrate and to its interface with the aluminum oxide. The high resistance of the Al_2O_3 and of the selenium

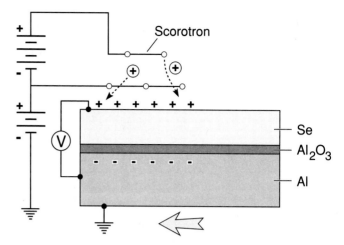

Figure 25–4. The xerographic plate, housed within a cassette during an exposure, plays the role that film assumes in standard radiography. The plate consists of a layer of photoconducting amorphous selenium, an electrical barrier of aluminum oxide, and an aluminum substrate. The exposed selenium surface is protected with an overcoating. This figure shows the sensitization of the xerographic plate, prior to exposure by a scorotron. The scorotron drives positive ions into the outer selenium surface. The plate is moved through the scorotron at constant speed, and a uniform positive surface charge density results. The "plate voltage" drop across the (normally highly resistive) selenium layer is typically 1000 to 1600 V everywhere, before exposure.

(when unexposed to radiation) prevents the electrons from neutralizing the positive ions. The situation is thus like that of a capacitor, in which opposite charges are stored on surfaces separated by insulating material. The charges now resident on the selenium and aluminum surfaces give rise to a "plate voltage" (typically between 1000 and 1600 V) across the selenium and a strong, uniform electrostatic field within.

Once prepared in this fashion, the plate is inserted into a cassette, and is ready for exposure to x-rays, Figure 25–5. A tube with a tungsten target is normally used, and a kVp somewhat higher than that for screen–film mammography. The ionization of a selenium atom by an x-ray photon leads to the creation of many electron–hole pairs. The electrons excited into the conduction band in the process are immediately swept by the electric field within the selenium to its outer surface, where they neutralize positive charges. Likewise, holes migrate toward the Al_2O_3 interface and are, in effect, neutralized by the electrons on the other side of it. The density of positive charge at a point on the surface is thereby diminished, during an exposure, by an amount proportional to the local x-ray intensity. The pattern of residual charge on the plate following the exposure forms an *electrostatic latent image* of the breast. (Note that "latent image" has a new meaning here.) Where few x-ray photons reached the cassette (such as behind a calcification), there remains a high concentration of positive charge. Where the beam was absorbed little, much of the positive charge may be gone. And the pattern of residual positive charges that makes up the latent image produces a corresponding varying electric field at the surface of the plate.

The electrostatic latent image on the plate is *developed* in a closed development chamber (Fig. 25–6). The chamber is filled, in some systems, with a powder cloud or aerosol of particles, 1 μm or so in dimension, of dark blue thermoplastic *toner* mate-

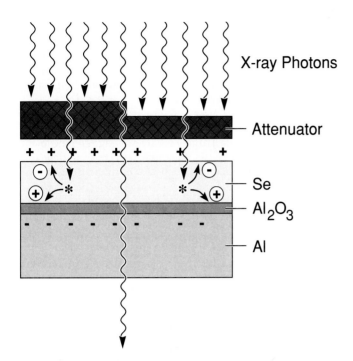

X-ray Photons

Attenuator

Se

Al₂O₃

Al

Figure 25–5. Exposure of a plate through an attenuating test object with a step discontinuity. X-ray photons that interact in the selenium cause a brief and localized increase in conductivity, so that the charge on the outer surface of the selenium decreases. After different parts of the plate have been exposed to different amounts of x-ray energy, the surface charge and the local plate voltage vary correspondingly.

rial. Other systems make use of a fluid developer containing finer, black pigment particles. (Many xerographic *copying machines* use finely powdered charcoal.) Either way, the particles are blown into the development chamber through a fine-bore nozzle and, in rubbing against the wall of the nozzle, many either lose or gain an electron, becoming charged.

After being removed from its cassette, the xerographic plate serves, with its selenium side facing down, as the lid of the development chamber. A set of wires, the development

electrodes, are suspended in a parallel plane nearby. The plate and the development electrodes are attached to the opposite poles of a voltage source, and create a strong electric field in the region between them. Toner particles of one charge or the other, depending on the polarity of the voltage source, will be drawn toward the plate.

For **positive development**, in which denser parts of the body will appear darker in the final image, a back bias voltage of 1000 to 2000 V positive (relative to the development electrodes) is applied to the aluminum backing of the selenium plate. Negatively charged aerosol particles are therefore swept toward it. The electric field near the development electrodes is nearly uniform, but as the toner particles approach the selenium plate, they feel the forces produced by the positive charges of latent image as well, and tend to aggregate in regions of greater local positive charge density. The concentration of toner ending up at any point on the plate is thus determined by the x-ray intensity originally incident there.

The final steps in the formation of an image are the *transfer* of the toner from the selenium plate onto a sheet of special, plastic-impregnated white *paper,* and then its heat *fixation* there. These involve charging up the plate again to loosen the toner, pressing the paper onto the plate hard enough to transfer toner particles to it, and baking the paper so as to bond the toner permanently.

All remaining electric charge and toner are removed from the selenium plate, and it is now ready to be sensitized again. The sensitization, x-ray exposure, and development must take place with the plate kept in complete darkness.

4. XEROGRAPHY ENHANCES EDGES AROUND CALCIFICATIONS

A xerographic image is characterized by large-area (i.e., low spatial frequency) contrast that is low and by edge (high frequency) contrast that is high (i.e., edge enhancement). Toward the anterior edge of the breast, where the thickness of tissue is decreasing relatively slowly, the intensity of transmitted x-ray energy increases; this kind of change shows up less in xerogra-

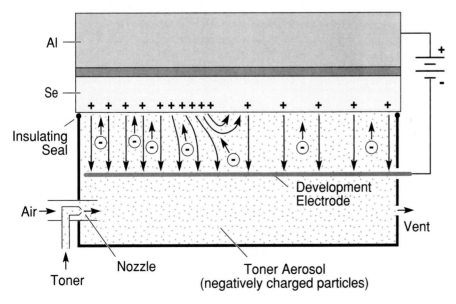

Al

Se

Insulating Seal

Air →

Nozzle

Toner

Development Electrode

Vent

Toner Aerosol (negatively charged particles)

Figure 25–6. Development of the image. The xerographic plate lies face-down and serves as the lid to the development chamber. The wire development electrodes (one of which is seen from the side) lie in a plane parallel to the lid. The xerographic plate and the development electrodes are attached across a source of high direct-current voltage (1000–2000 V), and create a strong electric field in the region between them. With the polarity adopted in this figure, negatively charged toner particles are drawn to the selenium surface. The greater the charge density remaining at a point on the surface following the exposure, the more toner particles that will be attracted there. Thus, the amount of toner landing anywhere is determined by the prior x-ray exposure. After toner has been deposited on the plate, it is transferred to a sheet of paper. The toner is then fixed to the paper by means of a heat treatment.

phy than in a screen–film mammogram, which is advantageous. But abrupt discontinuities in tissue composition or density, such as at a small calcification, fibril, duct, or blood vessel, appear more strongly (edge enhancement).

The explanation for this has to do with the electric field that sweeps toner particles toward the xerographic plate within the development chamber. The field is nearly uniform throughout most of the volume of the chamber. But a sharp discontinuity in the electrostatic latent image can result in a strongly distorted field very near the plate. In Figure 25–7, the portion of the plate to the left was partially obscured during exposure, and fewer x-ray photons arrived to cause the loss of positive charge from its surface. Near the discontinuity in surface charge, the electric field lines bend, and some even form closed loops. The charged toner particles are pulled along these field lines. More toner lands within the border of the electrostatic latent image than would do so if this edge effect did not occur. Also, somewhat less powder arrives at the plate just outside the edge, a phenomenon known as *deletion*. The excess pileup of toner inside the border of the latent image and the deletion just outside it together give rise to edge enhancement of the image. The magnitude of the edge enhancement effect depends on the amount of positive charge originally on the sensitized selenium plate, the strength of the electric field within the development chamber, and the inherent subject contrast and sharpness of the edge being imaged.

For a breast that contains a silicone implant or a large calcified mass, it is important to be able to visualize tissue at the interface. *Negative development*, a variation on the positive development theme of the last section, is helpful in such situations. The aluminum plate, in the development chamber, is attached to a source of negative back bias voltage. Now it is positively charged toner particles that are swept toward the plate. These are repelled from (rather than attracted to, as with positive development) regions of higher positive charge concentration on the plate surface, and the edge enhancement effect is slightly different: the deletion layer ends up on the silicone or calcification side of the interface and does not detract from the image of the tissue.

The diagnostic accuracy of xerography is comparable to that of screen–film mammography, and differences between their images are subtle. Largely because of edge enhancement, xerography is perhaps a little more effective at detecting cancers that manifest only as clusters of microcalcifications. Images of soft tumors may show up slightly better with a screen–film system. Recent improvements of the xerography technique, such as replacing the powder toner with a liquid and increasing the thickness of the selenium plate, have resulted in enhanced resolution and less patient dose. Still, the recent trend has been away from xerography and toward screen–film mammography.

5. MAMMOGRAPHIC DOSES AND RISKS

The possibility that a mammographic examination might itself cause cancer is an issue of clinical concern. Here we shall obtain a crude estimate of the magnitude of the risk associated with a typical screening mammographic examination.

It is normally assumed, for radiation safety purposes, that the probability of induction of a neoplasm in a tissue with ionizing radiation is linearly proportional to the average tissue dose:

$$risk = (risk/dose)(dose) \qquad (25.2)$$

For our risk estimate, the two pieces of information needed are

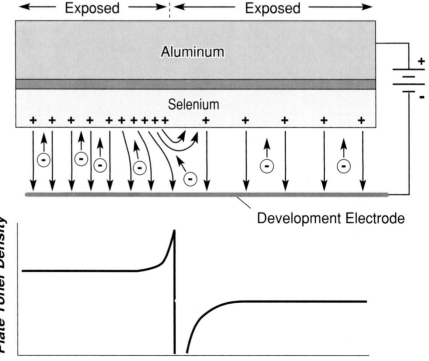

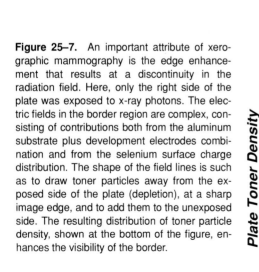

Figure 25–7. An important attribute of xerographic mammography is the edge enhancement that results at a discontinuity in the radiation field. Here, only the right side of the plate was exposed to x-ray photons. The electric fields in the border region are complex, consisting of contributions both from the aluminum substrate plus development electrodes combination and from the selenium surface charge distribution. The shape of the field lines is such as to draw toner particles away from the exposed side of the plate (depletion), at a sharp image edge, and to add them to the unexposed side. The resulting distribution of toner particle density, shown at the bottom of the figure, enhances the visibility of the border.

the expected dose and the likelihood per unit dose of inducing the disease.

The Conference of Radiation Control Program Directors (CRCPD) has recommended that the entrance skin exposure (ESE) from a single craniocaudal screen–film mammogram, with no grid, should be about 0.345 R. (The number is about the same when expressed in centigray of air kerma.) When a grid is used, which is normally the case, the ESE may be about twice that. Skin exposures between 0.7 and 0.9 R are acceptable for xeroradiography. This kind of information is meaningful, as the exposure from an individual mammography machine under clinical conditions can be measured easily.

The corresponding **average glandular tissue dose** depends also on the thickness of the compressed breast (typically 3 to 8 cm), its glandular tissue content, and the effective energy (or, equivalently, the HVL in Al) of the beam. The *mean glandular dose* per exposure to a 5-cm compressed breast from a properly operating mammography system with a grid might be of the order of 0.1 cGy (100 mrad). Screening mammography commonly involves two films, a craniocaudal view and a mediolateral oblique. (For the symptomatic patient, a straight lateral is normally also taken.) Let us assume, in this exercise, that a complete screening examination produces a mean glandular tissue dose of 0.2 cGy.

> The actual dose a particular patient receives can be estimated by repeating the examination (with the same technique factors) on an anthropomorphic **phantom**, within which are embedded dose-measuring devices such as thermoluminescent dosimeters (TLDs). Alternatively, the dose can be calculated from the entrance skin exposure (which can itself be estimated from the technique factors of the exposure) in ways that will be discussed in Chapter 31.

As noted in Chapter 2, Section 9, the lifetime risk that a 1-mSv uniform whole-body irradiation will induce a fatal cancer is estimated to be about 4 in 100,000, or 4×10^{-5}. For x-rays, this is equivalent to a risk per unit dose of 4×10^{-4} cGy^{-1}. Chapter 33 will demonstrate that the risk from irradiation of the breasts alone is of the order of 5% of that.

Therefore by Equation 25.2, the risk of inducing a fatal breast cancer with a typical mammographic examination is something like (0.2 cGy)(0.05)(4×10^{-4} per cGy), or about 5×10^{-6}. If the patient has several tens of mammograms over the course of a lifetime, the cumulative risk is about 1 in 10,000. This is orders of magnitude smaller than the probability that a woman will be stricken with a breast cancer that would be detected early by means of a mammogram.

In summary, the doses involved in mammography, and the associated risks, are so low that they can usually be considered inconsequential. The normal, asymptomatic woman significantly improves her overall survival odds by following the recommendations of the ACR and others on routine mammographic examinations. For a symptomatic or at risk patient, the benefits of having an examination are even greater.

6. OTHER METHODS OF BREAST IMAGING

Several other breast examination methods have been explored. None of them is at present a serious competitor to mammography, either for mass screening or for closer general examination of the symptomatic patient. But ultrasound has found certain clinical use, and magnetic resonance imaging may have the potential for it.

The propagation of *ultrasound* through a medium is sensitive to variations in its density and other physical properties, as will be seen in Chapters 45 to 47. Although not especially useful for initial detection of small lesions, ultrasound imaging can often distinguish cysts from solid masses in a breast, which x-ray often cannot do. The ACR has recommended, however, that ultrasound not be used either as a sole imaging modality or for screening purposes.

Early clinical results for magnetic resonance imaging are proving interesting, for reasons that will become apparent in Chapters 41 to 44.

Light diaphanography involves the transillumination of the breast with red light or infrared radiation. The transmitted light is picked up with a vidicon television camera, and a large or dense tumor may produce a detectable shadow irregularity. At the present time, diaphanography is still generally considered to be an experimental technique.

Thermography is the imaging of patterns of infrared radiation emitted from (indicating patterns of temperature on the surface of) the body. About half of the body's metabolic heat leaves by means of conduction, evaporation, and convection, but the rest escapes as infrared radiation. The rate at which infrared energy is thermally radiated from a particular region of skin depends on its temperature (Equation 5.6). A lesion not too deep within a breast may cause an irregularity in the temperature of the overlying skin of 1°C or even more, and this may show up as a difference between the infrared-images of the two breasts. The amounts of energy radiated are too small for direct photography with infrared-sensitive film, so thermography employs an electro-optical camera somewhat like early television cameras. Although thermography is still the subject of some research, the ACR currently takes the position that it is relatively ineffective at the detection of breast cancers.

Computed tomography has neither the resolution required to pick out microcalcifications nor sufficient contrast to detect some soft tissue lesions. It is expensive, moreover, and (unlike the modalities noted above) imparts a relatively high dose of ionizing radiation to the breast.

One final breast imaging modality of possible limited (because of cost) clinical significance is positron emission tomography. Positron emission tomography scanning, which also involves the use of ionizing radiation, will be discussed in Chapter 40.

Chapter 26 _____

Other Special Screen–Film Techniques

1. Conventional Tomography Blurs Out the Shadows of Tissues Everywhere but in One Plane
2. Film Subtraction Angiography Removes the Shadows of Tissues That Do Not Contain Contrast Agent
3. Stereoscopy Gives Some Impression of Depth
4. Assessment of Bone Demineralization

This chapter briefly describes several rather specialized techniques that may not be routinely employed at most clinics, but that do find some important uses.

1. CONVENTIONAL TOMOGRAPHY BLURS OUT THE SHADOWS OF TISSUES EVERYWHERE BUT IN ONE PLANE

Body section or **conventional tomography** (Fig. 26–1) images a planar section of the body, as does computed tomography (CT), but it acquires information in a totally different way: It removes the shadows from over- and underlying tissues by

blurring them out with intentional motion. What remains unblurred is an image primarily of tissues in the plane of interest.

In simplest form (Fig. 26–2), an x-ray tube and a film cassette move in opposite directions within parallel planes. They are attached to one another by means of a rigid lever pivoted at a fixed fulcrum point, so that their motions are completely linked. Consider any point, such as A, in the **focal plane**, which lies parallel to the planes of motion of the tube and cassette and which contains the fulcrum. If the tube and cassette (connected by the lever) are displaced during an exposure, the *image of point* A shifts by exactly the same distance that the film moves; that is, the image of A is projected always to the same spot (indicated as A′ before the move and A″ after) on the film. Hence there is no blurring, and the image of the tissues at point

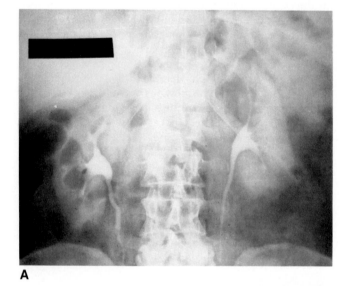

A

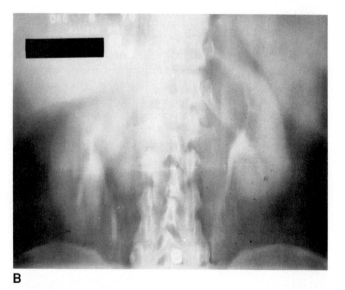

B

Figure 26–1. Example of conventional tomography imaging. **A.** Anteroposterior view of a 55-year-old woman with high blood pressure, taken 5 minutes after administration of contrast agent for an intravenous urogram. **B.** A 20-degree linear tomographic image with the plane of focus 8 cm above the table top. "A fairly well-circumscribed lucent mass measuring 7.0 by 6.5 cm is seen overlying the midcortex of the right kidney. This is a renal cyst arising from the anterior cortical surface. . . . Even though the location of the cyst is known from the tomogram, it cannot be seen on the plain film." *(From the American College of Radiology Learning File, courtesy of the ACR, Reston, VA.)*

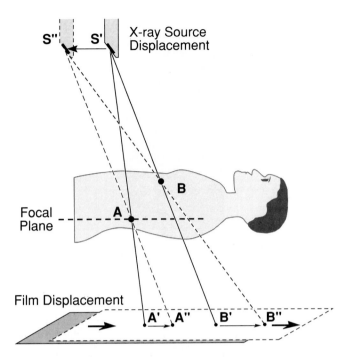

Figure 26–2. Conventional tomography, in which images of objects on the focal plane (inside the patient) are preserved, but those of objects away from the focal plane are blurred out. Imagine that a rigid lever attaches the source of the beam to the image receptor, with a fixed fulcrum somewhere on the focal plane. When the source of radiation moves the distance *S'S''*, the image of a small object at point A moves the distance *A'A''*. But because of the lever, the film moves exactly the same distance, so that the image stays at the same point on the film. The image of the object at point B, on the other hand, moves farther (*B'B''*) than the film, and blurs.

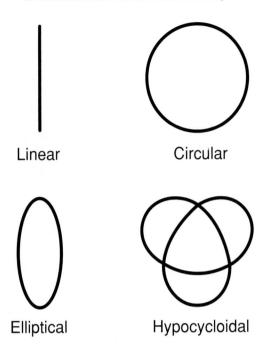

Figure 26–3. Some of the patterns in which the x-ray tube and film are made to move in conventional tomography.

A (and at every other point in the focal plane) remains in focus. But the image of the tissue at point B, which is *not* in the focal plane, will be blurred. And the extent of the blur will increase with its distance above or below the focal plane.

If the tube and cassette move little, nearly the entire body will be in focus. If the *exposure angle* (through which the x-ray tube travels during the exposure) is large, on the other hand, the section in focus will be relatively thin. Thus, one can reduce the thickness of the section imaged by increasing the exposure angle.

When the motions of the x-ray tube and cassette happen to be along a leg bone that is not in the image plane, say, the edge of the bone will suffer relatively little loss of sharpness. Motion perpendicular to the bone, on the other hand, will blur out its edge almost entirely. Moving the tube and detector in a circle (i.e., with a greater exposure angle) will yield something in-between. Motion in a larger circle will have more blurring effect, as will more complex paths (Fig. 26–3). Thus the effectiveness of motion in causing blur increases both with the exposure angle (which increases with tube velocity and exposure time) and with the complexity of the motion.

One can bring a different plane of tissue into coincidence with the focal plane by elevating or lowering the patient the appropriate amount and then shooting an additional film. Alternatively, you could shift the cassette a small distance closer to the patient, but cause it to move at exactly the same linear

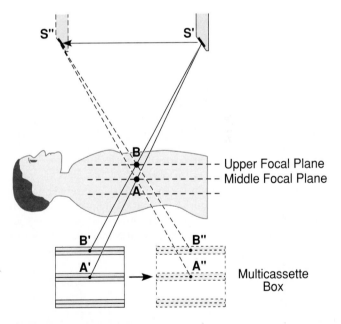

Figure 26–4. Imaging several planes within the body simultaneously by means of conventional tomography. The physical fulcrum is located somewhere on the middle focal plane, which also contains point A within the patient; the image of A at A' and A'' is unblurred for the middle cassette. The image of the point B, higher in the patient, blurs in the middle cassette, but not as B' and B'' in the *upper* cassette (which moves at the same speed as the middle cassette). In effect, the upper cassette images an upper focal plane, which lies parallel to, but above, the middle focal plane.

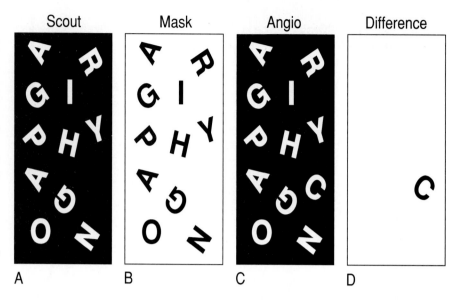

Figure 26–5. Film subtraction angiography. In this example, a number of small, lead letters are lying on the patient table. An additional letter "C" is added at a later time. The objective of the exercise is to find the "C". **A.** A scout film contains images of the irrelevant and interfering background material, patterns not of clinical interest. For our example, such material consists of the lead letters A, N, G, I, O, G, R, A, P, H, and Y before the "C" is added. **B.** A *mask* film is produced from the scout. Areas that were originally covered with letters, and are transparent to light in the scout, become opaque in the mask, and vice versa. **C.** A lead letter "C" is dropped onto the table, and the *angiographic* film produced. **D.** The angio and mask films are superimposed. The only area remaining translucent, where the two films differ, is at the letter "C". The *difference* image arising from superimposing the films can be captured by means of optical photography.

velocity as before. It will be traveling a bit too fast and far to focus the original focal plane, which contains the fulcrum. But it will be moving in just the right manner to bring into focus another plane of tissue, one lying slightly above the fulcrum. This suggests a way of imaging a number of slices simultaneously (Fig. 26–4): Replace the single cassette with a stack of them, and move them together, as a single rigid block. Screen–film combinations should increase in sensitivity with depth in the stack, to compensate for the attenuation of the x-ray beam.

2. FILM SUBTRACTION ANGIOGRAPHY REMOVES THE SHADOWS OF TISSUES THAT DO NOT CONTAIN CONTRAST AGENT

Subtraction radiography is another technique for removing irrelevant structural information from a film. It can be applied if the radiologic properties of the anatomic entity of interest can be altered while the rest of the imaged volume is left unchanged. Subtraction has long been used in angiography, where films are taken before and after radiopaque contrast agent is injected into a vein or artery.

Suppose that a handful of lead letters are thrown onto the patient table, and a "before," or *scout*, radiograph is shot. On development, the film reveals translucent letters against an opaque background (Fig. 26–5A). Then using light and special photographic film, a *subtraction mask* is prepared (Fig. 26–5B); in this "negative" of the scout film; it is now the letters that are opaque and the background that is translucent.

An additional lead "C" (for contrast agent) is now dropped somewhere on the patient table, and the "after" *angiogram film* (Fig. 26–5C) is taken and developed. Our objective is to locate the "C" in it. When the subtraction mask is placed on top of the positive angiogram film and correctly registered (lined up), light can pass through both films only at the "C" (Fig. 26–5D). In every other case, a transparent letter in the angio film is obscured by a corresponding dark letter in the mask. A record of the "C" *difference image* can be produced by exposing a fresh sheet of photographic film to visible or ultraviolet light through the superimposed mask and angiogram films.

The film subtraction angiography technique works essentially the same way in imaging a patient. A scout film is taken of the region of interest, and a negative mask prepared. Contrast agent is then injected, and the angiograph taken. When the mask and angiogram films are superimposed and in proper registry, the total optical density of the pair should be uniform, except where contrast agent is present. Suppose that, away from the contrast agent, 1% of light incident on the superimposed films is transmitted through both, so that the average optical density (OD) for the pair is 2.0; where the scout or angiogram film has an OD of 0.5, for example, the mask should be 1.5, and vice versa. This can happen if the film used to make

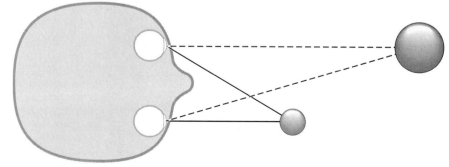

Figure 26–6. One ball is twice the size of the other, and twice as far from the eyes. Either eye alone sees two balls of the same apparent size, possibly side by side. The parallax phenomenon leads to a sense of depth with binocular vision, however, and one can easily determine the relative distances of the two objects.

the mask has a gamma of exactly 1 for exposure to light; the optical density of the developed mask will then be everywhere complementary to that of the scout and (away from vessels containing contrast agent) to that of the angiogram. Special subtraction film with a gamma of 1 has been created expressly for the purpose of making masks.

Subtraction angiography can be performed not only with film, but also with fluoroscopic image acquisition and computer-based subtraction. The rapidly developing field of digital subtraction angiography (DSA) and related modalities will be discussed in Chapter 36.

3. STEREOSCOPY GIVES SOME IMPRESSION OF DEPTH

Stereoscopy, which was widely employed in the past, is still useful as a simple method of resolving some kinds of three-dimensional image confusion.

With only one eye open, you can use perspective, apparent sizes and overlappings, and other forms of monocular information about objects to provide estimates of their absolute distances from you. With two eyes taking in slightly different views, the brain has the remarkable capability of rendering a single mental image with a sense of depth to it. This binocular depth perception does not allow you to judge absolute distances to objects much more accurately, but it does improve your ability to determine which of any two of them is closer.

One of the two balls in Figure 26–6 is twice as far from an observer as the other, and twice its size. Monocular vision provides no information on their relative positions. But with binocular vision, the right eye perceives one ball nearly behind the other, and the situation is quite different to the left eye, 4 in. or so away. Depth perception is based on the subconscious analysis of this **parallax**, or apparent displacement of objects relative to one another when viewed from different positions.

Stereoscopy mimics binocular depth perception, or *stereopsis*, with pairs of slightly different radiographs. Typically,

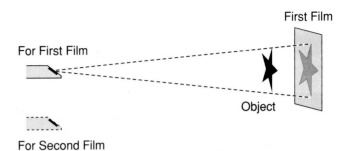

Figure 26–7. In stereoscopy, a first radiograph of an object is produced. The film is replaced with a fresh sheet, but the position of neither the cassette nor the object being imaged is altered. The source of radiation is displaced laterally, however, and a second film is shot. Displacing the source between films is like opening one eye, which had been held closed, and closing the other.

one film is taken at a distance of 100 cm (40 in.). Then, with the patient and cassette perfectly immobile, the x-ray tube is shifted laterally by 10 cm (10% of the source-to-image receptor distance). The cassette is replaced with a fresh one, at the same location, and a second film is shot (Fig. 26–7). Points at different depths in the patient will undergo different apparent displacements, or amounts of parallax, between the two films.

One cannot simply superimpose the films for viewing, but several devices have been invented to achieve the sense of perspective. The "binocular prism stereoscope" (Fig. 26–8), for example, fools the eyes into thinking that they are looking with depth perception at a three-dimensional scene when, in fact, the parallax is produced by the two films side by side. It is important to ensure that each eye is directed at the appropriate film and that the two films are oriented correctly, so that the surgeon doesn't end up operating on the wrong side of the patient.

Stereoscopy has found a promising new mammographic application in guiding percutaneous fine-needle aspiration biopsies of breast lesions, including those that are nonpalpable.

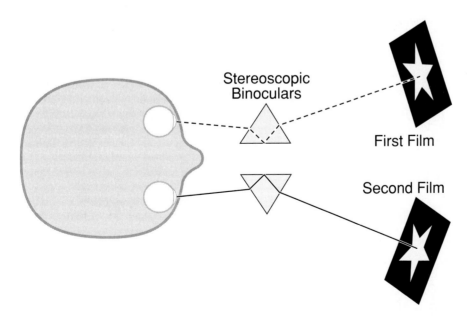

Figure 26–8. With this approach to stereoscopy, the brain thinks that the eyes are seeing a single film but with some sort of parallax built in. In reality, the eyes are viewing two separate films, but produced and displayed in such a fashion that together they capture the parallax.

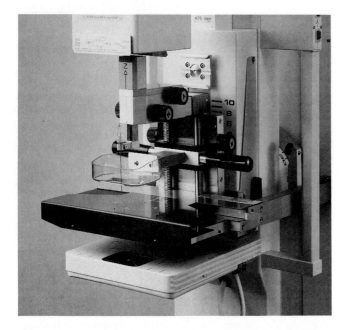

Figure 26–9. Needle placement assembly for use in mammographic percutaneous fine-needle aspiration biopsy of breast lesions. This apparatus is removed for normal mammography. *(Courtesy of the General Electric Company.)*

With the breast compressed, a scout film is taken to ensure proper positioning. A matched pair of mammograms are then taken, with the x-ray beam angled at +15 and –15 degrees on either side of vertical, for a total angular shift of 30 degrees. The cassette is moved one radiation field width between exposures, and only half the film is exposed with each view. After development, the film is displayed on a special light box, and the physician quickly indicates the position of the suspected lesion and a frame of reference with an electronic digitizer. A com-

puter calculates the necessary needle position and depth coordinates, and the needle is moved into place by means of screw micrometers (Fig. 26–9). The correct localization of the needle tip is confirmed (typically to within ±1 mm) with a second pair of stereotactic images. The breast must be kept compressed, of course, throughout the quarter-hour or so of the procedure.

4. ASSESSMENT OF BONE DEMINERALIZATION

Roughly 50,000 people die every year, in the United States, as a result of hip fractures attributable to osteoporosis. In addition to the personal suffering brought about by the disease, the nation is drained of some $10 billion of its resources because of associated medical and disability costs and lost workdays.

One simple method for following the bone mineral status of a symptomatic patient over time is based on film densitometry (Fig. 26–10). A radiograph is made of an arm and a reference step wedge of aluminum (which is radiologically similar to bone), side by side submerged in water. The water has about the same linear attenuation coefficient as soft tissue, and in effect removes all soft tissue from the picture, leaving behind only the bone and step wedge.

Attenuation of the x-ray or gamma ray beam along any particular path through the bone will depend on the mass attenuation coefficient and density of the bone and the total photon path length through it:

$$\text{attenuation in bone} = e^{-[\mu/\rho]_{\text{bone}} \cdot \rho_{\text{bone}} \cdot x_{\text{bone}}} \qquad (26.1)$$

Generally, neither $[\mu/\rho]_{\text{bone}}$ nor x_{bone} changes significantly as osteoporosis progresses, but ρ_{bone} will diminish. A decline in bone density will be revealed as a decrease in the peak height of the absorption curve and in the area beneath it.

The amount of attenuation by bone can be calculated from knowledge of the film's characteristic curve. Use of the aluminum step wedge to calibrate each measurement is a simpler approach that yields more reproducible results. The arm bone

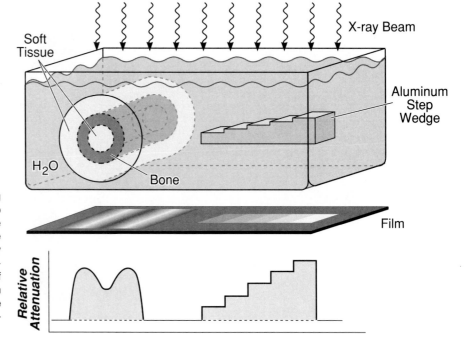

Figure 26–10. Simple system for measuring bone density. The arm and the aluminum step wedge are submerged in water so as to remove the effects of soft tissue. The image of the bone is scanned, and a graph of the optical density obtained, to provide a relative measure of attenuation. The step wedge allows a calibration of the optical density curve, that is, determination of the absolute amount of attenuation. Bone demineralization will cause that absolute attenuation by bone to decrease.

and step wedge will lead to the same film OD for a certain step thickness x_{Al}. A decrease, over time, in the thickness of the matching wedge step indicates a reduction in bone density. The same information can be obtained with an electronic x-ray detection system that circumvents the use of film.

The task of mass screening populations possibly at risk is more difficult. Complicating factors include the irregular sizes and shapes of bone and of the marrow cavities within and the nonmonochromatic nature of the x-ray beam. The use of radio-isotope sources of nearly monochromatic gamma ray photons and, more significantly, of dual-energy computed tomography (for examination, in particular, of the vertebral bodies) offers hope that such screening may still be efficacious and cost-effective.

_____ *Chapter 27* _____

Fluoroscopy

A modern x-ray imaging system is typically arranged so that, by moving the appropriate image receptor into place, it can be used for fluoroscopic, fluorographic, or screen–film imaging.

The essential new component is the image intensifier (II) tube, which transforms the spatial pattern of x-ray photons emerging from the patient into a small, bright optical image. Much of the time, that optical image is fed into a television camera or charge-coupled device (videofluoroscopy). Once a region of interest has been identified with TV, the optical output of the II tube can be filmed directly with a photospot camera (photofluorography) or, primarily with cardiac procedures, a motion picture camera (cinefluorography). Alternatively, a spot film device or film changer can bypass the II tube altogether and record radiographic images directly.

The television link will be discussed in the next chapter. Although it further degrades resolution, TV allows real-time observation of time-dependent processes that cannot be followed with standard radiography. It is useful in patient positioning and in the localization of areas to be explored in more detail by radiographic means. Television makes possible both the immediate transmission of images over great distances and their storage on videotape. Furthermore, the analog TV image signal can be sampled, digitized, and entered into a computer system for digital processing (digital fluoroscopy and digital subtraction angiography), analysis, communication, and archiving.

1. THE FLUOROSCOPIC SYSTEM

The image receptor of a fluoroscopic system is an *image intensifier (II)* tube, which transforms the slightly larger than life-size spatial pattern of x-ray photons emerging from the patient into

a small, bright optical image. For real-time viewing, this optical image can be fed into a TV camera or charge-coupled device (CCD—a recently developed solid-state device that, like a TV camera, transforms an optical pattern into an electronic signal). For better detail, the II tube output can be photographed directly with a photospot camera or, primarily for cardiac catheterization purposes, a cine camera (see Fig. 1–4B).

With some systems, the x-ray tube remains beneath the table, with the II tube above the patient. (The table itself must be uniformly transparent to the x-ray beam, and made of a strong material such as laminated wood or plastic reinforced with carbon fibers.) Alternatively, the x-ray tube and image receptor may be held by a rigid **C-arm** support (see Fig. 1–4C) that can be rotated about an axis or about any of several orthogonal axes. With a **biplanar** system a second x-ray tube (pointing at an angle to the first) can produce a nearly simultaneous second film or fluoroscopic image from a different viewpoint. One tube is usually turned off briefly while the other is being fired; this reduces the scatter to both image receptors and circumvents the need for a second high-voltage generator.

A mechanical linkage with the x-ray tube ensures that the II tube is centered on the x-ray beam. Both the x-ray tube and the **fluoroscopic tower** (which houses the II tube and the various cameras) can move inward and outward along the line joining their centers. This allows the accommodation of patients and body parts of all sizes, and is involved in zooming in on regions of interest.

A short exposure time may be required in conventional screen–film radiography, to freeze out motion blurring. Similarly, photospot and cine fluorography and some forms of digital fluoroscopy employ a pulsed x-ray beam, with short, rapid exposures and high x-ray tube currents. With standard fluoroscopy, by contrast, a primary objective may be long-term, continuous viewing. So although radiography and fluorography may push the x-ray tube briefly to its high current limit (hundreds of milliamperes), videofluoroscopy reduces the tube current to the lowest value that will produce diagnostically usable images (typically 1 to 3 mA with 80 to 100 kVp).

2. THE IMAGE INTENSIFIER TUBE TRANSFORMS A LIFE-SIZE X-RAY PATTERN INTO A SMALL, BRIGHT OPTICAL IMAGE

In the early days, fluoroscopy was performed in a dark room by projecting the x-ray beam emerging from a patient onto a fluorescent screen, and examining the resultant image directly with the eye (see Figure 1–4A). Because an image produced in this fashion is much dimmer than an object seen under daylight conditions, it could be observed only by means of the scotopic vision of the rods of the eye, which is a few thousand times more sensitive than normal photopic vision. It was necessary to dark-adapt the eyes for a half hour, and even then the images appeared faint and low in contrast. One's ability to resolve detail in these circumstances, moreover, was greatly diminished, as high-acuity vision is mediated by the cones, not the rods.

These problems vanished with the development of the image intensifier tube, Figure 27–1A, the heart of the modern fluoroscopic system. The II tube transforms an essentially life-size x-ray image into one that is of a small size suitable for direct input into the lens of a photospot, cine, or television camera and is 10,000 or more times brighter than that from a simple fluoroscopic screen.

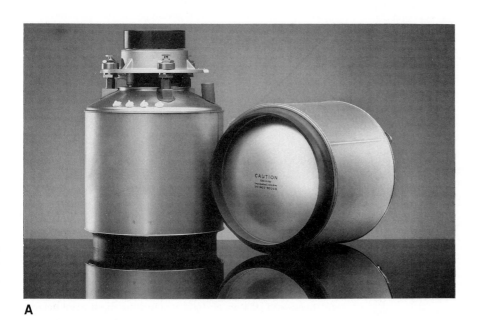

A

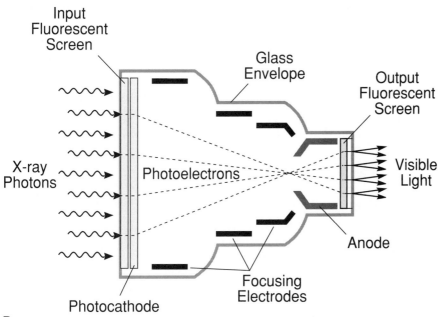

B

Figure 27–1. The image intensifier tube: **A.** Two II tubes without their shielding *(Courtesy of Philips Medical Systems,).* **B.** An image intensifier tube consists of a large (15- to 30-cm) input fluorescent screen plus photocathode combination, an anode and electron beam focusing electrodes (the electron optics), and a small (2.5- to 3.5-cm) output fluorescent screen. The optical image at the output screen is bright because of both minification and flux gain, as discussed in Section 3.

Figure 27–1B diagrams the anatomy of an II tube. The principal components are a large fluorescent input screen and photocathode combination, the electron optics electrodes, an anode, and a small fluorescent output screen, all within a glass envelope that maintains a high vacuum. (The thin-walled glass or metal front faceplate curves outward, for mechanical support against atmospheric pressure, and is very delicate.) A faint scintillation is created when an x-ray photon is absorbed by the input screen, and this light dislodges electrons from the adjacent photocathode; the photoelectrons are accelerated by the anode and, on striking the output screen, create a much brighter pulse of light.

The large *fluorescent input screen* of a typical II tube is a thin layer of cesium iodide deposited on the inside of the tube's faceplate. The photoelectric *K*-absorption edge of cesium occurs at 36.0 keV, and that of iodine at 33.2 keV. CsI is well suited, in terms of x-ray absorption, for procedures in the 80 to 120 kVp range, with photon effective energies of 30 to 40 keV. Because of its high mass attenuation coefficient, physical density, and intrinsic efficiency for converting x-ray photons into light, the CsI layer need be only 0.1 to 0.2 mm thick. As with the screen of a film cassette, the choice of thickness of the fluorescent screen involves a trade-off between x-ray capture efficiency and resolution.

The *photocathode*, a cesium and antimony (CsSb) metal alloy, is adjacent to the input screen, separated from it (to prevent chemical reactions) by a thin sheet of transparent, chemically inert material. Light produced by x-ray photon interactions in the CsI input screen ejects photoelectrons from the adjacent region of the photocathode. (The input screen and photocathode thus act together somewhat like the front end of a scintillation detector [see Chapter 16, Section 6].) The rate of release of photoelectrons from any point on the surface of the photocathode is proportional to the intensity of x-rays arriving at the input screen, so that the spatial pattern of electron emission is determined by that of the incident x-rays.

The photoelectrons are accelerated through 25 to 35 kV toward the *anode*, and focused closer together by *electrostatic lenses*. This is done in such a fashion that the spatial relationship among the electrons, which carry the image information, remains intact.

The accelerated electrons strike the silver-activated zinc–cadmium sulfide (ZnCdS:Ag) *output screen* at high velocity, producing a blue-green visible light image that is much smaller and brighter than that on the input screen. A very thin film of aluminum is deposited on the interior face of the output screen. Although it is almost entirely transparent to the incoming high-velocity electrons, the aluminum film provides them with a conducting path for leaving the output screen after they have given up their kinetic energy. It also prevents any light emitted by the output screen from heading back toward the photocathode; such "retrograde" light could randomly dislodge photoelectrons from the photocathode, which would result in reduced image contrast.

Most commercial II tubes have input screens between 30 cm (12 in.) and 15 cm (6 in.) in diameter, but up to 40-cm (16-in.) tubes are available. The output screen is 2.5 to 3.5 cm (1 to 1.5 in.) across. II tubes are surrounded by metallic shielding to exclude external magnetic fields (which could play havoc with the electron optics, introducing distortions and lessening resolution), and to prevent scatter x-rays from leaking out of the II

enclosure. A shielded 23 cm (9-in.) tube might be 30 cm (12 in.) in overall outer diameter and 25 cm (10 in.) tall, and weigh 15 kg (30 pounds).

Solid state and other alternatives to the II tube are being actively explored. Although none of them has yet achieved the widespread clinical acceptance enjoyed by the II, that may change over the next few years.

3. BRIGHTNESS AMPLIFICATION AND MINIFICATION

The light image on the output screen of an II tube is 5000 to 10,000 times brighter than that on the input screen, for two reasons.

The first, known as **minification,** is (like the inverse square law) purely a matter of geometry. If the diameter of the input screen, D_{in}, is 23 cm and that of the output screen, D_{out}, is 2.5 cm, then the ratio of their areas is 85:1. Suppose, for the moment, that each scintillation photon from the input screen caused the emission of exactly one light photon from an output screen 85 times smaller in area; then the light per unit area, or luminance (brightness), of the image would increase by a factor of 85. In general, the **minification gain** is

$$\text{minification gain} = (D_{in} / D_{out})^2 \qquad (27.1)$$

But each scintillation photon from the front screen will give rise not to one light photon at the output screen, as just assumed, but rather to many. This may be seen by keeping track of the energy from, say, a 50-keV x-ray photon after it is absorbed in the input screen (Fig. 27–2). Some 20% of the absorbed photon's energy is reemitted from the input screen in the form of 5000 visible light (about 2-eV) photons. These together may cause the ejection of a total of about 150 photoelectrons from the adjacent photocathode. Each such photoelectron acquires 25 keV of kinetic energy on the way to the anode, and produces 2000 or so light photons at the output screen. Thus, the II tube produces a visible **light photon flux gain,**

$$\text{flux gain} = \frac{\text{output screen light intensity}}{\text{input screen light intensity}} \qquad (27.2)$$

of $(150)(2000)/5000 = 60$: There is 60 times more light at the output screen, per original x-ray photon, than at the input screen.

The overall increase in brightness, or **brightness gain,** is determined by both the flux gain and the minification gain:

$$\text{brightness gain} = (\text{minification gain})(\text{flux gain}) \qquad (27.3)$$

EXERCISE 27–1.

What is the brightness gain for our 23-cm tube?

SOLUTION: With a minification gain of 85 and a flux gain of 60, the brightness gain is $(85)(60) \sim 5000$.

Another common, and related, measure of the efficiency of an II tube is the *conversion gain,* or conversion factor. The conversion gain measures the amount of output screen luminance obtained per unit of input x-ray exposure rate:

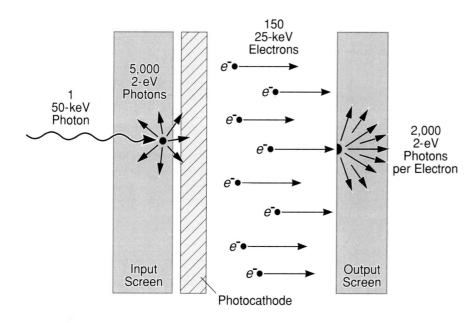

Figure 27–2. A hypothetical example of *flux gain* in an image intensifier tube: One 50-keV x-ray photon strikes the input fluorescent screen, and 5000 2-eV light photons are given off. These together manage to dislodge 150 electrons from a nearby portion of the photocathode. Each photoelectron gains 25 keV before hitting the output screen, and causes 2000 light photons to emerge from it. The flux gain is (150)(2000)/(5000) = 60.

$$\text{conversion gain} = \text{light}_{out}/\text{x-ray rate}_{in} \quad (27.4)$$

The standard unit for the conversion factor is the (candela/square meter)/(milliroentgen-second), abbreviated cd/m^2/mR/s. Typical values are listed in Table 27–1.

Most II tubes are designed to be operated with several different possible minification ratios. At greatest minification, the x-ray pattern that strikes the entire input screen appears at the output screen (Fig. 27–3). With a lower minification setting, only the more central portion of the input screen area is retained and projected onto the output screen. It's as if the diameter of the input screen, D_{in}, is reduced, but with the voltages on the focusing electrodes adjusted so that the image created at the smaller effective input screen again fills the output screen. The output image appears more magnified on the television monitor when less II tube minification is employed, but the field of view is smaller.

Suppose, for example, that you have an II tube with settings of 23 cm (9 in.), 16 cm (6 in.), and 11 cm (4.5 in.). You start out working with the 23-cm input screen setting, but in a particular situation you need to examine a part of the body only 15 cm in dimensions. To achieve better image quality, you switch the tube to the 16-cm mode, which automatically collimates the size of the x-ray beam down to 16 × 16 cm^2. There is less x-ray scatter degrading the contrast, the image appears larger on the display (whether on film or on TV), and, as less image minifi-

cation is less demanding of the electron optics system, resolution is better and there is less distortion. (The x-ray exposure within the beam is greater, but less volume is irradiated, so there is little difference from a radiation safety perspective.)

To reduce patient exposure and scatter, a *positive beam limitation (PBL)* system automatically limits the maximum possible opening of the x-ray beam collimators for any set of operating conditions. This ensures that the x-ray field is no larger than the input screen of the II, regardless of the distance between the x-ray tube and the II tube. (When the system is being used for radiography, PBL restricts the beam to the size of the screen–film cassette.) If several modes of minification are available, PBL limits the x-ray field to the II input screen size selected. If the region of interest is considerably smaller than the

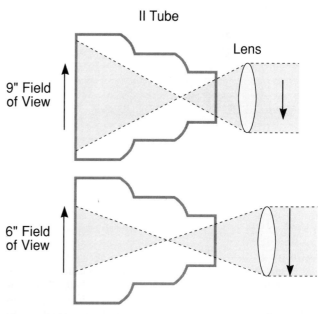

Figure 27–3. When the amount of *minification* is *reduced*, so that the field of view is smaller, the apparent size of the object being imaged increases.

TABLE 27–1. TYPICAL IMAGE INTENSIFIER TUBE PARAMETERS

	Input Diameter Used		
	36 cm	**23 cm**	**15 cm**
	14 in.	*9 in.*	*6 in.*
Output image diameter (cm)	2.5	2.5	2.5
Conversion factor (cd/m^2/mR–s)	150	75	30
Resolution (lp/mm)	3.6	4.2	5.0
10% Area contrast ratio	18:1	25:1	36:1
Pincushion distortion (%)	6	3	0

smallest selectable input screen size, one can manually collimate the x-ray field size down still further.

4. AUTOMATIC EXPOSURE CONTROL/ AUTOMATIC BRIGHTNESS CONTROL OF THE X-RAY TUBE OUTPUT

The light coming from the II tube is maintained at a level suitable for cine or TV camera use by means of an **automatic exposure control (AEC)** circuit, also known as **automatic brightness control (ABC)** circuit. AEC consists of a *feedback* system that samples the output of the II tube or of the TV camera, and uses the results to regulate the output of the x-ray generator. It thereby makes the average brightness of the II image relatively independent of patient thickness and composition and of the presence of contrast agent.

The average intensity of light at the II tube output screen can be monitored by way of a partially silvered mirror and a photosensor, such as a photomultiplier (Fig. 27–4). (Some workers reserve the name ABC for this particular kind of AEC.) Corrections can be brought about through automatic control of the kVp, the x-ray tube current, or both. If the x-ray tube is being

switched rapidly on and off, as in cinefluorography, relatively small changes may be made instantaneously by altering the duration of the x-ray pulses.

With videofluoroscopy, the AEC circuit usually monitors the average strength of the electrical video signal produced by the TV camera, rather than directly sensing the level of light from the II tube. In digital fluoroscopy, and in at least one conventional fluoro system, the AEC circuit controls not only the technique factors of the x-ray generator, but also the aperture size of a diaphragm at the input of the TV camera, as will be discussed in Chapter 36.

An additional, separate feedback loop, automatic gain control (AGC), used by the TV camera will be described in the next chapter.

5. IMAGE QUALITY AT THE OUTPUT OF THE IMAGE INTENSIFIER TUBE

The modulation transfer functions (MTFs) of the major components of a representative image intensifier tube are shown in Figure 27–5. The total system MTF at any frequency is obtained by multiplying the component MTFs at that frequency (Equa-

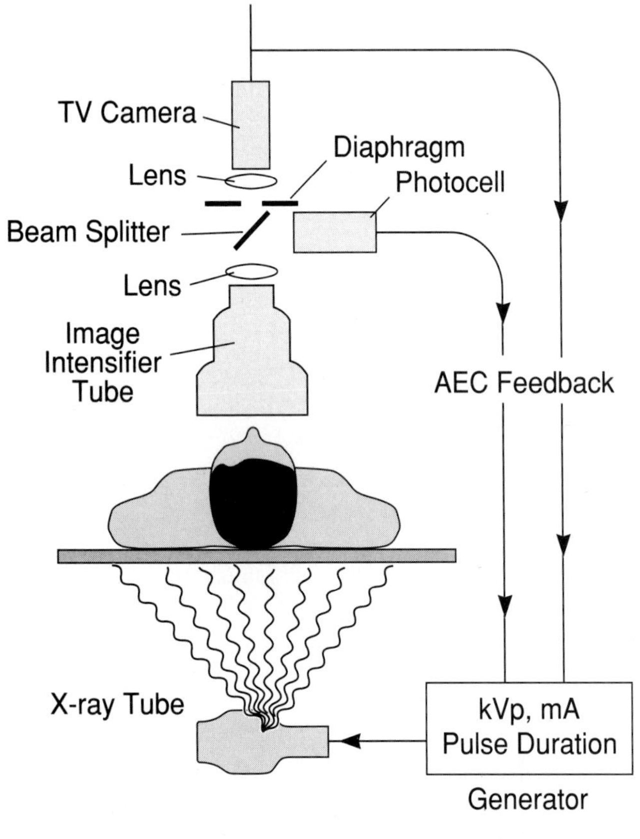

Figure 27–4. Automatic brightness control (ABC)/automatic exposure control (AEC). The intensity of the light emerging from the II tube is monitored by a beam splitter (a partially silvered mirror) and photocell, or from the average video signal of the TV camera. Should the average light level go down, a signal is fed back to the generator, which can increase the x-ray tube mA or kVp or, in cine, the x-ray pulse duration as well.

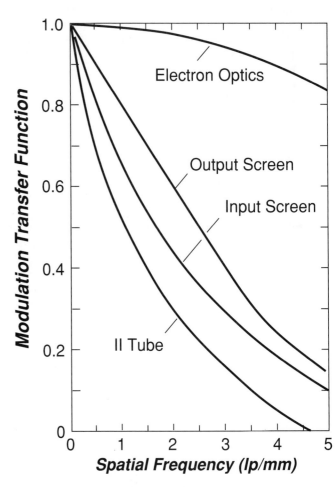

Figure 27–5. The modulation transfer function (MTF) of an II tube, at any spatial frequency, is determined by the separate MTFs of its constituent parts. The weak link in this chain is the input screen.

tion 24.5). The two components that most seriously degrade the system MTF are the input screen and, to a lesser extent, the output screen.

The resolution at the input screen (i.e., for a test bar pattern) and other specifications for a typical modern II tube are reproduced in Table 27–1. As a rule of thumb, a good CsI tube has an overall resolution of up to 4 or 5 lp/mm, but worsens when more minification is being used.

The curvature of the II tube's front faceplate and imperfections in the electron optics and in the associated optical lens systems give rise to pincushion distortion and vignetting. With **pincushion distortion,** the image of a straight object appears curved, primarily because different portions of the image experience slightly different degrees of minification. **Vignetting** is the decrease in brightness that occurs in the outer portions of the image, and is typically less than 25% or so. In a multimode tube, pincushion distortion and vignetting both improve, along with resolution, with less minification.

The capability of an II tube to reproduce subject contrast is commonly parameterized by means of a **contrast ratio**. This has been defined in various ways. Typically, a thick lead disk that covers 10% of the area of the input screen is centered on it, and the II is exposed to a low-intensity, uniform x-ray beam; the contrast ratio is the ratio of the average output brightness away from the disk to that under the disk.

Image contrast is diminished by any retrograde light that escapes in the reverse direction from the output screen and by x-ray photons that manage to pass through the II tube's input screen but interact with its output screen. Contrast is also reduced by **veiling glare**, light that is unintentionally scattered or reflected in an optical system. While it can occur in the camera lenses as well, most fluoroscopic veiling glare arises within the II tube itself.

6. FLUOROSCOPY IS QUANTUM LIMITED: THE QUANTUM SINK IS AT THE INPUT OF THE IMAGE INTENSIFIER TUBE

Quantum mottle is rarely very noticeable in radiography. The situation is quite different, however, in fluorography.

Whether a fluoroscopic system is used with a photospot camera, cine, or TV link, the x-ray exposure at the input screen of the II tube is normally determined by a trade-off: The degree of mottle must be acceptable with regard to low-contrast resolution, but the patient dose must not be unnecessarily high. The eye integrates, or averages, the image that it takes in over a period of about 0.2 second. This means that the exposure rate should be kept down to a level at which the apparent quantum mottle, as averaged over 200 milliseconds, will almost (but not quite) begin to diminish the clinical utility of the images. Fluoroscopy is thus said to be *quantum limited*. The radiation sufficient to produce mottle-free images would have to be much greater, and that would lead to an unacceptably high patient dose.

The maximum possible information content of an image is limited by the number of *quanta of information* it comprises. The numbers of information-bearing quanta (whether they be x-ray photons, visible light photons, accelerating electrons, or discrete points of light) that make up a fluoroscopic image at various stages of its existence are shown in Figure 27–6, assuming 10^6 x-ray photons originally incident on the II tube over each 0.2 second interval. The weakest link in the imaging chain, the

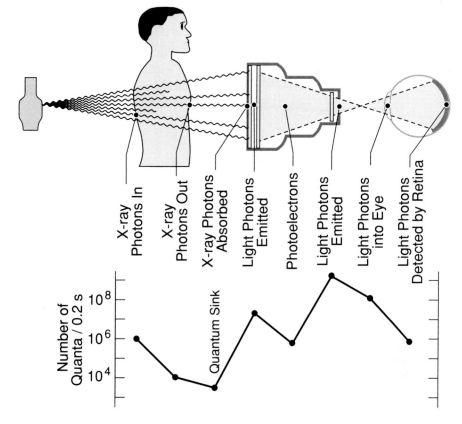

Figure 27–6. The degree of mottle in a fluoroscopic image is determined primarily by the number of individual quanta of information that it comprises. Here, 10^6 50-keV photons are incident on the patient every 0.2 second (the averaging time of the eye). About 10^4 photons emerge from the body as the primary x-ray image, and most of them are absorbed by the input screen of the II tube. Each absorption results in the generation of some 5000 visible light photons, but in the release of only about 150 photoelectrons from the photocathode. Every photoelectron causes 2000 light photons to emerge from the output screen (corresponding to a flux gain of about 60, as seen in Figure 27–2; minification gain is irrelevant, here.) There are further losses in the mirrors that bring the image to the eye and within the lens of the eye, and only a fraction of the light photons that reach the retina are used by it. The absolute low point in the number of information quanta, called the quantum sink, occurs at the II tube input screen. Nothing that takes place beyond that point can increase the amount of real information conveyed by the image (although various forms of image processing may improve its appearance.)

quantum sink, where the absolute number of such quanta is smallest, occurs at the II tube input. This establishes one kind of upper bound on image quality, and it can raised only by means of a greater x-ray exposure rate.

7. THE OUTPUT OF THE IMAGE INTENSIFIER IS COUPLED TO CAMERAS BY MEANS OF THE OPTICAL DISTRIBUTOR: LENSES

The output of an II tube is directed to the photospot, cine, or television camera by switching the orientations of mirrors within an *optical distributor.* (Fig. 1–4B). Some of the mirrors may be only partially silvered, so that at least a small fraction of the light can reach the TV camera at all times. (Highly efficient fiberoptic coupling between the II tube output and the input of the TV camera precludes, at present, the simultaneous direct use of a still or cine camera.) An adjustable optical lens system here can provide some zoom capability.

Light enters all three kinds of camera through lenses. Glass refracts light, and a convex *lens* is a piece of glass carefully sculpted so as to exhibit a remarkable property: All parallel rays of light (e.g., as emitted from a distant point source) converge to a single *focal point,* regardless of the part of the lens through which they pass (Fig. 27–7). The distance from the lens to its focal point is called the **focal length** and denoted *f,* and is a fundamental parameter that characterizes its imaging properties.

> Electromagnetic waves undergo *refraction* when passing from a vacuum or air into a transparent liquid (such as water) or a solid (e.g., glass), or in the opposite direction. The electric field of the wave interacts with the atomic electrons of the matter, because of which the wave travels more slowly. Since its frequency stays the same, at the interface there must result a discontinuous change in wavelength, by Equation 4.4, hence in the direction of propagation. A similar phenomenon occurs when ultrasound passes from one type of tissue into another, as will be described in more detail in Chapter 45.

Light emitted from different points on an object of finite size that is relatively close to the lens ends up at different places on an *image* or *focal plane* (Fig. 27–8), in such a manner that the resultant image is a realistic representation of the object. The image plane does not cut through the focal point of the lens in that case, but rather lies somewhat more distant from it. The distance from the lens to the image plane, S_{image}, is related to the distance from the object to the lens, S_{object}, according to the *thin-lens equation:*

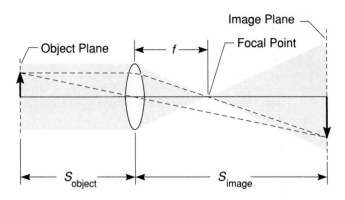

Figure 27–8. By following several rays, one can determine where the image of an object will be in focus and also the size of the image. The distances of the object and of the image from the lens and the focal length of the lens are related through Equations 27.5 and 27.6.

$$1/S_{object} + 1/S_{image} = 1/f \qquad (27.5)$$

The range in S_{object} over which an image remains in good focus is termed the *depth of field,* and the corresponding range in S_{image} is the *depth of focus.*

In Figure 27–8, the particular ray of light that passes through the center of the lens emerges traveling in the same direction as when it entered. This allows us to use similar triangles to determine the **magnification** produced by the lens:

$$\begin{aligned} \text{magnification} &= \text{image size}/\text{object size} \\ &= S_{image}/S_{object} \qquad (27.6) \end{aligned}$$

_____ **EXERCISE 27–2.** _____

A convex lens with a 2-cm focal length is 3 cm from an object. How far on the other side of the lens is the focal plane, and how great is the magnification?

SOLUTION: From Equation 27.5, $1/3 + 1/S_{image} = 1/2$, so the focal plane is 6 cm from the lens. As the magnification is $6/3$, the image will be twice the size of the object.

_____ **EXERCISE 27–3.** _____

A safe way to observe an eclipse of the Sun is to project its image onto a sheet of paper with a magnifying glass. Is the distance from the lens to the paper (imaging plane) equal to the focal length? In other words, can you set S_{object} in Equation 27.5 equal to infinity?

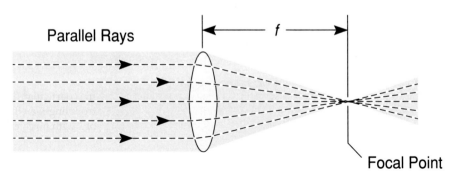

Figure 27–7. Parallel rays of light passing through a convex lens will converge at the focal point.

SOLUTION: No. The Sun may be 93,000,000 miles from Earth, but it is so large that it cannot be considered a point source—the optics are illustrated by Figure 27–8, rather than by Figure 27–7.

The *image* of an object formed by one lens may itself serve as an *object* for a second, following lens, and so on. The focal length of an entire optical system, usually taken to be the distance from the outermost lens to the focal point, is determined by the focal lengths and separations of the constituent lenses. Combination of Equations 27.5 and 27.6 suggests that by manipulating the focal length of an optical system, one can adjust the degree of magnification obtained.

Real lenses and lens systems display various *aberrations* (optical defects). **Chromatic aberration**, in which parts of an image that should be white come out in all the colors of the rainbow, occurs because a lens acts like a prism: There is a small dependence of the refractive index at the air/glass junction on the wavelength of light (Fig. 27–9). *Spherical aberration* refers to the inability of a lens to focus a point source as a perfect point image, even with monochromatic light. Both spherical and chromatic aberrations give rise to small amounts of blurring of optical images.

The larger the diameter of a lens, D, the more light that passes through it, and the greater the amount that will be focused to any point. The size of a lens may be expressed relative to its focal length, f, as its *f-number* (Fig. 27–10):

$$\text{lens } f\text{-number} = \text{focal length}/\text{diameter} \qquad (27.7a)$$

Larger lenses, with smaller f-numbers, pass much light and can expose film quickly, and are said to be fast. Neither the amount of anatomy being viewed nor the magnification of the image is affected by the diameter of the lens. But the resolution, depth of focus, depth of field, and contrast all tend to improve somewhat with smaller lenses, and there is somewhat less aberration, distortion, and vignetting.

The amount of light reaching a television camera or photographic film can be controlled by means of an iris diaphragm, or variable *aperture*, within a system of lenses. The size of an

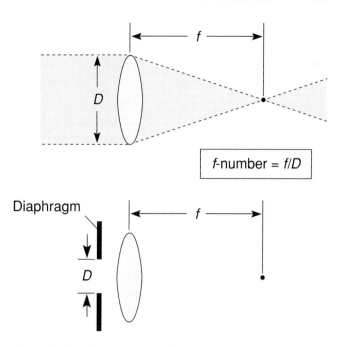

$$\boxed{f\text{-number} = f/D}$$

Figure 27–10. The *f*-number of a lens is defined as the quotient of its focal length and the diameter of the lens. Likewise, the *f*-number of a diaphragm in an optical system is found by dividing the system's focal length by the diameter of the aperture.

aperture may be expressed relative to the focal length of the entire optical system, in terms of f-numbers (Fig. 27–10B):

$$\text{diaphragm } f\text{-number} = \text{focal length}/\text{aperture diameter}$$
$$(27.7b)$$

Commonly used f numbers fall in the *f-stop* series 0.7, 1.0, 1.4, 2.0, 2.8, 4.0, 5.7, 8.0, 11.3, 16.0, . . . ; each f-stop is $\sqrt{2}$ times larger than the one preceding it, so that the *area* of the aperture (and the total amount of light passing through it) is less by a factor of 2. Optical systems are designed so that (as with the f-number of a single lens) neither the amount of anatomy being viewed nor the magnification of the image is affected by the aperture setting. The amount of light let through, however, will be proportional to the area of the aperture. The amount of distortion, the resolution, and the depth of focus and depth of field may worsen somewhat at the lower f-stops.

_____ **EXERCISE 27–4.** _____

The lens on one model of 35-mm (film width) camera has a 40-mm focal length and an f-number of 1.7. What is its diameter?

SOLUTION: By Equation 27.7a, diameter = 40/1.7 = 23.5 mm.

_____ **EXERCISE 27–5.** _____

In a particular fluoroscopic procedure, mottle in the image is troubling. Can the signal-to-noise ratio be improved by a factor of 2 with no change in average brightness?

SOLUTION: Quadrupling the mA of the x-ray tube for fluoroscopy (or the mA-s per frame of film for the cine or pho-

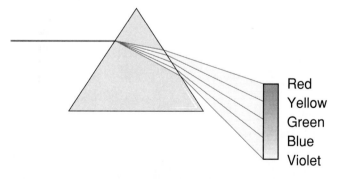

Red
Yellow
Green
Blue
Violet

Figure 27–9. A transparent material such as water or glass may not absorb light strongly, but it affects it in other ways. The electromagnetic interaction leads to a reduction in the speed of light in the medium; that, in turn, is responsible for the phenomenon of refraction. The extent of the interaction and the amount of refraction depend on the energy of the photons constituting the light—hence prisms and the chromatic aberration in a lens.

tospot camera) will bring about the desired improvement in x-ray photon statistics (Equation 18.5) at the input screen of the II. Increasing the *f*-stop of the aperture by two steps (reducing the optical aperture area by a factor of 4) then diminishes the amount of light allowed through (Fig. 27–11), to the previous level.

8. THE PHOTOSPOT CAMERA

A **photospot** or **photofluorographic camera** records the optical image on the output screen of the II as a photograph. A photospot camera uses 105-mm roll film or 100-mm cut film, with a frame rate of up to 6 to 12 images per second. The frame of film is large enough, for many purposes, to be observed directly, without projection or magnification.

Photospot photographs, produced by photospot cameras, are sometimes called "spot films." It is the cause of occasional confusion that the term is sometimes used to refer, as well, to the radiographic images produced on radiographic film by a "spot film device" or "spot film recorder," described below.

9. CINEFLUOROGRAPHY FOR CARDIAC ANGIOGRAPHY

In **cinefluorography,** the output of an II tube is photographed with a modified 35-mm motion picture camera. Over 90% of cinefluorography is performed in cardiac catheterization laboratories (CCLs) for coronary arteriography.

For a cine camera (Fig. 27–12), x-ray pulses are synchronized so as to occur only when the cine film is not moving. The camera contains a pulldown mechanism or arm to advance the film between x-ray pulses, and a pressure plate to hold it immobile during each exposure. There may (or may not) be a ro-

tating shutter that lets light from the II reach the film only while the x-ray tube is firing (or for a brief time thereafter, to capture the phosphor afterglow of the II tube output screen). Exposures (and film advancing) occur at rates of $7\frac{1}{2}$, 15, 30, 60, 120, or more frames per second. Exposure rate of 30 and 60 frames per second are commonly selected, typically for 10- to 20-second runs. To prevent blurring caused by cardiac motion, the individual x-ray pulses are typically 1 to 8 milliseconds in duration.

The usable portion of a frame of 35-mm (total width) film is a rectangle 24 mm wide × 18 mm high (Fig. 27–13). This must record, via a lens and diaphragm system, the circular output screen of an II tube. The effective diameter of the II tube output image, hence the degree of its overlap with a frame of film, can be selected by adjusting the lens system. The apparent size of the anatomic entity being filmed increases as one changes from *exact framing* to *total overframing*, (Fig. 27–14), but the field of view grows smaller. Optimal framing depends on the type of study, the size of the area of interest, and the size of the II tube. The Inter-Society Commission for Heart Disease Resources recommends*, for example, that *mean diameter framing* be used for general cardiac angiography and *maximum horizontal framing* (which gives 15% more magnification) for coronary arteriography. It is necessary also to ensure that the x-ray field covers the region of anatomy being imaged, but not much more. (These same framing considerations apply to the use of photospot and TV cameras, as well.)

To obtain the degree of spatial resolution required in coronary arteriography, the x-ray tube should have a 1.2-mm or smaller focal spot. It must also have an anode heat storage capacity higher than that of a conventional fluoroscopy tube. Constant potential or high-frequency generators with power

---

*M. P. Judkins et al. Report of the Inter-Society Commission for Heart Disease Resources. Circulation 1976; 53, No. 2.)

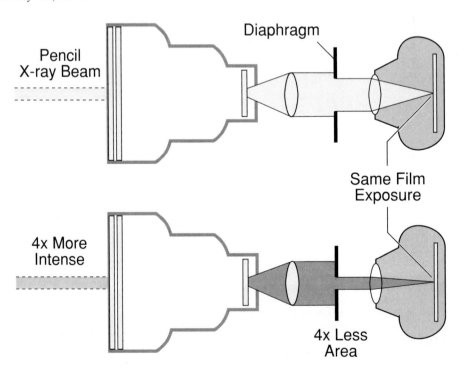

Figure 27–11. The intensity of an x-ray beam is increased by a factor of 4. To obtain about the same optical density of film within a camera, one can reduce the area of the diaphragm by the same factor. See Exercise 27–5.

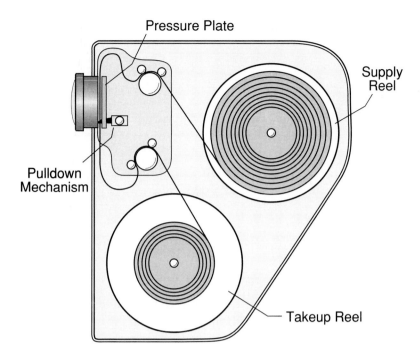

Figure 27–12. Schematic of a 35-mm motion picture camera used for cinefluorography. The pressure plate holds the film immobile during the brief time that the x-ray tube is firing, and the pulldown mechanism then advances it by one frame.

ratings in the 80 to 120 kW range are standard. Short x-ray pulses can be produced either with a grid-controlled x-ray tube or by means of a constant-potential or high-frequency generator with triode or tetrode (a vacuum tube with two grids) switching. Because of the brevity of the pulses, instantaneous tube currents of 500 to 1000 mA are commonly employed. The automatic brightness control circuitry can maintain a constant light output from the II tube by manipulating the x-ray tube potential and current and pulse duration or by varying the iris aperture.

_____ **EXERCISE 27–6.** _____

A 36-cm (14-in.) II tube is being used for cine in the 25-cm (10-in.) mode, with a resolution of 4.0 lp/mm. Will the resolution of an image be limited by the film?

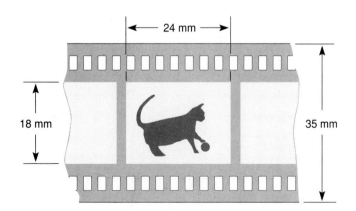

Figure 27–13. The usable area of a frame of 35-mm film is 24 × 18 mm.

SOLUTION: The image on film for maximum horizontal framing, say, will be about 24 mm in dimension. A 4.0 lp/mm pattern at the 250-mm input screen will be shrunk by a factor of 250 mm/24 mm ~ 10 at the output of the II tube, becoming a 40 lp/mm pattern. Film is easily capable of capturing a 40 lp/mm optical image. It is the 4 lp/mm capability at the II tube input that limits the resolving power of the system.

10. PATIENT ENTRANCE SKIN DOSES FOR PHOTOSPOT, CINEFLUOROGRAPHY, AND TV

There is a considerable range in the possible skin (and internal organ) doses delivered to a patient during the various fluoroscopic and fluorographic procedures. The following few examples are typical of what one might find for photospot, cine, and continuous viewing via television; doses to individual patients may differ significantly.

For a photospot camera image, the input to the air kerma _at the II tube_ should be on the order of 0.1×10^{-3} cGy (corresponding to an exposure of 0.1 mR) (Table 27–2). (Note from the table that the necessary II tube input exposure increases by a factor of about 4 if the input screen effective area is cut by a factor of 4; roughly the same amount of light arrives at a point on the film either way.) The table, patient, and grid together attenuate the beam by a factor of 300, say, and this corresponds to an air kerma _at the patient's skin_ of 30×10^{-3} cGy per film. (The air kerma at skin in centigray, the entrance skin exposure (ESE) in roentgens, and the skin dose in centigray are all numerically about the same.) A procedure may require some 30 photospot exposures, with a cumulative skin dose of something like 1 cGy. This is comparable to what a few radiographs of the abdomen might give.

Figure 27–14. Some of the "framing" modes for matching the II tube's output image to film. With exact framing, the entire image from the II barely fits within a frame of film. With total overframing, the entire frame is used to record only the interior portion of the II tube; as a consequence, objects seem larger, but the field of view is more limited. Choice of framing mode depends on the type of study, the size of the region of interest, and the diameter of the II tube input screen.

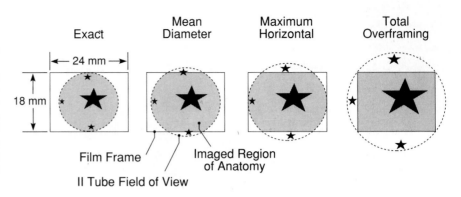

The mottle in a single cine frame can be somewhat worse than what would be considered acceptable in a still image: The eye is a relatively long-persistence receptor, and can integrate (or average out) the mottle over a period of about 200 milliseconds. This is the time it takes to view (and integrate over) five or ten adjacent cine frames. For an acceptable mottle level, an exposure rate of at least 20 μR per frame at the *input of the II tube* is recommended by the Inter-Society Commission for Heart Disease Resources. This might correspond to an air kerma rate *at skin* of, say, 5 to 15×10^{-3} cGy per frame. At 60 frames per second, this leads to a skin dose of the order of 50 cGy/min. For some procedures, the skin dose rate may be higher.

To image with fluoro and television, one might use an 80-kVp beam (2.5 mm Al total filtration) with a continuous 2- or 3-mA tube current and with the x-ray tube target 55 cm from the patient's skin. Under these conditions, the entrance skin air *kerma rate* will be something like 0.05 cGy/s, by Equation 19.1, or about 3 cGy/min. (The air kerma rate at the II tube input screen will be of the order of 1/300th of this, in agreement with the value listed in Table 27–2.) If the patient is viewed for several minutes, and if the tube is not moved over different parts of the body, this can result in a skin dose of tens of centigray. With improperly working equipment, the dose to the patient can be considerably more than that, possibly with high exposures to the medical staff, as well.

> Section 3.3.3 of NCRP Report No. 102 recommends that "The kerma rate, measured in air at the position where the center of the useful beam enters the patient, for all fluoroscopy units including those using TV systems under normal conditions (but including cine procedures), *should* be less than 5 cGy/min (5 rad/min) and *shall* be less than 10 cGy/min (10 rad/min) unless high level control is provided." (The Food and Drug Administration has regulations of a similar nature.) Many modern, properly maintained systems can operate well with significantly less than that amount of radiation.

11. SPOT FILM DEVICES AND FILM CHANGERS BYPASS THE IMAGE INTENSIFIER TUBE

A cine or photospot camera films the output of an II tube. Spot film devices and serial radiographic film changers, on the other hand, produce standard radiographs in the midst of otherwise fluoroscopic procedures.

A **spot film device** can quickly capture, with high resolution, images of a region of interest identified under normal fluoroscopy. A cassette, preloaded with film, is moved from its

TABLE 27–2. AIR KERMA RATES AT THE IMAGE INTENSIFIER TUBE INPUT SCREEN[a]

II Tube Size (cm [in.])	Photoscopy (10^{-3} cGy/fr [~mR/fr])	35-mm Cine (10^{-3} cGy/fr [~mR/fr])	Fluoroscopy (10^{-3} cGy/s [~mR/s])	DSA (10^{-3} cGy/fr [~mR/fr])
		II Input Air Kerma (Exposure) Rate		
30 [12]	0.06	0.006	0.06	0.6
23 [9]	0.1	0.01	0.1	1
15 [6]	0.2	0.02	0.2	2
NCRP	< 0.3	< 0.03		
ISCHDR		> 0.02		
		Resolution (lp/mm)		
	4	4	1.4–2.6	1.4–2.6

[a]Typical values of air kerma rate (per frame or per second) at the input screen of an image intensifier system (for several different screen diameters) needed to produce adequate photospot, 35-mm cine, fluoroscopy, and digital subtraction angiography (DSA) (static mode) images; Recommendations of the NCRP and of the Inter-Society Commission for Heart Disease Resources (ISCHDR) on exposure rates; and spatial resolutions. 1×10^{-3} cGy of air kerma corresponds roughly to 1 mR of exposure.
After Webster JG (ed): Encyclopedia of Medical Devices and Instrumentation *New York: Wiley, 1988 (Table 2, p. 692); and National Council on Radiation Protection and Measurements (NCRP):* Medical X-ray, Electron Beam, and Gamma-ray Protection for Energies up to 50 MeV (Equipment Design, Performance, and Use), *Report No. 102. Bethesda, MD: NCRP, 1989 (Section 3.3.3, and Table B.14).*

lead-shielded "park" or "ready" position and interposed briefly between the patient and the input of the II tube. Simultaneously, the technique factors are automatically switched from those appropriate for fluoro (typically 80 to 100 kVp and 2 to 3 mA, with the small focal spot) to those for conventional radiography (same applied voltage, but a hundredfold or so greater tube current and large focal spot). By collimating down to a small beam area and quickly displacing the cassette a single field width or length between exposures, one can obtain a rapid-fire series of many images on a single sheet of film. Formerly, cassettes were standardized at $9\frac{1}{2} \times 9\frac{1}{2}$ in., but spot film

devices are now available that accept a variety of cassette sizes and image multiformatting.

As a variation on that theme, in vascular angiography the dye-injection catheter is inserted into the patient under normal fluoroscopy. A *serial radiographic film changer* is then positioned in front of the II, to provide large area, high-resolution images. A pair of intensifying screens remains in the beam path and presses snugly against the film during an exposure; the screens are moved apart briefly as a sheet of film is transported into place between them or removed. A film changer may handle 30 frames at rates up to 4 per second.

Chapter 28

Fluoroscopic Television

1. **The Television Link in the Fluoroscopic Imaging Chain**
2. **The Television Monitor**
3. **The Plumbicon Camera**
4. **Storage of an Analog Signal on Videotape**
5. **The Resolution of a Television System Is Determined by the Raster Pattern**
6. **The Bandwidth of the Video Electronic Equipment**
7. **Automatic Gain Control of the TV Link**

It is with the introduction of the television link into the imaging chain that fluoroscopy reaches its full potential. Television makes possible the direct, real-time observation of a radiologic procedure on monitors inside the radiologic suite or even at great distances. It allows storage on videotape, with the capability of immediate playback. And it serves as an electronic conduit into the computer, allowing the combination of dynamic observation capability with digital image processing.

The use of television results in a further degradation of image quality, in addition to that caused by the image intensifier, but in many situations the price is small compared with the benefits.

1. THE TELEVISION LINK IN THE FLUOROSCOPIC IMAGING CHAIN

A television system consists typically of four components: a *camera* and camera control unit for image acquisition, a *channel* of transmission, *monitors* for image display, and a *videotape* or other image storage device (Fig. 28–1). There are two kinds of channels in common use: an electrical or fiberoptic *cable*, for close-circuit television (CCTV), or a transmitter, antennas (and perhaps an Earth orbital satellite), and receiver combination for *wireless* transmission.

In fluoroscopy, a *television camera* can view the output of the image intensifier (II) through a system of optical lenses, and thereby transform the image into an electronic **video signal**. The optical image from the II tube is focused onto a photosensitive target within the evacuated camera tube. A narrow beam of electrons, tracing out a raster pattern, rapidly and repeatedly scans the entire surface of this target (Fig. 28–2). The magnitude of the resultant video signal is, at any instant, proportional to the amount of light reaching the particular point on the target where the electron beam then happens to be striking. As the beam scans the various regions of the target, which are exposed to different levels of illumination, the video signal varies accordingly. A two-dimensional optical image is thereby transformed into a voltage signal that depends on a single variable, time.

The image is reconstructed at the TV *monitor* by, in essence, reversing the process. An electron beam within a cathode ray tube (CRT) scans its phosphorescent front screen, following the same raster pattern as is being used by the electron

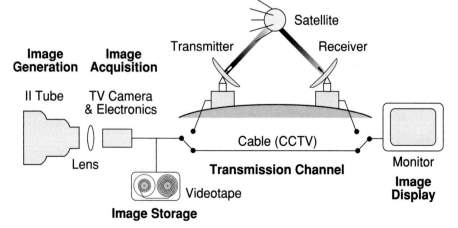

Figure 28–1. A television system (here being used to observe the output of an image intensifier [II] tube) consists of an image acquisition system, a transmission channel, and components for image display and storage. It may be advantageous to digitize the image information before transmission.

TV Camera

TV Monitor

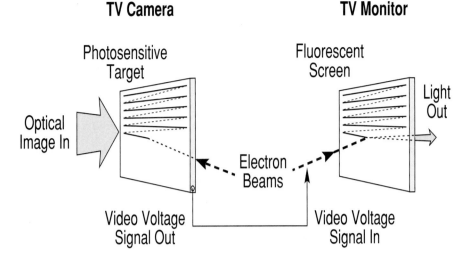

Figure 28–2. A TV camera views an optical image as being composed of a set of lines each of varying brightness, temporarily engraved on a photosensitive target. An electron beam in the camera scans these lines in a well-defined raster pattern; as the beam strikes any point on the target, it generates a video signal, the amplitude of which is proportional to the amount of illumination there. Simultaneously, and in a carefully synchronized fashion, the electron beam in the display monitor traces out the same raster pattern on a fluorescent screen. The number of electrons in the beam at any instant and the brightness of the resulting point of light are proportional to the amplitude of the incoming video signal.

beam of the camera. At the same time, the video signal transmitted from the camera and detected by the receiver is amplified and applied to the grid of the CRT; it thereby controls the brightness of the point of light produced, at that instant, on the monitor screen. The video signal voltage input, which varies with time, is thus translated back into a two-dimensional spatial pattern of brightness. Precisely timed voltage pulses generated by the camera control unit are used to ensure that the electron beam scanning raster patterns of the camera and of the display monitor are perfectly *synchronized.*

In summary, when the *camera's* electron beam encounters a brightly illuminated spot on its photosensitive surface, it tells the electron beam in the *monitor's* CRT to paint a bright spot at the corresponding point on the display screen. It is in this fashion that an optical image is captured by a TV camera, codified as a video voltage signal, and transformed back into a visual pattern at the display.

2. THE TELEVISION MONITOR

We shall begin our more detailed study of television with the monitor, which is a bit easier to describe than the camera.

The heart of a monitor is a specialized CRT (Fig. 28–3) (see

Chapter 8, Section 10). A tightly focused beam of electrons is accelerated through 20 to 25 kV, and strikes the phosphor of the viewing screen to create a point of light. The beam is deflected in a raster pattern by means of time-varying magnetic fields produced by the deflection coils. The point of light sweeps in a nearly (but not exactly) horizontal line across the screen, then snaps back (with the beam briefly **blanked,** or turned off), ready to begin the next lower line. Meanwhile, the incoming video signal controls the voltage on the control grid, hence the number of electrons in the electron beam, and thus the instantaneous brightness of the point of light on the phosphorescent screen. (The video signal also contains **synchronization pulses,** to ensure proper timing of the beam scanning process.) A picture is created out of closely spaced, parallel traces of light of varying intensity, somewhat like an engraving.

Color monitors are more complicated variations on this theme. Rather than being uniformly coated with fluorescent material that emits white light, the screen of a color monitor is covered with precisely situated triads of dots of three different kinds of phosphor that emit, respectively, red, yellow, and blue light. The dots are separated by less than a half millimeter, but the electron beam (or beams; some monitors use three) can be manipulated with sufficient fineness to excite each of the indi-

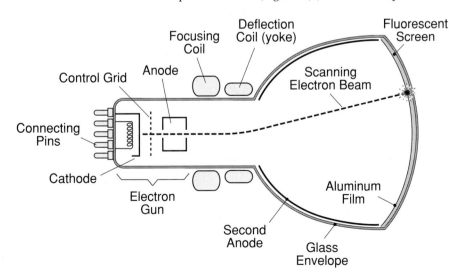

Figure 28–3. Schematic of a television monitor tube. An electron beam is focused and swept by means of magnetic fields produced by coils, and strikes a fluorescent display screen. (A thin layer of aluminum reflects any retrograde light toward the viewer and provides an escape route for the beam's electrons.) The instantaneous current in the beam and the brightness of the spot of light it produces are determined by the *video signal* voltage applied to the control grid.

vidual dots in a region by the amounts needed to produce the correct color and intensity.

_____ **EXERCISE 28–1.** _____

Does a TV monitor produce dangerous amounts of x-ray radiation?

SOLUTION: Not really. Because of the moderate atomic number of the phosphor and glass and the low energy of the electrons, bremsstrahlung radiation is produced at the screen with low efficiency. Nearly all the x-ray photons that are created, moreover, are absorbed by the glass.

_____ **EXERCISE 28–2.** _____

The width-to-height ratio of the TV screen was originally chosen to match the frames in 35-mm (wide) motion picture film. The usable area of a frame of cine film is 24 × 18 mm. What are the dimensions of a 25-in. (diagonal) screen?

SOLUTION: By the Pythagorean theorem, the diagonal of the usable area of film is $\sqrt{(18^2 + 24^2)} = 30$ mm. Scaling everything up by a factor of 25 in./30 mm, the TV screen is roughly 20 × 15 in.

Several different raster pattern conventions have been adopted in different parts of the World. With commercial television in the Americas and Japan, 30 complete pictures, or **frames,** are transmitted per second, each consisting of 525 parallel lines. The simple approach would be to draw the lines the way you read a book, starting at the top left corner and ending at the bottom right 1/30th second later. This is adequate to give the impression of *smooth motion*, but not rapid enough to completely eliminate *flicker*, or fluctuations in overall brightness, which can cause visual fatigue. Therefore, each frame is actually created out of two *interlaced* 262.5-line **fields.** The first field of a frame is drawn in 1/60th second, and the second field is then created out of lines laid down midway between the lines of the first (Fig. 28–4). The second field is displaced downward from the first by half the separation of neighboring lines in either field. The eye perceives the result as a nonflickering, 525-line image.

The commercial raster is found in many fluoroscopic television systems. Other scanning patterns (in particular, those used with high definition television [HDTV] and with digital imaging systems) employ more horizontal lines per frame, and may do away with interlacing. Whatever the method, of course, there must be compatibility between camera and monitor.

3. THE PLUMBICON CAMERA

Three kinds of vacuum tube cameras have been employed in broadcast television: the image-orthicon, the orthicon, and the vidicon. A particular kind of vidicon, known as the *plumbicon,* is widely used in fluoroscopy. It is small, relatively simple in construction and inexpensive, easy to operate, sensitive, and quicker to respond than other vidicons, so that there is less apparent "lag" in rapidly changing images.

The plumbicon of Figure 28–5 is viewing an object off to the left. A system of lenses projects an optical image through the front glass faceplate (window) onto the signal plate and target, which together transform the image into a spatial pattern of electric charges on the interior surface of the target. A

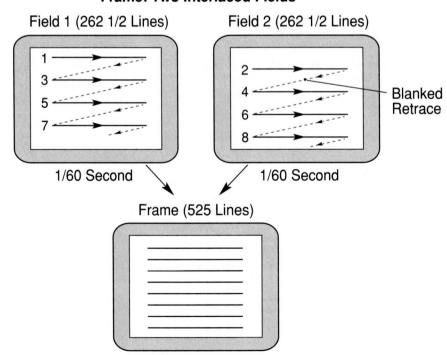

Figure 28–4. Raster pattern employed in commercial television in the United States, and normally for analog (nondigital) fluoroscopy, to yield a frame composed of two interlacing fields. A field consists of $262\frac{1}{2}$ lines and is displayed in 1/60th second. A new 525-line frame is thus produced every 1/30th second.

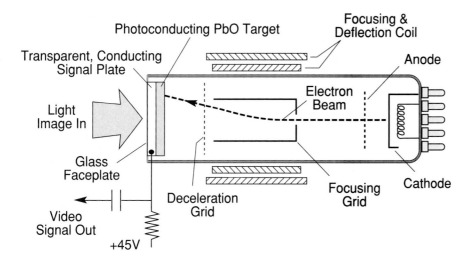

Figure 28–5. Schematic of a plumbicon TV camera tube. A constant-current electron beam, coming from the right, is focused to a point and swept in the standardized raster pattern by coils outside the tube. Light, incident from the left, passes through the transparent but electrically conducting signal plate and falls on the photoconducting lead oxide (PbO) target. The time dependence of the current that flows off the signal plate as video signal, as the beam follows its path, depends on the pattern of light illuminating the target.

scanning electron beam reads this distribution of charge, transforming it into a continuously varying electrical *video signal* output.

The *signal plate* is a thin layer of transparent but conducting tin oxide covering the interior surface of the glass faceplate. The *target* is a layer of semiconducting lead oxide (PbO), deposited directly on the interior surface of the signal plate.

The target, typically 1 to 4 cm in diameter, may be thought of as comprising a million or so tiny but separate capacitor–resistor circuits (Fig. 28–6A), each associated with a different point on the camera faceplate and corresponding to a different picture element (pixel) of any image being viewed. Let us restrict our attention to a single small region of the target, and to a single such capacitor–resistor combination. One plate of the "capacitor" is the conducting signal plate of the tube. The other side of the "capacitor" (i.e., a small portion of the interior surface of the target) will be charged up by the electron beam as it sweeps by. The voltages on the anode, the signal plate, and the various grids are so arranged that the electrons arrive at the target with only 45 eV of kinetic energy. The passing beam will therefore charge up the "capacitor" until there is a 45-V drop across it.

If the resistance of the "resistor" happens to be high, then the stored surface charge will leak off the "capacitor" very slowly (Figure 28–6B). (The time required for this discharge to occur [Equation 8.5] is proportional to the local "resistance.") So when the beam sweeps by the next time, 1/30th second later, almost no electrons will be required to charge it up again, and in the process of recharging it, almost none will flow off of the signal plate as video signal (Fig. 28–6A). If the resistance is low, on the other hand, so that the "capacitor" can discharge quickly, there will be a correspondingly large signal plate current when the electron beam sweeps by the second time and recharges it. So what determines whether the resistance in Figure 28–6A is high or low?

The lead oxide target* is a photoconductor: It is highly resistive in the dark, but becomes partially conducting when exposed to light, and its conductivity increases with the light intensity. For a point on the vidicon target that is not illuminated, the resistance of the "resistor" in Figure 28–6A is high, and almost no signal plate current will flow when the electron beam sweeps by. Where the target is well lit, however,

the video signal current resulting from the passage of the electron beam is relatively large. In this fashion, the variation of signal plate current over *time*, as the electron beam follows its raster path, provides a direct measure of the variation of signal plate illumination in two-dimensional *space*.

Note that the "capacitor" at a point on the target contin-

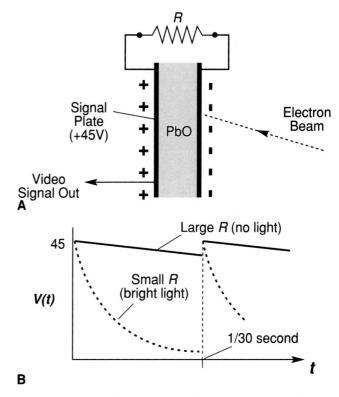

Figure 28–6. Generation of the video signal by the plumbicon. **A.** The lead oxide target may be thought of as consisting of hundreds of thousands of independent capacitor–resistor combinations. The "resistor" is a photoconductor, however, and its resistance, *R*, decreases when it is exposed to light. **B.** The rate at which a "capacitor" is discharged increases with the amount of illumination of its partner photoconductor. Bright light, hence low resistance, cause rapid discharge of the "capacitor." The amount of current required to charge up the "capacitor" again, when the electron beam next sweeps by 1/30th second later, is read out as the video signal.

---

*More precisely, the PbO layer acts as a reverse-biased semiconductor P-I-N diode, but explaining that would take us far afield.

ues to discharge the whole time over which that part of the target is illuminated. The signal plate current generated when the electron beam sweeps by is thus determined by the cumulative amount of charge lost (i.e., by the time integral of the photoconductivity) between consecutive passages of the beam, and not just by the instantaneous value of the photoconductivity (variations in which are much smaller, and harder to measure).

Finally, to summarize the preceding, the video signal occurring when the electron beam happens to strike a point on the target surface is determined by the local resistance, and that, in turn, is affected by the amount of illumination.

Recently, TV cameras built around solid state **charge coupled devices (CCDs)** have been developed. Doubtless they (or their solid state replacements) will soon find extensive use in fluoroscopy.

4. STORAGE OF AN ANALOG SIGNAL ON VIDEOTAPE

The electronic video signal generated by a TV camera and fed into a TV monitor can, at the same time, be recorded on videotape.

As noted in Chapter 4, Section 4, electric currents produce magnetic fields. The orbital and spin motions of the electrons in an atom or molecule, in particular, may produce such fields. In most substances, these individual atomic magnetic fields point in all different directions, and average to zero in bulk material. In a **ferromagnetic** substance, by contrast, interatomic forces cause the magnetic fields of a group of atoms to end up aligned parallel to one another. The fields add together, with the result that a piece of ferromagnetic material produces its own non-vanishing net magnetic field; that is, it is a *permanent* magnet.

Videotape is a thin ribbon of plastic coated with a fine powder of iron oxide or a similar ferromagnetic material. A single speck of iron oxide on the videotape surface is a tiny permanent magnet. The magnitude of its field normally does not change (nor does the physical alignment of the particle itself), but the orientation of the field can be affected relatively easily: The field of the iron oxide particle will line up nearly along any strong, externally applied magnetic field (Fig. 28–7) and remain frozen in that orientation. Until, that is, another, sufficiently strong external magnetic field realigns it.

Before videotape is written on, the permanent magnetic fields of the individual particles point in random directions. Anywhere along the tape, the local composite magnetic field that the separate particles together produce, their net **magnetization**, is zero. But sending a signal to the *write head* of a videotape machine changes that. The write head is an electromagnet that can produce a strong magnetic field, in the vicinity of the tape, in either of two opposite directions (Fig. 28–8). The video signal from the TV camera, after being amplified, is translated by the write head into a corresponding time-varying magnetic field. As the tape moves by, this causes the "permanent" fields of some of the magnetic particles to realign. The stronger the instantaneous field from the write head, the greater the number of particles in that portion of videotape affected, and the greater their local net magnetization. The time

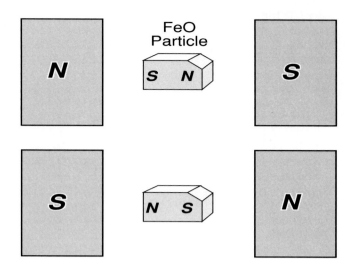

Figure 28–7. The *orientation* of the magnetic field within a small ferromagnetic particle, such as iron oxide, can be set by applying a sufficiently strong external magnetic field. Only the alignment of the magnetic field of the particle is affected, not the orientation of the particle itself.

dependence of the video signal is thus encoded as smooth variations in the amount and direction of the magnetization along the tape.

> A continuously varying voltage is known as an **analog** signal. As will be seen in Chapter 35, an analog signal can be digitized, and transformed into binary digital code, in which the voltage is either high or low, positive or negative, and so on, but nothing inbetween. When such a **digital** signal is stored on videotape, there are only two levels or directions of magnetization, rather than a continuum.

Conversely, information recorded on tape can be extracted with a *read head*. As the tape moves by, its varying magnetization induces a corresponding voltage in a pickup coil of wire (see Chapter 4, Section 5). This voltage is amplified, and can serve as the input to a TV monitor.

The electromagnet head of the videotape machine of Figure 28–9, which serves for both read and write purposes, revolves rapidly, on a horizontal plane, within a drum. Tape moves past the drum at 25 cm per second, typically, and its path is canted at a slight angle from the horizontal. As the electromagnet passes, it writes (or reads) closely spaced, parallel lines of magnetization. By recording on the diagonal this way, about 100 cm of lines of magnetization can be laid down per centimeter of tape length. The tape speed, rate of electromagnet rotation, and angle of tilt are chosen to optimize the trade-off between the quality of signal recorded and the duration of play.

Videotape can be played back immediately, and is reusable (although the quality of a recorded analog signal may deteriorate over time). But the image can be no better than that of the TV system feeding it. And without computer-based image enhancement, that will be considerably worse than what can be obtained with cinefluorography.

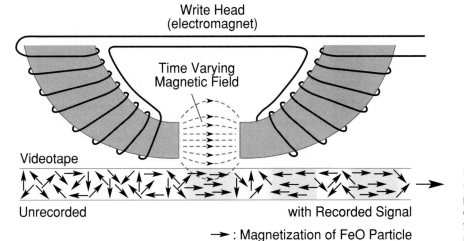

Write Head
(electromagnet)

Time Varying
Magnetic Field

Videotape

Unrecorded

with Recorded Signal

➔ : Magnetization of FeO Particle

Figure 28–8. The write head of a videotape machine is an electromagnet. As videotape passes by, the instantaneous magnetic field produced by the head affects the alignment of the fields of the particles in the tape and the local net magnetization.

5. THE RESOLUTION OF A TELEVISION SYSTEM IS DETERMINED BY THE RASTER PATTERN

Introducing television into the fluorescent imaging chain allows the performance of real-time procedures under direct radiologic observation, and lays the groundwork for both electronic communications and computer processing. But it involves a loss of image quality. Indeed, when a system includes television, the overall resolution is determined primarily by the electron beam scanning pattern.

The standard frame pattern commonly used in the United States consists of 525 lines. Of these, about 35 lines are blanked out and lost as the beam returns (twice per frame) from the bottom of the screen to the top. Resolution in the vertical direction is then limited by the fact that a single image is constructed out of the remaining 490 active lines, each of which is 1/490th of the image in width.

Four hundred ninety lines, each of which can be either dark or light, means at most 245 line pairs. One might suspect that, with 245 line pairs, it should be possible to faithfully capture an attribute of an object that changes in the vertical direction at a spatial frequency of less than 245 cycles (or line pairs) per image. A real television system is capable of providing a vertical resolution of only about 70% of that, or 170 lp/image. The ratio of the attainable resolution to the actual number of active line pairs per image is known as the **Kell factor.** With standard television,

$$\text{Kell factor} = (170 \text{ active lp/image})/(245 \text{ lp/image}) = 0.7 \quad (28.1)$$

The vertical modulation transfer function (MTF) correspondingly falls off rapidly in the region of 170 lp/image.

Suppose that an object that just fills the input screen of an image intensifier tube is D_{object} millimeters in diameter. If the image is represented and reconstructed out of 170 lp, the vertical resolution (in mm) will be (Fig. 28–10A),

$$\text{resolution (mm)} = (D_{object} \text{ mm})/170 \quad (28.2a)$$

Or, expressing this in line pairs per millimeter,

$$\text{resolution (lp/mm)} = (170 \text{ lp})/(D_{object} \text{ mm}) \quad (28.2b)$$

EXERCISE 28–3.

What resolution is achievable with a 36-cm (14-in.) II tube and a 525 line/frame TV raster pattern? What if the II tube is used in the 23 cm (9-in.) mode?

SOLUTION: A 360-mm object becomes a 170-lp image. The resolution is thus 170 lp/360 mm ~ 0.5 lp/mm. If the II tube is used in the 23-cm mode, the resolution improves somewhat, to 0.7 lp/mm.

Figure 28–10B and Exercise 28–3 demonstrate that one can improve resolution (at least, as affected by the TV link) by decreasing the minification mode of the II tube. A smaller part of

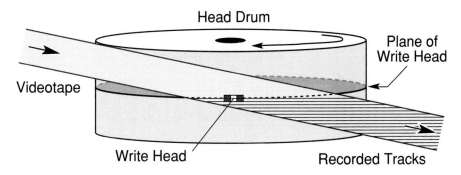

Head Drum

Plane of
Write Head

Videotape

Write Head

Recorded Tracks

Figure 28–9. High-density information storage is achieved by rotating the write head rapidly in a plane, within the head drum, and canting the tape by a few degrees relative to the plane of head rotation.

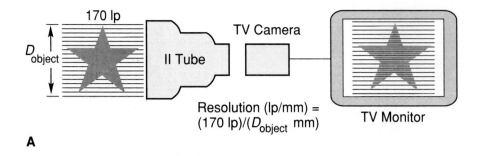

A

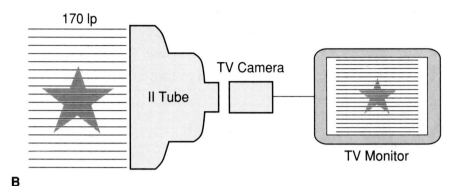

Figure 28–10. The vertical resolution of the television image of an object depends on the field of view. **A.** The resolution of a television image will be optimal if all 170 lp are used in its construction. **B.** With more minification, and a smaller image of the object of interest, the resolution will decrease.

B

the body is examined (and its apparent size is increased), but the number of scan lines remains the same. Hence better resolution. One can achieve the same effect with the *zoom* feature of the lens system at the input of the TV camera, enlarging the image after it has left the II tube but before it is scanned in the raster pattern.

Resolution in the *horizontal* direction is closely tied to the ability of the system to reproduce an abrupt change in the level of brightness along a scan line. Television systems are normally designed so that the horizontal resolution will be comparable to the vertical, which is to say something near 262.5 (= 525 vertical lines/2) line pairs per horizontal sweep.

The modulation transfer functions of a typical II tube, the television link, and a complete fluoroscopy/TV system are shown in Figure 28–11. The resolution of the II alone, or as captured on cine film, lies in the region of 4 lp/mm. That of an imaging system that includes TV is of the order of 1 lp/mm for a 525-line video system. This is adequate for many but not all diagnostic purposes.

6. THE BANDWIDTH OF THE VIDEO ELECTRONIC EQUIPMENT

The resolution requirements of television have implications for the **bandwidth** of the electronic equipment that processes the video signal.

The pattern of brightness along any horizontal sweep line can be Fourier represented as a sum that contains components with frequencies between 0 and 262.5 cycles per sweep. But the number of lines transmitted each second is (525 lines/frame)(30 frames/) = 15,750 lines/s. The amplifiers and other signal processing equipment must therefore be able to handle video signals with frequencies of a few kilohertz up to (262.5 cycles/line)(15,750 lines/s) = 4.1 MHz. The equipment

used for fluoroscopic TV is thus typically about 5 MHz in bandwidth, and is able to accommodate all electronic signals in the range 0 to 5 MHz. When resolution in each dimension is twice as great as that of current commercial TV, as is the case with some modern digital imaging systems and with high-def-

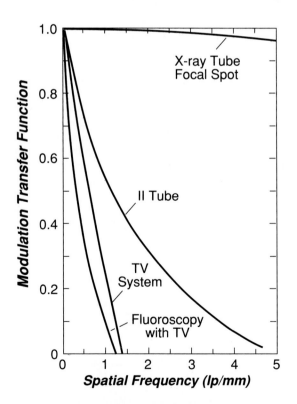

Figure 28–11. The modulation transfer function of a fluoroscopic system with a television link is limited primarily by the TV raster pattern.

inition television, a channel nearly 20 MHz or more wide would be required*. Sound information audible by humans, by comparison, can be adequately carried by a telephone channel less than 4,000 Hz wide.

7. AUTOMATIC GAIN CONTROL OF THE TV LINK

Automatic brightness control (ABC) for fluoroscopy was discussed in Chapter 27, Section 4. The television link employs an additional means, *automatic gain control (AGC)*, of stabilizing image brightness.

ABC is a *negative feedback circuit* that monitors either the current of photoelectrons through an II tube or the average

---

*Commercial HDTV systems in the United States will be required by the Federal Communications Commission (FCC) to stay within the current 5-MHz video bandwidth. Some will achieve this, at considerable cost and complexity, through digital image compression techniques (see Chapter 35, Section 10).

light coming out of it, and uses that signal to control the intensity of the beam produced by the x-ray tube. (As with a thermostat, negative feedback control tends to maintain something at a constant value.) AGC works further along the imaging chain. It follows the average strength of the video signal coming out of the TV camera over time, and adjusts the *gain* of the video signal amplifiers in the camera control unit to compensate for any changes. AGC is intended to act rapidly, to maintain a constant average monitor brightness for a constant radiation exposure level; ABC responds (typically more slowly) to changes in the intensity of x-rays emerging from the patient by varying the output of the x-ray tube.

There is a potential danger with an AGC system. Suppose the sensitivity of the light sensor in the ABC circuit happens to diminish somewhat over time. The ABC feedback circuit would increase the output of the x-ray tube to compensate. The brightness of the II tube would increase. But the TV system's AGC would simply reduce the overall level of brightness at the monitor, and the problem could go unnoticed. This kind of difficulty can be prevented by means of careful periodic quality assurance checks.

Chapter 29

Screen–Film and Fluoroscopic Quality Assurance and Radiation Safety

1. Image Quality Assurance and Radiation Safety Programs
2. Image Quality Assurance for Conventional Radiography: Does Your X-ray Machine Do What It Is Supposed to?
3. The Image Intensifier and Television System in Fluoroscopy
4. A Radiation Safety Program Protects the Patient, the Staff, and the Public
5. The Two Triads of Radiation Safety: Justification–Optimization–Limitation and Time–Distance–Shielding
6. Regulations on Emissions from Sources and on Doses to Individuals
7. Design of Shielding for an Imaging Suite
8. Surveying Imaging Equipment and Suites and Monitoring the Staff
Appendix 29–1. An Aside on Purchasing Equipment

A radiologic image quality assurance or quality control program is designed to ensure that equipment and procedures generate diagnostically useful images and pose little risk to the patient. A radiation safety program serves to keep radiation doses to medical staff and to the general public below certain specified *limiting values* and, beyond that, at levels that are *as low as reasonably achievable* (*ALARA*). The two kinds of programs will naturally overlap to some extent.

This chapter describes image quality assurance and radiation safety programs for a conventional radiography unit and additional requirements for fluoroscopic systems. Subsequent chapters on the other imaging modalities will contain brief sections on quality assurance that build on what is presented here.

1. IMAGE QUALITY ASSURANCE AND RADIATION SAFETY PROGRAMS

A comprehensive **radiologic quality assurance** (*QA*) or *quality control* (*QC*) program consists of (1) an **image quality assurance** program to maximize the likelihood of obtaining correct diagnoses; (2) a **radiation safety** program for minimizing the exposure of patients to nonproductive irradiation (and to other sources of risk in hazardous procedures) and for protecting medical staff and members of the general public from ionizing radiation; and (3) **administrative procedures** for keeping track of films and records, educating personnel, maintaining and upgrading equipment on a regular basis, minimizing patient discomfort, inconvenience, and cost, and other activities. Obviously there will be some degree of overlap among these programs.

This chapter is concerned with those aspects of such a gen-

eral QA program that pertain to image quality per se and to the doses of radiation delivered to people. It provides an outline and a brief overview of some of the more important image quality and radiation safety issues that a QA program should cover. It does *not* purport to serve as a blueprint for implementation of a comprehensive QA program in a planned or operating clinical facility.

The image quality assurance and radiation safety programs of a radiology department or other user of radiologic equipment should be designed by, and be under the immediate supervision of, a **qualified medical physicist**.* This medical physicist should be either a member of staff on-site or under long-term contract as a regular consultant, so that he or she can become intimately familiar with the equipment and the specific objectives of the facility, and thus be able to deal most effectively with its unique technical problems.

More extensive and detailed plans for radiographic and radiation safety QA programs are provided by a number of sources, most notably in publications of the American Association of Physicists in Medicine (AAPM), the American College of Medical Physics (ACMP), the American College of Radiology (ACR), the Center for Devices and Radiologic Health (CDRH; formerly the Bureau of Radiologic Health) of the Food and Drug Administration (FDA), the Conference of Radiation Control Program Directors (CRCPD), the International Commission on Radiological Protection (ICRP), the Joint Commis-

---

*Typical qualifications include a principal education in physics, radiologic physics, or engineering; either a masters degree plus 4 years of practical clinical experience or a doctorate plus 3 years of experience; and certification (or eligibility for certification) by the American Board of Radiology or the American Board of Medical Physics in any one or more of the subfields of medical physics.

sion on Accreditation of Healthcare Organizations (JCAHO), the National Council on Radiation Protection and Measurements (NCRP), the National Electrical Manufacturers Association (NEMA), the United States Nuclear Regulatory Commission (NRC), and the radiation safety branch of your own state's department of health.

Much of the content of this chapter, and of the QA sections of later chapters, is distilled from the sources in Table 29–1. Those documents include descriptions of the appropriate image QA and radiation safety checks, along with suggested schedules and performance criteria, for the major imaging modalities. Some of the tests should be performed at least once a year, and others as often as daily. The results of the more quantitative tests should fall within the ranges of values specified by the professional bodies or required by law.

There should be in place an *administrative mechanism* whereby QA procedures are carried out on a planned, systematic, and continuous basis. When problems are identified, the QA program should ensure that individuals with clearly assigned responsibility and authority undertake the appropriate remedial actions in a timely fashion. The results of *routine tests* and the reports of *changes or repairs* should be presented clearly and simply for final approval by the person with ultimate responsibility. As some problems can be detected most readily through slow drifts in measured parameters, it may be helpful to display quantitative results over time in graphic form. The use of a computer for test scheduling, data analysis, and record keeping can be a significant aid in keeping a comprehensive and integrated QA and radiation safety program running smoothly.

This all may sound both obvious and overly formal, but in the absence of such structured activity, important things don't get done. That can lead, in turn, to the use of unsafe procedures and the production of poor-quality images.

2. IMAGE QUALITY ASSURANCE FOR CONVENTIONAL RADIOGRAPHY: DOES YOUR X-RAY MACHINE DO WHAT IT IS SUPPOSED TO?

Do the various switch settings and meter readings on the console of your radiographic x-ray machine accurately determine and reflect the output of its generator and tube? Has the focal spot of the tube grown larger with use and age, with a resulting loss in resolution? Is the patient skin dose as low as it could and should be? An *image QA program* can ensure that these and a number of related questions all have the desired answers.

First, in addition to normal maintenance (repairing or replacing things when they are damaged or stop working), an entire system should be inspected periodically to confirm that everything is mechanically stable and electrically secure: Nuts are tight and nothing moves that shouldn't, and things that should move do; added beam filters are in place; light bulbs, motors, control switches, dead-man and safety interlock switches function correctly; high-voltage electric cables appear to be in good condition and ground wires are properly connected. Also, radiographic technique charts should be accessible (posted on the units or in the rooms), complete, and up to date.

It is prudent to ensure that the x-ray *tube protector circuit*, which prevents exposures with combinations of technique factors that could damage the tube, and the *tube heat sensor* are working properly (but don't fry the tube in the process).

Several important tests monitor the effectiveness of the control over the output of the tube–generator combination. If you shoot two films with the same technique settings, for example, the actual exposures should be very nearly the same. This *reproducibility* of exposures is tested by means of a procedure such as the following: Activate the x-ray tube and measure the air kerma, K_1, or exposure with an ionization chamber; change all the technique settings (and perhaps make another exposure), then return the controls to their original setting and take a second reading, K_2; repeat these steps and record K_3; finally, calculate the reproducibility, which might be defined simply as

$$\text{reproducibility} = (K_{\max} - K_{\min})/K_{\text{av}} \qquad (29.1)$$

where $K_{\max}$ and $K_{\min}$ are the largest and smallest of the three (or more) readings, respectively, and K_{av} is their average. (Alternatively, reproducibility could be reported in terms of the coefficient of variation, which is the standard deviation divided by the mean.) The test should be repeated with several different sets of technique factors, and the reproducibility should be less than 5% or 10% for all of them.

___ **EXERCISE 29–1.** ___

With a certain mA, kVp, and timer setting, a series of air kerma measurements yielded readings of 16.3, 16.4, 16.6, and 17.1 × 10^{-3} cGy, in that order. Is the reproducibility acceptable?

SOLUTION: By Equation 29.1, the reproducibility is (17.1 − 16.3)/16.6 = 4.9%. This closeness to the 5% action level, to-

TABLE 29–1. SOME SOURCES OF PROTOCOLS AND OTHER INFORMATION PERTAINING TO RADIOLOGIC IMAGING AND RADIATION SAFETY QUALITY ASSURANCE

AAPM	Report No. 25: Protocols for the Radiation Safety Surveys of Diagnostic Radiological Equipment (1988)
ACMP	Report No. 1: Radiation Control and Quality Assurance Surveys—Diagnostic Radiology. A Suggested Protocol (1986)
CRCPD	Suggested State Regulations for the Control of Radiation (SSRCR) (Obtain current regulations from your own state's department of health.)
FDA	Regulations published in the *Federal Register* and compiled in the Code of Federal Regulations (CFR) at 21 CFR 1000 and 21 CFR 1020 (1989)
ICRP	Publication 57: Radiological Protection of the Worker in Medicine and Dentistry (contains a separate report entitled Summary of the Current ICRP Principles for Protection of the Patient in Diagnostic Radiology) (1989)
NCRP	Report No. 49: Structural Shielding Design and Evaluation for Medical Use of X-Rays and Gamma Rays of Energies up to 10 MeV (1976)
NCRP	Report No. 99: Quality Assurance for Diagnostic Imaging Equipment (1988)
NCRP	Report No. 102: Medical X-ray, Electron Beam, and Gamma-Ray Protection for Energies up to 50 MeV (Equipment Design, Performance, and Use) (1989)
NCRP	Report No. 105: Radiation Protection for Medical and Allied Health personnel (1989)
NRC	Regulations at 10 CFR 20 (1991)

gether with the pattern of steadily climbing readings, suggests the need for closer study.

As you switch the tube current of your x-ray machine from the 100-mA station to 200 mA, with the timer setting unchanged, the exposure of a film should double. A test of *linearity* can confirm that the output rate of the system is proportional to the mA-s selected and shown on the tube ammeter (Fig. 29–1).

Likewise, it is necessary to ensure the accuracy and reproducibility of the manually set *exposure timer*. The traditional method is to expose a film beneath a top with a pinhole through it; the top is made to spin at a determinable rate, and the exposure time is readily obtained from the length of the pinhole's trail on film. There are now available electronic, radiation-activated stopwatch-like instruments that are much simpler to use: when placed in the beam path, such a device counts time only when the x-ray tube is switched on. There are a dozen or so additional tests of the operation of the *phototimer*.

Among the most important QA tests are those of *peak potential (kVp)* of the generator and the *half-value layer (HVL)* of the beam in a reference medium (such as aluminum or water), since beam quality has strong influence on film contrast and overall darkening and on patient dose. Devices have been developed to allow quick checks on these and other beam parameters. The Wisconsin cassette determines the kVp of a beam and the HVL by comparing the relative amounts of radiation that pass through different fixed thicknesses and types of metals, exposing a test film. Several electronic instruments (Fig. 29–2) can do essentially the same thing rapidly and automatically, using photodiodes or other radiation detection devices rather than film. The measured HVLs in aluminum, for different kVp settings, and the amounts of total beam filtration that should be in place should not be less than the values indicated in Table 29–2.

The voltage applied across the x-ray tube can be measured directly (and somewhat more accurately) with a specialized voltmeter (voltage divider). But that involves an invasive measurement, mucking about inside the generator, and is normally

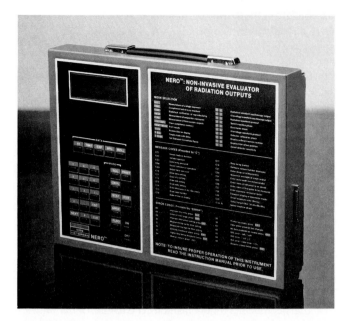

Figure 29–2. A device for noninvasive determination of x-ray beam parameters. This automated electronic beam quality analyzer measures kVp, HVL, exposure in milliroentgen, exposure duration, and fluorographic exposure rate. (The radiation detector, which connects by wire, is not shown.) A sequence of measurements can be made under computer control, and a preformatted report (covering beam quality, exposure reproducibility, exposure linearity, etc.) generated automatically. *(Photo courtesy of Victoreen, Inc., Cleveland, Ohio.)*

required only at the time of major generator repair or installation of a new tube.

The *output* of the system can be checked for various combinations of technique factors with a calibrated ionization chamber or semiconductor diode detector and an electrometer. Air kerma rate (or exposure rate) at tabletop should be in at least rough agreement with Equation 19.1. The signal produced by a diode detector and fed directly into an oscilloscope, moreover, allows a visual inspection of the *output waveform* (Fig. 29–3) for any irregularities and as a separate check on timer accuracy.

Focal spot size and shape for an x-ray tube can be estimated by means of a pinhole camera (see Fig. 10–5). A more commonly employed method involves forming the image of the *star test pattern* (Fig. 29–4), which consists of converging thin wedges of radiopaque material. The distance between the lines where a part of the image blurs can be related by simple geometry to the corresponding dimension of the source of the beam. (The elongation of the region of blur in the image reflects the noncircular shape of the focal spot.) Suppose that for a star pattern with the standard 90 lead spokes (each of which subtends an angle of 2 degrees), the lines are found to blur, at some part of the image, at a distance r_{blur} (in mm) from its center. The corresponding dimension of the focal spot, F (in mm), is approximately

$$F = r_{blur}/14.33(M - 1) \qquad (29.2)$$

where M is the magnification of the image (see Equation 22.1).

As the dimensions of a focal spot depend on the mA and

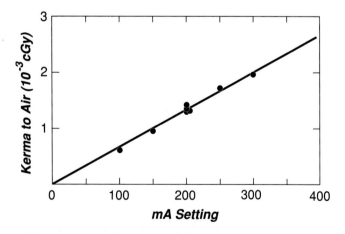

Figure 29–1. Test of linearity, demonstrating that for a fixed exposure duration, the output of the x-ray tube tracks with the tube current (mA) setting.

TABLE 29–2. MINIMUM ACCEPTABLE VALUES FOR MEASURED BEAM HALF-VALUE LAYER (HVL) IN ALUMINUM (IN MM) AND REQUIRED AMOUNTS OF TOTAL BEAM FILTRATION (MM AL)

	kVp						
	30	*50*	*70*	*90*	*110*	*130*	*150*
HVL (mm Al)							
One-phase	0.3	1.2	1.6	2.6	3.1	3.6	3.9
Three-phase	0.4	1.5	2.0	3.1	3.6	4.2	4.8
Filtration (mm Al)	0.5[a]	1.5			2.5		

[a]Or 0.03 mm Mo for molybdenum-target tubes.

From National Council on Radiation Protection and Measurements (NCRP): Medical X-ray, Electron Beam, and Gamma-ray Protection for Energies up to 50 MeV (Equipment Design, Performance, and Use), *Report No. 102. Bethesda, MD: NCRP, 1989 (Table 3.1), with permission.*

kVp, the National Electrical Manufacturer's Association (NEMA) has specified operating conditions under which measurements should be made. NEMA has also published "tolerance limits," or amounts by which measured focal spot dimensions may exceed the *nominal size*. The most recent set of these is reproduced in part in Table 29–3.

_____ **EXERCISE 29–2.** _____

The (magnified) image on film of a 4.5-cm-diameter star pattern is 7.2 cm across. The diameter of the blur region is measured to be 3.1 cm along the direction of the anode–cathode line and 2.6 cm in the perpendicular direction. Each spoke subtends a 2-degree angle. What is the size of the focal spot?

SOLUTION: The 2-degree angle means that there are 90 lead spokes, so Equation 29.2 may be used. The magnification M is 72 mm/45 mm = 1.6. Along the tube axis, $r_{star} = 31/2$ mm = 15.5 mm, so that the length of the focal spot is $15.5/(14.33)(1.6 - 1) = 1.8$ mm. Likewise, the width of the focal spot is 1.5 mm.

_____ **EXERCISE 29–3.** _____

A tube with a 1.0-mm nominal focal spot has a measured spot 1.8×1.5 mm. Is it within NEMA specs?

SOLUTION: No. By Table 29–3, the length is OK, but the width is not.

The overall resolution of a radiographic system, including the effects of both focal spot size and screen blur, may be determined directly by means of a parallel line (bar) test pattern.

The indicator (whether mechanical, that is, a built-in tape measure, or optical) of the *source-to-skin distance (SSD)* from the focal spot to the patient should be checked. The location of the focal spot is usually marked on the tube housing, and it can be verified easily by triangulation: Place a radiopaque object of dimension OB the distance SOD' from some reference mark on the tube housing, and measure the dimension IM of the image at the distance SID' from the same reference point. By similar triangles, the true source of the beam is the distance y above the reference mark, where

$$IM/OB = (SID' + y)/(SOD' + y) \qquad (29.3)$$

The *light field* used for patient setup should coincide with the radiation field, and both should be centered relative to the image receptor (whether film cassette or image intensifier). The *positive beam limitation (PBL)* circuits should automatically restrict the beam collimators to a size no greater than that of the film (or the input of the image intensifier [II] for fluoro).

All *grids* should be in good physical condition, aligned, and, for Bucky grids, moving properly. Problems with focused grids are not uncommon. Likewise, the inner surfaces of *cassettes* should be clean and undamaged and make close physical contact with film. When a new type of either cassette or film is introduced, it must be demonstrated that the match between film and cassette is acceptable.

It is necessary to ensure that *film processing chemicals and equipment* and *film* itself are in good condition. The concentrations and temperatures of chemicals in automatic processors

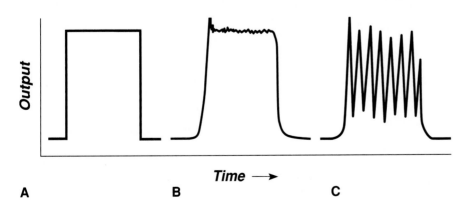

Figure 29–3. Waveform (intensity-versus-time relationship) for an x-ray generator-plus-tube combination. **A.** An ideal radiation output waveform. **B.** A realistic radiation output waveform for a three-phase generator. Because the beam does not turn on and off instantaneously, one can specify the exposure time only approximately. **C.** This radiation output waveform indicates that one of the three voltage phases is missing.

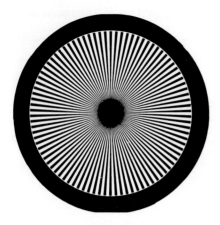

Figure 29–4. Star test pattern for determining the dimensions of the focal spot. *(Photo courtesy of RMI.)*

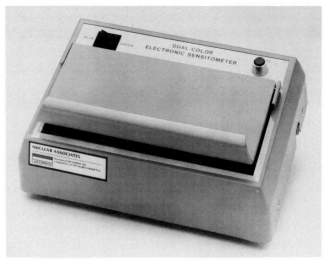

A

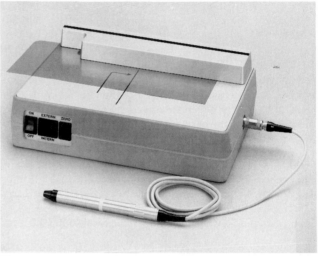

B

Figure 29–5. Film QA involves careful control over both the film itself and the processor. One aspect of this is the frequent determination of the characteristic curve by way of a sensitometer and an optical densitometer. **A.** A sensitometry exposes undeveloped film to precisely controlled (through a multiple-step optical density wedge) amounts of light. The film is then developed, and the steps of optical density are measured with an optical densitometer. **B.** When connected to a personal computer, this model of optical densitometer can automatically display or print the measured characteristic curve, and enter parameters such as base fog, speed, and gamma into the permanent QA record. *(Photos courtesy of Nuclear Associates.)*

have a significant effect on film speed, contrast, granularity, and fog level. It is critically important that they be monitored frequently, particularly after solutions have been changed or replenished. A *sensitometer* (a device that produces a calibrated set of levels of light exposure [Fig. 29–5A]) and an optical densitometer (Fig. 29–5B) together allow one quick and convenient check of film and processor stability.

Undeveloped film should be stored standing on edge at a temperature in the range 15 to 21°C (60 to 70°F). It should be subject to no chemical fumes and exposed to no more than a negligible amount of ionizing radiation. Darkroom fog is a widespread problem, and *darkrooms* must be protected against the surreptitious entry of white light. Spent chemicals should be disposed of in a legal and environmentally safe fashion. Improperly maintained processors or films can give rise to a variety of artifacts such as blotches, streaks, and patterns from static electricity.

A number of variations on the preceding themes, and additional tests, are required for QA of mammographic and other specialized systems. *Mammographic QA,* in particular, has become a refined business, with its own specialized procedures and tools.

TABLE 29–3. FOCAL SPOT SIZE ACCEPTANCE LIMITS

Nominal Size (mm)	Maximum Dimension (mm)	
	Width	*Length*
0.05	0.075	0.075
0.10	0.15	0.15
0.15	0.23	0.23
0.20	0.30	0.30
0.30	0.45	0.65
0.40	0.60	0.85
0.50	0.75	1.10
0.70	1.10	1.50
1.00	1.40	2.00
1.50	2.0	3.00
2.00	2.6	3.70

From NEMA, 1979.
From National Electrical Manufacturers Association (NEMA): Test Methods for Diagnostic X-ray Machines for Use During Initial Installation (Standards Publication No. XR 8–1979).

3. THE IMAGE INTENSIFIER AND TELEVISION SYSTEM IN FLUOROSCOPY

Most of the image QA for conventional radiography carries over into fluoroscopy. But in addition, it is necessary to consider a number of factors related to the performance of the image intensifier, the cine and spot film cameras and film changers, the automatic brightness and gain controls, and the equipment for producing, displaying, and recording the video image. (*Caveat:* With some of these tests, one can damage the TV camera by exposing the image intensifier directly to the x-ray beam, without adequate beam attenuation.)

The *high-contrast spatial resolution* of the II can be measured by means of lead bar patterns, like those used in radiography, or copper wire mesh patterns. The same test devices can then be used for the II plus the TV link. Also of interest is the ability of the system to image larger, low-contrast objects, as revealed by *contrast-detail* studies like that of Figure 18–14 (again, both without and with TV).

Some other aspects of a fluoroscopic system that require monitoring are the accuracy, flexibility, and stability of the automatic brightness and gain control systems; *lag*, or the inability to follow a fast-moving x-ray pattern (such as may arise by rapidly displacing the fluoroscopic tower); *flare* (also called *veiling glare*), which refers to light that scatters within an optical system and (like scatter x-rays created in the patient) reduces contrast; image *distortion* (pincushion effect or barrel effect), which arises because of imperfections in the electron optics of the II tube, that is, when patterns of x-ray energy falling on different regions of the input screen are not minified by exactly the same amount; and *vignetting*, or reduction in image brightness away from the center of the II or TV camera.

One can check TV monitors, videotape recorders, and hard copy devices with electronic signals produced by a video test pattern generator (Fig. 29–6) or by a video test pattern videotape.

To minimize dose to the staff and nonproductive dose to the patient, it is prudent to check tube output regularly, at least annually, and after any significant maintenance work. A fluoro system should be able to produce good images of an anthropo-

morphic (human-equivalent) phantom (composed of plastic and aluminum) with a "skin" entrance air kerma rate of under 5 cGy/min (about 5 R/min of exposure). Improper functioning of either the automatic brightness control or the TV link can lead to higher than necessary exposures.

EXERCISE 29–4.

An improperly functioning fluoroscopic system is producing air kerma at the patient's skin at a rate of 25 cGy/min, and is on for 4 minutes. What is the patient's skin dose?

SOLUTION: If a single region is being imaged, the skin dose will be of the order of 100 rem. If the beam is being moved around, skin dose at any point will be less. But as will be seen in Chapter 33, that does not necessarily diminish the total risk to the patient.

4. A RADIATION SAFETY PROGRAM PROTECTS THE PATIENT, THE STAFF, AND THE PUBLIC

Medical imaging accounts for more than 90% of the human-made ionizing radiation dose to which people are exposed.

Some irradiation of the patient is obviously unavoidable, but it is a primary objective of a radiation safety program to keep *nonproductive* exposure to a minimum. Some obvious, but sometimes overlooked, ways to do this are to eliminate diagnostically unnecessary examinations, such as in routine screening for employment or hospital admission; to involve radiologists, whenever possible, in medical decisions involving the prescription of x-rays; to allow only properly qualified staff to operate the equipment; to ensure, through regular QA activities, that the imaging equipment is functioning optimally; and to include dose considerations in the choice of technique factors.

Medical staff involved with imaging spend much time in the vicinity of active radiologic equipment (and, in the case of nuclear medicine, near radioactive materials). Although their dose rates are almost always exceedingly low, dose does accumulate over time. It is therefore essential that, as they carry out their tasks, staff keep their exposures *as low as reasonably achievable* (*ALARA*). This can be achieved through proper control and radiation surveys of work areas and through monitoring and training of the staff.

5. THE TWO TRIADS OF RADIATION SAFETY: JUSTIFICATION–OPTIMIZATION–LIMITATION AND TIME–DISTANCE–SHIELDING

When a medical exposure is to be made, there should always be the expectation that some benefit will come of it; that the doses to everybody involved (patient and staff) are as low as can reasonably be achieved; and that in any case, the doses are not so high as to pose unacceptable levels of risk. These three

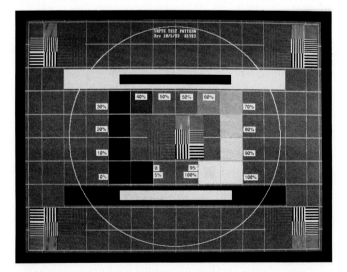

Figure 29–6. QA test pattern for television monitors, videotape devices, and hard copy recording cameras, recommended by the Society of Motion Picture and Television Engineers (SMPTE). This pattern, produced by an electronic signal generator, may be used for evaluation of a video system's ability to handle resolution, contrast, uniformity, distortion, and so on. *(Photo courtesy of Nuclear Associates.)*

TABLE 29–4. RADIATION PROTECTION PRINCIPLES

Justification
Optimization (ALARA)
Limitation

ideas are known as the principles of **justification, optimization,** and **limitation** of radiation exposure, respectively (Table 29–4). The second of them, optimization, is also called the **ALARA** principle.

An effective radiation safety program ensures the justification, optimization, and limitation of all exposures. Although all three are indispensable, the most visible and the easiest to put into effect is limitation. If limits are expressed in doses to individuals, it is relatively straightforward to determine quantitatively (with calculations, measurements, or both) whether or not the limits are being met.

Fortunately, good radiation control practice depends largely on common sense. To protect yourself from something harmful, you will spend as little time as possible around it, stay as far from it as you can, and separate yourself from it by means of an effective barrier. Minimizing exposure **time,** maximizing the **distance** from the source, and establishing adequate **shielding** are the primary actions for protecting patients, staff, and members of the public against the possible hazards of x-rays (Table 29–5).

The next few sections will demonstrate how restriction of access to sources of ionizing radiation (time and distance) and the judicious use of shielding can help keep exposures ALARA, and in particular can prevent the doses to individuals from even approaching the legal limit. The regulatory basis underlying this approach to radiation safety will be discussed in more detail in Chapter 34. For the time being, we shall simply state and make use of a few of the most important *recommendations* from advisory bodies, such as the National Council on Radiation Protection and Measurements [NCRP], and *legally binding* rules, and dose limits promulgated by agencies such as the Nuclear Regulatory Commission (NRC) and your state's Department of Health.

6. REGULATIONS ON EMISSIONS FROM SOURCES AND ON DOSES TO INDIVIDUALS

Regulations for protecting people from ionizing radiation fall into two quite different general categories: those that govern the *emission* of radiation *from sources,* and those that limit the *doses actually received* by those who are potentially exposed.

Federal agencies and states have established protective regulations governing the manufacture and operation of equipment. Regulations issued by the Food and Drug Admin-

TABLE 29–5. RADIATION PROTECTION ACTIONS

Minimize exposure time
Minimize distance
Sufficient shielding

istration (FDA) in 1986, for example, require that the *maximum air kerma rate* (at the point of entry into the patient) from a manually operated fluoroscopic system be less than 5 cGy/min (5 R/min of exposure), and less than 10 cGy/min when operated in the automatic exposure rate mode. The actual exposure rate from a machine that is not operating properly can be several times the limit. Also, there must be a timer that produces an audible signal after 5 minutes of continuous exposure. And federal standards have stipulated minimum source-to-skin distances (SSDs) of 15 in. (38 cm) for stationary fluoroscopic systems and 12 in. (30 cm) for mobile units (but there may be exceptions for some specific surgical procedures if necessary).

Radiation that leaks out of the housing of the x-ray tube can expose both the patient and the medical staff. A worst-case scenario of **leakage radiation** occurs when the generator is set to its highest kVp, and the tube current is the greatest that the anode can tolerate for nonstop operation, according to the anode thermal characteristics charts. Under those conditions, air kerma from leakage radiation should be under *0.1 cGy/h* when measured *at distance of 1 m* from the source.

Some states call for routine inspections of x-ray machines, whether in hospitals or in private clinics, but such efforts may be hampered by the large number of units in operation and the limited number of qualified inspectors. It is generally agreed that the anticipation of inspections by the JCAHO every few years is a driving force for the implementation and proper maintenance of comprehensive QA programs in hospitals.

The second group of radiation safety regulations deal with the maximum permitted doses that may be received by individuals. There are no rules limiting the dose that a *patient* can receive during the course of a medical examination. (To maintain patient doses ALARA, radiographic exposures should generally be made with the highest kVp and the fastest screen–film combination that will yield a diagnostically adequate image, and with the smallest possible field size.)

There are, however, limits on the exposures that medical *staff* and members of the *general public* may receive (Table 29–6). Various limits are issued (and revised from time to time) by different federal, state, and advisory organizations, as will be discussed in Chapter 34. But for all intents and purposes, the occupational exposure of medical *staff* is limited to an annual effective dose equivalent (EDE) of *50 mSv* (5 rem) per year. (The EDE is a risk-weighted dose equivalent averaged over the entire body, and will be described in Chapter 33.) This limit can be met easily with proper shielding of radiographic suites, reasonable behavior around activated sources of radiation, and monitoring of individual staff and of the work area. Staff working around a fluoroscopic unit, in particular, should wear lead aprons and gloves, as appropriate, and make use of mobile shields; exposure should be diminished by lead drapes hanging from the fluoro tower, when possible, by cover shields on cassette holders, and by table end shields.

The International Commission on Radiation Protection (ICRP) and the NCRP have recommended a *1-mSv* (0.1-rem) annual limit on the exposure of *members of the general public,* and this limit is being adopted by the relevant United States regulatory bodies. Exposure of the public from radiographic sources can be limited by means of proper shielding and by preventing public entry into *controlled areas,* which are areas (legally under the supervision of a radiation safety officer) in which there is a possibility of significant exposure.

TABLE 29–6. ANNUAL DOSE LIMITS

	Annual Limit (EDE)[a]	
	mSv/y	*rem/y*
Patient	—	—
Occupational	50	5
Public	1	0.1

[a]Effective dose equivalent.
From National Council on Radiation Protection and Measurements (NCRP): Recommendations on Limits for Exposure to Ionizing Radiation, *Report No. 91. Bethesda, MD: NCRP, 1987 (Table 22.1).*

7. DESIGN OF SHIELDING FOR AN IMAGING SUITE

Some ionizing radiation will pass through the walls, ceiling, floor, windows, and doors of any imaging suite. The amount that passes through a wall, for example, depends on its thickness and attenuation characteristics, on the amount of shielding material (such as lead sheeting) covering it, on its distance from the source of radiation, and on the energy and intensity of the source. The cost of protective walls, on the other hand, increases with the area (hence with the size of the suite), the density and thickness of the concrete, and the amount of lead sheeting needed. The design of shielding for an installation is based largely on the trade-off between the amount of protection desired and the cost.

If ever you are responsible for the design (or design approval) of a shielding project, you should obtain the services of an experienced medical or health physicist. For a minor job on a small imaging suite, the solution may be simple (such as $\frac{1}{16}$ or $\frac{1}{8}$ in. of lead or the equivalent on a few surfaces), but bigger projects can be detailed and tricky. And the end result usually must meet state and/or federal standards.

The construction of shielding involves three steps. First, the barrier thicknesses are computed, taking into account the room layout and dimensions, the nature and quantity of the radiation to be produced by the equipment, and assumptions about who might be exposed and how. Second, after construction is completed, the adequacy and integrity of the barrier are verified with extensive field radiation surveys. Finally, comprehensive documentation is prepared on the specifications, acceptance testing, and plans for routine future checking of the shielding.

To illustrate the first of these considerations, let us determine the amount of shielding needed for one particular wall of a room that contains an x-ray machine (Fig. 29–7). Our immediate objective is to calculate the *attenuation factor, A,* by which

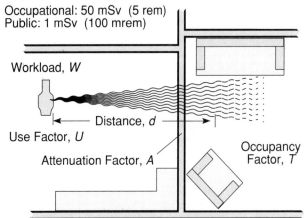

Figure 29–7. Factors to be considered in the calculation of the attenuation factor, *A*, for a barrier that provides radiation protection of a room adjacent to the imaging room: the workload of the x-ray tube during the course of a week, *W* (in mA-min), and the range of kVp's employed; the directions that the beam is angled, which determines the use factor, *U*; the amount of time people spend in the adjacent room, hence the occupancy factor, *T*; the distance from the tube to the interior of the adjacent room, *d*; and the dose limits for occupants of the adjacent room.

a protective barrier must reduce the amount of radiation passing through the unshielded wall. But it is first necessary to find the answers to a number of important questions:

1. How much radiation does the imaging machine actually produce? As a general rule of thumb, corroborated by Equation 19.1, a diagnostic x-ray tube puts out less than 0.01 Gy air kerma per milliampere-minute (about 1 R/mA-min) at a distance of 1 m:

$$\text{tube output} < 10^{-2}\,\text{Gy/mA-min} \quad \text{at 1 m} \quad (29.4)$$

The output of the machine is then proportional to the time the tube is on and to the current through it. Also of critical importance is the maximum operating potential (kVp). Table 29–7 lists, for a busy installation, the typical weekly **workload**, *W* (in mA-min), at several different potentials.

2. Can the x-ray beam expose the wall directly? A **primary barrier** that protects against direct exposure by the beam itself must be much more attenuating than a *secondary barrier* that protects only against scatter radiation and leakage through the shielding within the x-ray tube housing. The **use factor, *U*,** is a measure of

TABLE 29–7. TYPICAL WEEKLY WORKLOADS FOR BUSY INSTALLATIONS

	Daily Patient Load	Typical Weekly Workload, *W* (mA-min)		
		≤100 kVp	*125 kVp*	*150 kVp*
General radiography	24	1000	400	200
Fluoroscopy with II, including spot films	24	750	300	150

From National Council on Radiation Protection and Measurements (NCRP): Structural Shielding Design and Evaluation for Medical Use of X-rays and Gamma-rays of Energies Up to 10 MeV. *Report No. 49. Bethesda, MD: NCRP, 1976 (Table 2), with permisison.*

TABLE 29–8. USE FACTORS FOR PROTECTIVE BARRIERS

Barrier	Primary Barrier Use Factor, U	Secondary Barrier Use Factor, U
Floor	1	1
Wall	$\frac{1}{4}$	1
Ceiling	Very small	1

From National Council on Radiation Protection and Measurements (NCRP): Structural Shielding Design and Evaluation for Medical Use of X-rays and Gamma-rays of Energies Up to 10MeV. Report No. 49. Bethesda, MD: NCRP, 1976 (Table 3), with permission.

the relative amount of *time* the primary beam points toward the wall (Table 29–8).

3. How much *time* do people spend just outside the wall? The ICRP has recommended relative **occupancy factors**, T, for different uses of that space (Table 29–9).
4. What is the minimum **distance**, d, that people on the other side of the wall can be from the machine?
5. Who is on the other side of the wall? If there is a pediatrics department secretary at a desk (i.e., not a radiation worker), the shielding should meet the 1-mSv (0.1-rem) annual limit for the *general public*. If the space is the control room for another radiographic unit, the 50-mSv (5-rem) annual limit for *occupational* exposure in a controlled area would apply (see Table 29–6). The exposure to the control area from its own unit, of course, must also be taken into account.

Without shielding, that is, with $A = 1$, the expected weekly exposure of people just beyond the wall would be proportional to the output of the tube, the workload, and the use and occupancy factors, and inversely proportional to the square of the distance from the tube:

$$\text{weekly air kerma (no shielding)}$$
$$= \text{output} \cdot \text{workload} \cdot \text{use} \cdot \text{occupancy}/(\text{distance})^2$$
$$= (10^{-2}\,\text{Gy/mA-min}) \cdot (W\,\text{mA-min/wk}) \cdot U \cdot T/d^2$$
$$(29.5a)$$

TABLE 29–9. OCCUPANCY FACTORS

Occupationally exposed persons

   $T = 1$

Nonoccupationally exposed persons

   $T = 1$ Full occupancy: work areas such as offices, laboratories, shops, wards, nurses' stations; living quarters; children's play areas; and occupied space in nearby buildings

   $T = \frac{1}{4}$ Partial occupancy: corridors, rest rooms, elevators using operators, unattended parking lots

   $T = \frac{1}{16}$ Occasional occupancy: waiting rooms, toilets, stairways, unattended elevators, janitors' closets, outside areas used only for pedestrians or vehicular flow

From National Council on Radiation Protection and Measurements (NCRP): Structural Shielding Design and Evaluation for Medical Use of X-rays and Gamma-rays of Energies Up to 10MeV. Report No. 49. Bethesda, MD: NCRP, 1976 (Table 4), with permission.

The amount of attenuation, A, provided by the shielding should be sufficient to reduce the exposure to the limiting value, or less:

$$1 \times 10^{-3}\,\text{Gy/wk (staff)} \quad \text{or} \quad 0.02 \times 10^{-3}\,\text{Gy/wk (public)}$$
$$\geq A \cdot (10^{-2}\,\text{Gy/mA-min}) \cdot (W\,\text{mA-min/wk}) \cdot U \cdot T/d^2$$
$$(29.5b)$$

This makes use of the numerical near-equivalence of the gray of air kerma and the sievert of dose equivalent (or of the roentgen of exposure and the rem) for x-rays. Thus, $1 \times 10^{-3}\,\text{Gy}$ (100 mrad) and $0.02 \times 10^{-3}\,\text{Gy}$ (2 mrad) per week correspond to 1/52nd of the annual limits for occupational exposure and exposure of members of the public, respectively (see Table 29–6). As everything else in it is known, Equation 29.5b can be solved for A.

Once A has been obtained, the corresponding thicknesses of various shielding materials can be determined easily from standard tables, such as Table 29–10. A is not a simple exponential function of the thickness of the barrier, because this is *not* a situation of *good geometry*. A large portion of wall may be irradiated, and scatter from different parts of it is significant. As you would expect, A does depend strongly on the kVp.

_____ **EXERCISE 29–5.** _____

Records indicate that a general radiography unit is used about 800 mA-min each week, nearly all at 100 kVp. It is 2 m from a wall that separates it from a formerly inaccessible room that is to become the radiation physics work area. The wall consists of 5.5 cm of ordinary (2.2 g/cm^3) concrete against plywood. Should there be additional lead shielding? The head of the department wants an ample margin of safety for his people.

SOLUTION: The acceptable level of occupational exposure is 1 mSv/wk, but the designer of the shielding decides to include another factor of 1/10 or so for extra safety. With use and occupancy factors of unity, Equation 29.5b becomes

$$(1/10) \cdot (1 \times 10^{-3}\,\text{Gy/wk})$$
$$\geq A \cdot (10^{-2}\,\text{Gy/mA-min}) \cdot (800\,\text{mA-min/wk}) \cdot 1 \cdot 1/2^2$$

from which $A = 5 \times 10^{-5}$. In other words, the beam has to be attenuated by a factor of $1/A = 20{,}000$. It would take four tenth-value layers (TVLs) and 1 half-value layer (HVL) to achieve this. By Table 29–11, about $(4 \times 0.88\,\text{mm}) + (1 \times 0.27\,\text{mm}) = 3.8$ mm of lead would be needed if there were no concrete present.

By Table 29–11, the 5.5 cm of concrete already in place corresponds to about 1 TVL at 100 kVp; it is therefore necessary to decrease the beam intensity by a further factor of 1/2000. This can be achieved with 3 TVLs plus 1 HVL of lead, or a sheet at least 2.9 mm thick. One-eighth-inch lead sheeting should be adequate.

Walls and other surfaces that are never exposed directly to the primary beam still must be adequately protective against the transmission of *scatter radiation* from the patient's body or *leakage radiation* escaping through the housing of the tube. Generally much less shielding is necessary. The calculations are somewhat like those for the primary beam, but a little more

Virtually all the energy removed from the beam by means of *photoelectric* interactions is absorbed locally, $\{E/hf\}_{photo} = 1$, so that

$$[\tau/\rho]_{ab}(Z, hf) = [\tau/\rho](Z, hf) \qquad (30.6)$$

The photoelectric mass *energy absorption* coefficient is therefore practically equal to the photoelectric mass *attenuation* coefficient which, in turn, was seen in Equation 14.8 to be proportional to $(Z/hf)^3$ (except near absorption edges). This is demonstrated for water in curve A of Figure 30–2.

The *Compton* contribution to $[\mu/\rho]_{ab}$, curve B in Figure 30–2, is a bit trickier. $[\sigma/\rho]_{ab}(Z, hf)$ depends on the Compton mass attenuation coefficient which, as discussed in Chapter 14, Section 5, varies very slowly with photon energy, curve C, and (except for hydrogen) with atomic number. But $[\sigma/\rho]_{ab}(Z, hf)$ is also a function of the fraction of the photon's energy that is imparted to the Compton electron:

$$[\sigma/\rho]_{ab} = [\sigma/\rho] \cdot \{E_{ab}/hf\}_{Compt} \qquad (30.7)$$

Figure 12–3 (where E_{ab} was called KE_e) plotted $\{E_{ab}/hf\}_{Compt}$ against photon energy for several photon scatter angles. Averaging Equation 30.7 over all possible scatter angles leads to the *Compton mass energy absorption coefficient*, $[\sigma/\rho]_{ab}(hf)$, curve B.

The total mass absorption coefficient, $[\mu/\rho]_{ab}(hf)$, for water is plotted with a solid line in Figure 30–2, along with the total attenuation coefficient, $[\mu/\rho](hf)$.

A simple argument suggests why the Compton mass energy absorption coefficient of Figure 30–2, curve B, passes through a maximum at an energy of about 500 keV. In a collision, one object transfers energy to another most efficiently when their masses are equal—Think of a pair of billiard balls, as opposed to a bowling ball banging into a tennis ball or vice versa. By Equation 7.6, a 511-keV photon has an effective mass equal to the rest mass of an electron; energy is transferred most readily (i.e., the energy absorption cross section exhibits a peak) for such a photon.

3. IN PRACTICE: ONE MEASURES OR ESTIMATES THE EXPOSURE OR AIR KERMA AT A POINT, RATHER THAN THE PHOTON ENERGY FLUENCE

In their present form, Equations 30.4 are not of much practical use. Photon energy fluence is no easier to measure in the clinic than is dose itself. (But do not worry that the first two sections of this chapter were wasted time; we shall soon make good use of them.)

Radiation *exposure* and *air kerma*, on the other hand, are measures of the ability of a photon beam to ionize air. Although perhaps not too exciting in and of itself, a knowledge of the exposure or air kerma at a point in the beam allows inference of the dose to any material that happens to be at (or very near) the same point. Which is exactly what we *do* want. So let us shift attention, briefly, to the exposure.

When air is irradiated with x-rays, every high velocity photoelectron or Compton electron produced in a photon interaction will ionize hundreds or thousands of nitrogen and oxygen molecules. Each such ionization event liberates a new electron and leaves behind a cation. The hundreds or thousands of electrons freed in this process dissipate their kinetic energy in causing further ionizations. After having slowed down sufficiently, the electrons attach onto neutral air molecules, forming anions. Nearly equal numbers of positive and negative ions are thereby created, and almost all of them are singly charged. (Later, the anions and cations find one other and *recombine*, neutralizing their charges, but that is not of interest to us here.)

The exposure from a beam of ionizing photons, X, was defined in Figure 11–3 and in Chapter 16, Section 2, as the quantity of x-ray or gamma ray energy that causes total charge q of either sign to be produced anywhere as a consequence of irradiating a block of air of mass m:

$$X \rightarrow charge/mass = q/m \qquad (30.8)$$

We use an arrow here rather than an equal sign, as exposure refers to an attribute of the *beam* at a point in the beam path, whereas the charge per mass is a measure of what the beam would do to air at that point.

The conventional unit of exposure is the *roentgen*, denoted

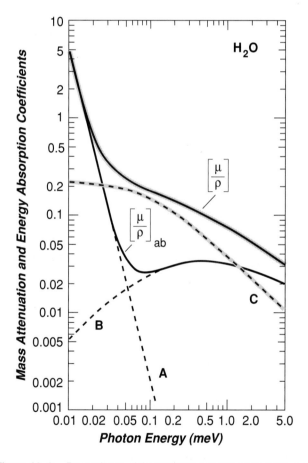

Figure 30–2. Dependence of the total mass energy absorption coefficient, $[\mu/\rho]_{ab}(hf)$, on photon energy for water. Curve A is the photoelectric mass energy absorption contribution (which is nearly identical to the photoelectric mass attenuation coefficient). Curve B is the Compton mass energy absorption coefficient. Also shown are the Compton mass attenuation coefficient, curve C, and the total mass attenuation coefficient, $[\mu/\rho](hf)$.

TABLE 30–1. CONVENTIONAL AND SI UNITS OF EXPOSURE

SI units	C/kg	1 C/kg = 3.876×10^3 R
Conventional units	R	1 R = 2.58×10^{-4} C/kg

R. An exposure of 1 R is the amount of ionizing radiation that gives rise to the liberation of exactly 2.58×10^{-4} C of charge of either sign in a kilogram of irradiated gas (Table 30–1). The SI unit of exposure, the C/kg, has no special name.

_____ **EXERCISE 30–2.** _____

A certain brief exposure of a volume of air 5 cm on a side results in the ionization of 6×10^{10} molecules. What was the exposure in SI units and in roentgens? The density of air at standard temperature and pressure (STP = 0°C, 1 atm of pressure = 1.013×10^5 N/m^2), is 1.293 kg/m^3.

SOLUTION: A block of air of volume 1.25×10^{-4} m^3 is of mass 1.6×10^{-4} kg. If the 6×10^{10} molecules are nearly all singly ionized, then the charge of either sign liberated is $(1.6 \times 10^{-19}$ C/ion)$(6 \times 10^{10}$ ions$) = 9.6 \times 10^{-9}$ C. The exposure is $(9.6 \times 10^{-9}$ C$)/(1.6 \times 10^{-4}$ kg$) = 6.0 \times 10^{-5}$ C/kg. In roentgen, this is $(6.0 \times 10^{-5}$ C/kg$)[(1$ R$)/(2.58 \times 10^{-4}$ C/kg$)] = 0.23$ R $= 230$ mR.

It is found experimentally that over a wide range of x-ray energies, approximately the same amount of energy, 33.7 eV, is expended, on average, for each pair of ions that is produced in air, (Table 30–2). This 33.7 eV per ion pair accounts for all possible ionizations of inner- and outer-orbital electrons and for the energy that excites but does not ionize molecules. The energy per ion pair for air is commonly designated W. W happens to have the same numerical value when expressed in SI units of energy per charge.

_____ **EXERCISE 30–3.** _____

How many anions are produced if the energy of a 67-keV photon is completely absorbed in air?

SOLUTION: 67,000 eV/33.7 eV per ion pair = 2000 anions and 2000 cations, nearly all of which are singly charged.

_____ **EXERCISE 30–4.** _____

Show that $W = 33.7$ J/C.

SOLUTION: Expand (energy/charge) as the quotient (energy/ion pair)/(charge/ion pair). The numerator and denominator can, in turn, be expressed as (energy/ion pair) = (33.7

TABLE 30–2. AVERAGE ENERGY PER ION PAIR TO IONIZE AIR, W

SI units	$W = 33.7$ J/C
Conventional units	$W = 33.7$ eV/ion pair

eV/ion pair)$(1.6 \times 10^{-19}$ J/eV) and (charge/ion pair) = 1.6×10^{-19} C/ion pair, respectively. Divide out, and keep careful track of the units.

In the next section we shall need to know the *dose to air*, D_{air}, arising *from an exposure X*. Dose is defined as the ionizing energy deposited per unit mass, which can be expressed as

$$(\text{energy/mass}) = (\text{energy/charge})(\text{charge/mass}) \quad (30.9)$$

As the dose is being deposited in air, by Equation 30.8 and Exercise 30–4, this becomes

$$D_{air}(\text{Gy}) = W \cdot (q/m) = 33.7 \cdot X \text{ (C/kg)} \quad (30.10a)$$

in SI units (Gy and C/kg) and

$$D_{air} \text{ (rad)} = 0.873 \cdot X(\text{R}) \quad (30.10b)$$

in conventional units* (rads and roentgens). As indicated by Equation 30.3, at diagnostic energies D_{air} = air kerma.

4. DETERMINING DOSE IN TISSUE FROM EXPOSURE IN AIR—THE *f*-FACTOR

Exposure or air kerma at a point in the path of an x-ray beam can be determined easily in either of two ways:

- Directly from an exposure measurement with a calibrated ion chamber, as will be discussed in Sections 6 and 7.
- From knowledge of the technique factors employed and tabulated output characteristics of the x-ray machine. The tables of machine outputs, in turn, were based on earlier exposure measurements with calibrated ion chambers.

Either way, the dose to nearby tissues can easily be learned from the value of the exposure.

Suppose that two different materials experience the *same photon energy fluence*, Ψ. The dose in the first medium, D_1, is related to the energy fluence through Equation 30.4b as

$$D_1 = [\mu/\rho]_{ab,1} \cdot \Psi \quad (30.11a)$$

So, too, in the second medium,

$$D_2 = [\mu/\rho]_{ab,2} \cdot \Psi \quad (30.11b)$$

By our design the two regions receive the same energy fluence, so that division of one equation by the other yields

$$D_1 = ([\mu/\rho]_{ab,1}/[\mu/\rho]_{ab,2})D_2 \quad (30.12)$$

Suppose that the second medium is air. Equation 30.10 related the dose in air to exposure. Inserting Equation 30.10 into Equation 30.12 reveals that the dose to the first medium (designated "med") can be determined from a measurement of exposure in air (the second medium) at the same point in space:

$$D_{med} = 33.7 \, ([\mu/\rho]_{ab, med}/[\mu/\rho]_{ab, air}) \cdot X \quad (30.13)$$

in SI units.

It simplifies things to separate Equation 30.13 into two

_____

*Some older books use a value of 0.869 rather than 0.873.

terms that relate, respectively, to the strength of the radiation field and to the energy absorption process:

$$D_{med} = X \cdot f_{med} \qquad (30.14a)$$

where

$$f_{med} = 33.7\ \{[\mu/\rho]_{ab,\ med}/[\mu/\rho]_{ab,\ air}\} \quad \text{Gy}/(\text{C}/\text{kg}) \quad (30.14b)$$

In conventional units,

$$f_{med} = 0.873\ \{[\mu/\rho]_{ab,\ med}/[\mu/\rho]_{ab,\ air}\} \quad \text{rad}/\text{R} \quad (30.14c)$$

f_{med}, the *exposure-to-dose* or *roentgen-to-rad* conversion factor, or simply the *f-factor*, of the medium, was introduced briefly in Chapter 16, Section 2. Numerical values for f_{med} will be tabulated in the next section.

_____ **EXERCISE 30–5.** _____

The entrance skin exposure (ESE) for a diagnostic procedure is 100 mR. The *f*-factor is about 0.92 rad/R. What is the skin dose?

SOLUTION: $(0.92\ \text{rad}/\text{R})(0.1\ \text{R}) = 92\ \text{mrad} = 92 \times 10^{-3}\ \text{cGy}.$

_____ **EXERCISE 30–6.** _____

How do you relate tissue dose to air kerma?

SOLUTION: Use Equation 30.12, but substitute air kerma for D_2.

5. THE *f*-FACTOR DEPENDS ON THE PHOTON ENERGY AND ON THE NATURE OF THE IRRADIATED MEDIUM

The *f*-factor depends on the nature of the material irradiated and on the energy of the x-ray photons. As the compositions of the irradiated medium (such as soft tissue) and air differ from one another, the details of the photon interaction and energy deposition processes in them will not be identical. $[\mu/\rho]_{ab,\ med}(hf)$ and $[\mu/\rho]_{ab,air}(hf)$ are therefore dissimilar functions of photon energy. As a result, their ratio, f_{med} of Equation 30.14, is energy dependent.

f_{med} is presented, in conventional units, as a function of monochromatic photon energy for water, muscle, bone, and air in Figure 30–3 and Table 30–3. Table 30–3 also shows the *f*-factors for several (three-phase) x-ray machine generating voltages, obtained by averaging Equation 30.14 over the filtered (2.5 mm Al) photon energy spectrum.

_____ **EXERCISE 30–7.** _____

During a 90-kVp diagnostic procedure, an ionization chamber inside the beam field and held near the body determines the exposure to be 0.05 R. What is the skin dose?

SOLUTION: By Equation 30.14a and Table 30–3, the dose is about 50 mrad, corresponding to a dose equivalent of 50 mrem.

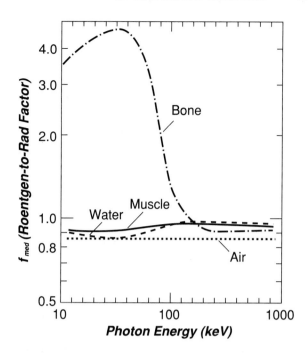

Figure 30–3. *f*-factor (or roentgen-to-rad conversion factor) as a function of energy for water, muscle, bone, and air. At any energy, $f_{med}(hf)$ compares the mass energy absorption coefficient, $[\mu/\rho]_{ab}$, of a medium with that of air, a convenient reference material. The magnitude of $f_{med}(hf)$ at low photon energies depends strongly on the rate (relative to that for air) of photoelectric events occurring in the medium. At high energies, it is the Compton effect that dominates.

In SI units, this is 50×10^{-3} cGy of dose and 0.5 mSv of dose equivalent.

The effective atomic numbers (Z) of water (7.5) and muscle (7.4) are similar to that of air (7.8), and values of $f_{med}(hf)$ for both are close to 0.873. Because of its greater hydrogen content and consequent higher electron density, fat has an *f*-factor above that of water at high energies, where the Compton effect dominates, and water has an *f*-factor above f_{med} for muscle for the same reason. $f_{bone}(hf)$, on the other hand, strongly reflects the photoevents involving calcium at low energies and, at high energies, the relative paucity of hydrogen.

The *f*-factor for air itself, $f_{air} = 0.873$ rad/R = 33.7 Gy/(J/C), is independent of photon energy. This is so not because of any unique physical properties of air; indeed, the tendency of the gas to absorb photons does depend on their energy. f_{air} is constant, rather, simply because air was chosen to serve as the reference material against which all others are compared: The *f*-factor for any substance is a relative measure of the extent to which its radiologic properties differ from those of air.

The dose to a medium depends on $[\mu/\rho]_{ab}$ and on the photon energy fluence, Ψ, (see Equations 30.4). Each of these, in turn, depends on photon energy. The definition of exposure, on the other hand, is concerned with the amount of charge liberated in air, but not at all with the energy of the photons doing the job. It may be a bit surprising, then, that the dose deposited in a tissue, which depends on photon energy, can be determined from a measurement of exposure, which does not. The

TABLE 30–3. THE f-FACTOR (ROENTGEN-TO-RAD FACTOR)[a]

Source	Effective Energy (keV)	f_{med}				
		Water	Muscle	Fat	Bone	Air
20 keV	20	0.89	0.92	0.51	4.3	0.873
60 keV	60	0.92	0.94	0.74	3.0	0.873
100 keV	100	0.96	0.96	0.91	1.5	0.873
150 keV	150	0.97	0.96	0.96	1.1	0.873
60 kVp	30	0.88	0.92	0.53	4.4	0.873
80 kVp	32	0.88	0.92	0.54	4.4	0.873
100 kVp	34	0.89	0.92	0.55	4.3	0.873
120 kVp	37	0.89	0.93	0.57	4.2	0.873
Density (kg/m^3)		1000	1040	916	1650	1.293
Electron density (x 10^{26} electrons/kg)		3.343	3.31	3.34	3.19	3.006
Effective Z		7.5	7.6	6.5	12.3	7.8

[a]Values of the f-factor, f_{med}, for various media and photon energies, in conventional units. The physical and electron densities and effective atomic numbers are reproduced from Table 14–1. Air density at STP.
After Johns, HE, Cunningham JR: The Physics of Radiology, *4th ed. Springfield, IL: Charles C. Thomas, 1983 (Appendix A), with permission.*

explanation is that all the energy dependence of the situation is contained in the "constant" of proportionality, $f_{med}(hf)$, which connects the dose and exposure through Equations 30–14.

_____ **EXERCISE 30–8.** _____

How is the energy fluence, Ψ, related to the exposure X in air that it produces?

SOLUTION: $D_{air} = 0.873 \cdot X$ and $D_{air} = [\mu/\rho]_{ab,air} \cdot \Psi$, so $\Psi/X = 0.873/[\mu/\rho]_{ab,air}$

Because f_{med} is generally quite close to unity, the dose and exposure at a point often are numerically similar, and rads, rems, and roentgens are sometimes used interchangeably. The difference between the three constructs, however, should be borne in mind.

6. INSTRUMENTATION: CLINICAL ION CHAMBERS

The standard instrument for making measurements of exposure is the calibrated ion chamber, attached to an electrometer. Clinical ion chambers come in a variety of sizes and shapes, but most are cylindrical, spherical, disk-shaped, or "well" chambers. Each of these consists of two electrodes, electrically insulated from one another and attached to the opposite poles of a source of high direct-current voltage. One of these connections is made by way of a sensitive electrometer, which is capable of detecting the flow of small amounts of charge (typically 10^{-15} C or less). When the chamber is irradiated, the reading of the meter, q (in C), reports the charge of either sign produced in the air between the electrodes and swept to them by the high voltage. q is directly proportional to the exposure, X:

$$X = N_c \cdot q \qquad (30.15)$$

Once the ion chamber's **calibration factor** N_c is known, it is possible to determine the exposure at a point directly from the electrometer reading from an ion chamber situated there. A similar expression (with a slightly different calibration constant) relates air kerma to electrometer reading.

The calibration constant N_c of a chamber can be obtained or checked by comparing its response to that of a reference chamber, whose constant is known and was obtained earlier at (or can be traced reliably to) the National Institute of Standards and Technology (NIST). (Formerly the National Bureau of Standards; NIST houses a highly accurate *free air* chamber that serves as the primary reference.) The *chamber calibration* process consists of taking readings of q with the chamber of interest exposed to a steady photon beam for a specified period of time, followed by readings q_{ref} (under identical conditions) with a reference chamber of known calibration constant, N_{ref}. As the two chambers receive the same calibration exposure X, the constant N_c for the chamber being calibrated can be extracted from $X = N_c \cdot q = N_{ref} \cdot q_{ref}$ and from the experimental readings of q and q_{ref}.

Solid-state diode detectors have to some extent replaced ion chambers for many routine diagnostic radiology measurements. Because the density of silicon is 2000 times that of air, and because only a tenth as much energy is needed to create an ion pair in it, the sensitivity of a solid state diode detector is between 1000 and 10,000 times that of an ion chamber of the same size. Its response is fast enough, moreover, for it to follow the rapid changes of beam output as an x-ray tube is switched on and off. The principal drawback of a diode is its stronger dependence on photon energy, which precludes its use for high accuracy (but not all) dosimetry.

7. ELECTRON EQUILIBRIUM

The simplicity of the definition of exposure (see Equation 30.8) is deceptive. Photoelectrons and Compton electrons can be liberated anywhere along the x-ray beam path through the air-filled ion chamber of Figure 30–4. Each of these can, in turn, ionize many other molecules, and the resulting secondary electrons and ions may be swept up by the

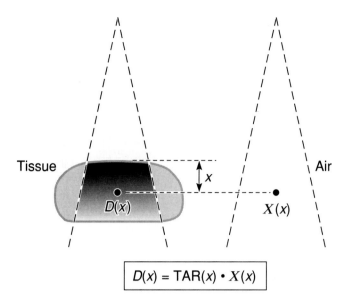

$$D(x) = TAR(x) \cdot X(x)$$

Figure 31–4. The TAR relates the *dose* at depth x in a body to the exposure one would find at the same point but in the absence of the body. TAR(x) depends on photon energy and on field size, but is independent of the beam source-to-skin distance, SSD.

(Future TAR tables may make use of SI units.) TAR(x) is a function of the quality of the beam and of its dimensions A at the point of interest,

$$TAR(x) = TAR(x, hf, A) \qquad (31.1b)$$

but is nearly independent of the source-to-skin distance. Figure 31–5 offers a sampler of TAR values for a 40×40-cm field and typical diagnostic energies, with 2.5 mm Al equivalent total beam filtration.

The TAR for the point at $x = 0$, on the skin surface, TAR(0), in particular, is known as the "backscatter factor." It is somewhat different from f_{med} in Equation 30.14, which related dose in a small volume of tissue at a point of interest to the exposure there: The TAR accounts for the effects of radiation scattered back from within the patient and reaching the calculation point, and the f factor does not.

_____ **EXERCISE 31–3.** _____

What is the dose to an organ 10 cm deep in a patient from a 40 x 40-cm² (at the organ) 80-kVp beam? From the previously measured output characteristics of the tube, the exposure *in air* at the location of the organ (but in the absence of the patient) is known to be 150 mR, under otherwise identical conditions.

SOLUTION: From Figure 31–5, TAR (10 cm, 40×40 cm², 80 kVp) = 0.35, so that by Equation 31.1, the dose is 50 mrad.

TAR tables can be obtained from *Monte Carlo* calculations, in which a computer creates and keeps track of thousands of hypothetical x-ray photons as they pass through hypothetical matter and undergo random interactions, with probabilities determined by the photoelectric and Compton mass attenuation and energy absorption coefficients. Alternatively, they can be based on experiments involving irradiation of an anthropomorphic, tissue-equivalent phantom. More commonly, the closely related percent depth dose (PDD) is measured in a water tank (see Fig. 15.11) and the TAR(x) is then calculated directly from that.

TAR and PDD values usually refer to measurements on the central axis of a rectangular beam, but both can be extended so as to allow the determination of dose at other points in or outside a beam of any shape. The next section will define

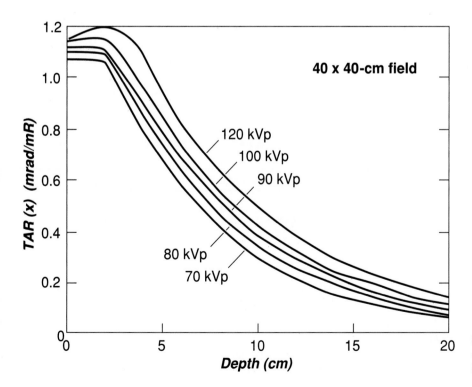

Figure 31–5. Typical values of TAR(x) for 40 × 40-cm (at depth x) beams of various kVps, with 2.5 mm Al equivalent total filtration.

a partial TAR, which reveals the dose (from direct exposure, scatter, or both) to an organ anywhere in the body caused by the irradiation of any small-volume element of tissue.

4. CALCULATION OF ORGAN DOSE, OR DOSE TO A FETUS, FROM A RADIOGRAPH

To learn the dose at a certain depth within a body and at the center of the radiation field, the TAR is all you need. Most interesting clinical problems, however, are not that simple.

Two publications of the Center for Devices and Radiological Health (CDRH, a part of the Food and Drug Administration), provide information that is useful in estimating organ doses for standard procedures. *Organ Doses in Diagnostic Radiology* and *Handbook of Selected Tissue Doses for Projections Common in Diagnostic Radiology* contain tables of average doses to certain organs and tissues per unit of entrance skin exposure (in rads/R).

An example of this kind of information, for lumbar spine, is reproduced in part in Table 31–1. The table relates organ dose (in mrad), for different beam qualities, per roentgen of *entrance skin exposure* (*ESE*). Organ doses for a particular real exposure also depend, of course, on the dimensions of the patient and on the choice of technique factors, grid, screen–film combination, and so on.

_____ EXERCISE 31–4. _____

An anteroposterior (AP) examination of the lumbar spine of an average size female patient is performed with a 7 × 17-in. beam with a half-value layer (HVL) in aluminum of 3.0 mm, and a 400-speed screen–film system with a grid. Estimate the dose to a first-trimester fetus.

SOLUTION: By Table 30–4, the ESE should be of the order of 330 mR. By Table 31–1, the dose to the uterus would be about (0.33 R)(279 mrad/R) ~ 90 mrad.

You will usually be able to read the organ dose per unit of entrance skin exposure directly from these tables. If the tables do not contain the organ or procedure of interest, you can easily obtain the dose from a user-friendly, two-step calculation:

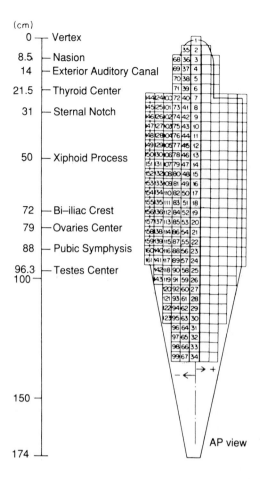

Figure 31–6. Mathematical phantom for use in the CDRH method of computing effective TARs. *(From Rosenstein M. Organ Doses in Diagnostic Radiology. HEW Publication (FDA) 76-8030, 1976 [Fig. 5].)*

- From the technique factors selected, the output tables for the x-ray machine, and the distance from the focal spot to the organ of interest, calculate the exposure at beam-center and in the plane of the organ.
- Employing tabulated "partial" TAR values appropriate for the beam position, dimensions, and quality, calcu-

TABLE 31–1. TYPICAL DOSES (mrad) TO ORGANS FROM AN ANTEROPOSTERIOR LUMBAR SPINE EXAMINATION OF A FEMALE PATIENT, PER ROENTGEN (1 R) OF ENTRANCE SKIN EXPSOURE (ESE)[a]

	HVL (mm Al)			
	2.0	**3.0**	**4.0**	**5.0**
	Organ Dose (mrad) per Roentgen of ESE			
Lungs	22	34	43	50
Active bone marrow	12	23	34	44
Thyroid	0.1	0.3	0.5	0.5
Trunk Tissue	58	80	97	110
Breasts		Negligible		
Ovaries	98	157	202	236
Uterus	180	279	352	404

[a]Beam quality expressed in terms of half-value layer (HVL) in aluminum. The source-to-image receptor distance (SID) is 40 in., and the field is 7 × 17 in. at the film.
Rosenstein, M: Handbook of Selected Tissue Doses for Projections Common in Diagnostic Radiology (HSS Pub. [FDA] 89–8031). Washington, DC: US Dept. of Health and Human Services (FDA), 1988 (Table 38).

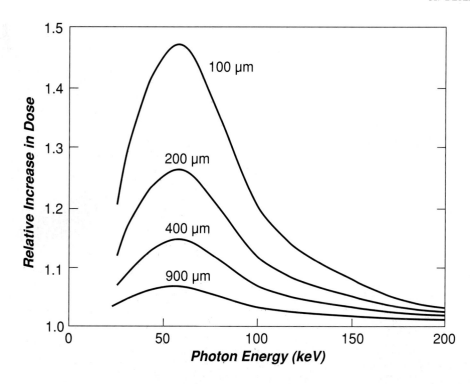

Figure 31–7. Increases in dose to soft-tissue inclusions of various diameters in bone, relative to the bone dose.

late the effective TAR, then the dose at the organ within the patient.

In calculating the effective TAR, the patient is represented by a computational phantom composed of several hundred volume elements (Fig. 31–6). The method relates, by means of a table of *partial TARs,* the amount of dose to the organ of interest that results from the irradiation of each particular small volume element. One must thus determine which volume elements are irradiated and add up the corresponding partial TARs to obtain the composite, effective TAR. This yields the dose to the organ (in rads) per unit exposure (in R). The organ of interest need not itself be in the beam path; the approach works just as well for an organ subject only to scatter radiation.

5. DOSE TO SOFT TISSUE IN BONE CAVITIES

All of the preceding assumed the condition of electron equilibrium in tissue (see Chapter 30, Section 7). But electron equilibrium breaks down in the vicinity of an interface between materials with different radiologic properties. This phenomenon has particular significance for the osteocytes housed in small

cavities within a bone and for tissues lining its inner and outer surfaces.

Figure 31–7 indicates the increase in dose deposited as photon beams of various energies pass from bone into soft tissue inclusions. The number of photoelectrons and Compton electrons liberated per cubic centimeter is greater in bone than in soft tissue. So more electrons spill across a bone surface downstream into soft tissue than would have been produced in soft tissue under electron equilibrium. Hence the elevated dose, at least over the distance required for equilibrium to be reestablished in soft tissue. The excess dose to soft tissue encapsulated within, or adjacent to, bone is greatest for those energies at which the *f*-factor for bone is maximum.

The volume of soft tissue taken to elevated dose increases with the bone surface area. The average dose is therefore greater for soft tissue housed in many small cavities than in one large one. Over the diagnostic range, the dose to soft tissue inclusions in small (10-µm) bone cavities can be as much as a factor of 4 times what the soft tissue dose would be in the absence of the bone. The dose in trabecular spaces averaged over the entire skeleton, however, is only 10% to 15% greater than the dose to nearby muscle.

Effects of Ionizing Radiation on Tissue

If our only concern were the x-ray shadows cast by bones and contrast agents, then physicians could focus complete attention on the ways that various materials attenuate x-ray beams and on the extent to which Compton scatter photons degrade the resultant images.

But in clinical practice it is necessary also to take into account the possible hazards associated with x-irradiation. The problem is clear but inescapable: The very photoelectric and Compton events that remove photons from the beam, and are responsible for image formation, also produce photoelectrons and Compton electrons. And as these high velocity electrons course through tissue, they ionize molecules within the cells, inducing chemical changes that can lead, occasionally, to carcinogenesis, genetic harm, or other severe health effects.

1. RADIOLYSIS OF WATER

The typical mammalian cell is 80% to 90% water and, as a consequence, soft tissue has radiologic properties similar to those of water. Water is considerably easier to work with in the lab, of course, and a much more amenable starting point for theoretical study. Substantial amounts of time and effort have therefore gone into examining the effects of ionizing radiation on water.

The x-irradiation of water will send photoelectrons and Compton electrons speeding through it. In some encounters, the close passage of such an electron will transfer energy to a water molecule and excite it, or even ionize it:

$$H_2O + energy \rightarrow H_2O^+ + e^- \qquad (32.1a)$$

H_2O^+ is an *ion radical*: Not only is it an ion, but also, because it contains an *odd number of electrons* in the outer molecular orbitals, it is a **free radical**. It is therefore chemically highly reactive.

> Atoms and molecules generally try (for non-obvious quantum mechanical reasons) to have all their orbital electrons paired up. A free radical has an odd number of outer-orbital

electrons, one of which must therefore be unpaired. The odd electron out would feel more comfortable with a partner, even if it has to be taken away from another molecule. As a consequence, radicals are very reactive.

H_2O^+ combines with a water molecule, within about 10^{-10} second, to form a H_3O^+ ion and the neutral hydroxyl free radical, $OH^\bullet$:

$$H_2O^+ + H_2O = H_3O^+ + OH^\bullet \qquad (32.1b)$$

The **hydroxyl radical** has eight paired electrons and one unpaired electron, which is indicated by the dot.

By similar reactions, the hydrogen radical, $H^\bullet$, and other reactive species are produced. Also, because water molecules are polar with a slight excess of electron charge on the oxygen and a deficit on the hydrogens, a free electron may draw several of them to itself, creating a short-lived, reactive *aqueous* or *solvated electron* cluster, before attaching to one of them.

Free radicals survive in a cell typically for 0.1 to 1 microsecond before reacting. If any of them happen to diffuse into the vicinity of a DNA molecule during that time, they are capable of reacting with it and inflicting damage on it. It is estimated that perhaps 75% of the damage to mammalian cells from x-irradiation is mediated by hydroxyl radicals.

2. THE BIOLOGIC EFFECTS OF IONIZING RADIATION COME PRIMARILY FROM DAMAGE TO DNA

A dose of several thousand rads, which is usually sufficient to kill nearly all the cells in a culture or an organ, ionizes only about 1 in 10^7 molecules. That is, even high doses affect only a very small fraction of the molecules of any particular type. This suggests the presence within a cell of a number of specific targets, damage to any one (or a few) of which results in cell sterilization (which may be expressed sooner or later as cell death).

Much research suggests that virtually all biologic radiation effects that occur at relatively low (diagnostic-level) doses are attributable to damage to DNA. Striking cellular evidence of DNA involvement is found in the radiation induction of chromosomal aberrations (Fig. 32–1). Chromosomes examined at the first metaphase or anaphase of the mitotic cycle following irradiation may reveal fragments of chromosomes, single or double rings, dicentrics, interchanged parts, and other abnormal forms. The various types of abnormalities that occur and the likelihood that they will do so depend on the stage of the cell cycle during which irradiation takes place.

> Recall that the mitotic cell cycle consists of five general phases. During the long, "resting" *interphase*, when the DNA is replicated, the chromosomes are uncoiled and invisible. In *prophase*, the DNA begins condensing into tight, stainable coils, and the nuclear membrane and nucleoli disappear. During *metaphase*, each chromosome appears as a pair of chromatids joined at the centromere; the spindle forms and links the cell's poles, and the chromosomes align along its equator. In *anaphase*, the chromosomes move along the fibers of the cell's spindle to the poles. And at *telophase*, the chromosomes unwind, the nuclear membrane and nucleoli reappear, and the cell divides into two new daughter cells that enter interphase.

At the molecular level, damage to DNA can occur by means of either of two general processes (Fig. 32–2). With a *direct attack*, a high-velocity electron ionizes or excites part of the DNA molecule itself into a chemically unstable state:

$$\text{DNA} + \text{energy} \rightarrow \text{DNA}^{\bullet} \qquad (32.2a)$$

Alternatively, the damage can be caused in *indirect* attacks by chemically reactive free radicals that exist briefly, but long enough to diffuse into the vicinity of DNA. The radiolysis

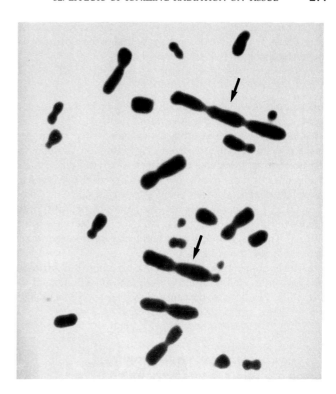

Figure 32–1. Direct evidence of the ability of ionizing radiation to cause genetically based biologic harm. Chinese hamster lung fibroblast cells were exposed to 8 Gy, and chromosome spreads were prepared 15 hours later. The arrows indicate two radiation-induced dicentric chromosome aberrations. *(Photo courtesy of James B. Mitchell, National Cancer Institute.)*

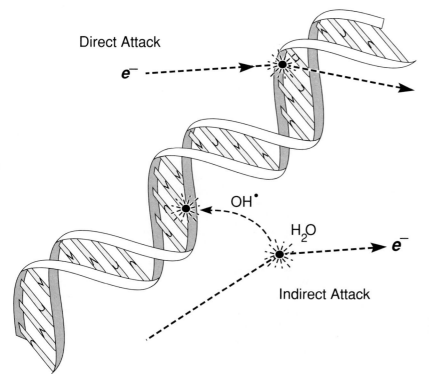

Figure 32–2. A fast-moving electron can cause damage to a DNA molecule by ionizing it directly, in a so-called direct attack. Alternatively, in a two-step indirect attack, the fast electron ionizes water, thereby creating hydroxyl (OH$^{\bullet}$) or other free radicals that subsequently migrate through the cellular soup and disrupt the DNA.

product most effective in damaging DNA molecules is the hydroxyl radical. It is an oxidizing agent that in the hydrogen extraction reaction,

$$DNA–CH_3 + OH^• \rightarrow DNA–CH_2^• + H_2O \qquad (32.2b)$$

for example, leaves behind a radical site which can undergo a subsequent, self-destructive reaction.

Damage to DNA resulting from either direct or indirect attack may consist of a localized point mutation in which the composition or geometry of a purine or pyrimidine base is changed. Or it may involve a break in one of the two sugar–phosphate chains or even a double-strand scission. Such alterations may be reparable; if not, they may be of little consequence (leading to nothing more than individual cell death at mitosis). They may, on the other hand, transform a normal cell into one that is cancerous.

The entire process, from initial x-ray photon–electron interaction in the cell, through subsequent ionizations and the formation of radicals, to damage to DNA and eventual biologic expression, is summarized in Figure 32–3.

3. LINEAR ENERGY TRANSFER AND THE SPACING OF IONIZATION EVENTS

A typical diagnostic energy photoelectron or Compton electron generates clusters of several ionizations every 100 Å (every 10^{-8} m) or so in water or soft tissue (Fig. 32–4). The rate per unit distance along its path at which the electron transfers energy to the surrounding medium, or **linear energy transfer (LET)**, ranges from about 0.3 to 10 keV per micrometer, depending on its velocity. This is significantly less than what one finds with heavy charged particles (such as alpha particles).

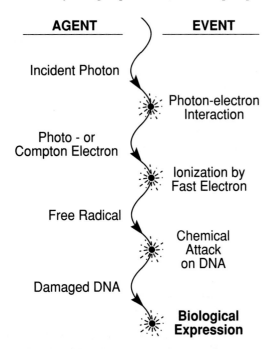

Figure 32–3. Summary of the events leading from an initial high-energy photon–electron interaction to biologic expression of harm.

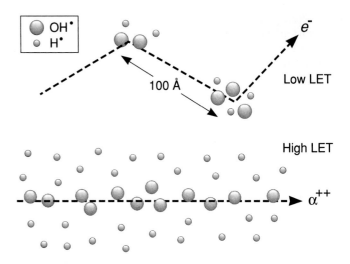

Figure 32–4. Linear Energy Transfer (LET) is an important determinant of the ability of ionizing radiation to cause biologic damage. A fast-moving electron (and, by association, the x-ray photon that liberated it) gives rise to small, widely separated clusters of ions, and is said to be of relatively low LET. An energetic alpha particle, by comparison, leaves a dense trail of ions in its wake and is high LET. In general, high-LET radiation is more biologically harmful, per gray, than is low-LET radiation.

For that reason, electrons (and the x-ray photons that set them in motion) are called *low-LET* particles.

_____ **EXERCISE 32–1.** _____

What is the range of a 100-keV electron in soft tissue, if the average LET for the electron is 1 keV/μm?

SOLUTION: For a very rough calculation, we assume that the electron dissipates its energy at a constant rate over its range, and stops when the energy is gone,

$$(\text{range})(1 \text{ keV}/\mu m) = 100 \text{ keV}$$

from which the range = 0.1 mm. Thus even the most energetic electrons liberated by diagnostic x-rays travel only a millimeter or so in biologic tissues. Their range is even less in solid detector materials. How does this compare with the mean free path of 100 keV photons?

Because of its much greater mass, an alpha particle moves at only about 1% of the speed of an electron of the same kinetic energy. It exerts disruptive electric forces on any atom in its path for longer periods and, therefore, has a greater opportunity to excite or ionize it. The density of local ionizations along its path is considerably greater, typically on the order of 250 keV/μm. Alpha particles are *high LET*.

An alpha particle passing through water generates a dense line, along its trajectory, of hydroxyl and hydrogen free radicals spaced only a few angstroms apart. The much lighter hydrogen radicals diffuse rapidly outward, forming an H$^•$ sheath about the line of OH$^•$. Because of their proximity, the hydroxyl radicals tend to recombine among themselves:

$$OH^• + OH^• \rightarrow H_2O_2$$

This leaves the hydrogen radicals to recombine among themselves, as well:

$$H^{\bullet} + H^{\bullet} \rightarrow H_2$$

Indeed, hydrogen gas sometimes evolves from water irradiated with high-LET particles such as alpha particles.

The formation of hydrogen peroxide may contribute to the effectiveness of high-LET radiation in causing both cell mutations and cell death.

4. RELATIVE BIOLOGIC EFFECTIVENESS OF RADIATION

A number of parameters affect the response of cells or tissues to irradiation. Some of these are the normal rate of cell turnover (i.e., frequency of mitosis), the state of cell differentiation, the stage of the cell cycle at the time of irradiation, and the presence of naturally occurring or synthetic chemical radiation sensitizers (in particular, oxygen) and protectors. Among the most important are the LET and the detailed pattern of the ionizations produced by the radiation.

When a low-LET particle, such as a fast electron, passes close to a DNA molecule, ionizations of the medium will occur at points far enough apart that damage will almost always be confined to only one base or one sugar–phosphate strand. And cells usually can **repair** many of such faults.

> The trail of ions and free radicals left by a typical high-LET particle such as an alpha particle, by contrast, is a thousand or so times denser. The odds are therefore much greater that radicals will be available to attack both DNA strands at proximate sites, severing the molecule. Double-strand breaks are much less likely to be repaired or to be repaired correctly. (This explains the efficiency of high-LET radiation in cell killing; its effectiveness at transforming a cell into a malignant one is not as well understood.)

The **relative biological effectiveness (RBE)** is a measure of the ability of a particular kind of ionizing radiation to cause damage to a specific tissue, cell, or organism. The RBE of a radiation is defined as ratio of two doses,

$$\text{RBE(LET)} = D_{\text{ref}}/D_{\text{rad}} \qquad (32.3)$$

and it is written in this form as a reminder that it is a function, in particular, of the LET of the radiation of interest. D_{ref} is the dose of a reference type (typically 250-kVp x-rays or cobalt-60 gamma rays) that gives rise to some particular biologic effect, and D_{rad} is the dose of the radiation under study required to achieve the same biologic endpoint. The more effective the radiation in question, the less the dose required to reach the biologic endpoint and the larger the RBE. The RBE depends on the entity irradiated and its physiologic status, the biologic endpoint chosen, and the patterns of ionization produced by the radiation.

Figure 32–5 illustrates a typical RBE(LET) function, with 50% cell killing in a colony as the biologic endpoint. X-rays and electrons of all energies have roughly the same LET, hence an RBE of 1. Alpha particles are significantly more efficient at cell killing. The peak in RBE(LET) for alpha particles occurs when energy is deposited along the tracks of the ionizing particles with an LET of about 100 keV/μm. (At higher values of the LET, such as can be obtained with accelerated heavy ions, the spacing of ionizations is so close that

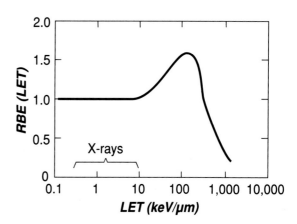

Figure 32–5. Relative biologic effectiveness (RBE) is defined, (Equation 32.3) for a specified biologic endpoint (e.g., death of 50% of the cells in a colony). This is a typical graph relating the RBE of radiation to its linear energy transfer (LET). Up to a point, the damage per gray increases as the spatial density of ionization events increases; above 100 keV/μm or so, however, diminishing returns sets in.

a sizable fraction of the dose energy is wasted; the inefficiency of this overkill situation is reflected in a falling RBE(LET) curve.)

———— **EXERCISE 32–2.** ————————

Nine grays of 250-kVp x-rays will kill 99% of the hamster fibroblast cells in a Petri dish. Three grays of 3-MeV neutrons will do the same. What is the RBE?

SOLUTION: By Equation 32.3, RBE = (9 Gy)/(3 Gy) = 3.

5. THE SIEVERT TAKES THE *Q* INTO ACCOUNT

The main message of the last section is that all grays and rads are not created equal. A centigray of alpha particles will generally cause much more biologic harm than will a centigray of x-rays.

Dose equivalent is a practical measure of quantity of ionizing radiation that takes into account its effectiveness (relative to that of x-rays) in causing biologic harm. Dose equivalent, *H*, is related to dose, *D*, by means of a **quality factor, *Q*:**

$$H = D \cdot Q \qquad (32.4)$$

The traditional unit of dose equivalent is the rem. The SI unit that is replacing it is the sievert, where 1 Sv = 100 rem.

> The quality factor *Q* is like, but not the same as, the RBE. RBE usually refers to cell killing studies; *Q* refers primarily to carcinogenesis and mutagenesis. And whereas RBE(LET) is sensitive to the precise value of the energy, the type of cells being irradiated, and the biologic endpoint, *Q* is a coarse, average measure. These differences are reflected in the use of the RBE in sophisticated radiobiology research and the *Q* for practical, applied radiation protection (health physics) purposes.

For the electrons set in motion by x-rays and gamma rays and for beta particles (all of which are low-LET forms of radiation), Q is taken to be unity,

$$Q = 1 \quad \text{(photons, beta particles)} \quad (32.5a)$$

so that the gray and the sievert are numerically equal,

$$\left.\begin{array}{l} 1\,\text{Gy} \rightarrow 1\,\text{Sv} \\ 1\,\text{rad} \rightarrow 1\,\text{rem} \end{array}\right\} \quad \text{(photons, beta particles)} \quad (32.5b)$$

The arrow is intended to suggest that a gray of dose gives rise to, or is responsible for, a sievert of dose equivalent.

Alpha particles, which are encountered in uranium mines, nuclear weapons production facilities, and houses with high radon content, have a Q of about 20:

$$Q = 20 \quad \text{(alpha particles)}$$

A 1-Gy dose of alpha particles deposits the same ionizing energy per gram in a person as does 1 Gy of x-rays, but the risk is believed to be 20 times or so greater:

$$1\,\text{Gy} \rightarrow 20\,\text{Sv} \quad \text{(alpha particles)}$$

For historical reasons, radiotherapists almost always talk in terms of centigrays (or rads), and radiation safety people prefer millisieverts or (millirems). The two sets of units are frequently employed interchangeably in imaging, but the difference in their meanings should be kept in mind. A gray of dose refers to density of ionizing energy deposited in anything (including tissue). A sievert of dose equivalent relates more specifically to risk of carcinogenesis in humans.

In the following chapters, we shall usually (but not always) follow the common and simplifying practice of letting the symbol D and the term *dose* refer both to real, physical dose (Gy or rads) and to dose equivalent (Sv and rem). The context will invariably make clear which construct is applicable and, because $Q = 1$ for radiologic purposes, the quantities will always turn out numerically right.

6. IONIZATION OF RADIATION-RESPONSIVE MATERIALS

This chapter has focused on the effect of a dose of ionizing radiation on biologic tissues. But recall from Chapters 16 and 17 that the responses of detectors also depend largely on ionization and excitation events.

Fluorescence, for example, is initiated when an x-ray photon imparts some or all of its energy to an electron in a photoelectric or Compton collision. The resultant high-velocity liberated electron then dissipates its energy in exciting hundreds or thousands of other electrons from the valence into the conduction band of the fluorescent material. Similarly, for radiographic film exposed directly to x-rays, the photographic process begins with the ejection of an electron from an atom or ion of a silver halide crystal by an x-ray photon.

Vastly different endpoints from the consequences of damage to DNA, but similar beginnings.

APPENDIX 32–1. Cell Killing with High Linear Energy Transfer Radiation

Closely related to the issue of radiation-induced carcinogenesis is that of the sterilization, or outright killing, of cells with radiation.

According to *target theory* models of cell killing, lethal damage occurs if ionizing radiation strikes certain radiosensitive sites a certain, cell-specific number of times or more. When the conditions of biology and irradiation are such that a *single hit* to a *single target* (there may be many such targets in a cell) causes cell death, then the survival curve will be purely exponential.

Consider, for example, the effect of alpha particles on a colony of actively dividing mammalian cells in a Petri dish. These high-LET charged particles leave dense trails of ionization in the cells they traverse, and DNA molecules are likely to experience either lethal double-strand breaks or no effects at all. Cell killing is therefore, under these conditions, an all-or-nothing affair, and surviving cells retain no "memory" of any irradiation which, indeed, affected only their less fortunate neighbors.

Suppose our colony originally consists of $n(0)$ cells. After a dose of D Gy of ionizing radiation, only $n(D)$ of them remain capable of dividing. With a further dose increment, ΔD, the number of "surviving" cells diminishes by an additional

$$\Delta n = -D_{37} \cdot n(D) \cdot \Delta D \quad (32.6)$$

where

$$D_{37} = -\Delta n / n \cdot \Delta D$$

is the constant (independent of previous irradiation) probability per unit dose of cell death. The relative number of survivors, $S(D)$, is given by

$$S(D) = n(D)/n(0) = e^{-D/D_{37}} \quad (32.7)$$

illustrated as the straight line in the semi-log cell *survival curve* of Figure 32–6.

The survival curve for cells exposed to low-LET radiation

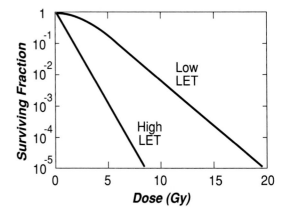

Figure 32–6. The cell survival curve for high-LET radiation tends to be nearly exponential in dose (Equation 32.7), suggestive of a single-target, single-hit model of cell killing. (Note the use of semilog graph paper.) The presence of a shoulder at low doses for low-LET radiation implies a more complex cell killing process. The reasons that high-LET radiation is more effective than low-LET radiation at killing cells are related to, but different from, the reasons why it more readily causes cancer.

such as electrons and x-ray photons normally will display an initial *shoulder* (see Fig. 32–6). In this case irradiation begins having a significant effect only after several tens or hundreds of centigray have been deposited, as with a pump that must be primed. The kill probability per unit dose depends on the amount of dose already delivered, and Equation 32.6 is replaced by

$$\Delta n = -c(D) \cdot n(D) \cdot \Delta D \qquad (32.8)$$

The independent variable in $c(D)$ implies a survival probability that is not perfectly exponential in dose. This situation might arise if each photon caused a single strand break, but cell death occurred only if there were two such events sufficiently close to one another. (Most cells have mechanisms for repairing single-strand breaks over time.)

A further aside for the mathematically inclined: It is not difficult to determine the general shape of the survival curve for the *multitarget, single-hit* model, in which there are M equally sensitive, independent, targets in a cell, and its death occurs if and only if all M targets are hit at least once. As with the single-target, single-hit situation, no detailed knowledge of radiobiology is required.

Let $p(D)$ be the probability that any particular target remains *un*hit after the cell population has received the dose D of radiation. The probability of hitting all M targets is $[1 - p(D)]^{M}$. The likelihood that at least one of the targets in a cell will be missed, such that the cell survives, is thus

$$S(D) = 1 - [1 - p(D)]^{M} \qquad (32.9a)$$

Now we employ Poisson statistics to find an expression for $p(D)$. The expected or average number, μ, of times that any given target will be struck should increase linearly with dose D delivered,

$$\mu = kD \qquad (32.9b)$$

for some constant k. By Equation 18.11a, the likelihood of a target remaining unhit (i.e., being struck zero times) when the average target receives μ hits is

$$p(D) = P_{\mu}(0) = e^{-\mu} = e^{-kD} \qquad (32.9c)$$

Insertion of Equation 32.9c into Equation 32.9a finally yields the cell survival curve for a multitarget, single-hit cell population:

$$S(D) = 1 - (1 - e^{-kD})^{M} \qquad (32.9d)$$

This expression reduces to the exponential survival curve of Equation 32.7 for the single-target, single hit case.

Carcinogenesis and Other Radiation Hazards

A fundamental objective of imaging must be to strike the soundest possible balance between the potential benefits of correct diagnosis and the risks involved in obtaining that diagnosis. This is the case both for the individual patient, whose medical situation may be unique, and in the formulation of general policies, such as on breast or chest mass screening. And the safety of the medical staff providing the diagnostic services must always be taken fully into account.

A central, and difficult, part of this optimization process is the quantification of the hazards associated with low levels of radiation exposure. This chapter covers some of the biology and epidemiology that underlie our understanding of radiation carcinogenesis and other radiation-induced health effects, with some consideration of the implications for radiation safety programs. Finally, it is noted that when one is making or implementing a policy that involves both benefits and risks, effective communication with those who will be affected can be critically important.

1. RADIOGENIC HEALTH EFFECTS

The earliest experimenters with x-rays were largely unaware of the hazards and were not overly worried about personal safety. The major side effect of irradiation commonly observed was a reddening of exposed skin; some radiologists even used this *erythema* to gauge x-ray beam strength. But many cases of severe and irreversible *radiogenic* (radiation-induced) injury, including a number of carcinomas of the epidermis, were reported in the first few decades of the century. Over the years radiologists, radium dial painters, uranium miners, atomic bomb survivors, and many others have provided tragic and extensive evidence of the dangers of ionizing radiation.

Serious radiation effects are of four general types:

1. *Acute* effects, seen after high, brief exposures. A whole-body dose of a few sieverts (a few hundred rems) delivered over a short period may lead to death within several months or less.
2. *Degenerative* damage to organs following exposures to lower doses (hundreds of millisieverts, tens of rems), such as opacification of the lens of the eye and loss of fertility.
3. *Stochastic* effects, such as carcinogenesis, or genetic effects (expressed in offspring). These can arise, many researchers believe, even at very low doses (tens of millisieverts, rems, or less).
4. *Teratogenic* effects from exposures in utero, and a lowering of intelligence or even severe mental retardation (tens of millisieverts).

At the exposure levels encountered in imaging with ionizing radiation (on the order of tens of millisieverts or less), only stochastic effects and possible harm to the fetus need be of concern (Fig. 33–1).

2. ACUTE AND OTHER NONSTOCHASTIC (DETERMINISTIC) EFFECTS OCCUR AT RELATIVELY HIGH DOSES

The word **stochastic** means that events occur randomly, and only their probabilities of occurrence can be estimated.

Acute radiation responses and the degenerative damage of organs, by contrast, are said to be **nonstochastic** or **deterministic** health effects. A nonstochastic effect will occur when the dose imparted to an organ or tissue is high enough to reduce significantly its ability to function, or in other ways to impair the individual's state of being. As such, it will occur, with

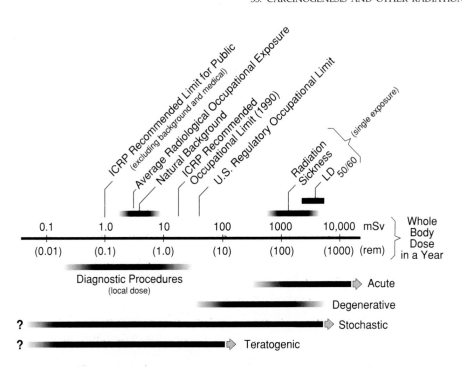

Figure 33–1. Summary of several different kinds of dose information discussed in this chapter and the next. The typical exposures and the recommended or legal limits on annual dose (all listed along the top) do not include contributions from natural background radiation nor, for a medical patient, from intentional exposure. Estimates of the $LD_{50/60}$, from which one-half a human population would die within 60 days, refer to a single, whole-body dose, as does that for radiation sickness. "Average Radiological Occupational Exposure" refers to an average among United States radiologists, cardiologists, orthopedic surgeons, general practitioners, radiologic and dental technologists, nurses, and other health care workers, along with others in medically unrelated fields, who make use of ionizing radiation in the course of their work. "Diagnostic Procedures" refers to the range of local doses to the region under examination (rather than whole-body dose) during a single procedure. At the bottom of the figure are shown the dose ranges over which the four general types of radiogenic health effects are of concern. There is no unequivocal direct evidence of the occurrence of stochastic effects in humans at very low doses (1 mSv or less), but some consider it prudent to assume that the risk is proportional to dose there. Annual exposure to natural background radiation in the United States averages about 3 mSv/y (300 mrem/y), of which 2 mSv/y is attributable to indoor radon.

a reasonable degree of certainty, if an organ-specific threshold dose level is exceeded. And the severity of the response increases with dose once the threshold is exceeded.

An acute effect in an organ is commonly a consequence of radiation-induced death of many of the organ's cells, occurring either soon after irradiation or at mitosis ("reproductive death"). As a general rule, the higher the rate of cell turnover, the more radiosensitive the organ. In 1904, Bergonie and Tribondeau noted that "The higher the reproductive activity of the cell, the longer the period of its mitosis, and the less the degree of its differentiation, the greater the biological action of Roentgen rays." The highly radiosensitive lymphocyte, which normally divides infrequently if at all, provides an interesting exception to this rule.

The deterministic category includes a wide variety of radiation sequelae among the various organs, ranging from the barely noticeable to the catastrophic. Erythema or desquamation of the skin, temporary or permanent sterility, opacification of the lens of the eye, fibrosis of the lung, ulceration of bowel and esophagus, renal failure, severing of the spinal cord, and other consequences of overexposure of parts of the body have been studied extensively, particularly in connection with cancer radiotherapy. (Indeed, it is the tolerance levels of the surrounding normal tissues that limit the aggressiveness with which a tumor can be treated with radiation.)

The disaster at Chernobyl in 1986 and the specter of Hiroshima and Nagasaki are everpresent reminders that people occasionally receive excessive whole-body exposures. The resulting radiation sickness may manifest as elevated temperature, fatigue, and nausea and vomiting, and may be followed by death. The single, whole-body dose at which 50% of a human population will die within 60 days, $LD_{50/60}$, is of the order of 3 to 5 Sv (300 to 500 rem) for individuals who receive no medical care and as high as 8 Sv for those who have excellent supportive care.

A whole-body acute exposure of 2.5 to 5 Sv may lead to the *hematopoietic syndrome* (*bone marrow death*) as a result of sterilization of the precursor cells. Death may occur within weeks or months, when the circulating cells die out and are not replenished. An exposure of 5 to 12 Sv gives rise to the *gastrointestinal (GI) syndrome*, with extensive bloody diarrhea and destruction of the GI mucosa. Depletion of the stem cells that generate the epithelium of the gut leads to death within days or weeks. Above 100 Sv, the neurologic and cardiovascular systems break down, and death by way of the *central nervous system (CNS) syndrome* follows within hours.

The hematopoietic, GI, and CNS syndromes are seen at high levels when the dose is imparted in a single exposure and at high dose rate. The body can stand high doses more readily when their delivery is spread out over time. Partly because of this, radiotherapy treatments can be *fractionated*, with certain beneficial results, into many small daily doses. If the volume undergoing treatment receives only a few hundred rads each day, the cumulative dose that a healthy tissue can stand will be much greater than its single-exposure tolerance; the same is not true, presumably, for the malignancy.

Acute effects are not observed at the dose levels encountered in diagnosis. Even low doses, however, may give rise to radiation-induced cancers.

3. RADIATION CARCINOGENESIS AND MUTAGENESIS (DELAYED, STOCHASTIC EFFECTS) MAY OCCUR AT LOW DOSE

It is generally believed that cancer in an individual results from the introduction of certain kinds of misinformation into cellular DNA, causing the failure of mechanisms that regulate cell proliferation. Similarly, hereditary effects may be expressed in offspring when the DNA of a parent's germ cells contains significant informational errors. While such failures can be a consequence of normal aging, they also may result from exposure to naturally occurring or synthetic carcinogens and mutagens.

Radiation has been called the "universal carcinogen." The cellular barriers and transport mechanisms that confine or exclude chemical and biologic agents cannot prevent the entrance of high-energy photons and electrons, and all organs and tissues are vulnerable to their effects. The evidence is convincing that a trail of ionizations through a cell can give rise to alterations of base sequences or other damage to its DNA. This can cause (or switch off the suppression of) uncontrolled mitosis.

Although ionizing radiation is perhaps the most extensively studied cancer-initiating agent, the multistage process by which it transforms a normal cell into one that is neoplastic is not fully understood. It does appear that the initial event is *stochastic* in nature; that is, a high-velocity electron or diffusing free radical interacts with cellular DNA in a random fashion, as discussed in Chapter 32. Thus, the greater the amount of radiation imparted to an organ or tissue, the larger the likelihood that at least one of its cells will undergo such a change. It is the *probability* that a cell will switch into a cancerous form that *is dose dependent*, and *not the severity* of the consequences. There is *no known threshold* below which stochastic effects do not occur, nor, on the other hand, is there certainty that a stochastic effect will show up at relatively high doses.

Because carcinogenesis and genetic effects may not become evident until years after the irradiation, these are commonly known as *delayed* effects.

4. EPIDEMIOLOGIC BASIS FOR THE LINEAR, NO-THRESHOLD CARCINOGENESIS DOSE–RESPONSE MODEL AND FOR RADIATION RISK ESTIMATES

To formulate radiation protection policy, estimates are needed of the probabilities of induction and mortality for various cancers and for severe genetic and teratogenic effects as functions of absorbed dose. While useful insights have been provided by animal and in vitro cell studies, the most important information has come from epidemiologic studies of cancer incidence and mortality among Hiroshima and Nagasaki A-bomb survivors, patients of therapeutic (e.g., for ankylosing spondylitis) and diagnostic (e.g., multiple fluoroscopy for tuberculosis) radiologic procedures, and uranium miners and other occupationally exposed groups. The results of these studies are summarized in a series of reports from the United Nations Scientific Committee on the Effects of Atomic Radiation (UN-SCEAR) and from the Committee on Biological Effects of Ionizing Radiation (BEIR) of the National Research Council (NRC) of the National Academy of Sciences. The most recent BEIR report, entitled *Health Effects of Exposure to Low Levels of Ionizing Radiation* and referred to as *BEIR V*, appeared in 1990.

Analysis of the available data is difficult, and few of the conclusions drawn from it can be accepted unquestioningly. First, there are obvious possible problems with the quality of the raw data, such as the reliability of death certificate information in some study groups. This is complicated by the *latency period* of cancer induction. While leukemias (especially childhood leukemias) may show up within a few years of exposure, solid tumors take typically one or two decades, making it hard to establish a link with any potential causal agent.

Also, the probabilities of occurrence of "natural" (and radiogenic?) cancers may depend strongly on factors such as age, sex, diet, race, nationality, socioeconomic level, and occupation. There may also be various selective biases in the data: Studies of radiation workers may be influenced by the *healthy worker effect.* (Individuals in dangerous or demanding jobs tend to be fitter than others and inherently less prone to some sickness; also, they are usually kept under more careful medical surveillance, which helps to maintain their state of well-being.) Similar considerations may apply to the long-term survivors of the atomic bomb blasts.

There is little direct evidence of carcinogenesis at less than 100 mSv (10 rem) or so (although data exist suggesting the induction of cancers by exposures in utero of less than 10 mSv). Therefore risks at low doses, in the region of clinical interest, must be estimated by interpolating down from the higher doses where the data do exist. Figure 33–2 illustrates some of the problems that arise in constructing such a *dose–response* or *dose–effect* curve. The curve is obtained by observing people exposed to various amounts of radiation and counting the relative number of cancers of a particular type found at each dose level. Radiogenic cancers are not distinguishable from others, however, and the very few radiation-induced cancers that result from low doses are totally swamped by statistical fluctuations in the orders-of-magnitude larger background number of "natural" cancer deaths. Thus, the most statistically significant data points are for individuals who received doses of the order of 100 to 200 mSv (10 to 20 rem) or more.

Unfortunately there are no certain signs from epidemiology, animal studies, or theory as to the shape of the low-dose portion of the dose–response curve. But it is reasonable to assume that at relatively low exposure levels, the probability of cancer induction is a smoothly varying function of dose. Even complicated functions seem simple and smooth when the independent variable is confined to a relatively small domain. It is therefore to be expected that at low doses, the probability of occurrence of a stochastic effect will involve a function, $f(D)$, that is either linear in dose equivalent, D,

$$f(D) = \alpha_1 D \qquad (33.1a)$$

nal may have been 01010000, for example, or 11111100. But if the odds of there being one mistake are small, which is usually the case, the chance of there being two errors is *very* small.

2. A COMPUTER IS A MACHINE THAT PROCESSES INFORMATION ACCORDING TO A PROGRAM

A computer accepts **input information** from a source, acts on it in a way determined by a *stored set of instructions,* or **program**, and generates an **output**. (This output might be displayed as print or images, or might control a machine or process, or serve as the input for another program or another computer.) The physical components of the computer constitute the **hardware**. The set of stored (by the hardware) programs is called the **software**. And the information actually operated on is the *data*. Blocks of software that can be accessed separately are known as program (instruction) **files** and data files.

Programs fall into two general categories: operating system programs and applications programs. The **operating system** is the set of programs that keep the computer itself running—managing the disks, keyboard, and other physical devices and performing a variety of necessary housekeeping functions. The operating system programs are not immediately related to the details of the specific task at hand, and a "user-friendly" operating system is largely invisible (transparent) to the user. The choice of operating system for a computer depends on the power of the computer and on the complexity of the jobs that it must confront. MS-DOS, for example, is well suited for running small personal computers, with one user carrying out a single task at a time; UNIX is a more powerful operating system commonly employed with sophisticated computers that can serve many users performing different tasks simultaneously.

Particular **applications programs** that perform image manipulation, statistical analyses, word processing, and so on, are usually written by a vendor or the user in a programmer-friendly **higher level language** (e.g., ADA, BASIC, C, FORTRAN, PASCAL).

A computer is designed to think in bits and bytes. It consists of tremendous numbers of microscopic, solid-state devices that, in effect, act like switches. These are *binary* switches, with only two possible states: shut and open. Such a pair of physical conditions can be used to represent the two possible *states* that a bit can assume, namely, 1 and 0. The computer's *memory*, for example, includes *registers*, banks of such electronic switches used to store sequences of bits. When the computer *writes* the byte 01011100 into an 8-bit register, for example, its eight switches are left in the configuration shown in Figure 35–1. The computer can later *read* the register by trying to send currents through all eight switches and seeing which ones conduct. It can use other kinds of switchable, binary physical processes to represent 0 and 1 bits, too, such as high and low voltages or microscopic regions of magnetic material whose magnetization can be aligned in either of two directions. In any of these fashions, a computer can store numbers and other symbols and reveal them on demand.

A computer is also capable of performing arithmetic and logical operations involving numbers and symbols. As a very simple example, let's devise a combination of switches to test

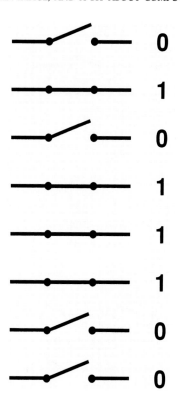

Figure 35–1. One byte of information can be stored in an 8-bit register that consists, in essence, of eight switches. An open switch corresponds to a 0 and a closed switch to a 1. The content of this register is the byte 01011100.

the truth of the compound statement "it is cool and sunny," where each of the two component statements, "it is cool" and "it is sunny," may be either true or false. An AND circuit might consist of a battery, a light bulb, and two switches in series (Fig. 35–2A). Suppose "it is cool" is represented by a switch that is *closed* when the statement is *true,* and open when the statement is false (Fig. 35–2B), and so also for "it is sunny." Current flows around the complete circuit (causing the bulb to light and indicating that the compound statement "it is cool and sunny" is true) only when the component statements are both true (Fig. 35–2C).

EXERCISE 35–4.

Devise an OR system of switches that can determine if at least one of two statements is true.

SOLUTION: A pair of switches in parallel (Fig. 35–3A) will conduct current in three of the four possible configurations. Its truth table is shown in Figure 35–3B.

Much of the work of a computer can be carried out by means of combinations of simple AND, OR, and the closely related NOT and NAND circuits. An adder that sums two bits, for example, can be built out of 11 AND circuits, 5 ORs, and 3

"AND" Logic

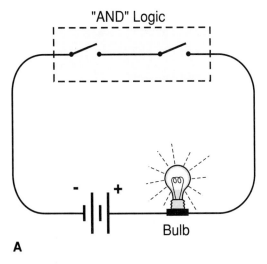

A

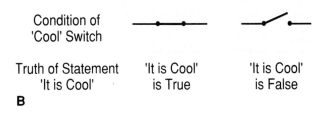

B

Cool	Sunny		Cool & Sunny
False	False		False
False	True		False
True	False		False
True	True		True

C

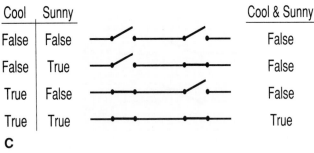

Figure 35–2. Processing information with switches. **A.** A simple "AND" logic circuit. **B.** A statement is true if the corresponding switch is closed. **C.** The AND circuit will conduct only if both switches are closed, just as a compound statement is true only if the first AND the second constituent parts are separately true.

NOTs, and requires 21 separate transistors. A byte-adder that sums two bytes is made up of eight such bit-adders. More involved mathematical operations, such as multiplication and integration, can be performed by multiple use of these simple circuits; the product 17 × 9 may be evaluated by adding 17 to itself 9 times.

What makes this rather tedious and simpleminded approach feasible is the phenomenal speed with which a computer takes its tiny steps. Individual switches can be made to

"OR" Logic

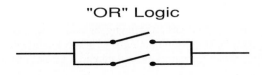

A

Cool	Sunny	Cool or Sunny
False	False	False
False	True	True
True	False	True
True	True	True

B

Figure 35–3. A pair of switches in parallel constitute an "OR" circuit. Current can flow if either one OR the other of them is closed or if both are closed.

open and close tens or hundreds of millions of times a second, in synchrony with the computer's internal master clock. So even an operation that requires a hundred thousand separate switchings may still be carried out in under a millisecond.

The wizardry of the computer stems ultimately from the fact that the very commands that tell switches to open and close can themselves be represented by combinations of bits. A program is a sequence of such commands that together lead to the performance of some logical or arithmetic task, and the program itself is stored in the computer's memory. The computer has ways, of course, of knowing which strings of bits constitute the operating system and applications programs and which are data.

The architecture of a digital computer is shown, in most rudimentary form, in Figure 35–4.

The **central processing unit (CPU),** is the part that actually performs logical and arithmetic calculations and, in other ways, directly processes information. The CPU for a micro- or minicomputer employed in clinical imaging is often constructed on a single wafer, or *chip,* of silicon (Fig. 35–5) known as a **microprocessor**.

> In carrying out highly specific image processing operations, such as those involved in CT image reconstruction, the system might also make use of an *array processor*. This idiot-savant of the computer world is something like a CPU, but is designed and hard-wired to undertake only one or a few highly specific tasks; it lacks the flexibility of a CPU, but can perform its highly specialized jobs at much greater speed.

Memory usually refers to the large numbers of sets of solid-state switches that store the operating system and the ap-

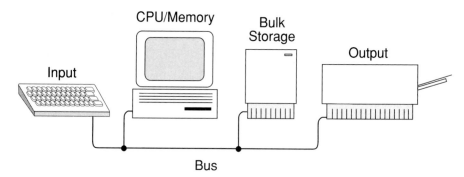

Figure 35–4. Rudimentary block diagram of a computer system. The central processing unit (CPU) and its immediately accessible (random access) memory are connected to the input and output devices, and bulk memory, by means of buses.

plications program that are currently directing the CPU, and the data that the system is manipulating. The CPU chip itself contains some memory, and has immediate access to thousands or millions of bytes of additional memory on separate memory chips. *Bulk storage* consists of the hard disks, floppy disks, optical disks, tape, or other devices used to store information for intermediate or long periods. (Long-term storage is also known as *archiving*.)

The *input* device consists of a keyboard and cathode-ray tube (CRT) display, perhaps, or a medical imaging machine. *Output* information might be fed to a TV monitor and multiformat camera, a laser printer, or a telephone line or radio transmitter.

The four main components are linked together by collections of electrical cables, or *buses*. The CPU and memory together are commonly referred to as "the computer," the various input, output, and bulk memory devices as "peripheral devices," and the whole thing as the "computer system." Several independent computer systems in a hospital or region can be linked together to makeup a **local area network (LAN).**

3. MOVING INFORMATION AROUND WITHIN A COMPUTER SYSTEM

A computer is continually moving information around within itself, back and forth with its peripheral devices, and perhaps even with other computer systems. It can transmit bits one at a time, somewhat like Morse code, as a temporal sequence of low and high voltages that correspond to 0 and 1 bit. The byte 01011100 would appear on a wire as the sequence of voltages

(relative to ground) in Figure 35–6A. Such serial transmission is commonly used for communication between the CPU and relatively low-speed peripheral devices such as keyboards, printers, and modems. Alternatively, a computer can transmit all the bits of an entire byte simultaneously, through a parallel channel that consists of eight separate wires, as in Figure 35–6B. Either way, there are only two possible voltages on a wire, "low" and "high," and if the difference between the two is sufficiently great, the introduction of errors into a message becomes very unlikely. *Analog* signals (in which the voltage varies smoothly and continuously over some range), by contrast, are easily subject to distortion and the injection of noise, as is readily apparent on your TV whenever a plane flies by.

Communication among chips within a computer may be via short pieces of ordinary wire. Signals between a computer and its peripheral devices are commonly carried on *coaxial cable* (in which the two conductors are a hollow tube of wire braid and a single central wire, separated from one another by insulating material), which is relatively resistant to electrical noise. Megabits of information per second can be transmitted on coax over short distances with an error rate of under 10^{-9} (one error per billion bits transmitted).

Information may also be transmitted within or among

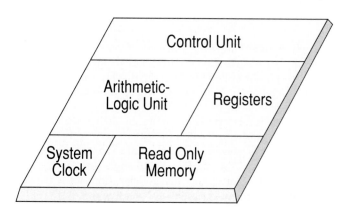

Figure 35–5. A typical microprocessor, the "brains" of a computer, is 1 cm or so on a side.

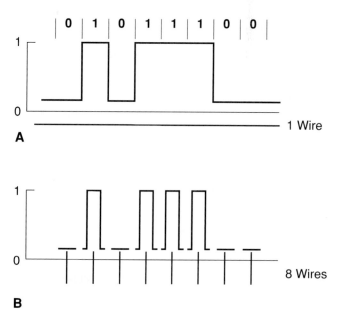

Figure 35–6. Transmission of the byte 01011100. **A.** In series, on one wire (voltages being taken relative to that on a "ground" wire). **B.** In parallel, on eight wires.

computer systems by means of *fiber optics*. Light-emitting diodes (LEDs) transform digital electronic signals into pulses of light. These are conducted along fine filaments of glass or plastic (coated with a material that refracts and reflects escaping light back into the fiber), switched by electro-optic devices, and detected by photoelectric diodes. Fiberoptic systems can transmit at very high rates (2,000 Mbit/s or more) and are totally insensitive to electrical noise. Also, it is possible to pass several messages simultaneously through a single channel ("multiplexing") by using a different color of light for each.

4. DIGITAL REPRESENTATION OF AN IMAGE: EXAMPLE OF THE DIGITIZED RADIOGRAPH

Let us return briefly to the process, introduced in Chapter 1, Section 3, and Chapter 24, Section 1, of digitizing a radiograph. Recall that the film is partitioned into an imaginary matrix, or grid, of pixels. A computer directs a laser beam to the pixels one at a time and, for each, a photodetector produces a voltage proportional to the amount of light transmitted through the film. (Alternatively, a film mounted on a light box can be viewed by a TV camera.) The analog voltage from the photodetector (or TV camera) (Fig. 35–7A) is *sampled*, and then *digitized* by means of an *analog-to-digital* (A/D) converter (sometimes written ADC) (Fig. 35–7B). The image can then be represented as a matrix of binary pixel *addresses* and *values*. There are some losses of information in sampling and digitizing, and our system must be designed to ensure that the image is not degraded beyond its level of usefulness.

> You and a mercury thermometer together constitute an analog sensing device and an A/D converter. The length of the mercury column is a continuous function of temperature, but you read and report it only to the nearest tenth of a degree.

The spatial frequency (samples per centimeter) with which the system must sample the analog voltage coming from the photodetector or TV camera is inversely related to desired pixel size. The smaller the pixels and the greater their number (and the greater the number of gray levels employed), the more faithfully can the representation capture the original image. It should be self-evident (and it reflects the important Nyquist Sampling Theorem of Information Theory) that a pixel should be smaller than half the size of smallest detail that needs to be resolved. Similar considerations arise with television raster patterns (see Chapter 29, Section 5).

> Digitization of an image that happens to be spatially periodic may give rise to an interesting interference phenomenon called *aliasing*. If the pixel dimension is comparable to the spatial period of the object being imaged, a "beat" interference pattern may appear. This is similar to the moiré pattern that appears when two sheets of silk lie flat on one another.

To redisplay the image, it is necessary to select a suitable **gray scale**, or relationship between the pixel value at any address and the corresponding pixel brightness (and/or color) in the physical display. The number of different gray scale val-

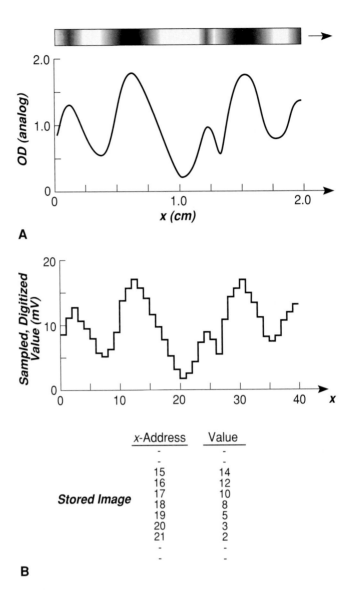

Figure 35–7. Digitization and digital representation of an image. **A.** A laser scans a film, moving in the *x* direction, and generates a continuously varying (analog) voltage in a photodetector. **B.** The analog voltage is sampled every 0.5 mm, and reported to the nearest millivolt. The information is stored as a listing of all spatial addresses and corresponding voltages. The image can be displayed by reversing the process.

ues, which determines the fineness of possible shading, is called the *image depth*. One might choose to have a pixel value of 0 correspond to pitch black on the display, and some suitably large value (such as 255) to white, but other choices of gray scale depth may be preferable.

The gray level step size generally should be less than what can be distinguished visually. But little is gained by making the separation of gray levels correspond to an intensity difference smaller than the random fluctuations in intensity that occur naturally. Thus, the "noise" level imposes a natural lower bound on the useful intensity level step size. At the other extreme, too small a number of gray scale levels can give rise to artifacts, such as the appearance of false sharp edges.

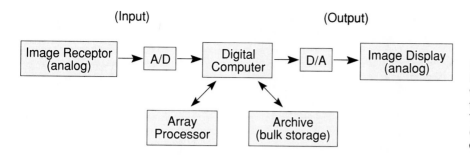

Figure 35–8. Typical imaging system. The image receptor generates an analog voltage which, after passage through an analog-to-digital converter (A/D), is entered into a computer. The image is processed, and the output voltage (after digital-to-analog conversion) controls the display device.

____ EXERCISE 35–5. _____

How many bits are required to represent a 280-level gray scale?

SOLUTION: 9 bits. An 8-bit system can handle at most only 256 levels of gray (typically designated levels 0 through 255).

____ EXERCISE 35–6. _____

What is the *precision* in gray scale *depth* that a system with a 10-bit gray scale can achieve?

SOLUTION: $2^{10} = 1000$, approximately. A 10-bit deep gray scale can provide 1/1000 or 0.1% precision.

In the preceding example, the film plus the laser optical densitometer served as an image acquisition system. As the laser scanned the film, an analog voltage signal proportional to the transmitted intensity or optical density was produced, along with corresponding address information. Other digital imaging systems begin the same way, with the generation of a continuous or pulsed signal voltage by a receptor (Fig. 35–8). In digital angiography, for example, the detector system consists of an image intensifier optically coupled to a TV camera; in CT, it is an array of xenon gas ionization detectors or solid-state fluorescent x-ray detectors; in MRI, a radio-frequency pickup coil (rf antenna). In each case, there is produced an analog voltage that is a measure of tissue characteristics at points within the patient that can somehow be located or identified. The analog signal voltage is digitized (as are voltages that keep track of the pixel addresses, if need be), subjected to image reconstruction or other image processing techniques, and stored in memory. For subsequent display, addresses and signal values are transformed back into analog voltages, and fed into the display device. The resulting array of pixel intensities relates to tissue parameters at the corresponding points in the body.

5. ONE (1024 × 1024) IMAGE IS WORTH A MILLION (8-BIT) WORDS

The potential **information content** of an image depends on the size and amount of spatial detail and on the subtlety of the gray scale shading. Unfortunately, the amount of computer time and/or power required to process the image and the cost both increase with the information content.

The number of pixels required to represent the image increases with both the dimensions of the region of interest and the desired spatial resolution:

$$\text{number of pixels} = (\text{image area})(\text{pixels/area}) \quad (35.2a)$$

This can be expressed in an equivalent form involving the pixel size:

$$\text{number of pixels} = \text{image area/pixel area} \quad (35.2b)$$

The number of bits required to address any particular pixel depends, in turn, on the total number of pixels. If an image is electronically partitioned according to a 1024 × 1024 grid, for example, the intensity is determined at a million (approximately) sites. The x and y coordinates can each be expressed as a 10-bit binary number, so that every site can be accessed by a single 20-bit address.

Likewise, the number of bits required to represent the image intensity at each pixel depends on the maximum number of gray levels that the system is designed to accommodate. If every picture element is to display 256 levels of gray (requiring an 8-bit deep value system), then the image is fully described in a listing of a million bytes, one for each address. For greater contrast resolution or dynamic range, more than one byte (e.g., 10 bits) would be used per address.

____ EXERCISE 35–7. _____

A laser beam 100 μm in diameter is used to digitize a 14 × 17-in. film. What is the pixel format?

SOLUTION: 14 × 17 in. = 355,600 × 431,800 μm. If each pixel is to have dimensions comparable to that of the laser beam, the pixel format will be something like 3600 × 4400.

6. MAKING BEST USE OF THE GRAY SCALE: WINDOWING AND COLOR

A variety of computer-based techniques have been developed to enhance the diagnostic utility of digital images. Perhaps the most widely employed of these is **windowing** (Fig. 35–9).

Also known as *contrast enhancement, contrast stretching,* or *gray level mapping* (because every gray level value in an image is mapped to a new value according to some prescription), *windowing* refers to the manipulation of the gray scale to improve image appearance. The objective is generally to force the *full* range of display brightness levels (from pitch black to pure white) to correspond to only the most interesting portion of the range of values that the physical parameter being imaged can assume.

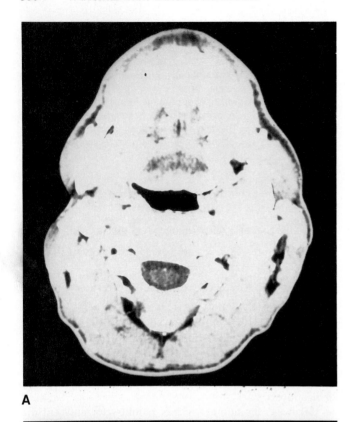

A

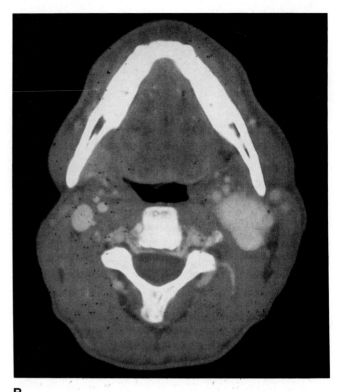

B

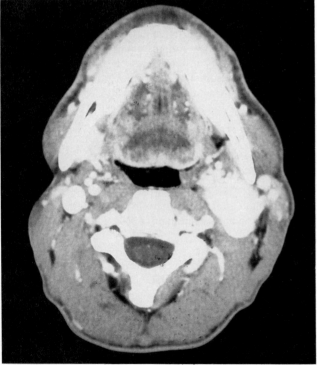

C

Figure 35–9. Effect of windowing. Shown are three computed tomography (CT) images of a contrast-enhanced neck. **A.** This image is too narrowly windowed; that is, the full display scale, from black to white, corresponds to only a small range of the measured CT numbers (amounts of x-ray attenuation). As a result, tissues that happen to lie outside that range appear all black or all white. **B.** With windowing that is too wide, large differences in tissue characteristics appear as small differences in shades of gray, and contrast is too low. **C.** Proper windowing. *[Photos courtesy of GE Medical Systems].*

Suppose, for example, that in a digitized radiograph, the region of interest (ROI) is much brighter, on average, than the rest of the image. The relevant physical parameter is the optical density (OD) of the film (and, indirectly, the attenuation of the x-ray beam within the patient). The **display window level** can be set so that the middle of the gray scale corresponds to the middle of the exposure range of interest, and the **display window width** is adjusted to cover that range adequately (Fig. 35–10). In effect, one can alter the effective speed and gamma of the system (after completion of the exposure) to optimize the average level of brightness, and the amount of contrast, in the ROI.

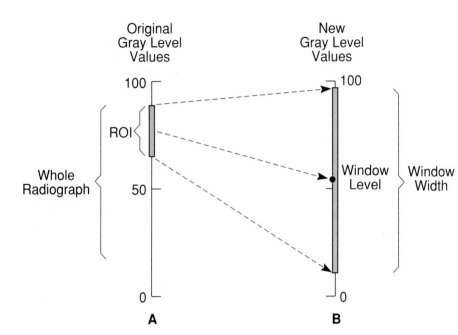

Figure 35–10. Example of window selection. **A.** Suppose the region of interest (ROI) within an image makes use of only a fraction of the available gray scale. **B.** Through a "mapping," the gray scale is stretched and shifted until nearly the entire range of intensities (or shades of gray from black to white) corresponds to the range of image/tissue values found in the ROI.

This kind of operation can be carried out automatically by the computer, by means of *histogram windowing*. A histogram (see Chapter 18, Appendix 18–1) is constructed out of the relative numbers of pixels with the different starting gray scale values. In the simplest form of histogram windowing, the gray scale is then adjusted so that pure white corresponds to one end of the histogram, and pure black to the other. More complex approaches have been developed to make even better use of the information content of the histogram.

Another way to increase the effectiveness of display may be to introduce color. *False colors* can draw attention to regions of special interest. In nuclear medicine, for example, areas of high and low radionuclide concentration might appear red and blue, respectively. Alternatively, different colors can be assigned to different physical characteristics in one image or in a set of simultaneously displayed monochromatic images. It should be noted, however, that some physicians tend to find coloration, in some situations, more distracting than helpful.

7. MAKING THE IMAGE MORE MEANINGFUL TO THE EYE: AVERAGING AND OTHER FILTERING

Once in the computer, an image can be processed in other ways as well. Parts or all of the image can be blown up in size or minified, rotated, inverted, or stretched in various ways. The computer can enhance edges or draw line borders where the gray scale values are rapidly changing. A series of still images can be run in rapid sequence, to yield a cine effect. If three-dimensional image display capability is available, as with MRI or multislice CT, the possibilities for image manipulation increase manyfold.

Digital filters may be used to reduce noise, correct some inherent inadequacies of the imaging system, or in other ways improve image quality. Like an audio low-pass filter, which removes high-frequency random electrical noise, a *smoothing program* diminishes random fluctuations in the pixel values

among neighboring pixels. Suppose, for example, that in a nuclear medicine study, the gray level value of a pixel is the count of detected gamma rays coming from the corresponding part of the body. Even with a uniform spatial distribution of radionuclide, there will be naturally occurring variations in the numbers of counts in adjacent voxels, as described by Equation 18.11, purely because radioactive decay is a Poisson statistical process. One simple smoothing algorithm replaces the number N_1 in pixel 1 with something like

$$\text{new } N_1 = (4 \cdot N_1 + N_2 + N_3 + N_4 + N_5)/8 \qquad (35.3)$$

where $N_2, \dots, N_5$ are the original numbers of counts in the four nearest-neighbor pixels. The computer then does the same for pixel 2, and so on. This spatial blurring represents a real loss of information, in particular of pixel-sized detail, but the resulting smoother image may nonetheless be clinically more meaningful to the eye. Other algorithms can subtract the average background from throughout the image. Others yet can amplify small differences in contrast between adjacent regions and/or emphasize the edge between them.

Some clinical procedures are followed as functions of time, with the same region of interest imaged in a temporal sequence of distinct *frames*. If the image does not change too rapidly over time, the value at a particular pixel address may be *frame averaged* over several consecutive frames. As suggested by Equation 18.5, the signal-to-noise will increase with the number of frames used, N, as

$$\text{SNR}(N) = \text{SNR}(1) \cdot \sqrt{N} \qquad (35.4)$$

The temporal resolution will decrease accordingly. Alternatively, the computer can subtract sequential frames from one another, thereby highlighting the changes that have occurred over the times between them.

___ **EXERCISE 35–8.** ___

In MRI, it is common practice to create two separate versions of each image, with all imaging parameters held the same, and average them. How much does this improve the ability of the system to reveal low-contrast lesions?

SOLUTION: According to Equation 35.4, averaging two images improves the SNR, compared with that of a single image, by a factor of $\sqrt{2} \sim 1.4$. By Equation 18.6, an irregularity with 1.4 less contrast would now be detectable.

Finally, it is becoming apparent that computers can do more than just process images for better use by the eye and brain of the physician. A computer itself may be able to search images for clinically significant patterns. Such *pattern recognition* and *image analysis* capabilities are still in their infancy, but *expert systems* that can detect spatial patterns characteristic of certain pathologic conditions in liver, lung, breast, and other organs have already been reported. More about this exciting and demanding area of research in Chapter 48.

8. THREE-DIMENSIONAL DISPLAY

A form of display that is finding increasing use (such as in pre-operative planning for neuro-, facial, and orthopedic surgery) is the three-dimensional **surface rendering** of organs and bones. The skull in Figure 35–11, for example, was constructed out of a number of adjacent CT cranial slices. The computer finds the interface between bone and soft tissue in each slice, where the x-ray linear attenuation coefficient (and CT number) changes abruptly, and draws a contour line there. A program then "tiles" the bone surface area defined by the stack of contours, and modulates the shading so as to give the impressions of overlap and depth.

The **volume-rendered** heart in Figure 35–12A was generated with CT by, in effect, assigning to each voxel of the display an optical transparency that is determined by the x-ray linear attenuation coefficient of the tissue in the corresponding

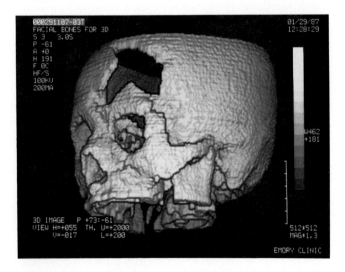

Figure 35–11. Surface rendering of a skull, constructed out of a set of separate computed tomography slices. A software program automatically draws a contour along the outer surface of the bone in each slice. The set of individual contours then makes up a "wire-frame" image of the skull. Finally, a "paving" program covers the wire-frame image with a surface. *(Photo courtesy of Philips Medical Systems.)*

volume element of the body. In Figure 35–12A, the image display parameters have been set to create a heart that is nearly transparent everywhere, except in the coronary arteries, which contain contrast agent. A readjustment of the display parameters, so as to cause all tissues to appear opaque, yields an image (Fig. 35–12B) that gives the impression of surface rendering, although it was produced in a very different fashion.

Holographic technology, using lasers, can provide a truly three-dimensional aspect to images. Perhaps as significant will be the impact of computer-based *virtual reality* interactive display systems. Virtual reality would allow the physician to, in effect, shrink to microscopic size and move about within the three-dimensional region of interest, viewing parts of it from any desired vantage point. Until recently the stuff of science fiction, such display may come to play important roles in surgical planning and elsewhere.

9. IMAGE DISPLAY HARDWARE

An image generated by computer may be viewed directly in real time, as on a TV monitor, or after production of a hard copy. Either way, each address of the image in memory is *bit-mapped* to a unique pixel location of the display.

A modern computer monitor used for imaging is essentially a TV monitor, but with significantly greater resolution capability. The display consists typically of 1024 lines, with 1024 distinct points (pixels) per line, yielding a 1-million-pixel image. This is comparable to the images attainable with high-definition television (HDTV). (The difficulties with HDTV have had to do not with the monitor tube, but rather with the need to *compress* information extremely rapidly, for transmission through a relatively narrow bandwidth channel, and then decompress it at the receiver end.)

Many CRTs employed as high-quality computer monitors do not interlace lines of two fields to create a new frame every 1/30th second. Although interlacing works well for commercial television, for static images it can lead to some impression of flicker. One solution for computer display is to scan the entire frame 60 times per second. Alternatively one can select a CRT with a phosphor of longer persistence; this may produce annoying lag effects, however, when parts of an image do move rapidly.

Other possibilities being considered for video viewing are liquid crystal, fluorescent, gas plasma, or other flat panel displays, if the brightness and resolution can be improved adequately.

The CRT coupled to a multiformat film camera is widely used as a source of hard copy. With a laser camera (or laser printer), by contrast, a laser beam of variable intensity scans film (or paper) directly; it is not necessary first to produce an optical image on a CRT, as a separate step, to be photographed. With a laser beam about 100 μm diameter, the resolution can approach 10 lp/mm, which is considerably better than what can be achieved by photographing a CRT.

The resolution inherent in a digital image and that of the available display device are not necessarily mutually compatible. Nuclear medicine is an inherently low resolution modality, and a 128 × 128-pixel matrix is adequate to represent most information that can be obtained. A standard TV monitor, with 525 raster lines per frame, would be more than sufficient for the

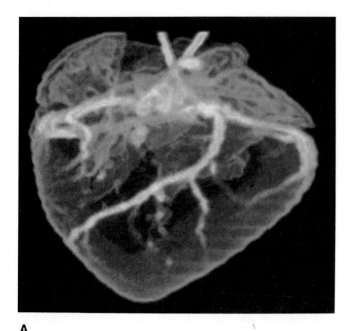 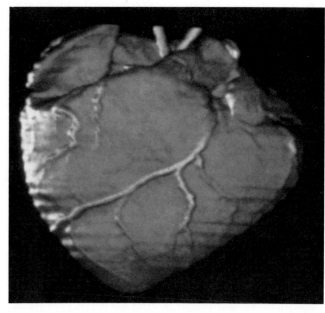

A   B

Figure 35–12.   Volume rendering of an image of an hog heart, from data obtained by multislice computed tomography. **A.** The display parameters are adjusted in such a manner that all voxels are nearly transparent, except for those corresponding to volume elements in the heart that contain contrast agent (i.e., the coronary arteries). **B.** With a readjustment of the display parameters, so that all voxels appear opaque, the image resembles one that is surface-rendered. *(Photos courtesy of B. Knosp, R. Frank, M. Marcus, and R. Weiss, University of Iowa Image Analysis Facility and Department of Internal Medicine, and Vital Images, Inc. Fairfield, Iowa.)*

job. High-resolution digital radiography, on the other hand, may employ a matrix as fine as 4096 × 4096, and standard TV technology is inadequate. Such differences must be taken into account in the design of display hardware and software.

10. DATA COMPRESSION: STORING MORE INFORMATION IN LESS MEMORY

It can become extremely expensive and time consuming to store or transmit large volumes of data, such as the tens of megabytes of information involved in producing the single three-dimensional image in Figure 35–11. But image **data compression** techniques, going by such esoteric names as "discrete cosine transform" and "fractal compression," can in a few seconds of computer time reduce the number of bits required to represent an image by an order of magnitude (factor of 10) or more. The process of compression is known as *encoding,* and the reverse process, restoration of image to near- or perfect original form, as *decoding.*

A very simple example: Suppose we are using a 10-bit gray scale, with possible values running between 0 and 1023. The computer discovers, in some image, that pixels at the adjacent addresses 5283 through 5288 happen to have the same gray level, namely, 5 (Table 35–3A). We could store this information as is. But we could also cleverly define a special command that lets the computer drop all but the first and last addresses for a series of identical gray level values: We remove the particular value 1023 from the gray scale itself, and reserve it as a "flag", which indicates that all the addresses from the flagged one to the next one listed contain the same pixel value (in this example, 5) (Table 35–3B).

This is an example of perfect or *noiseless* encoding, in which there is no loss of information or introduction of noise. It may be possible to obtain more (or cheaper or faster) compression with noisy methods, in which there is some loss of information and degradation of image quality, but such methods can be adopted only if images that are decompressed and redisplayed remain clinically adequate.

11. IMAGE STORAGE HARDWARE

Most computer-based imaging systems use magnetic hard disks for intermediate-term data storage and magnetic floppy

TABLE 35–3. A SIMPLE EXAMPLE OF DATA COMPRESSION[a]

A. Original Data		B. After Compression	
Address	*Value*	*Address*	*Value*
5281	620	5281	620
5282	623	5282	623
5283	5	5283	1023 (flag)
5284	5	5288	5
5285	5	5289	614
5286	5	5290	612
5287	5		
5288	5		
5289	614		
5290	612		

[a]The particular pixel value 1023 is reserved, as a flag. It indicates that the addresses between the current one and the next one listed all contain the same pixel value.

TABLE 35–4. TYPICAL STORAGE PARAMETERS (AS OF 1991)

	Capacity (Mbyte)	Access Time	Cost ($/Mbyte)
Semiconductor memory	1–20	μs	300
Magnetic hard disk	20–1200	50 ms	20
Optical disk	2000	100 ms (same platter) 10 s (different platter)	0.05
Magnetic floppy disk	1	sec	0.50
Laser card	10	sec	
Magnetic tape	20–200	min	0.20
Optical tape	125,000	min	

disks and tapes for long-term archiving. For all three, as with videotape (see Chapter 29, Section 4), information is encoded on a magnetizable medium that moves relative to write and read heads. But although the magnitude and orientation of the magnetization change continuously along analog videotape, it assumes only two values (representing "1" and "0") on digital tapes and disks, and a small physical gap is inserted between adjacent bit locations (Table 35–4).

A *disk* allows rapid **random access** to data files. Like the needle of a phonograph player, the read head can be moved almost instantaneously to the appropriate sector of the disk. A "Winchester disk" drive contains several rigid magnetic platters permanently mounted within an airtight, mechanically secure housing. Other, generally more expensive, drives use hermetically sealed but removable packs of disks. A single hard disk stores 10 or 20 megabytes of data, and a disk pack may contain 20 or more platters (Table 35–4). That may seem like a lot of information, but bear in mind that one $1024 \times 1024 \times 8$ image (1 million addresses, with a gray scale value 8 bits deep) consumes 1 Mbyte of memory, and that a single study may use tens of images.

A rapidly gaining competitor to the magnetic hard disk is the **optical disk**, which is similar to the audio compact disk (CD). A laser writes by burning microscopic pits through the metal film coating on a plastic optical platter, and reads by sensing reflected laser light. A platter may store 3 gigabytes (Gbyte, 3×10^9 bytes), and a mass storage optical disk *jukebox* might hold a hundred or so platters. Unlike a magnetic disk or tape, which can easily be erased and reused many times, most currently available optical disks are *write once, read many* times (WORM) devices. Erasable optical storage disks, however, are also commercially available.

> One form of write many, read many optical storage makes use of a laser–magnet combination. The magnetization of a region of the magnetizable material can be changed by an applied field only when heated. A laser, in turn, can provide the necessary heating and confine it to an extremely small area.
>
> Electron trapping optical medium (ETOM) storage also holds promise for rapid access to vast amounts of information. A disk is coated with a material that contains many electron traps per unit volume. Writing and reading involve exciting electrons into and out of these traps with laser light of different colors.
>
> As of this writing, 4-Mbyte LSI large-scale integration (LSI), transistor-based memory chips are available.

Hard disks may be necessary for rapid image acquisition and processing, but there is need for another, less expensive approach for long-term archiving. *Magnetic tape* provides only *serial access* to information—one may have to spool through great lengths of irrelevant material before coming to the file that is needed—but it is capable of storing vast amounts of data relatively cheaply. A 1200-ft-long, nine-track tape that takes 1600 bits per inch (bpi) on each track holds 23 Mbyte, and a 2400-ft-long, 6250-bpi tape holds 180 Mbyte. *Optical tape* works essentially like the magnetic variety, but uses a laser to burn a permanent record into the plastic and to read it. It has significantly greater storage capacity than a piece of magnetic tape of the same length, but it cannot be reused.

The removable *floppy disk* or diskette and the *laser card* are intermediate between disk and tape in terms of access time and cost, but are of limited storage capacity. They allow easy storage or local transfer of relatively small amounts of information.

12. HOW NOT TO PICK UP A COMPUTER VIRUS

We shall conclude this introduction to computers on a note of caution. Any computer, or network of interlinked computers, is a system, to a large extent built on trust, for processing and probably sharing information. The users must be able to assume the basic integrity of the data being exchanged and of the system itself.

It is regrettable but to be expected, however, that some individuals may try to find ways to cause disruptions. It is therefore necessary, in the interest of security, to restrict access and to limit the free flow of information. **Passwords** and other such measures are minor nuisances, compared with the havoc the malicious misuser can wreak.

> An insidious source of problems is the *computer virus*. (A "worm" is practically the same thing.) A virus is a segment of code, intentionally inserted into an applications program, that gains entry to a computer under false pretenses and then "crashes" the system and perhaps other systems linked to it. Or it might be designed to destroy certain programs or data files. Or, perhaps worst of all because it is so hard to detect, it could cause certain programs to make occasional but critical errors. A virus can go to work right away, or after any incubation period chosen by its creator.

There are no ways to protect completely against viruses, but practicing the computer equivalent of safe sex can reduce the likelihood of infection. First, abstain if you can. Don't enter outside programs into your system unless you really need them. Obtain the programs that you do require from reputable sources that are unlikely to be carriers. Borrowed or inexpensive "pirated" software packages, in particular, are poor and perhaps catastrophic investments. You should never let unauthorized users into your system, either directly or via a local area network (LAN). Back up your programs and data on floppy or tape; the number of layers and frequency of needed backup depend on how valuable and rapidly changing your files are. Check your system frequently with a virus detection program. And if your system does come down with a virus, immediate use of a virus-removal program may be able to remedy the problem.

Chapter 36

Digital Angiography and Radiography

Computers are finding important roles in radiography and, even more so, in fluoroscopy.

With digital subtraction angiography, the computer stores images of a region before and after contrast material is injected into the patient, subtracts the one from the other, and displays the difference between the two as an image in its own right. That task can be performed, albeit with much less flexibility and ease, by means of film subtraction radiography; but rapid, multiple-image subtraction imaging would be impossible without the computer's storage and arithmetic capability.

The use of the laser/computer combination for digitizing developed radiographic film has already been discussed. *Digital radiography* (DR), also called *computed radiography* (CR), replaces the screen and film with a special photostimulable phosphor plate instead; after x-ray exposure, the plate can be read directly into the computer via laser scanning. An advantage of DR is the broad range of x-ray exposures that a photostimul-able phosphor plate can accommodate, allowing images to be produced with wide latitude as well as high contrast.

1. DIGITAL FLUOROSCOPY AND DIGITAL SUBTRACTION ANGIOGRAPHY

Several forms of computer-based radiography and fluoroscopy have been devised, but *digital fluoroscopy* (DF) is the most widely used. The block diagram in Figure 36–1 indicates that a digital fluoroscopic system results from the union of an image intensifier and television-based fluoroscopic unit with a digital computer. Although a digital system might not offer the resolution achievable with a photospot camera or screen–film, the image processing capability may more than compensate (Figs. 36–2 and 36–3). The computer can be bypassed, of course, for normal fluorographic operation.

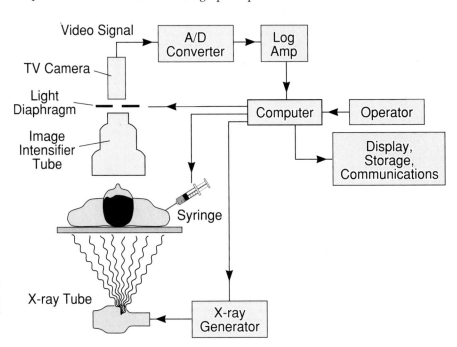

Figure 36–1. Block diagram of a digital fluoroscopic system as used for digital subtraction angiography. After being digitized, the video signal from the TV camera passes through a logarithmic amplifier into the computer for processing.

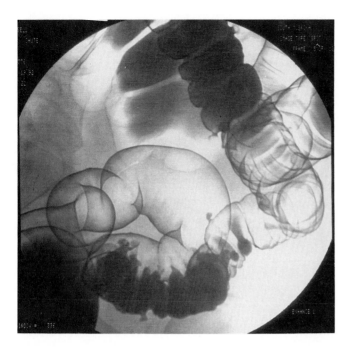

Figure 36–2. Digital fluoroscopic spot film (double-contrast barium enema) of a 35-year-old woman with diverticular disease. The image processing capability, dynamic range, and immediate display may more than compensate for the lower resolution. *(Courtesy of W. McCann, South Muskoka Memorial Hospital, Bracebridge, Ontario, Canada.)*

DF is employed largely for *digital subtraction angiography* (*DSA*). DSA is conceptually similar to its analog predecessor, the film subtraction technique discussed in Chapter 26, Section 2. In simplest form, a digital *mask* image of the region of interest is made *before* the injection of contrast agent into a vein or artery (see Fig. 1–6A). An *angiogram* image is obtained a suitable time *after* the injection (see Fig. 1–6B). If the only difference between the two pictures arises from the presence of the contrast medium in the second image, then the subtraction process eliminates practically all the shadows from the background tissues, leaving behind a remarkably clear view of the blood vessels (see Fig. 1–6C). Various forms of filtering may enhance the contrast or other desirable aspects of the difference image, and it may help to incorporate some familiar background anatomic reference structures, or landmarks, by adding a faint overlay of the original mask image (see Fig. 1–6D). A number of variations and refinements on this general theme are possible, and some are discussed later.

DSA offers several significant advantages over film subtraction. First, the response of the image intensifier (II)–TV system is nearly linear over a much wider range of x-ray exposures than is film, so there is little likelihood that important regions in either the mask or the angio image will be over- or underexposed. Second, computer processing can amplify very small differences between regions, or changes over time, in x-ray intensity picked up by the image receptor; while a radiologist may miss differences in x-ray attenuation of 2% to 3% in a film, a DSA system allows the detection of structures with a subject contrast of 1% or less. Third, because image acquisition, image processing, and image display are controlled by essentially independent components of the system, each can be opti-

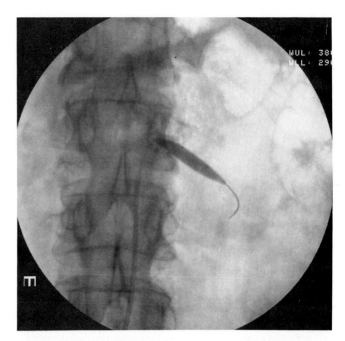

A

B

Figure 36–3. Certain attributes of an image can be enhanced, and its diagnostic usefulness thereby perhaps increased, through digital processing. **A.** Digital spot film of the inflated balloon in renal angioplasty, with optimal technique factors and laser camera display. **B.** High-pass digital filtration brings out edge effects and other high-spatial-frequency-phenomena. *(Courtesy of Gary Hartwell, University of Virginia Medical Center.)*

mized separately. Fourth, DSA is relatively easy to perform, and one can view the final product immediately, rather than having to wait for film development and subtraction. And finally, because of the improved contrast, it may be possible to image with less contrast agent; for an arterial injection, a relatively small amount of contrast agent can be introduced through a fine catheter, at less patient discomfort and risk (e.g., from arterial spasm or damage, from the effect of iodine on the kidneys, or from stroke).

A disadvantage of some DSA systems is the limitation of field of view to that of the II tube input screen, although 36 cm (14″) II tubes are not uncommon now. Another possible problem is lower resolution. Sharpness is clearly critical in the examination of fine blood vessels. The resolution obtainable with film-based angiography is of the order of 6 to 8 lp/mm, which is needed to see fine-structural defects (ulcerations, etc.) inside small vessels. The resolution of a high-quality image intensifier tube is typically 4 to 6 lp/mm, and that of the entire DSA may be lower by a factor of 2 or more because of the television system. (Some DSA systems in the United States still use a 525 line/frame television system and a 512×512-pixel matrix.) But the move is on toward higher-resolution television and a finer pixel matrix (up to 4096×4096 pixels), enabling DSA to image ever smaller vessels.

2. STANDARD DIGITAL FLUOROSCOPY/DIGITAL SUBTRACTION ANGIOGRAPHY HARDWARE

It is essential that the mask image and subsequent angio images be nearly identical, aside from the presence of the contrast agent. The imaging parameters should, therefore, not change appreciably between exposures in a series, and random noise should be minimized. (Some forms of *systematic* noise, such as interfering visual patterns from overlying tissues, are largely removed by the subtraction process.)

A standard fluoro *x-ray tube* and *generator* may be employed, but must be of high capability and quality. Up to 7 exposures per second may be called for, and as many as 30 for cardiac DSA, typically at 70 to 75 kVp, 200 mA, and 25 mA-s (although appropriate technique factors may differ greatly from these values). The need for a small focal spot for high resolution (especially when using a pixel matrix finer than 512×512 or when employing radiographic magnification), together with a high heat tolerance for short multiple exposures, places severe demands on the x-ray tube, as with cinefluoroscopy. And since a series of as many as 100 images may have to be produced with the same exposure parameters, the generator must be stable and able to maintain a virtually constant tube current and kilovoltage. Modern constant-potential or high-frequency generators can do the job.

The *optical link* in a DF system consists of an image intensifier tube, an electronically controlled diaphragm, and a TV camera.

A DSA system may use a conventional high-quality II tube, but special tubes with thicker phosphors (to increase quantum detection efficiency, at the cost of some resolution) are available. A large field of view, up to 36 to 40 cm (14 to 16 in.) in diameter, is desirable for the imaging of chest or abdomen or the extremities, but 30 cm (12 in.) is more common.

The optical *diaphragm* must be capable of regulating the amount of light that enters the TV camera over a two-decade range of output intensities from the II tube. Normal fluoroscopy and continuous fluoro mode DSA make use of currents of the order of several milliamperes. To achieve adequate photon statistics (i.e., a sufficiently low degree of quantum mottle) in pulsed mode DSA operation, however, the tube current will be perhaps 100 times that; so also will be the instantaneous intensity at the output screen of the image intensifier. The diaphragm must therefore be able to fine-tune the light throughput at both ends of this range.

The *TV camera* must produce a very low level of electronic noise. Although such noise is fully obscured by quantum mottle under normal fluorographic operation, the quantum statistics are much better for DSA, and any excess electronic noise could become distractingly apparent in low-contrast images. The television link must be considerably more stable than for conventional fluoroscopy or commercial TV, moreover, so that instabilities over time do not disrupt the proper registration of DSA frames. The standard fluoroscopic (and DSA) television camera is the plumbicon, a form of vidicon that employs lead oxide as the target material. The saticon is a vidicon that uses selenium as the target. It is capable of finer resolution than the plumbicon, and may replace it in digital systems as the 512×512-pixel matrix is replaced by 1024×1024-pixel and finer formats.

A possible future alternative to the television camera is the *charge-coupled device* (CCD), which may be linked to the II tube by means of fiber optics. The CCD is a two-dimensional array of several hundred thousand tiny (5 to 20 μm on a side), independent photodiodes on a semiconductor chip. Each of these corresponds to a single pixel. The CCD exhibits low electronic noise, virtually no lag, and a resolution better

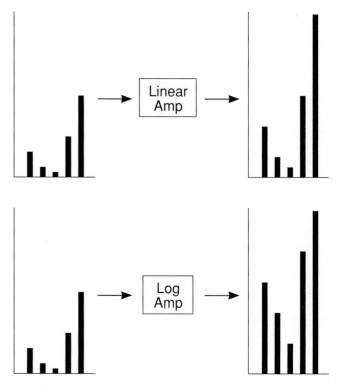

Figure 36–4. Passage of a signal through a logarithmic converter or amplifier, in which the gain decreases as signal strength increases. This compresses the signal range, and helps to ensure that weaker signals are not lost amid the stronger.

than that of the II tube itself, and its response is linear over a much wider dynamic range.

The continuous analog voltage corresponding to a single TV frame is sampled and transformed into digital form by an *analog-to-digital (A/D) converter.* Ten-bit A/D converters, which can express an analog voltage as one of $2^{10} = 1024$ digital values, are sufficient for the assignment of video signal gray levels and, for a 1024×1024 matrix, the pixel addresses. The A/D converters must be able to operate at 10^7 conversions per second to accommodate 30 525-line frames, or 7.5 1050-line frames, per second. Further possible constraints on the rate of image acquisition come from the computer hard disk's data transfer speed and storage capacity.

After analog-to-digital conversion, the video signal is normally passed through a digital *logarithmic converter* or *log amplifier.* This device amplifies the weakest signals the most (Fig. 36–4), and thereby reduces the likelihood of losing the subtleties among the fainter signals. Also, a log amplifier makes the apparent contrast of a contrast material-filled vein largely independent of the thickness of under- and overlying body tissues (Fig. 36–5). As suggested in Figure 36–5B, if images coming straight from the video camera are subtracted from one another, the contrast will be greater for a vessel surrounded by less tissue. That artifact largely disappears if it is the logarithm of the strength of each signal that is subtracted (Fig. 36–5C). (In film subtraction angiography, the intrinsic logarithmic response of the film achieves a similar result.)

The *computer* controls the firing of the x-ray tube and the exposure parameters, and handles image data acquisition and image processing. It may be faster and more cost-effective to perform some aspects of image processing, such as subtraction and filtering, on an array processor rather than within the central processing unit (CPU). Iodine-based contrast agent is injected into the patient intravenously or intraarterially by means of a motor-driven syringe; the amount, rate, and timing of injection can be controlled by the computer.

3. SCAN MODES

The standard raster of commercial television and analog fluoroscopy (interlaced line, 30 frames/s) may be used for **continuous fluoro mode** DSA. With a tube current of only 5 to 10 mA, as many as 20 or 30 television frames may have to be averaged to produce a single DSA frame with adequate photon statistics and signal-to-noise ratio (SNR). Because of the length of the exposure, temporal and spatial resolution is relatively poor. The advantage of the approach is that a standard TV system can be used; the DSA system is hardly more than a simple plug-in connection to the video signal processor.

Much more commonly, however, the radiation is delivered in short, high-intensity pulses, typically at a rate of 1 per second. With the **pulsed interlaced scan mode**, the TV camera acquires several frames of video signal (two interlaced 1/60th-second TV fields each) while the x-ray tube is firing. This approach leads to significantly better resolution and signal-to-noise than can be obtained with continuous digital fluoro, and often at a lower dose to the patient.

With **pulsed progressive scan mode**, the TV lines are scanned in natural, rather than interlaced, sequence. Some manufacturers, moreover, *blank* the TV camera during the exposure itself; that is, an electric charge image is accumulated on the target of the camera (see Chapter 28, Section 3), but the electron beam is suppressed until after the x-ray beam has been turned off. At the beginning of the next normal TV frame, the electron beam is restored and scans the completed charge pattern stored on the target. (With this approach, a pulse can be of any desired length, not just 1/30th of a second, the duration of a TV frame.)

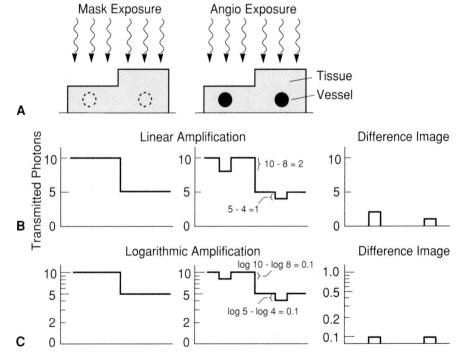

Figure 36–5. Another advantage of log amplification in digital subtraction angiography. The contrast in the difference image is less dependent on the thickness of the over- and underlying tissues. **A.** During the *mask* exposure, twice as many x-ray photons pass through the thinner block of tissue, to the left. During the *angio* exposure, the photon intensity directly behind the iodine-filled vessel is 20% down, regardless of the tissue thickness. **B.** With linear amplification of the mask image, the intensity of the photon beam emerging from the thin block of tissue is 10 units, and that for the thick block, 5 units. In the angio image, the intensities are 8 and 4 units directly behind the two vessels. In the difference image, the contrasts of the two vessels are (10 – 8) = 2 and (5 – 4) = 1. **C.** The effect of logarithmic amplification can be seen by redrawing the mask and angio portions of (B) on semilog paper. This transformation renders the vessel contrast independent of tissue thickness. *(After Curry et al.,* Christensen's Physics of Diagnostic Radiology. *4th ed., Philadelphia: Lea & Febiger, 1990, Fig. 22–11.)*

In the **slow scan mode**, 7.5 1050-line frames are scanned per second. This allows a doubling of the resolution, in both vertical and horizontal directions, as would be appropriate for a 1024 × 1024-pixel matrix, without having to widen the bandwidth of the electronic gear.

> Most electronic equipment is designed to accommodate only a limited range, or band, of signal frequencies. This usually simplifies the circuitry and allows rejection of noise with frequency components outside the passband.
>
> Instead of adopting the slow scan mode, one could process 30 1050-line frames per second by quadrupling the bandwidth of the video signal and of the equipment. This would allow in a correspondingly greater amount of random noise, however, and would require more extensive equipment redesign.

Information obtained by any of these modes can be presented in **freeze-frame** display, in which the image remains on the TV monitor after the exposure is over, as long as the viewer wishes. This can lead to considerable reduction of dose below what the patient would receive with conventional fluoroscopy.

4. OVERCOMING MOTION ARTIFACTS: MASK RE-REGISTRATION AND DUAL-ENERGY SUBTRACTION

The form of DSA described earlier, in which a mask made before the arrival of contrast is subtracted from a postinjection image, is known as **temporal mask subtraction**. A refinement of the technique involves frame-averaging several mask images and subtracting the resulting mask from the average of several postinjection images. (This approach can be optimized by means of sophisticated averaging approaches such as *matched filtering*, in which the relative contributions to the postinjection frames are weighted according to the instantaneous concentration of iodine in the vessels [Fig. 36–6].)

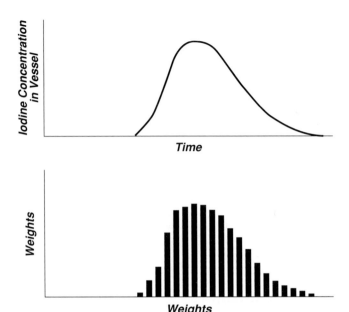

Figure 36–6. A digital subtraction angio image may be improved by averaging contributions from several postinjection frames. With matched temporal filtering, the weight (i.e., relative contribution) of each frame is proportional to the iodine concentration in the vessel at the time.

Patient motion is an important source of image degradation with mask subtraction. The injection of iodine contrast agent, for example, may elicit a swallowing reflex, and also peristalsis can be significant. Even with small motions, misregistration of the mask and angio images gives rise to a difference image that contains a characteristic form of noise (Fig. 36–7A). If the entire region of interest moves rigidly between exposures, then either manual or computer-determined *re-registration* of the two images can eliminate the problem (Fig. 36–7B); the images are

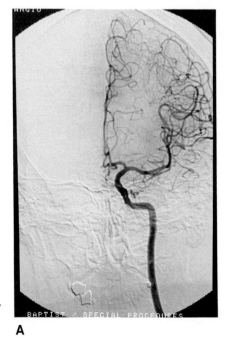
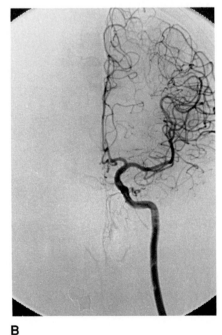

Figure 36–7. Effect of patient motion. **A.** The result of misregistration of mask and angio images on the difference image. **B.** After pixel shifting one image relative to another. *(Courtesy of Siemens Medical Systems, Inc.)*

A   **B**

moved relative to one another until the presence of streaks and other noise in the difference image is minimized. The salvage job cannot be complete, however, when some parts of patient in the field of view move more than others, or if movements occur that are not in-plane.

> Motion effects can be diminished also by means of *time interval difference subtraction*. Images A, B, C, . . . , are obtained at equally spaced times postinjection. A is subtracted from B to produce the first difference image, B from C to form the second, and so on. This may also allow the identification of certain pathologic vascular conditions from irregularities in the advance of the contrast agent over time.

An alternative to mask subtraction is **dual-energy subtraction.** The attenuation coefficients of soft tissue and bone decrease relatively gently with increasing energy in the region of 33 keV, but iodine exhibits an absorption edge there. Two images, one created with monochromatic x-rays just below 33 keV and the second with slightly more energetic x-rays, would therefore display significant differences where iodine is present. In practice, one uses a continuous bremsstrahlung beam with quite different kVp settings, but the basic idea is the same. The generator kVp and the x-ray tube filtration are switched quickly while a nearly constant exposure is maintained. This can usually be performed rapidly enough to eliminate all motional effects.

It is possible to adjust the images so that either bone shadows or soft tissue shadows are removed from the difference. But since the photoelectric and Compton attenuation coefficients do not change with energy at the same rates, over the bremsstrahlung spectrum, one cannot (with only two different kVp settings) eliminate both bone and soft tissue at the same time.

Other forms of subtraction are being developed. Among these are **hybrid subtraction**, which combines the temporal and dual-energy techniques, and *three-energy subtraction*, by means of which both bone and soft tissue shadows are largely removed, ideally leaving only contrast-enhanced vessels.

5. DIGITAL (COMPUTED) RADIOGRAPHY

Digital fluoroscopy employs the standard analog fluoroscopic image receptor—the image intensifier tube plus TV camera combination—with the work of the computer coming largely after image acquisition. **Digital radiography (DR)** does not even employ the analog radiographic image receptor (screen-plus-film).

With the **stimulated luminescence** DR system, the screen–film cassette is replaced with an *imaging plate* coated with a *photostimulable heavy-metal phosphor* (e.g., certain europium-activated barium fluorohalide compounds). X-irradiation disrupts the balance in the number of electrons inhabiting electron traps. This imbalance, in turn, affects the amount of luminescence light given off later (and detected by a photomultiplier tube) when the plate is subsequently read by scanning with a laser beam in a raster pattern (Fig. 36–8).

With some stimulated luminescence DR systems, the imaging plate is moved into place for exposure, laser-read following exposure, and erased in preparation for the next image, all

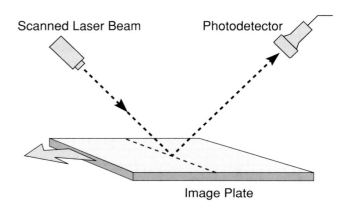

Figure 36–8. Detecting (with a photomultiplier tube) the stimulated luminescence light given off as the imaging plate of a digital radiography system is scanned with a laser beam.

automatically. There is no need for a technologist to shuffle cassettes about, and several images can be taken per second.

Stimulated luminescence DR tolerates an extremely *wide latitude* of x-ray exposures. With screen–film radiography, the range of exposures that lead to acceptable optical densities is relatively limited. The characteristic curve of the screen–film combination is sigmoidal, as was seen in Chapters 17 and 21. At exposures below the toe of the curve, the developed film is all clear, and above the shoulder, the film is totally opaque. For both very low and very high exposures, the optical density is nearly independent of exposure, hence incapable of capturing much image information. With DR, on the other hand, the output of the radiation detector is nearly linear over a much greater dynamic range of exposures; information that would be totally lost with film may therefore be retained with DR.

The computer provides the ability to manipulate separately the acquisition, processing, and display aspects of DR. Figure 36–9A presents two of the dozen or so different effective characteristic curves that a commercial DR system has stored, and that are available for selection by the operator. The curve marked "A" is similar to that of a typical screen–film system used for chest radiography, and gave rise to Figure 36–9B. The curve labeled "B", produced (from the same x-ray exposure of the patient) the strikingly different Figure 36–9C. The physician may find it helpful to view several images from the same patient raw data, but as produced by means of different characteristic curves.

Film digitization (rather than DR) is used as an intermediate step in many departments that are going digital. Although the computer can help out with a somewhat over- or underexposed film, film digitization offers neither the wide latitude of DR nor the resolution of film. But film digitization does provide a way to enter an analog image (if that happens to be the clinical information available) into a computer system for electronic processing, storage, and communication.

Both DR and film digitization involve the acquisition and temporary storage of the x-ray image on an intermediate medium (an image plate or film), with subsequent transfer of image information into the computer. It is also possible to enter the information into the computer in a single step as, for example, with **slit** or **line-scanning radiography:** A narrowly colli-

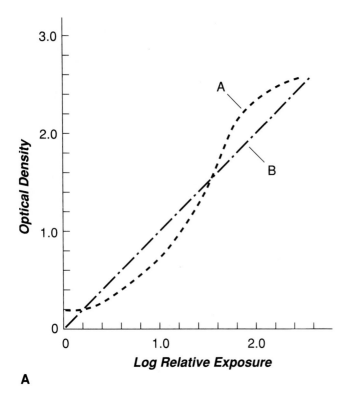

A

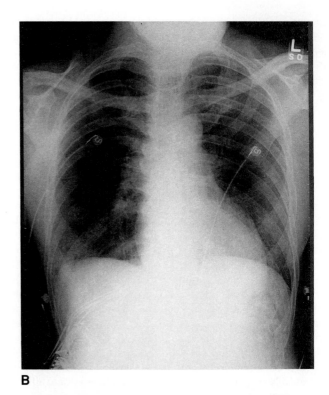

B

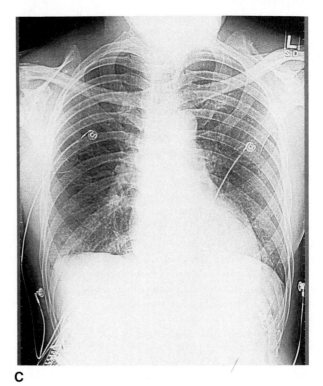

C

Figure 36–9. Digital (computerized) radiography (DR). **A.** Two of the several dozen prestored, available effective characteristic curves for a DR system. **B.** The image corresponding to characteristic curve A is similar to that of a typical screen–film system. **C.** Image produced through use of curve B. *(Courtesy of Fuji Medical Systems U.S.A., Inc.)*

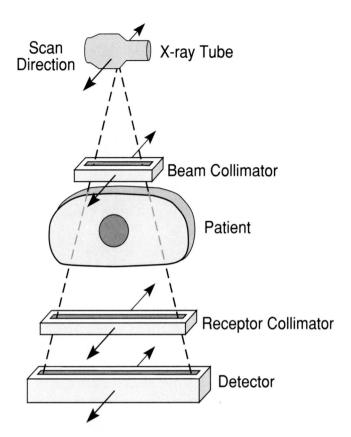

Figure 36–10. Scanning slit radiography as a means of reducing contrast degradation by scatter. This is one of several ways in which a radiographic image can be entered directly into a computer without going through the intermediate step of forming an image on film or on a photostimulable phosphor plate.

mated sliver of x-rays, or *fan beam*, is moved along the body, as with a computed tomography scout scan. The beam transmitted through the body is monitored by a similarly moving, long and narrow fluorescent screen, observed by a linear array of 1024 or so photodiodes or other detectors (Fig. 36–10). As with computed tomography, the use of the fan beam radically reduces the contrast degradation resulting from scatter, as the x-ray field at any instant is only a few square centimeters in area.

Computed Tomography I: Creating A Map of CT Numbers

1. **Computed Tomography Maps the Linear Attenuation Coefficient Throughout a Transverse Slice of Tissue**
2. **Hounsfield Numbers**
3. **A First-Generation Computed Tomography Scanner**
4. **The Ray Sum Is the Logarithm of the Attenuation Along the Ray**
5. **A Simple Algorithm for Reconstructing $\mu(x, y)$ from a Complete Set of Profiles**
6. **Filtered Back-Projection Is Much Faster**

By eliminating the confusion caused by the overlapping of tissues in three dimensions, computed tomography (CT) allows superb clarity and tissue contrast in two. This has lead to a revolution in the way radiologists, surgeons, radiotherapists, and other physicians view, and perhaps even think about, the body.

In conventional fluoroscopy, nuclear medicine, and ultrasound, computers are not needed for the actual formation of images. A computer may enhance image quality by means of averaging and other filtering techniques, allows the following of time-dependent phenomena, and can improve image appearance through gray scale windowing, but fluoroscopic systems, gamma cameras, and ultrasound devices were producing diagnostically useful pictures long before digital technology came on the scene. With CT (and magnetic resonance imaging [MRI] and the tomographic forms of nuclear medicine: single-photon emission computed tomography [SPECT] and positron emission tomography [PET]), on the other hand, the computer is absolutely essential for the numerical reconstruction of the image itself out of un-image-like raw data.

This chapter describes CT imaging and reconstruction computations. The next focuses on hardware and image quality.

1. COMPUTED TOMOGRAPHY MAPS THE LINEAR ATTENUATION COEFFICIENT THROUGHOUT A TRANSVERSE SLICE OF TISSUE

With conventional radiography, information on three-dimensional anatomy is projected onto a two-dimensional plane. Subtle irregularities easily become lost in the superpositioning of the image patterns produced by overlapping tissue structures. Soft-tissue lesions within the lung, for example, can be obscured by the large and complex variations in beam attenuation caused by the ribs and air spaces. Similarly, most photons entering the head are absorbed or scattered by cranial bone, rendering difficult the imaging of the gray or white matter within.

Computed tomography involves irradiation of one transverse slice of tissue at a time, and yields a *two-dimensional map of the linear attenuation coefficient*, μ, throughout that slice. It thereby preserves much of the information that is lost by radiography, while improving the soft-tissue contrast sensitivity tenfold or more.

The mapping process involves mathematically partitioning the slice under examination into a square **matrix** of thousands of small tissue *volume elements*, or **voxels** (Fig. 37–1). The matrix size is commonly expressed in terms of the number (M) of voxels in each dimension: A square 256×256 matrix, for example, contains about 65K (65,000) voxels. Voxels in CT are on the order of 1 mm² in cross-sectional area and several millimeters in depth (the thickness of the slice of tissue irradiated and imaged). The matrix size, $M \times M$, the in-plane dimension of a voxel, d, and the linear dimension of the field of view (FOV) are related as

$$M \cdot d = \text{FOV} \qquad (37.1)$$

which is similar to Equation 35.2b. Voxels are square, but the field of view need not be.

The **image reconstruction** process involves the determination of the *linear attenuation coefficient* μ associated with every voxel. The computed map of attenuation coefficients is eventually displayed as a *matrix* of **pixels** of various shades of gray, with one pixel normally corresponding to each voxel. The gray scale is usually arranged so that regions of greater μ appear lighter, but this is a somewhat arbitrary convention, and flicking the *polarity* switch will reverse it. Indeed, CT images can be presented with variations in attenuation coefficient

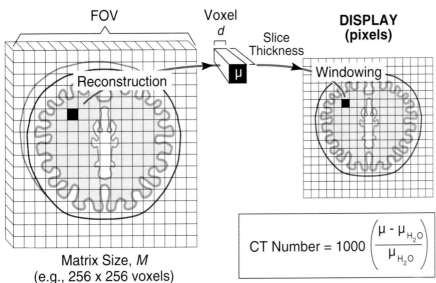

ANATOMIC SLICE (voxels)

FOV

Voxel *d*

Slice Thickness

DISPLAY (pixels)

Reconstruction

μ

Windowing

Matrix Size, *M* (e.g., 256 x 256 voxels)

$$\text{CT Number} = 1000 \left(\frac{\mu - \mu_{H_2O}}{\mu_{H_2O}} \right)$$

Figure 37–1. An overview of computed tomography (CT). A transverse slice of anatomy is mathematically partitioned into thousands of *voxels*. Numerous x-ray transmission measurements, together with the image *reconstruction* process, allow the determination of the linear attenuation coefficient, μ, of the material in each voxel. CT numbers express these μ values relative to μ_{H_2O}, the attenuation coefficient of water (a useful reference material). The displayed image is an array of *pixels*, each with a degree of brightness (shade of gray) related (by means of a gray scale *windowing* transformation) to the CT number of the corresponding voxel. FOV, field of view.

represented with gradations of *false colors*, rather than shades of gray.

2. HOUNSFIELD NUMBERS

As discussed in Chapter 14, the attenuation coefficient of any material depends on x-ray beam energy. CT normally uses relatively high energy (120 to 140 kVp) x-rays (with an effective energy of 70 to 80 keV), which interact with soft tissues primarily by means of the Compton effect. A CT image of soft-tissue structures therefore reflects primarily their physical and electron densities.

The energy dependence of the attenuation coefficients normally is not of direct clinical interest, however, and it simplifies matters to be rid of it. The **CT number** of a tissue at a point is therefore defined as

$$\text{CT number} = 1000 \cdot (\mu - \mu_{H_2O})/\mu_{H_2O} \qquad (37.2)$$

where μ_{H_2O} is the linear attenuation coefficient of water at the effective energy of the beam, and μ is that of the tissue in the voxel of interest. (The quotient of Equation 37.2 does not cancel out the energy dependence of μ completely—it would do so only if μ and μ_{H_2O} changed with photon energy at exactly the same rate—but it does remove a good bit of it, particularly for soft tissues.) Display then consists of a map of pixel values that indicate *relative* (to water), rather than *absolute*, linear attenuation coefficients. Water is chosen as the reference material because it constitutes 80% to 90% of soft-tissue mass, it is a convenient and absolutely reproducible material for use in CT machine calibration, and the gentle variation of its attenuation coefficient with photon energy is similar to that for soft tissues.

For the scaling constant in Equation 37.2, 500 was originally used, but 1000 has become the accepted convention. CT numbers with this normalization (1000) are expressed in **Hounsfield units** (*H*). CT numbers above and below 0 H correspond to tissues of attenuation coefficient greater or less than μ_{H_2O}. One Hounsfield unit represents a 0.1% difference in linear attenuation coefficient from that of water.

Typical values of CT numbers, in Hounsfield units, are shown in Table 37–1 for an x-ray beam in the range 120 to 140 kVp. Note, in particular, that the CT number of water is zero, and that those for air (for which the linear attenuation coefficient is nearly 0) and bone are −1000 and about +1000, respectively.

Computed tomography is normally used to examine soft tissues, which (apart from lung) do not differ radically from one another in CT number. When examining such tissues, it is

TABLE 37–1. REPRESENTATIVE COMPUTED TOMOGRAPHY (CT) NUMBERS

Tissue	CT Number, *H*
Water	0
Air	−1000
Dense bone	~1000
Blood	42–58
Hemorrhage	60–110
Blood clot	74–81
Heart	24
Cerebrospinal fluid	0–22
Gray matter	32–44
White matter	24–36
Astrocytoma	54
Muscle	44–59
Normal liver	50–80
Fat	−20 to −100
Lung	−300

From Webster JG, ed. Encyclopedia of Medical Devices and Instrumentation. *New York: Wiley, 1988, p. 834.*

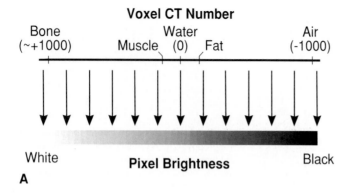

Voxel CT Number

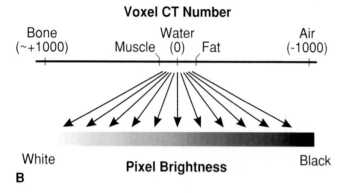

Figure 37–2. Windowing. **A.** Computed tomography (CT) numbers range from –1000 H, for air, to about +1000 H, for bone, but there is rarely any need to display the entire range in an image. **B.** It is generally preferable to cause the range of gray scale values to correspond only to the range of CT numbers of the tissues of interest.

therefore desirable that most of the gray scale variation of the display, from black to white, should correspond to this rather narrow range of CT values (Fig. 37–2). The *display window level* (see Chapter 35, Section 6) can be set by the technologist so that the middle of the gray scale corresponds to the middle of the CT number range for the region of interest. The *display window width* is simultaneously adjusted to cover that range adequately.

Intracranial tissue CT numbers, for example, might range from 0 to +80 H. Setting the display window level at +40 H and the width at 120 H would be appropriate, so that the entire gray scale corresponds to CT numbers from –20 H to +100 H. Windowing in CT was illustrated in Figure 35–9.

3. A FIRST-GENERATION COMPUTED TOMOGRAPHY SCANNER

In 1971, Godfrey Hounsfield and a British company, EMI Ltd., unveiled the first commercial CT head scanner.

The x-ray tube and the signal detector of this *first-generation scanner* are mounted on a **gantry**. Their positions are fixed relative to one another, but they are allowed both *linear* and *rotational* motion relative to the patient. In a scan, the tube/detector assembly (and the narrowly collimated x-ray beam) are swept laterally across the patient's head (Fig. 37–3A), cutting out a transverse plane. The gantry is then rotated through 1 degree about the patient (Fig. 37–3B), and the beam is swept again. This procedure is repeated 180 times.

The beam is collimated so as to irradiate a region of tissue, at any instant, only a centimeter or so high (the slice thickness) and several millimeters wide. Such a pencil-like beam is called a *ray*. The tube is turned off during gantry rotation, but left on continuously while the attenuation is sampled for 160 adjacent and parallel but separate rays during each transverse sweep. The $160 \times 180 = 28,800$ ray measurements for a single trans-

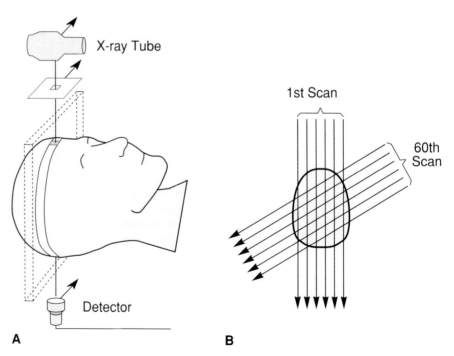

Figure 37–3. Operation of a first-generation scanner. **A.** The tightly collimated x-ray beam and the detector are swept across the patient. **B.** The gantry is rotated slightly, and a new sweep begun. Shown here is the beam after 60 such sweeps and rotations.

verse slice provide more than enough information to allow the reconstruction of a 160×160-pixel matrix of values of the attenuation coefficient.

4. THE RAY SUM IS THE LOGARITHM OF THE ATTENUATION ALONG THE RAY

Suppose, to simplify the numbers, that the collimated ray beam is 1 mm wide and the slice thickness is 10 mm. We shall mathematically partition the transverse slice of tissue under examination into square voxels of comparable dimensions (1 mm on a side, 10 mm deep) and give them addresses according to an (x, y) coordinate system (of the same scale) embedded within the slice. The ray that happens to lie parallel to the x axis and at $y = 7$ mm is shown in Figure 37–4.

How much attenuation does the ray at $y = 7$ suffer before exiting the patient? It passes through voxels at addresses $(x, y) = (5,7), (6,7), (7,7)$, and so on, where the linear attenuation coefficients are $\mu(x, y) = \mu(5,7)$ mm^{-1}, $\mu(6,7)$ mm^{-1}, $\mu(7,7)$ mm^{-1}, ..., respectively. In the first voxel in the body, the ray is attenuated by the amount $e^{-\{\mu(5,7) \cdot 1\}}$. It is further diminished by a factor of $e^{-\{\mu(6,7) \cdot 1\}}$ in the second, so that the net attenuation in the first two voxels is $e^{-\{\mu(5,7) \cdot 1 + \mu(6,7) \cdot 1\}}$. The total cumulative attenuation of the ray along the entire length of its path in tissue is obtained by continuing this process in the same fashion:

$$I/I_0 = e^{-\Sigma \mu_i \cdot \Delta s_i} \qquad (37.3a)$$

where μ_i is the coefficient in the ith voxel, Δs_i is the distance the ray travels through it, and sigma notation was introduced in Equation 18.8a.

It is inconvenient to work with exponentials, so one takes the logarithm of both sides of Equation 37.3a and defines a *ray sum* or **ray projection** p for this ray* as

$$p = -\ln I/I_0 = \Sigma \mu_i \cdot \Delta s_i \qquad (37.3b)$$

We have been talking of calculating the ray sum p from knowledge of the values of μ_i along a path (see Equations 37.3). In practice, it is the converse process that occurs: One *measures the ray sums, p*, by means of the radiation detector, for each of a large number of rays, and then *computes*, by means of a reconstruction calculation, *the set of μ_i values* that would give rise to the measured set of ray sums.

In the example in Figure 37–4, the process begins with a measurement of the ray sum for the ray at $y = 1$. The beam then steps up to $y = 2$, and the new ray sum is acquired. A complete set of such ray sums at any particular gantry angle is called a *projection*, or *profile*. (In the case of the EMI Scanner and for the particular profile shown in Figure 37–4, this consists of the set of separate ray sums for the 160 rays running parallel to the x axis.) The production of a single-slice image involves measurement of 180 profiles, one for each of the 180 values of the gantry angle. The image is *reconstructed* by extracting the attenua-

---

*For rays not parallel to the x and y axes, the computer must take account of the fact that Δs_i is not necessarily equal to the length of the side of a voxel, and that a ray will cover only parts of voxels. If the voxels are allowed to grow infinitesimally small, Equation 37.3b becomes the *ray-integral*, $\int \mu \cdot ds$.

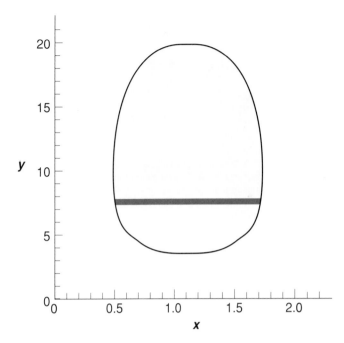

Figure 37–4. It is necessary to embed an x, y coordinate system within the transverse slice of tissue under examination and to establish a corresponding coordinate system for display. Shown here is the ray at $y = 7$.

tion coefficients for all voxels from the $160 \times 180 = 28{,}800$ resulting ray sums; this reconstruction would involve manipulation of 28,800 equations of the form of Equation 37.3b, in effect, each with a unique, measured, and stored value of p. Read on!

5. A SIMPLE ALGORITHM FOR RECONSTRUCTING $\mu(x,y)$ FROM A COMPLETE SET OF PROFILES

Conceptually the easiest way to reconstruct the pixel map of CT numbers is to *solve the set of linear equations*, each of the form of Equation 37.3b, that correspond to a complete set of ray sums. This section will work through an especially simple example.

Suppose we are imaging a body slice that consists of four voxels of unit dimension ($\Delta s = 1$). To simplify the notation, we shall label the voxels 1 through 4 and the rays A through D, as indicated in Figure 37–5A.

The ray sum for ray A is related to the attenuation coefficients in the voxels through which it passes as

$$p(A) = (\mu_1 \cdot 1) + (\mu_2 \cdot 1) \qquad (37.4)$$

Suppose that, in our example, $p(A)$ is *measured* by the CT machine to be of magnitude 5, so that

$$p(A) = \mu_1 + \mu_2 = 5 \qquad (37.5a)$$

Similarly, the other ray measurements yield

$$p(B) = \mu_3 + \mu_4 = 2 \qquad (37.5b)$$
$$p(C) = \mu_1 + \mu_3 = 3 \qquad (37.5c)$$
$$p(D) = \mu_2 + \mu_4 = 4 \qquad (37.5d)$$

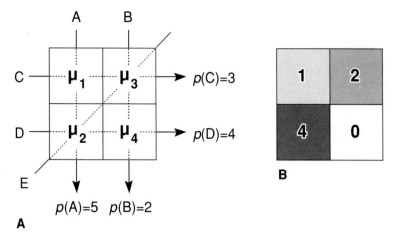

Figure 37–5. The "body" for this simple exercise has been partitioned into four voxels. **A.** The labeling of the four voxels by way of the subscripts and of the five measured ray sums A through E. **B.** The set of attenuation coefficients that gave rise to the ray sums measured in (A).

Innocently assuming that we shall have no trouble in solving these four equations for the four unknowns μ_1 through μ_4, we subtract Equation 37.5c from 37.5a and find

$$\mu_2 - \mu_3 = 2 \tag{37.6}$$

So far so good. We need a second equation involving μ_2 and μ_3, so we subtract Equation 37.5b from 37.5d. What we get is Equation 37.6 again, indicating that we do *not* yet have a complete solution to our problem.

Somewhat nervously, now, we make one more ray projection measurement, with the gantry angled at 45 degrees, and obtain

$$p(E) = \mu_2 + \mu_3 = 6 \tag{37.7}$$

This does, indeed, provide additional information which, together with Equation 37.6, allows unequivocal determination of all four attenuation coefficients (Fig. 37–5B) and the construction of the corresponding map of pixel CT numbers for this slice of tissue.

___ **EXERCISE 37–1.** _____

Confirm the correctness of Figure 37–5B.

SOLUTION: From Figure 37–5B, $\mu_1 = 1$ and $\mu_2 = 4$. Then $\mu_1 + \mu_2 = 5$, in agreement with Equation 37.5a and with $p(A)$ in Figure 37–5A. So also for Equations 37.5b, 37.5c, 37.5d, and 37–7.

> Why were the first four equations not enough? A glance at Figure 37–5B reveals that the combined sum of the ray projections for the two vertical rays (5 + 2 = 7) will be the same as that for the two horizontal rays (3 + 4 = 7), namely, $\mu_1 + \mu_2 + \mu_3 + \mu_4$. Although this is not physically significant, it does mean that Equations 37.5a through 37.5d are not mathematically completely independent of one another, and therefore do not provide sufficient information for their simultaneous solution.

6. FILTERED BACK-PROJECTION IS MUCH FASTER

The simple algebraic method just described (known as matrix inversion, after the mathematical tool normally involved) for determining the matrix of attenuation coefficients becomes ex-

tremely cumbersome and time consuming when the number of voxels grows large. Complications arise, moreover, when the linear equations are not all mutually consistent; such a situation might arise, for example, if a patient moved slightly in the midst of a measurement. Other approaches to the general reconstruction problem have been explored, some originally in connection with radioastronomy and electron microscopy imaging and in early attempts at nuclear medicine (emission) CT. The methods found to work best fall into two general categories, the iterative and the analytic.

An *iterative* algorithm produces, for a slice, a sequence of "images," each of which is a refinement over its predecessor. (An **algorithm** is a specific, step-by-step recipe for performing a mathematical calculation.) It begins typically by setting all entries in the pixel matrix equal to the same value of μ. In the first iteration, the algorithm calculates the complete set of ray sums from this matrix, compares these calculated ray sums with what is actually measured, and adjusts the matrix of pixel μ values accordingly. This new set of μ's should be closer to reality than was the original guess. In the second iteration, the algorithm recalculates the ray sums from the revised pixel matrix, recompares with the original set of ray measurements, and thereby obtains a better approximate map of the μ's. This procedure is repeated until the calculated pixel map no longer changes appreciably with further iterations.

Faster still are the **analytic** methods that are currently used today in commercial CT machines. The two most commonly employed analytic methods are *Fourier reconstruction* and *filtered back-projection*. The two are related, but filtered back-projection has the advantage that calculations can begin after a single profile is obtained, rather than having to wait for completion of all profile measurements on a slice.

The mathematical details of **filtered back-projection** are complex, but the basic idea is quite simple. The approach employs a modification of the back-projection method, so we will start by describing that.

Suppose we are scanning a phantom that is radiotransparent, except for a single radiopaque voxel at an unknown location. Our objective is to determine and display the position of the opaque voxel. Back-projection does this by repeating many times a three-step procedure (described below) with the x-ray pencil beam aligned with some fixed orientation; the beam angle is then changed, and the repetitive three-step procedure

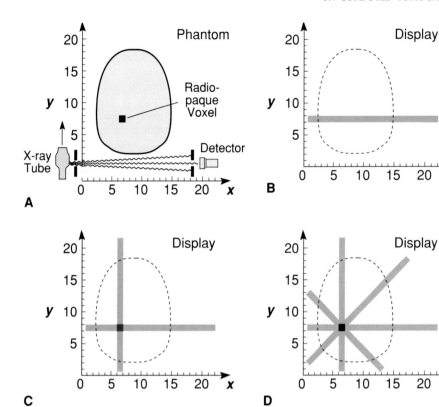

Figure 37–6. Back-projection reconstruction of the image of a phantom that is transparent except for one radiopaque voxel. **A.** The process begins with the x-ray beam oriented horizontally within the *phantom*, and readings at *y* = 1, 2, 3,.... **B.** Back-projection on *display* of a horizontal stripe, corresponding to the radiopaque voxel at *y* = 7. **C.** Back-projections from two angles are enough to localize a single voxel. **D.** With many back-projections in the display, the individual stripes are much fainter than is the pixel where they all intersect.

is carried out again. Typically, 180 or more different angles of the beam are required to generate an image, but for locating a single opaque voxel, as in the following simple example, two angles will do.

We begin by orienting the x-ray beam parallel to the *x* axis of the phantom coordinate system, and position it so that it passes through the voxels at *y* = 1 (Fig. 37–6A). At the same time, we define a corresponding *y* = 1 on the display which, for our purposes, can be simply a piece of graph paper. With this first beam angle,

- *Step 1:* Measure the transmission and ray sum along the ray.
- *Step 2:* Paint (back-project) a stripe, one pixel wide and parallel to the *x* axis, along the corresponding ray on the

display graph paper. The darkness of the stripe is to be proportional to the ray projection of the x-ray beam; that is, the greater the amount of beam attenuation by the phantom along the ray, as determined in step 1, the darker the stripe to be laid down in the display.

- *Step 3:* Move one voxel up, then return to step 1.

That is, after completion of the first cycle, move the x-ray beam to *y* = 2 in the phantom and the paint brush to *y* = 2 on the graph paper, and carry out the three-step procedure again. And repeat the process until the entire phantom is covered for this orientation of the x-ray beam. With our example of the single radiopaque voxel, the display will (at this time) show a single stripe at *y* = 7 (Fig. 37–6B).

Now rotate the x-ray beam through an appropriate angle

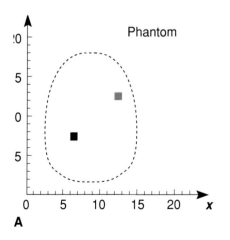

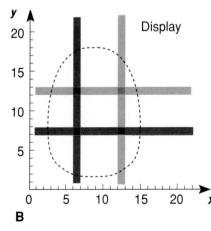

Figure 37–7. To locate two voxels, three back-projection angles are required. Two of them are shown.

(90 degrees here) and go through the whole process again. A second, vertical stripe will eventually appear on the graph paper, at $x = 6$, and intersect the first at the pixel that corresponds to the opaque voxel in the phantom (Fig. 37–6C). Thus two x-ray beam alignments are enough to locate unambiguously a single point opacity. The part of the display that represents the region of high CT number, moreover, is twice as dark as elsewhere along the individual back-projection slices. Back-projecting at a number of additional gantry angles enhances this difference (Fig. 37–6D) so that eventually the back-projections are not too noticeable, except where they intersect.

But one pixel does not an image make. Let's try this again with a more challenging phantom that contains two voxel non-uniformities, the CT number of one being twice that of the other. The back-projections obtained from two profiles intersect at four places (Fig. 37–7) and are thus not sufficient to image the phantom unambiguously. A third profile resolves the issue, however, as the three back-projections intersect at only two places.

Expanding this argument, so as to cover more than two attenuating voxels, leads eventually to the conclusion that 180 back-projection profiles are sufficient to generate a 256×256-pixel matrix. (Commercial units now employ typically 720 or 1440 profiles.) The computer doesn't actually paint back-projection stripes on paper, of course, but its memory does keep track of where the stripes should be. It can then display them or, rather, the overall image they generate on a TV monitor.

Image quality can be significantly enhanced through use of a suitable mathematical *filter*. A filter, in essence, replaces a single back-projected stripe (one voxel wide) with a bundle of several stripes, of nonuniform darkness. In fact, some of the stripes are of "negative darkness"; they actually subtract from other bundles, coming in at other angles, that they may overlap. The overall effect of replacing back-projection with *filtered back-projection* is to render the stripes vanishingly faint everywhere except where they intersect. Because incorporating the filter involves the mathematical process of convolution (see Chapter 24, Section 7), filtered back-projection is sometimes called the *convolution* algorithm.

This business may all sound somewhat involved, and the reader may be surprised to learn that the whole filtered back-projection image reconstruction process can be accomplished with only a few dozen lines of computer code.

The Fourier reconstruction approach will be discussed later, in connection with the generation of magnetic resonance images.

Chapter 38

Computed Tomography II: Hardware and Image Quality

Computed tomography (CT) differs radically from screen–film radiography and fluoroscopy in that it is absolutely dependent on the computer for the performance of image reconstruction calculations.

CT hardware is also quite different. Rather than collecting information from the entire region of interest at one time, as in analog or digital fluoroscopy, an individual CT detector samples a portion of the x-ray beam only a few square millimeters in area. The entire region of interest can be examined by various configurations of x-ray tube and detectors, and five of these have come to define distinct generations of CT scanners. The evolution has been toward a larger number of detectors, greater simplicity of x-ray tube and detector motion, and much greater speed of data acquisition.

Although the image quality issues for CT will be familiar from the study of radiographic and fluoroscopic systems, some of the trade-offs required, and problems that arise, are new.

1. FIVE GENERATIONS OF COMPUTED TOMOGRAPHY SCANNERS

CT scanners have been evolving continuously since the early 1970s. A few of the changes, however, have been sufficiently radical to demarcate what are now known as the five "generations" of CT machines. Machines currently being manufactured are of the third, fourth, and fifth generations, and there are pros and cons to each of these.

The design of a **first-generation** machine (Fig. 38–1) was sketched in the last chapter. In simplest form, a single x-ray tube and collimator produced a pencil beam, and one signal detector monitored the intensity transmitted through the patient. (Another detector sampled the beam before it entered the patient, to allow compensation for fluctuations in tube output.) One hundred and sixty separate attenuation data readings

were taken as the tube and detectors were translated continuously sideways. At the end of this transverse linear sweep, the gantry that supports the tube and detectors was rotated through 1 degree, and a new sweep begun. A complete scan, consisting of 180 repetitions of these two steps, took up to 5 minutes.

The **second-generation** machine (Fig. 38–2) was some-

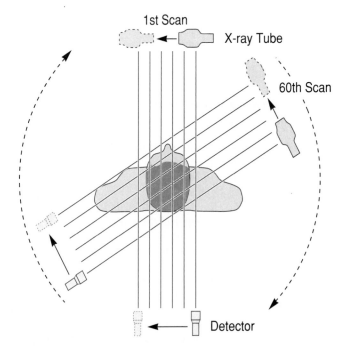

Figure 38–1. *First-generation* scanner. The tightly collimated pencil beam and detector sweep together across the patient, cutting out a transverse pancake slice; the gantry then rotates through 1 degree about the longitudinal axis of the patient, and the next sweep begins.

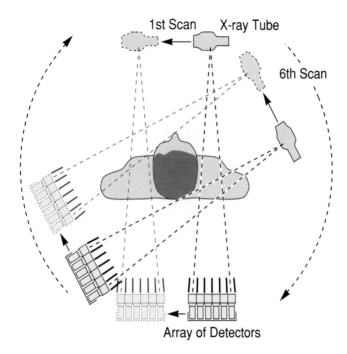

Figure 38–2. *Second-generation* scanner. The fan beam is wide enough to cut through only part of the patient's anatomy. The x-ray tube and a bank of several dozen detectors sweep across the patient; the gantry rotates through 10 degrees, typically, and the next sweep begins.

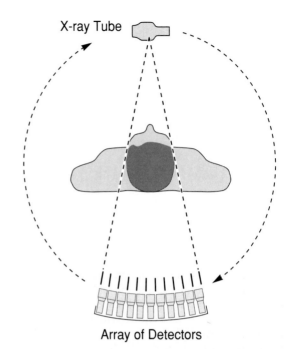

Figure 38–3. *Third-generation* scanner. The fan beam is wide enough to encompass the region of interest. The x-ray tube and an array of several hundred detectors rotate smoothly about the patient; there is no linear motion of tube and detectors.

what like the first, but a fan-shaped beam was used, as was a linear *array* of separate detectors. With 30 detectors, for example, measurements were taken with the tube and detector array at a half-dozen different positions across the patient for each gantry angle; this had the same effect as making 180 measurements with one detector. Because the fan beam covered much more of the patient than did a pencil beam, it was possible to rotate the gantry through larger angle steps, somewhere between 10 and 30 degrees per step. A drawback was that a little more scatter struck the detectors than with the narrow-beam geometry of a first-generation machine; the great advantage was the considerably shorter scan time, down to 15 seconds.

With the introduction of the **third-generation** scanner in 1976, the linear motions of the tube and detectors have been completely eliminated. A fan beam wide enough to completely cover the patient and a linear array of 250 to 900 separate detectors, spread out so as to intercept the entire fan (Fig. 38–3), are employed. The only motion of the gantry is a single 360-degree rotation about the *isocenter*. Because this takes as little as 1 second, artifacts that arise from respiratory motion can be eliminated almost entirely.

The **fourth-generation** machine has a stationary ring of 600 to 4800 detectors, and only the tube and fan beam rotate (Fig. 38–4). Scan times are comparable to those of third-generation machines. The detectors are calibrated twice during each rotation. (In a third-generation machine, calibration is performed only once every several hours and is therefore somewhat more critical.) Both third- and fourth-generation machines have proven to be highly successful, and neither has revealed itself to be of unequivocally superior design.

The **fifth-generation** machine has a fixed array of detectors and a mechanically fixed but electronically movable x-ray source; that is, *nothing* physically moves. One machine design makes use of a set of individual x-ray tubes fired rapidly in sequence. Another employs a radically new x-ray tube design

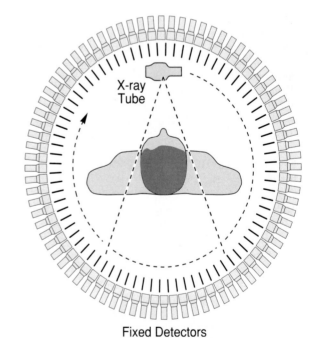

Figure 38–4. *Fourth-generation* scanner. Only the x-ray tube and fan beam rotate about the patient. The thousand or so detectors surrounding the patient are stationary.

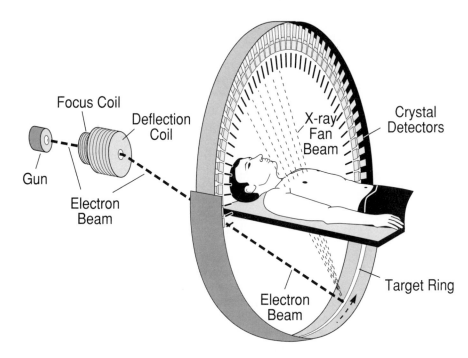

Figure 38–5. *Fifth-generation* scanner. In one design, an array of x-ray tubes fires in rapid enough sequence to freeze the motion of the heart. As with a fourth-generation scanner, the detectors do not move. Shown here is a single x-ray beam–source system. The target is a continuous tungsten strip that makes a 210-degree arc around the patient, and the electron beam and focal spot are caused to swing along that arc in 50 to 100 milliseconds. The electron beam and target reside together within a single evacuated chamber, not shown here. Opposing the target ring, and constituting its own 210-degree arc, is an array of 400 to 800 individual detectors. With four separate, closely spaced target rings, the system can image four adjacent slices in rapid succession. *(Drawing based on diagrams and information kindly provided by Imatron, Inc.)*

in which the electron beam is swept along a curved tungsten strip anode that partially circumscribes the patient (Fig. 38–5). (The envelope that maintains the high vacuum is not shown.) Either way, the source of the x-ray beam swings around the patient fast enough to freeze all significant motions, including those of the heart.

2. X-RAY TUBES, COLLIMATORS, AND DETECTORS

Although some CT scanners are pulsed, most generate x-rays continuously. The tube, which may conduct a good fraction of an amp, is oil-cooled, and uses a rotating anode typically with a small focal spot, down to 0.6 mm. (Fifth-generation machines move the electron beam rather than the anode.) So as to not exceed the heat capacity of the tube, a cooling period between scans or sets of scans may be required.

The anode–cathode axis is aligned along the patient, perpendicular to the plane of the patient slice being irradiated, eliminating complications from the heel effect. More filtering is employed than with radiography because of problems introduced into the reconstruction calculations by beam hardening within the body. A filter is sometimes "scooped out" toward the middle, a crude form of tissue compensation that makes the beam emerging from the patient's body more uniform.

Most of the Compton photons coming from the irradiated thin slice scatter away from the detectors. The beam may be collimated at the detectors, moreover, as well as at the x-ray tube. As a result, nearly all the radiation that reaches the detectors carries primary x-ray image information. Energy windowing of the detector output (see Chapter 16, Section 6), which is a primary means of removing scatter radiation in nuclear medicine, is not needed.

Commercial scanners currently employ either scintillation or gas-filled ionization detectors. Primary design considerations are detector efficiency, a short response time (no afterglow), stability of operation, low dependence of detector response on x-ray energy (to reduce the effects of beam hardening), and cost.

The great advantage of **scintillation detectors** is their high density and nearly 100% detection efficiency. Bismuth germanate (BiGeO) and calcium fluoride (CaF_2) have replaced sodium iodide and cesium iodide because of their shorter fluorescence decay times.

Ionization chamber detectors, filled with the inert gas xenon, are operated in a voltage range for which the current

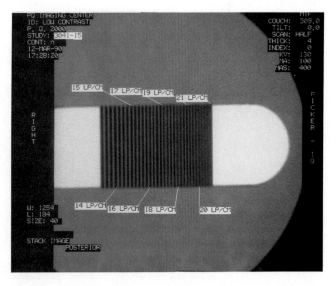

Fig. 38–6. Image of an in-slice resolution test pattern. *(Courtesy of Picker International.)*

through the detector is proportional to the radiation exposure. For greater detection efficiency, the xenon is pressurized to 25 atm (thereby increasing its density), and the chambers are long in the direction of travel of the x-ray photons. Although less efficient than a scintillation detector, an ion chamber is easier to manufacture in small sizes, its response is linear with exposure, and it costs less. This last point is important, given that some CT scanners may use a few thousand detectors. Other detectors, in particular semiconductor photodiodes, also have attractive characteristics, and are under development.

3. IMAGE QUALITY: RESOLUTION

The resolving power of CT, which generally refers to the ability to distinguish adjacent small, high-contrast objects, must be considered from two perspectives—resolution within each transverse plane and resolution in the direction perpendicular to those planes.

Within a plane (Fig. 38–6), a high-contrast resolution of 0.3 mm is normally achievable, with commercial manufacturers' claims ranging from about 0.25 to 0.6 mm. This is limited by detector aperture size, the image spatial sampling rate, the x-ray tube focal spot size, and the reconstruction algorithm (including, for filtered back-projection, the mathematical enhancement filter), and is considerably poorer than that of conventional radiography. The displayed resolution depends, of course, on achievable pixel size. The dimension of a pixel should be about a half or less of the system's required in-plane resolution to make full diagnostic use of its inherent capabilities. Thus with a 512×512-pixel matrix, a system may be able to display a 25×25-cm^2 region of interest at 1-mm resolution, in accord with Equation 37.1. But "hardware-zoom" can concentrate all the available pixels of the matrix into a smaller subregion of the original field of view (FOV), resulting in pixels of reduced effective size and a display with improved resolution.

Slice thicknesses down to 1 mm can be obtained, with slices taken every 1 to 10 mm. If coronal and sagittal plane views are constructed out of many transverse slices, slice thickness is what limits longitudinal resolution.

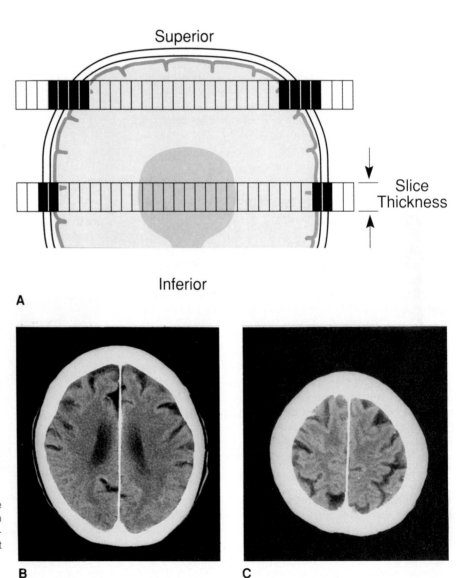

Fig. 38–7. A. The apparent thickness of the cranial wall depends on the angle it makes with the computed tomography slice. **B, C.** Transverse slices of the same head taken at different latitudes. *(Courtesy of GE Medical Systems.)*

CT machines allow the user to choose from among a few slice thicknesses, and in making this selection, several factors should be kept in mind. Doubling the slice thickness has the effect of averaging the measurement of the attenuation coefficient over a voxel twice as long. In a region where tissue characteristics change rapidly (e.g., at a bone–soft tissue interface), slice *thickness* may have a significant effect on *transverse* resolution and contrast (as well as on longitudinal resolution). This phenomenon is responsible, in part, for the apparent dependence of cranial wall thickness on axial position (Fig 38–7).

Also, as the attenuation of a ray by a voxel depends on an average of the radiologic properties of all the tissues in it, even a speck of high-atomic-number and/or high-density material within a voxel can significantly bias the calculated average CT number of the corresponding pixel. It is this *partial volume effect* that causes small calcifications, which might well be invisible in radiography, not only to show up clearly in CT, but even to appear significantly larger (pixel sized) than they really are.

4. IMAGE QUALITY: SCAN NOISE AND CONTRAST

When a uniform water bath is scanned (Fig. 38–8A), not all the pixels will exhibit a CT number of exactly 0 Hounsfield units. There will be a small spread, rather, in the relative numbers of pixels exhibiting different CT numbers near zero (Fig. 38–8B). This naturally occurring statistical variability is known as **scan noise**. Images from modern scanners are primarily *quantum* limited (see Chapter 27, Section 6), and the most significant random variations in voxel CT numbers are due to fluctuations in the number of x-ray photons passing through tissue and eventually striking the detectors. A simple Poisson statistics argument explains the dependence of the magnitude of this scan noise on slice thickness, deposited dose, and pixel size.

Consider the situation in which we choose to measure the same single-ray sum a number of times; that is, we repeat the experiment without moving the x-ray beam. Suppose that after passing through a water bath, 10,000 photons, on average, activate the detector. Then, by Chapter 18, Section 5, and Equation 18.11, the probability of finding any particular number (such as 10,783) of such photons in any one measurement will be Poisson distributed about $N = 10,000$, with a standard deviation of $\sqrt{N} = 100$. The relative width of the distribution in Figure 38–8B is proportional to this standard deviation. The signal-to-noise ratio (SNR) (see Equation 18.5) is then $N/\sqrt{N} = \sqrt{N} = 100$.

If we double the *dose* deposited in a slice during the measurement, or double the *thickness* of the slice (either of which will double the number of photons reaching the detector), the signal-to-noise will improve by a factor of $\sqrt{2}$. Equivalently, the scan noise, which can be defined as the relative variation (see Equations 18.4c and 18.5),

$$\text{scan noise} = 1/\text{SNR} = \sqrt{N} \qquad (38.1)$$

diminishes by a factor of $\sqrt{2}$.

Pixel signal-to-noise depends also on the choice of *pixel size*. Doubling the dimensions of a pixel means quadrupling its area and the count of x-rays passing through the corresponding voxel of the patient, hence doubling the signal-to-noise. (Averaging the counts over groups of four pixels of the original size would have the same effect.) We are not getting something for nothing here, of course: What is gained in noise reduction is lost in resolution.

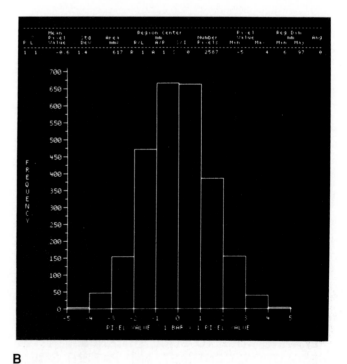

A   **B**

Figure 38–8. Computed tomography (CT) noise. **A.** Image of water phantom. **B.** The associated scan noise histogram, plotting the number of voxels against CT number. Modern scanners are quantum limited; that is, this spread in CT numbers is attributable primarily to natural, random variations in the number of detected x-ray photons, as described by Poisson statistics. *(Courtesy of GE Medical Systems.)*

In soft tissues, where the subject contrast is inherently low, the imaging ability of CT depends on the magnitudes of differences in attenuation coefficient (which may be slight), on the sizes of the objects of interest (if comparable to voxel size), and on the noise level. It is therefore necessary to hold the level of noise down. But important objectives of CT are to make the scan time short and to keep the patient dose low, both of which may diminish the SNR. In resolving the dose–noise trade-off, the designs of commercial scanners have evolved to a point where the exposure per scan results in a scan noise (Equation 38.1) of about 0.5% or less or, equivalently, an inherent signal-to-noise ratio of the order of 200.

That still allows a capability for imaging soft tissue that is, compared with standard radiography, quite remarkable. With 0.5% of noise, in which brightness varies randomly by 5 H or so from pixel to pixel, the eye may be able (barely) to distinguish a small region that differs from background by 5 H—the contrast that would be produced by a real 0.5% difference in tissue attenuation coefficient. It is left as an exercise to show that such a 0.5% difference, which is detectable by CT, corresponds to a change in the optical density of a radiographic film a factor of 10 or so times too slight to be seen.

> Noise is introduced into CT images in a number of other ways, as well. Electronic noise arises spontaneously in the preamplifiers of the x-ray detectors, and this will be amplified along with the true signal by the rest of the electronic circuitry. Information is lost (and the signal-to-noise ratio thereby reduced) also in the process of digitizing the continuous electrical signals coming out of the preamplifiers and through approximations made in the mathematical reconstruction.

_____ **EXERCISE 38–1.** _____

The attenuation coefficient of a 1-cm organ differs from that of its surroundings by 1%. In a part of the body 20 cm thick, will the organ be seen on a radiograph?

SOLUTION: This is like the example worked out in Chapter 19, Section 4. Most of the beam passes through x cm of tissue of attenuation coefficient μ cm^{-1}. A small part of it goes through $x - \Delta x$ of tissue at μ, and then Δx at $\mu + \Delta\mu$. The rays are attenuated by amounts $e^{-\mu \cdot x}$ and $e^{-(\mu \cdot x + \Delta\mu \cdot \Delta x)}$, respectively. The difference yields a subject contrast (see Equation 19.2) of $0.434 \cdot \Delta\mu \cdot \Delta x = 0.434 \cdot (\mu)(\Delta\mu/\mu)(\Delta x)$.

For soft tissue, μ is typically 0.2 cm^{-1}; the relative difference in the transmitted intensity is thus $0.434 \cdot (0.2 \text{ cm}^{-1})$ $(0.01)(1 \text{ cm}) = 0.1\%$, which is much too small to be seen on a radiograph. And this doesn't even consider scatter or the obscuring effects of patterns in the overlying tissues!

5. DOSE, AND A USEFUL EXPRESSION RELATING DOSE TO SLICE THICKNESS, RESOLUTION, CONTRAST, AND PATIENT SIZE

The doses delivered in a single CT slice tend to be in the range 1 to 4 cGy at skin surface and to fall off somewhat in the middle of the head or body (Fig. 38–9). Dose in a slice increases by a

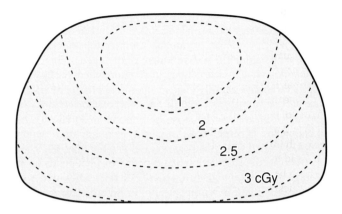

Figure 38–9. Typical distribution of the doses deposited in a single-slice computed tomography examination. For multiple contiguous slices, the doses might be twice these values.

factor of between 1.2 and 2.5 for a set of contiguous CT slices, however, because of overlap and scatter, as should be evident from the single-slice dose profile in Figure 38–10.

The dose, D, and a number of the imaging parameters are interconnected, and we shall present without proof a simple, approximate expression relating them:

$$D \cdot R^3 \cdot h/(\text{SNR})^2 \cdot e^{-p} = \text{constant} \qquad (38.2)$$

R is the resolution in millimeters (not lp/mm), and h is slice thickness. The signal-to-noise ratio (SNR) is a primary determi-

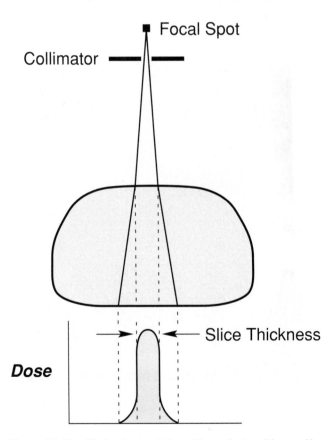

Figure 38–10. Single-slice irradiation of the patient and the resulting dose profile.

nant of the amount of contrast required for detection of a pattern in an image. And e^{-p}, where p is a typical ray sum for the patient, is a direct measure of patient size.

Equation 38.2 suggests that to reduce the level of noise by a factor of 2 while keeping the resolution and slice thickness the same, it is necessary to increase the dose fourfold. Likewise, to improve the resolution by a factor of 2 with no increase in dose or loss of possible contrast, one could switch from a slice thickness of 2 mm to one of 16 mm, assuming no loss of resolution through the partial volume effect. So also, when passing from the head to the body, resolution and/or signal-to-noise would have to be sacrificed to maintain the same skin exposure and slice thickness. Some of the other possible trade-offs described by the equation were discussed in previous sections.

6. RING, STAR, STREAK, AND OTHER ARTIFACTS

CT images occasionally display various kinds of **artifacts.**

Aberrations arise at the interfaces of materials of significantly different radiologic properties. Surgical clips and other *metallic objects*, in particular, will lead to *star artifacts* (Fig. 38–11), as may pockets of gas. In early head imaging, with iterative reconstruction algorithms, this effect caused a narrow ring to appear within and adjacent to the skull. This problem normally does not arise with analytic algorithms.

If the efficiency of one detector is significantly different from that of the rest, all the ray sums that it picks up will be irregularly large or small. The effect of this *detector imbalance* on an image is the appearance of a *ring artifact*, whose diameter depends on position of the detector in the array.

Motion of the patient may lead to loss of resolution and,

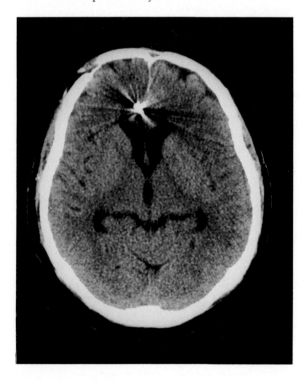

Figure 38–11. Star artifact caused by a metal clip. *(Courtesy of GE Medical Systems.)*

sometimes, even to streaks in the image. Such motion artifacts occur when an algorithm tries to assemble an image out of pieces of data that are not mutually consistent. They may be caused by respiration or even peristalsis, when involving the movement of bowel gas. Solutions include instructing the patient to remain still and using immobilization devices, antiperistaltic drugs, and sedation; most important of all has been the advent of faster scanners.

When an x-ray beam enters tissue, the lower-energy photons interact with matter and are attenuated more readily than are those of higher energies. As the beam hardens, the effective attenuation coefficient for a tissue decreases. The CT number of a voxel thus depends on its position in the body. This effect can easily lead to 10-H nonuniformities in the image of a homogeneous tissue. It can be especially troublesome in the head, because of the high calcium content of the skull. Thick copper beam filters and mathematical corrections of detector output (based on expected effects from beam hardening in typical patients), however, greatly reduce the seriousness of this *beam hardening* artifact.

7. QUALITY ASSURANCE

The ordinary imaging problems one has with scanners are usually much less severe than any of the artifacts, noted above, and can be prevented with a simple routine quality assurance program. Many of the kinds of tests used for radiography and fluoroscopy carry over to CT. In addition, the scale of CT numbers can be *calibrated* by ensuring that those of water and air are 0 ± 1.5 and -1000 ± 3 H, respectively. The *constancy* of the CT number for water should be checked daily, along with the *uniformity* and *scan noise* of the image of a large (20-cm-diameter) water phantom. Other checks with test phantoms confirm low- and high-contrast resolution (see Fig. 38–6), image linearity, slice thickness, and so on. Many of these tasks can be carried out by radiologic technologists. More extensive quality assurance should be performed periodically by a qualified medical physicist or engineer.

8. FUTURE DEVELOPMENTS

Although the period of most rapid growth and development of CT may be past, there is still much to look forward to.

High-speed fifth-generation machines, already discussed, are under continuing development. For third- and fourth-generation machines, in which the gantry rotates, much faster throughput times may be achieved with *slip-ring* technology and *helical scanning*. Previously, the gantry would have to reverse direction after each rotation, to untwist the power cables. With slip-rings, power is supplied to the x-ray tube by way of electrically conducting brushes making contact with grooved rings, and no twisting of cables occurs at all. The gantry rotates continuously in one direction and the patient table moves through the donut at constant speed, with the x-ray beam sweeping out a spiral or helix within the patient.

Dual-energy scanning has also been the focus of active research. The region of interest is imaged at two different kVp's, one immediately after the other (or by interlacing x-ray pulses of different energies). Alternatively, one can measure each ray sum simultaneously with two separate detectors, such as NaI and CaF$_2$, that have dissimilar energy responses. Either approach makes possible (because of the energy dependence of the tissue attenuation coefficients) separate estimates of tissue density and atomic number.

Image display technology has recently been undergoing considerable evolution. Surface and volume renderings of three-dimensional objects are finding increasing numbers of applications in the clinic (see Figs. 35–11 and 35–12), and the technologies of holography and virtual reality, as well, may soon be exploited for display purposes.

Finally, one can expect that our reliance on the computer will expand considerably along the lines of image interpretation. Artificial intelligence and computer-based pattern recognition capabilities will doubtless assume an ever-increasing role in diagnosis.

Part 8

Gamma Ray Imaging

Diagnostic nuclear medicine provides information on patient physiology by providing images of the in vivo uptake and distribution of administered radiopharmaceuticals.

There are three essential ingredients to a nuclear medicine study: (1) a pharmacologic agent that is taken up preferentially by an organ or biologic compartment of interest; (2) a radionuclide that can be attached to the agent and that emits gamma rays of sufficient energy to escape the body; and (3) a device to detect or image these gamma rays. An irregularity in the rate of uptake or washout of the radiopharmaceutical or in its spatial distribution may be indicative of a pathologic condition.

This chapter is concerned with the characteristics of the radiopharmaceuticals of choice. The next focuses on the detection of gamma rays from outside the body and on imaging technology.

Radioactivity and the products of nuclear decay were described in Chapter 7.

1. DESIRABLE CHARACTERISTICS OF A RADIOPHARMACEUTICAL

A nuclear medicine uptake or imaging study exploits the tendencies of certain radioactive materials to concentrate within specific organs or biologic compartments and to release a form of radiation that can be detected from outside the body. While the atoms of a few elements naturally go to a particular tissue, as with iodine to the thyroid, more generally the **radionuclide** must be attached to an organ-seeking **agent**. (As discussed in Chapter 7, "nuclide" refers to a nuclear species with well-defined characteristics, including a particular value for the _atomic number, Z,_ and for the _mass number,_ the total number of nucleons: protons plus neutrons. The prefix "radio-" implies that the nuclide is unstable.) The resulting radionuclide–agent combination, or **radiopharmaceutical**, must be not only diagnostically useful, but also safe and affordable.

The ideal _radionuclide_ (Table 39–1) releases _only gamma rays_ and has a _convenient half-life and chemical properties._ Particulate emanations expend all their energy in traveling through a few millimeters (beta particles) or a few micrometers (alpha particles) of tissue, and are therefore doubly undesirable: they cannot be detected from outside the body, and they deposit a potentially harmful dose in the patient. Gamma ray photons in the region 70 to 500 keV, on the other hand, stand a good chance both of escaping the body and of subsequently being detected by suitable instrumentation. It is helpful for the gamma emissions to be _monochromatic,_ since scatter radiation can then be largely eliminated through energy windowing (Chapter 16, Section 6). The half-life (the time it takes for half the remaining radionuclei in a sample to undergo decay) should be comparable to the time required to prepare the radiopharmaceutical and perform the examination: long enough to allow for the radiochemistry and for physiologic uptake and distribution, but short enough for the irradiation of the patient

TABLE 39–1. THE IDEAL RADIOPHARMACEUTICAL[a]

Radionuclide properties	
Gamma ray emission	140 keV, monochromatic
Particulates (beta, alpha)	None
Half-life	6 hours
Toxicity	Nontoxic
Radionuclide production	
Source	On-site, molybdenum-99 generator
Source replacement	Weekly
Cost	Low
Preparation	Elution, in minutes
Purity	< 0.1% Mo breakthrough, etc.
Agents	
Availability	In kits
Specifity	Specific to variety of organs
Preparation	In minutes
Binding to technetium	Stable
Quality assurance	Instant thin-layer chromatography, etc.

[a]Technetium-99m, which can be readily attached to various organ-specific agents, comes close to being an ideal radionuclide for nuclear medicine imaging.

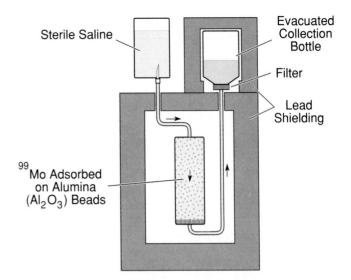

Figure 39–1. A generator for the daily production, in the clinic, of technetium-99m. Molybdenum-99, adsorbed to the surfaces of beads of alumina, undergoes beta decay with a 66-hour half-life. During daily elution with sterile saline, daughter technetium atoms dissolve into the solution and are flushed into the collection bottle.

to diminish rapidly after completion of the study. The radionuclide must be readily attachable to the agent, and it generally should be producible on-site, in the nuclear medicine department, in a **generator**.

The essential characteristic of an *agent* is that it be *organ/compartment specific*, preferably with a *differential uptake* between normal and pathologic tissues. There are a number of processes by which agents concentrate in organs. Iodine is drawn into thyroid cells by active transport. Reticuloendothelial cells take up sulfur colloid by phagocytosis, and lung scanning is made possible through temporary capillary blockade by macroaggregated albumin. Injected serum albumin simply dilutes to fill the blood pool.

Recently there has been great interest in the use of *monoclonal antibodies* as agents. With the other agents of nuclear medicine, concentration in a tissue is determined by the tissue's overall physiologic status, by the general level of functioning of its parenchymal cells. Some monoclonal antibodies, by contrast, are disease specific, and could provide information on the nature of a disorder, as well as on its location.

An agent plus radionuclide combination must be *nontoxic* (in the very small amounts administered), and the binding between them must be adequately *stable* both in vitro and in vivo. A number of agent-containing **kits** are commercially available that allow quick preparation of the radiopharmaceutical, simply by adding the locally generated radionuclide.

While several dozen radionuclides have found one use or another in nuclear medicine, by far the most widely employed is the metastable (excited) form of technetium-99. ^{99m}Tc has a half-life, $t_{0.5}$, of 6 hours, and it can be made to combine fairly easily with a variety of agents. Its complete decay scheme is complex, but only the 140-keV gamma ray is of significance, and one may think of the entire process that occurs within the patient as

$$^{99m}\text{Tc} \rightarrow {}^{99}\text{Tc} + 140 \text{ keV gamma}$$
$$\text{(in patient, } t_{0.5} = 6 \text{ hours)} \qquad (39.1)$$

The technetium-99m is either delivered from a commercial radiopharmacy or produced locally in the nuclear medicine department in a ^{99m}Tc **generator**, also known as a molybdenum

cow (Fig. 39–1). The manufacturer binds the radioactive *parent* ^{99}Mo to an alumina (Al_2O_3) or resin exchange column. There it transforms, with a half-life of 67 hours, into metastable technetium:

$$^{99}\text{Mo} \rightarrow {}^{99m}\text{Tc}$$
$$\text{(in generator, } t_{0.5} = 67 \text{ hours)} \qquad (39.2)$$

The daughter technetium is held chemically much less tightly than molybdenum to the column material, and can be *eluted* (washed) out of the cow with oxidant-free physiologic saline solution. The elutant, which consists of nearly pure sodium pertechnetate in water, is then ready for combination with the agent in a kit.

The time required for the regrowth of technetium, after a cow is milked, is determined largely by its own (6-hour) half-life (Fig. 39–2). Following an elution, *transient equilibrium* between parent (Mo) and daughter (Tc) radionuclides is nearly reestablished after several daughter half-lives, and it is therefore possible and efficient to milk the cow once a day. The initial specific activity (activity per unit of solution) of the technetium solution declines with the molybdenum activity, and the cow becomes useless after about a week.

The molybdenum parent can be prepared by the manufacturer in either of two ways. The nonradioactive isotope ^{98}Mo can be bombarded with a high flux of neutrons in a nuclear reactor,

$$^{98}\text{Mo} + n \rightarrow {}^{99}\text{Mo} \qquad (39.3a)$$

a process known as *neutron activation*. Such reactor-produced ^{99}Mo cannot be separated from the residual ^{98}Mo *carrier* that failed to become radioactive, and which competes for sites on the exchange column of the cow.

^{99}Mo can also be produced in the fissioning of uranium reactor fuel:

$$^{238}\text{U} \rightarrow {}^{99}\text{Mo} + \text{other fission by-products} \qquad (39.3b)$$

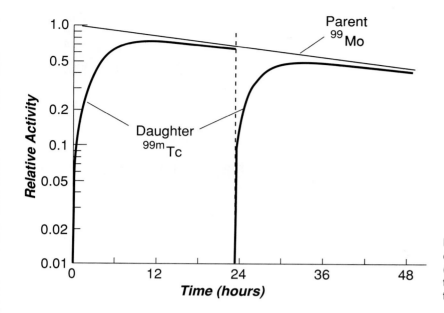

Figure 39–2. Activities within a molybdenum-99 generator of the ^{99}Mo parent and ^{99m}Tc daughter over time (on semilog graph paper). The regrowth of the technetium activity is controlled by its own 6-hour half-life, and the cow can be milked daily.

The radioactive molybdenum can be separated chemically from the other fission by-products, and is prepared in highly pure form.

Some of the radionuclides commonly employed in conventional nuclear medicine are listed in Table 39–2. As suggested by their half-lives, ^{60}Co and ^{137}Cs are used primarily for instrument calibration purposes. ^{99m}Tc, ^{113m}In, and ^{87m}Sr come from generators; the rest must be ordered directly from the producer, and suffer the loss of activity that occurs during transportation and storage. The positron-emitting radionuclides employed in positron emission tomography (PET) scanning constitute a totally separate list, and will be discussed in the next chapter.

2. ACTIVITY (Ci OR Bq) AND HALF-LIFE

The **activity** of a sample of radioactive material is defined as the number of decay events per unit time. The SI unit of activity is the **becquerel** (Bq),

$$1 \text{ Bq} = 1 \text{ decay event/s} \qquad (39.4a)$$

The perhaps more familiar **curie** (Ci) is related to it through

$$1 \text{ Ci} = 3.7 \times 10^{10} \text{ Bq} \qquad (39.4b)$$

Two convenient relationships between the sets of units are

$$1 \text{ mCi} = 37 \text{ MBq} \qquad (39.5a)$$

and

$$1 \text{ MBq} = 1/37 \text{ mCi} \qquad (39.5b)$$

where 1 megabecquerel (MBq) = 10^6 Bq.

The activity of a sample is not necessarily the same as the count rate obtained with a detector. If every nuclear decay resulted in the emission of exactly one ionizing particle, and if the detector were capable of sensing each of them, then the number of counts per second would be the sample's activity. But some gamma ray photons are absorbed by the sample material itself, and the detector is not 100% efficient; detector readings must be modified correspondingly.

TABLE 39–2. PROPERTIES OF SOME OF THE RADIONUCLIDES USED IN STANDARD CLINICAL NUCLEAR MEDICINE[a]

Z	Nuclide	Half-life	Principal Photon Energy (keV)
24	Chromium-51	28 d	320
27	Cobalt-57	270 d	122
	Cobalt-60	5.27 y	1332
31	Gallium-67	79.2 h	92, 184, 296
34	Selenium-75	120 d	265
38	Strontium-87m	2.8 h	388
43	Technetium-99m	6 h	140
49	Indium-111	2.8 d	173, 247
	Indium-113m	1.73 h	393
53	Iodine-123	13.3 h	159
	Iodine-125	60 d	35, 27
	Iodine-131	8.04 d	364
54	Xenon-133	5.3 d	81
55	Cesium-137	30 y	662
80	Mercury-197	2.7 d	77
81	Thallium-201	73 h	135, 167

[a]Does not include positron-emitting radionuclides used for positron emission tomography.

From Simmons GH, Sodd VJ. Physics of Nuclear Medicine (Table 1). In Doi K, Lanzl L, Lin P (eds): Recent Developments in Digital Imaging (Monograph No. 12). New York: American Institute of Physics, 1984, with permission.

_____ **EXERCISE 39–1.** _____

An imaging study makes use of 100 MBq of ^{99m}Tc. What is that in curies?

SOLUTION: By Equation 39.5b, 100 MBq = 2.7 mCi.

_____ **EXERCISE 39–2.** _____

A renogram (renal uptake and clearance) study requires the use of 50 to 300 µCi of ^{131}I (depending on the age and medical status of the patient) attached to a suitable agent such as ortho-iodohippurate (OIH). What is the activity range in SI units?

SOLUTION: By Equation 39.5a, 100 µCi = 0.1 mCi = 3.7 MBq. The range is thus 2 to 10 MBq.

As discussed in Appendix 39–1, the activity of a sample of radionuclide diminishes over time exponentially with a **half-life**, $t_{0.5}$, characteristic of the isotope:

$$A(t) = A(0) \cdot 2^{-t/t_{0.5}} \qquad (39.6a)$$

This is seen more commonly in the form

$$A(t) = A(0) \cdot e^{-\lambda \cdot t} \qquad (39.6b)$$

where the *transformation constant* λ is related to the half-life through

$$\lambda \cdot t_{0.5} = 0.693 \qquad (39.7)$$

Equation 15.8 presented a similar link between the linear attenuation coefficient of photons in matter and their half-value layer (HVL).

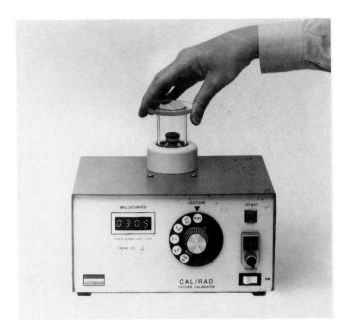

Figure 39–3.   A well counter used, among other things, to confirm the activity of every shipment to the department from the radiopharmacy and to check the amount of any radiopharmaceutical to be administered to a patient. *(Courtesy of Nuclear Associates.)*

3. RADIOPHARMACEUTICAL QUALITY ASSURANCE

An important activity of a nuclear medicine facility is the maintenance of a rigorous quality assurance program for preparation of the radiopharmaceuticals. The radionuclide itself must be sufficiently pure. In the case of ^{99m}Tc, *molybdenum breakthrough* must be less than 0.1%, according to the rules of the Nuclear Regulatory Commission (NRC); that is, 1 mCi (37 MBq) of ^{99m}Tc must be accompanied by less than 1 µCi (37 kBq) of ^{99}Mo. And the total amount of ^{99}Mo injected into the patient must be under 5 µCi (about 0.2 MBq). Actual breakthrough is typically 1% to 10% of the allowed limit. It is necessary to test for other radionuclide impurities, as well, and for aluminum from the ion exchange column. The binding of radionuclide to agent may be checked with instant thin-layer chromatography (ITLC). Also, conditions of sterility and pyrogenicity must meet the requirements of the United States Pharmacopeia (USP).

The activity of the material eluted from a generator, or of that to be injected into a patient, may be determined by means of a gas ionization or crystal scintillation **well counter** (Fig. 39–3). The accuracy of the counter itself at different gamma ray energies must be checked regularly with sealed, long-lived calibration sources such as ^{57}Co, ^{60}Co, and ^{137}Cs.

_____ **EXERCISE 39–3.** _____

Is more molybdenum likely to appear in the elutant from a cow containing molybdenum produced by neutron activation of ^{98}Mo or that produced by separation of uranium fission by-products?

SOLUTION: By neutron activation. But much of the dis-

solved molybdenum will be the stable isotope, which is not considered in assessing breakthrough.

_____ **EXERCISE 39–4.** _____

A molybdenum-cow yields 10 mL of elutant with a specific activity of 3 kMBq/mL (80 mCi/mL) of ^{99m}Tc. Part of it is needed for imaging 9 patients, each of whom will receive 5 mCi in a 0.5-mL bolus. How should these injections be prepared?

SOLUTION: The desired specific activity for injection is 5 mCi/0.5 mL, or 10 mCi/mL. Diluting 1 mL of the elutant with 7 mL of sterile saline solution would do the job.

4. THE RADIATION SAFETY PROGRAM FOR RADIONUCLIDES

Many aspects of nuclear medicine radiation safety are similar to those for diagnostic radiology. The ultimate objective is to keep doses to staff and the public, and nonproductive dose to the patient, as low as is reasonably achievable (ALARA) and far below any applicable legal limits. Time of exposure to radiation should therefore be minimized, and distance and shielding from the source should be maximized, all within reason. Syringes and vials of elutant, for example, should be kept within lead or lead–glass sheaths and behind lead bricks.

In the handling of radiopharmaceuticals, there is an additional need to prevent, to the extent possible, the inadvertent transfer of radionuclides into or onto the body. The primary line of defense against such contamination is not to allow its spread in the first place. Food, drink, and smoke should be kept out of the work area, and pipetting should never be done by mouth. Workers should wear coveralls and disposable gloves. Work areas should be covered with paper towels and always kept clean and neat. Some volatile materials require handling under a fume hood or within an airtight box. Workers should be monitored with film or other badges, worn on the lapel and finger. And areas where radionuclides are handled should be surveyed regularly with a sensitive contamination detector, such as a Geiger counter.

The NRC and the states have spelled out detailed rules designed to ensure that the risk of radioactivity contamination is minimized. There are prescribed procedures (in 10 CFR 20) for opening the boxes in which radionuclides are shipped, for storing the material before use, for disposing of that which is not employed (As noted in Chapter 34, Section 5, you cannot just flush it down the drain), for labeling work areas, samples, and waste, for educating and monitoring personnel, and for surveying work areas. And it is necessary to keep accurate, comprehensive records on all of this.

There must also be a clearly understood, standard procedure for handling spills: Nearby workers should be notified promptly; the radioactive material should be isolated, contained, and mopped up with disposable towels (which must, themselves, then be disposed of properly); and the area should be cleaned and surveyed. For larger accidents, the hospital's Radiation Safety Officer must be contacted immediately.

A final caveat. Most nuclear medicine uptake and imaging studies involve the use of 1 to 10 *milli*curies (about 40 to 400 MBq) of radiopharmaceutical. One important exception is the radionuclide ^{131}I, which is unusual in two respects: (1) 100 or 200 *micro*curies (4 to 8 MBq) is commonly employed for diagnosis, and (2) ^{131}I is used not only for diagnosis, but also for therapeutic purposes, such as in the treatment of hyperthyroidism and metastatic thyroid carcinoma. A typical therapeutic dose is 100 *milli*curies (4 kMBq), enough to cause complete ablation of the thyroid. Incidents have occurred in which a patient in a clinic for diagnosis was inadvertently given a therapeutic dose of ^{131}I, with severe consequences. This could happen because of failures of the responsible technologists to assay the shipments received from the manufacturer with a survey meter, to check the shipping papers, to assay the amounts being given patients with a well counter, or to label bottles and other containers clearly—because of a breakdown in the normal radiation safety program. Hence the need for unflagging attention to QA and radiation safety procedures, and the importance of maintaining good ALARA techniques.

5. THE GEIGER COUNTER COUNTS INDIVIDUAL NUCLEAR DECAY EVENTS

A nuclear medicine department employs a variety of devices not only for imaging, but also for quantifying the amount of radionuclide present. Ion chamber or scintillation detector well counters are in constant use, for example, to assay and confirm the activities of radionuclides to be administered to patients and for the performance of in vitro clinical tests. The operation of such devices has been described in earlier chapters.

The **Geiger counter** (see Fig. 29–8B), which is the standard *survey* instrument for detecting trace amounts of radioactive contamination on work benches, floors, sinks, etc., works somewhat differently. Like an ion chamber, a Geiger counter consists of a gas-filled chamber containing two electrodes attached to an electronic charge-sensing device (Fig. 39–4). But the potential difference between the electrodes is significantly higher, typically 1000 V or so. When x-rays or gamma rays interact with the chamber wall, they liberate photoelectrons and Compton electrons, which then enter and ionize the gas within. The resultant cations, anions, and electrons are rapidly accelerated to high velocities by the strong electric field between the electrodes. They themselves cause further ionizations, and the process snowballs. This *cascade* is augmented by the emission of ultraviolet (UV) light from deexciting gas molecules. The result is an intense electrical discharge throughout the gas and a pulse of current through the attached electrometer. When amplified and passed into a small loudspeaker, this gives rise to an audible click.

Once started, such an avalanche will continue indefinitely, unless intentionally stopped. The discharge can be *quenched*, to ready the chamber for the next incoming gamma ray, either electronically or chemically. A special electronic circuit can turn the high voltage briefly off, after a discharge has begun. Alternatively, a discharge will quickly die out if the chamber gas contains molecules that can absorb a sufficient amount of the liberated ultraviolet and ionic kinetic energy. Earlier Geiger counters of the latter type contained ethers and alcohols that dissociated permanently on absorbing a UV photon. The obvious problem with those chemical quenchers was the finite useful lifetime. Modern devices contain organic halogen compounds that can recombine into their original form after dissociation.

The time it takes to quench a discharge, known as the system's *resolving time*, or **deadtime**, is of the order of 100 mi-

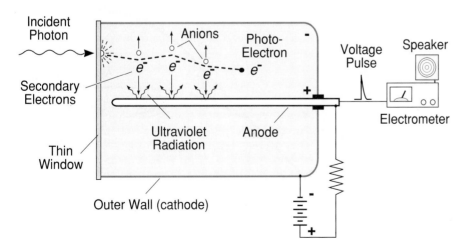

Figure 39–4. Discharge of a Geiger counter, triggered by a photoelectric event in its window. The photoelectron ionizes some of the gas molecules it passes near; these are accelerated through a large potential, and they too cause ionizations. This charge amplification process leads to the creation of a voltage pulse that is readily detected by the electrometer.

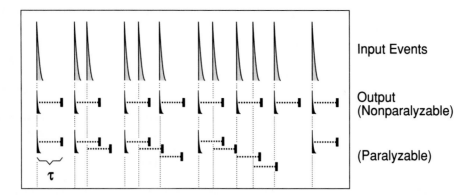

Figure 39–5. Paralyzable versus nonparalyzable devices. After any input event that triggers the instrument, there occurs a *deadtime* of duration τ, during which it cannot register again. A *nonparalyzable* device simply disregards input events that occur during the deadtime. A *paralyzable* device, however, begins its deadtime clock anew after every input event, whether or not it registers; that is, it must experience a quiet period, free of any input events, at least τ long before it is primed to register again. In the period of time covered here, there were 12 events, any one of which could, in the absence of other events, trigger the device. A nonparalyzable device with a deadtime of τ would be triggered eight times. A paralyzable device would count five events.

croseconds. You are doubtless wondering what happens if a gamma ray interacts with the chamber during the dead period from a preceding gamma event: No pulse is registered, but the cascade (and the dead time clock) are started anew (Fig. 39–5). This leads to the problem that at high *true count rates*, the *observed count rate* may actually decrease rapidly with increased sample activity (Fig. 39–6). Geiger counters (and most other radiation detectors) are thus said to be *paralyzable* devices. With a deadtime of the order of 100 microseconds, a Geiger counter is useful only up to a few thousand counts per second; above that, the observed count rate may differ significantly from the true count rate.

The scaler (counter) and other kinds of electronic gear to which a Geiger chamber is attached, by contrast, may be *nonparalyzable*. After one pulse registers, a subsequent pulse that

occurs during the device's deadtime is simply ignored altogether. It does not register, but it does not extend the deadtime initiated by the previous pulse, either.

To arrive at the true count rate R_t, it is clearly necessary to correct the observed count rate, R_o, from a detector so as to take its deadtime, τ, into account. A nonparalyzable device that actually observes and counts R_o pulses in a second, for example, will be nonfunctional for the total time $R_o \cdot \tau$ during that second. But during the functional (*non*-deadtime) portion of the second, of total duration $1 - R_o \cdot \tau$, it registers the R_o pulses. The *true* rate is thus

$$R_t = R_o/(1 - R_o \cdot \tau) \quad \text{(nonparalyzable)} \quad (39.8)$$

The process of correcting for deadtime in a paralyzable system is similar.

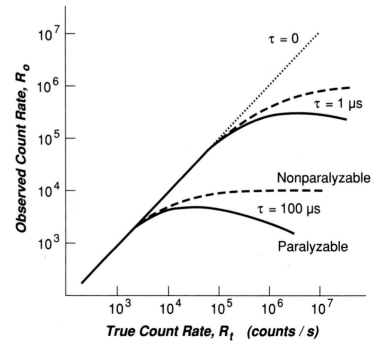

Figure 39–6. The relationship between observed count rate, R_o, and true count rate, R_t. For the ideal instrument, $R_t = R_o$ (dotted line). For a nonparalyzable device of deadtime τ, according to Equation 39.8, the observed count rate levels off to a value of $1/\tau$ for large R_t (dashed lines). For a paralyzable device, R_o actually begins declining above true count rates of about $1/\tau$ (solid lines).

6. THE WIDTH OF A RADIONUCLIDE'S PHOTOPEAK, AND ENERGY WINDOWING THE OUTPUT OF A SCINTILLATION DETECTOR

Geiger counters are the most sensitive of the gas-filled detection devices. They are easy to operate, stable, reliable, and relatively inexpensive. They are used extensively in radiation protection work to survey radionuclide contamination of personnel and the environment.

But despite their virtues for radiation surveys, Geiger counters are orders of magnitude too slow for sample calibration, and they cannot discriminate among photons of different energies, a capability essential to the operation of most gamma ray imaging devices. The scintillation detector, commonly used in well counters, survey meters, and gamma cameras, suffers neither of these deficiencies.

Chapter 16, Section 6, noted that in the energy spectrum obtained by a properly calibrated scintillation detector, the position of a radionuclide's photopeak is determined solely by the energy of its gamma rays. The *width* of the photopeak is something else again. The width of a spectrum is usually expressed as the full width at half-maximum (FWHM) in keV, or, equivalently, as the *percentage energy resolution*, defined as

$$\text{\% energy resolution} = 100 \cdot \text{FWHM/peak energy} \quad (39.9)$$

One might expect a very narrowly peaked pulse height spectrum from monochromatic gamma rays. But with a sodium iodide plus photomultiplier tube (NaI/PMT) scintillation detector, the FWHM for ^{99m}Tc gamma rays is about 20 keV, corresponding to an energy resolution of 14%, as shown by the solid curve in Figure 39–7. The 1332-keV gamma ray of cobalt-60, by contrast, is about 80 keV wide for a NaI/PMT detector, with an energy resolution of 6%. When obtained with a germanium–lithium (written Ge(Li), and pronounced "jelly") semiconductor diode detector, however, the photopeaks of both radionuclides are nearly 20 times narrower—the case of ^{99m}Tc appearing as the dashed line in Figure 39–7. Thus, the width of

a photopeak depends on both the energy of the gamma rays and the nature of the detector material. How come?

The height of a voltage pulse caused by a photoelectric event in a detector is determined primarily by the number of electrons initially liberated with the absorption of the gamma ray. This is the case both for scintillation detectors and for semiconductor diode detectors.

With a NaI/PMT detector, between 1 and 5 photoelectrons are ejected from the photocathode of the PMT, on average, for every 1000 eV of gamma ray energy absorbed by the scintillation crystal, depending on the nature of the crystal and the design of the PMT. The number of electrons eventually reaching the final dynode of the PMT may be a million times greater, but the critical issue is what happened at the photocathode.

Suppose, for example, that an average of 3 photoelectrons are released from the photocathode of a NaI/PMT detector for every 1 keV of absorbed gamma ray energy. For ^{99m}Tc, then, about 420 photoelectrons will be produced with the complete absorption of a 140-keV photon:

$$(3 \text{ electrons/keV})(140 \text{ keV}) = 420 \text{ electrons} \quad (39.10)$$

This is only a rough figure, and the number of electrons released with the absorption of a particular 140-keV gamma ray will most likely be somewhat above or below 420. The actual distribution of the numbers of such electrons liberated is described closely by *Poisson statistics* (see Equation 18.11). The standard deviation in number of photoelectrons liberated is $\sqrt{420} = 20.5$, with a corresponding energy standard deviation of $(20.5) \cdot (1\text{keV}/3 \text{ electrons}) = 6.8 \text{ keV}$.

> A reminder: If there are N photoelectrons freed from the photocathode of the PMT, on average, then the standard deviation in that number (an appropriate measure of the width of the distribution) is given by $\sqrt{N}$. The exact number of electrons produced will be somewhere between $(N - \sqrt{N})$ and $(N + \sqrt{N})$ 69% of the times it is measured, and there is a 96% chance that the number of electrons will fall in the range $N \pm 2\sqrt{N}$, by Table 18–1.

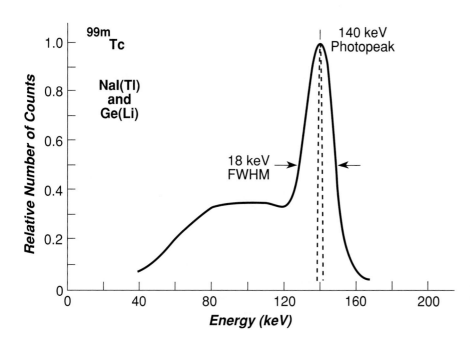

Figure 39–7. Gamma ray spectra of ^{99m}Tc obtained with NaI[Tl] (solid line) and Ge[Li] (broken line) detectors. The great difference in full width at half-maximum (FWHM) occurs largely because for the Ge[Li] detector, much less energy is required to excite electrons into the conduction band, so many more of them are liberated per incident gamma ray—hence (by Poisson statistics) the smaller relative variation. The photon spectrum obtained with the NaI[Tl] detector displays, in addition to the photopeak, structures attributable to Compton scatter of the gamma rays and to other instrumental effects.

For ^{99m}Tc gamma ray photons absorbed by a sodium iodide detector, the (Poisson) distribution of voltage pulse heights is the one shown as the photopeak in Figure 39–7. The FWHM happens to be a bit more than two standard deviations.

Random variations in the number of light photons created, and in the amount of light energy escaping from the crystal, and other aspects of pulse height determination increase the measured percentage energy resolution somewhat beyond this. But when all is taken into account, statistical arguments like the preceding can accurately explain the dependence of the photopeak FWHM on photon energy and detector design.

_____ **EXERCISE 39–5.** _____

It takes, on average, 3 eV to liberate an electron–hole pair in a Ge(Li) diode detector. How will the FWHM compare with that for a NaI scintillation detector?

SOLUTION: By Equation 39–10, 1 keV of photon energy produces 3 photoelectrons in NaI. The same energy releases 333 electrons in Ge(Li)—about 100 times as many—and the relative variation in that number will be less by a factor of $\sqrt{(100)}$ = 10. The FWHM for the Ge(Li) detector will be less by that amount.

_____ **EXERCISE 39–6.** _____

It takes, on average, 33.7 eV to liberate an ion pair in air. Considering only the counting statistics aspect of the difference, how will the FWHM for an ion chamber compare with that for a NaI scintillation detector?

SOLUTION: As there will be 333/33.7 times as many electrons involved, the FWHM will be $\sqrt{10}$ = 3 times narrower.

It is generally advantageous (and sometimes necessary, as in the case of imaging with a gamma camera) to be able to count or process only those pulses that lie close to the center of the photopeak. This can be achieved by means of an electronic pulse height analyzer (PHA) and energy discriminator (see Chapter 16, Section 6) that are set to accept only those pulses that lie within a certain prescribed energy range. Such **energy windowing** can be of benefit in two quite different ways: (1) With a gamma camera, it greatly reduces image degradation from Compton scattered photons. (2) Only those counts that correspond to decays of the nuclei of interest, and not to other radioisotopes or electronic noise, are accepted. It is common practice to set the width of the window equal to one or two times the FWHM, but the best choice depends on the photon energy and the application.

The photopeak, incidentally, is not the only significant structure to show up in gamma ray spectra. The low-energy Compton plateau in Figure 39–7 is attributable to Compton events occurring either in the patient or in the scintillation crystal. In the latter case, some of the energy of an incident gamma ray escapes the crystal as a scatter photon, after one or multiple scattering events, and only the amount imparted to the Compton electron(s) can be transformed into visible light energy. The Compton electrons themselves are produced with energies ranging from near 0 eV (for a glancing collision) to a maximum value somewhat below the photopeak energy (see Fig. 12–3).

A radionuclide spectrum may display a "backscatter peak" attributable to photons that have been Compton scattered through large angles and into the detector crystal by something outside of it, such as the protective metal shield. Some spectra contain structure at lower energies, such as peaks from characteristic x-rays produced by the iodine of the detector crystal or by the lead shielding, and peaks from the coincident detection of gamma rays emitted nearly simultaneously by two different radionuclide atoms.

7. ORGAN UPTAKE STUDIES

Studies of the rate or completeness with which a biologic compartment or organ takes up certain ingested, inhaled, or injected materials can shed light on the physiologic status of the compartment.

The plasma volume of the blood pool, for example, may be learned from an _activity dilution_ study: 0.4 MBq (10 μCi) of radioiodinated serum albumin (RISA), labeled with ^{125}I, is injected intravenously (Fig. 39–8). After 10 minutes of mixing with the patient's blood, a sample is removed and spun down in a centrifuge. The activity, A_{sample}, of the volume, V_{sample} (typically 1 mL), of plasma is measured in a well counter, and the result is adjusted to compensate for the background counts that register even when the instrument is empty. To the extent that the _concentration_ of RISA in the sample is the same as that in the rest of the patient's blood, the patient's total plasma volume V may be found from

$$A_{sample}/V_{sample} = 0.4 \text{ MBq}/V \qquad (39.11)$$

Rather than measuring activity of the radioiodine actually injected, in practice one sets aside exactly the same volume of RISA at the outset and dilutes it 3000:1 (which is about what happens to the RISA in the patient's blood pool). A sample of this diluted reference solution is then compared with what is taken from the patient. In that way, the same well counter settings may be used for both measurements, eliminating one source of inaccuracy.

The extreme sensitivity of nuclear medicine tests may be gauged by noting that the mass of the iodine is a factor of 10^{-13} less than that of the blood pool in which it dilutes.

A similar, but completely in vivo, study may be used to assess thyroid function: 0.4 MBq (10 μCi) of ^{131}I in the form of the sodium salt is administered orally, and the same amount is set aside in a sealed test tube for comparison. A day later, the activity from the throat of the patient and that from the reference sample (in the throat of an anthropomorphic phantom) are compared by means of a scintillation detector probe. (To account for background counts from iodine in parts of the body other than the thyroid, separate measurements are also made with the thyroid region itself blocked with a piece of lead.) And again, a simple ratio yields the percentage uptake.

A _renogram_ is a _dynamic_ study, in which the time development of radiopharmaceutical uptake, rather than the absolute amount taken up, is of interest. Figure 39–9 suggests that while the left kidney excretes ^{131}I-labeled Hippuran normally, there appears to be an obstruction preventing clearance from the

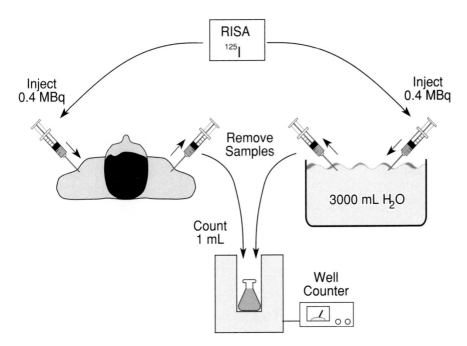

Figure 39–8. Isotope dilution study to determine the volume of the blood plasma pool. To compare the dilution of a certain amount of radionuclide in the patient's blood compartment with its dilution in a known volume of water, samples from both are counted in a well counter.

right kidney. Tests of this type are commonly performed with a gamma camera.

A *whole-body counter* is a room containing a number of NaI detectors arrayed so as to give a reasonable estimate of the total amount of a radionuclide in the body. The amount of potassium-40 (which constitutes 0.01% of naturally occurring potassium), for example, is a measure of lean soft-tissue mass, which can be a function of the state of health. Whole-body counters can also monitor the uptake of radionuclides in the workplace or following nuclear accidents. Shielding a whole-body counting room with thick plates of steel can reduce 50-fold the background counts from cosmic rays and environmental radioactivity. Care must be taken in the selection of the shielding materials, however, as trace amounts of radionuclides are commonly added to molten steel for production control purposes.

If the thousands of tons of lightly contaminated scrap copper, nickel, steel, and other metals from decommissioned nuclear power plants, nuclear weapons facilities, and the like, throughout the world are improperly re-cycled and released for unrestricted general commercial use, low but ubiquitous levels of radioactivity could become a major problem for the microelectronics, photography, and nuclear counting industries, and perhaps even a threat to health.

8. PHARMACOKINETICS: BIOLOGIC COMPARTMENT MODELING

Tracer kinetics studies are usually interpreted in terms of physiologic or anatomic compartment models. In the simplest situation, the concentration of a tracer in a compartment, $C(t)$, decreases exponentially with time as the tracer material is cleared from it. If the rate of washout is proportional to the concentration remaining in the compartment,

$$\Delta C(t)/\Delta t = -\lambda_b \cdot C(t) \qquad (39.12)$$

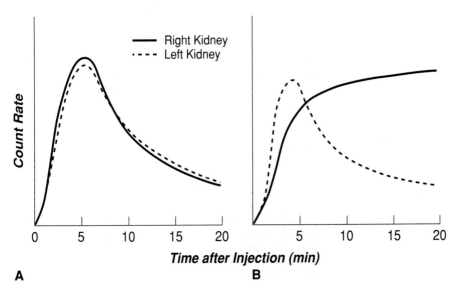

Figure 39–9. A renogram, in which uptake and excretion of Hippuran by each kidney are monitored separately. This kind of study is performed easily with a gamma camera. **A.** A pair of normal kidneys. **B.** The right kidney takes up the radiopharmaceutical fairly well, but fails to clear it, possibly because of an obstructed ureter.

and characterized by the biologic decay constant λ_b, the remnant concentration is then described by

$$C(t) = C(0) \cdot e^{-\lambda_b \cdot t} \tag{39.13}$$

Nuclear medicine makes use of radioactive tracers. The activity of such a tracer in a compartment decreases with time not only because of its removal from the compartment, but also because of physical decay of the isotope. The two processes are competing, in the sense that once a nucleus is removed from the compartment by one mechanism, it can no longer be removed by the other. By the general law of addition of probabilities for mutually exclusive events (see Equation 13.8) the total effective probability per unit time that a radionucleus will be removed from the compartment (by one mechanism or the other) is

$$\lambda_{\text{eff}} = \lambda_b + \lambda_p \tag{39.14a}$$

where λ_p is the physical decay transformation constant for the radioisotope. (In Chapter 14, Section 1, the same kind of argument legitimizes the separation of the mass attenuation coefficient into photoelectric and Compton components.) The activity in the compartment under examination will diminish exponentially with overall effective characteristic time $1/\lambda_{\text{eff}}$. By Equation 39.7, this expression can be rewritten in the form of half-lives as

$$1/t_{0.5,\,\text{eff}} = 1/t_{0.5,\,b} + 1/t_{0.5,\,p} \tag{39.14b}$$

APPENDIX 39–1. The Exponential Decay of Radionuclide Activity

A radiochemist prepares a pure sample that consists, at time $t = 0$, of $N(0)$ radioactive atoms. Some of the nuclei in the sample "disintegrate" (i.e., emit alpha or beta particles or gamma rays), such that at the later time t, only $N(t)$ nuclei are still intact. An additional $-\Delta N$ decay over the subsequent, relatively short interval Δt. The number of decays per second at time t is proportional to the number remaining, or

$$\Delta N/\Delta t = -\lambda \cdot N(t) \tag{39.15}$$

The *physical decay constant* or *transformation constant*, λ, is specific to the radioisotope under examination and depends on nothing else. In particular, it does not vary with time. This is so because radionuclei have no individual histories; every nucleus is oblivious to the decays of the other nuclei in the sample and to the span of time that has passed since its own creation. The probability per second of its decay or, equivalently, the fraction of remaining nuclei that decay per second,

$$\lambda = -\Delta N / N(t) \cdot \Delta t \tag{39.16}$$

is therefore perfectly constant. The probability rate will be exactly the same tomorrow, or next year, as it is now. (The number of radionuclei remaining intact in a sample and still available to undergo decay may be smaller, but that's a totally different issue.)

By the arguments in Chapter 15, the number of surviving radionuclei diminishes exponentially:

$$N(t) = N(0) \cdot e^{-\lambda \cdot t} \tag{39.17}$$

The units of λ are "per second" or (s^{-1}). In the characteristic time of $1/\lambda$ seconds, the number of remaining radionuclei in a sample will decrease by a factor of 0.37.

The *activity*, $A(t)$, of a sample of radioactive material is defined as the number of decays per (relatively short) unit of time:

$$A(t) = -\Delta N/\Delta t \tag{39.18}$$

From Equations 39.16 and 39.17, the activity of a sample is proportional to the number of radionuclei remaining in it, and the constant of proportionality is λ:

$$A(t) = \lambda \cdot N(t) \tag{39.19}$$

The activity of the sample, which can be determined with a suitable counting device, also decreases exponentially with time, with the same time constant as in Equation 39.17:

$$A(t) = A(0) \cdot e^{-\lambda \cdot t} \tag{39.20}$$

_____ **EXAMPLE 39–7.** _____

One millicurie of technetium is injected into a patient Monday at noon. What is the residual activity at 12:01 AM Thursday?

SOLUTION: The half-life of ^{99m}Tc is 6 hours, so the time span amounts to 10 half-lives. If, but only if, none of the sample leaves the body in urine, feces, perspiration, breath, or in other ways, the activity will decrease by a factor of $(\frac{1}{2})^{-10} = 0.001$. That is, 1 μCi will remain.

_____ **EXAMPLE 39–8.** _____

Demonstrate that the half-life, $t_{0.5}$, of a radiopharmaceutical is related to the transformation constant λ through Equation 39.7, $\lambda \cdot t_{0.5} = 0.693$.

SOLUTION: Set $t = t_{0.5}$ in Equation 39.20, and use $A(t_{0.5})/A(0) = \frac{1}{2}$.

_____ **EXERCISE 39–9.** _____

A certain radionuclide has a half-life of 1 week. A series of measurements on a sample of it reveal that 4.7 decays occur per second now, on average. How likely is it that 8 decays will occur during the next second? What about during 1 second exactly 2 weeks from now?

SOLUTION: See Exercise 18–5. The probability that 8 decays will occur in a particular second 2 weeks from now is determined the same way, but with an average activity of 1.175 Bq.

_____ **EXERCISE 39–10.** _____

One thousand identical pacemakers are given apparently identical new batteries. Do they fail (i.e., the output falls below some specified level) exponentially?

SOLUTION: The relative number of batteries "surviving" over time, $n(t)$, and the relative failure rate, $(\Delta n/n)/\Delta t$ (corresponding to λ), are revealed in Figure 39–10. Failure is not exponential because the physical characteristics (in particular, the exact rates of power consumption, at any instant, and the

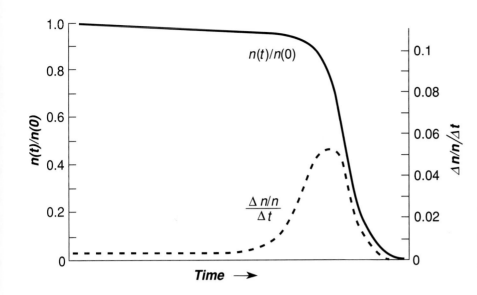

Figure 39–10. Unlike a radionucleus, a battery *does* have a history, and its state-of-being changes with time. The decline over time in the number, $n(t)$, of remaining batteries in a sample population is therefore not exponential, and $(\Delta n/n)/\Delta t$ is not constant.

amount of remaining energy) of a battery *do* vary over time. What would you expect to find for electronic component failure among the pacemakers themselves? What about when either battery or component failure might occur?

_____ **EXERCISE 39–11.** _____

It was claimed in Section 7 that the mass of the iodine is a factor of 10^{-13} less than that of the blood pool in which it dilutes. Confirm the 10^{-13} figure.

SOLUTION: By Equation 39.19 and the 60-day half-life, there are 3×10^{12} atoms of ^{125}I in a 0.4-MBq sample. The mass of 6×10^{23} (Avogadro's number) atoms of ^{125}I is 125 g. The mass of the 0.4-MBq sample is thus $(3 \times 10^{12}/6 \times 10^{23}) \cdot (125) = 6 \times 10^{-10}$ g, or 2 parts in 10^{13} of the 3000-g blood pool.

_____ **EXERCISE 39–12.** _____

Show that the discharge of a capacitor through the resistor of an RC filter circuit (see Chapter 8, Section 6) occurs exponentially with time.

SOLUTION: By Ohm's law, the current through R is proportional to the voltage across it: $\Delta q/\Delta t = V/R$. But the voltage across the capacitor is proportional to the charge remaining on it: $V = q/C$. Combining these, $\Delta q/\Delta t = -q/RC$, where the minus sign accounts for the flow of charge *off* of the capacitor. The solution to this (differential equation, when Δt becomes vanishingly small) is $q(t) = q(0) \cdot e^{-t/RC}$.

_____ **EXERCISE 39–13.** _____

Why would the intensity of light emitted by a fluorescent material diminish nearly exponentially with time following excitation with a pulse of x-rays?

SOLUTION: The rate at which electron traps are depopulated, with the emission of light, is proportional to the number that still contain electrons (see Chapter 16, Section 5).

Chapter 40

Nuclear Medicine II: Imaging

In the organ uptake studies described in the preceding chapter, it is the accumulation of radiopharmaceutical by a whole organ that is followed, either as a function of time or after physiologic equilibration.

Imaging literally adds new dimensions (two or three) to the information content of such studies, revealing the differential uptake of a radiopharmaceutical by different parts of the organ. If the radiopharmaceutical concentrates preferentially in one region, there occurs a correspondingly brighter area in the display. If, on the other hand, a portion of the organ is missing, or fails to take up the gamma emitter, or is obscured by overlying tissues, the region appears dark.

The imaging procedures performed in a nuclear medicine department depend on the size, experience, and interests of the department staff, the availability of nonstandard radionuclides and sophisticated technology (and computer expertise), and the accessibility of competing diagnostic modalities.

Two important offshoots of planar nuclear medicine are single-photon emission computed tomography (SPECT) and positron emission tomography (PET), both of which allow the imaging of individual slices of tissue, like computed tomography (CT), and the presentation of that information in a three-dimensional format.

1. THE RECTILINEAR SCANNER . . .

Before the advent of the gamma camera, radionuclide differential uptake images were produced with the *rectilinear scanner* (Fig. 40–1). Only those high-energy photons that pass along the single, narrow channel of the *collimator* can reach an otherwise shielded sodium iodide crystal and photomultiplier tube (PMT). The detection head is swept in a raster pattern: back and forth across, and slowly down, the patient. A point of light is made to appear at the corresponding place on the screen of a cathode-ray tube (or a dot is made on paper by a printer) each time a gamma ray is detected, and the screen is photographed. The density of points on the film or paper is thus a measure of the intensities of gamma rays emerging from the various regions of the body.

Figure 40–2 suggests a fundamental and important image quality trade-off found with the rectilinear scanner and with the gamma camera as well: A larger-diameter collimator channel will pass more gamma rays, but it will be less clear where any one of them came from. Thus, improvements in detector *sensitivity* must be paid for in loss of *resolution*.

The gamma rays detected by the scanner in Figure 40–1 could originate from radionuclei at any depth in the patient's body. But the image manifests a quasi depth dependence: The shallower the point of origin of the gamma ray in tissue, the more likely it is to reach the detector. A *focusing multihole collimator* (Fig. 40–3A), on the other hand, allows attention to be focused on tissues lying at any depth of interest beneath the surface. The collimator contains a number of channels, all converging to a *focal point*. Gamma rays coming from the vicinity of the focal point can reach the detector through all of the channels; fewer avenues are available to those emitted above or below it. Thus somewhat like conventional tomography (not CT) or an optical lens system, a focusing collimator selects out a single plane of tissue, several centimeters thick, for special consideration. The relative response of the system as a function of the distance of radionuclide above or below the focal plane may be seen from a set of *isoresponse curves* (Fig. 40–3B).

There are problems with the rectilinear scanner. Its head must move slowly enough for a statistically adequate reading of activity to be made at each position. But although increasing the amount of radionuclide (hence radiation dose) given to the patient can offset the problem of slow data acquisition, there is no way the system can be used to simultaneously follow rapid changes in different parts of an image over time. Both efficient

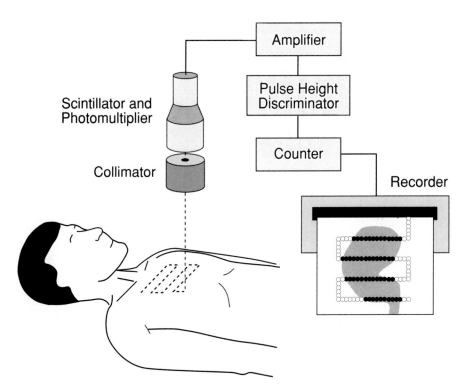

Figure 40–1. By means of a rectilinear scanner, mapping the spatial distribution within the body of a gamma-emitting radionuclide. The two-dimensional motions of the scintillation detector are mimicked by those of the recorder, and the output of the recorder is proportional to the count rate sensed by the detector.

data acquisition and the performance of dynamic studies call for the services of a gamma camera.

2. ... HAS LARGELY BEEN REPLACED BY THE GAMMA (ANGER) CAMERA

The **gamma camera**, designed by H. Anger in the late 1950s, works somewhat like an eye (Fig. 40–4).

Gamma rays cannot be focused, so the role of the lens is played by a **multihole collimator**, consisting of hundreds of small-diameter channels, separated from one another by thin lead foil septa. A gamma ray that does not travel along the straight and narrow is absorbed in the lead, as with a radiographic grid. Most commonly used is the *parallel-hole* collimator (Fig. 40–5A). A *converging-hole* collimator (Fig. 40–5B) produces magnified images. A *diverging-hole* collimator minifies (Fig. 40–5C) and allows the imaging of large organs by a camera with a smaller-diameter detection head, such as on a mobile gamma camera. Some collimators are invertible and can be used in either the converging or diverging mode. Finally, the *single-pinhole collimator* (Fig. 40–5D) will either magnify or minify, depending on the closeness of the organ of interest to the camera. The de-

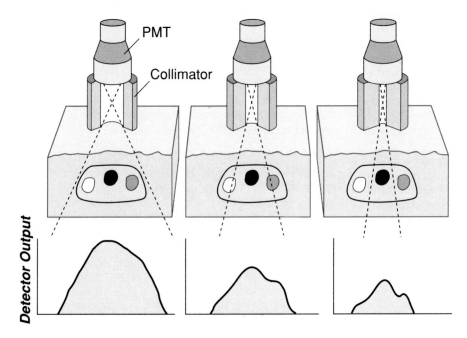

Figure 40–2. A basic trade-off in radionuclide imaging: The wider the collimator channel(s), the greater the sensitivity of the instrument, but the lower its resolving capability. PMT, photomultiplier tube.

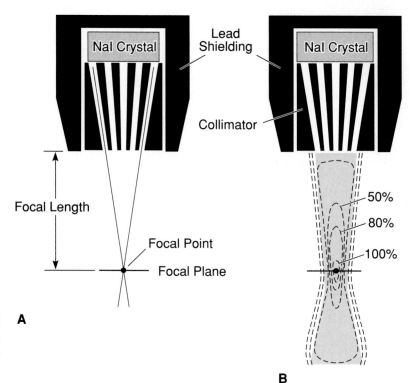

Figure 40–3. With a focusing collimator, the detector is most sensitive to radionuclide concentrated near the focal plane, in this case several centimeters beneath the skin surface. Percentages refer to detector sensitivity relative to that at the focal point.

tails of collimator design strongly affect image quality, as will be seen in Section 4.

Behind the collimator is a 1-cm ($\frac{3}{8}$-in.)-thick or, for better resolution on newer machines, 0.6-cm ($\frac{1}{4}$-in.)-thick single crystal of NaI[Tl], some 25 cm (10 in.) to 60 cm (24 in.) in diameter. This scintillation crystal is observed (usually through a *light pipe*, an optical coupling device) by a close-packed hexagonal array of 37, 61, 75, or 91 hexagonally shaped photomultiplier tubes.

The outputs of the PMTs feed into an analog **position-logic** or *scintillation-location* **circuit** that determines the position coordinates within the crystal of each scintillation event. (The crystal, PMT array, and scintillation-location circuit together act like the retinal photoreceptors and associated neural network of an eye.) Any gamma ray that makes it through the collimator and interacts with the crystal creates a scintillation. That burst of light produces voltage pulses in all the nearby PMTs (Fig. 40–6), and the nearer a photomultiplier tube to the scintillation, the larger the pulse. The scintillation-location circuit knows where every PMT is, and juggles the responses of all of them to arrive at a best estimate of where in the crystal the burst of light occurred.

The circuit outputs three voltage pulses for every scintillation. A pair of them, V_x and V_y, correspond to the event's x and y coordinates relative to the crystal (see Fig. 40–4B). The third, V_z, is proportional to its brightness, hence to the energy of the responsible gamma ray. This allows energy windowing; events are retained only if they belong to the photopeak. It is important to reject scintillations from Compton scatter photons created either in the patient or within the detector crystal, as they are informationally useless and reduce subject contrast.

In older machines, the x and y coordinate voltage pulses for each accepted scintillation went directly to the display, and

a pinpoint of light was produced at the appropriate place on the screen of a cathode-ray tube (CRT). The thousands of equally bright, fine-focused dots appearing briefly on the CRT were accumulated on film, commonly with a Polaroid camera. (A *multiformat camera* allows a number of images to be recorded on one large sheet of film.) To achieve a clinically useful image, consisting of several hundred thousand counts, the patient is viewed (and the shutter is held open) for a good fraction of a minute, or more.

In newer systems, the x and y pulses for each accepted photopeak scintillation are fed, via their respective analog-to-digital converters (ADCs), into a computer. Interfacing the gamma camera with a computer opens the system to the entire realm of dynamic and gated studies and image processing and display possibilities.

Several devices that provide information like that from a gamma camera are under development. Although gas-filled multiwire proportional chambers and various semiconductor imaging machines offer certain advantages, as of yet none of them has had much success in replacing the large scintillation crystal plus multiple PMT combination in the clinic.

3. LIST AND FRAME MODES OF IMAGE STORAGE IN THE COMPUTER

Computers are indispensable for the acquisition and processing of dynamic images, as in nuclear cardiology, and for the generation of SPECT or PET (tomographic) images.

A commercial gamma camera is normally supplied with its own dedicated computer system attached. An interface between the two, with fast, high-accuracy analog-to-digital converters for digitizing the voltage pulses corresponding to the x

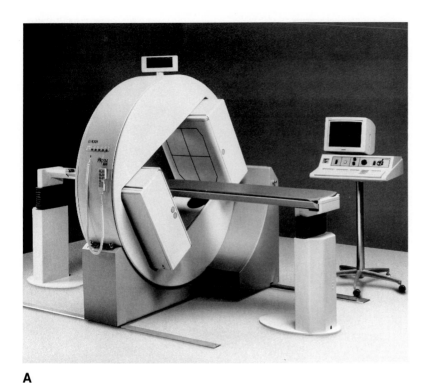

A

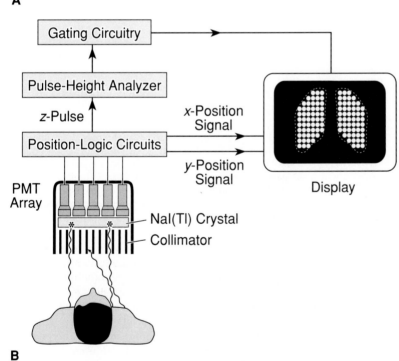

B

Figure 40–4. A modern gamma camera. **A.** A two-headed SPECT machine. Either head alone can serve as a simple gamma camera. **B.** The imaging head contains a collimator, a large-diameter, thin single crystal of thallium-doped sodium iodide, and an array of photomultiplier tubes (PMTs). With a gamma ray interaction, the resulting scintillation of light in the NaI(Tl) crystal is sensed by all the nearby PMTs. Its position is worked out by the position-logic circuit, and the corresponding pixel of the display becomes brighter. *(Photo courtesy of Picker International.)*

and y coordinates of scintillations, must be included. The computer's operating system should be capable of inputting and storing the scintillation data (high-priority task) and, at the same time (but with lower priority), creating an image out of those data.

Information is stored in the computer in either of two quite different general formats. In the **list mode**, the x and y coordinates and time of every photopeak scintillation go directly to memory as a separate (x, y, t) data triad (Fig. 40–7A). This allows complete retention of *all* the raw data accumulated,

making it of use for some types of research. It can also be useful in following rapidly changing processes, as in first-pass cardiac studies.

Static frame mode is more like photographing a nuclear medicine CRT screen with a Polaroid: The region being imaged is partitioned into a square matrix, consisting of from $64 \times 64 = 4K$ (4000) to $512 \times 512 = 262K$ voxels, each with its own (x, y) address. Every gamma ray event simply increments (increases in a step) by one the number of counts at the corresponding pixel (Fig. 40–7B). Much less memory is required than for list

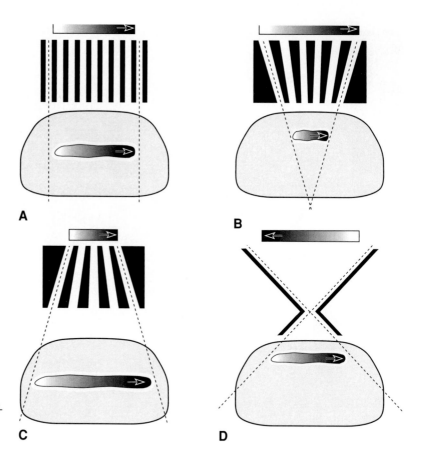

Figure 40–5. Gamma camera collimators. **A.** Parallel-hole. **B.** Magnifying. **C.** Minifying. **D.** Pinhole.

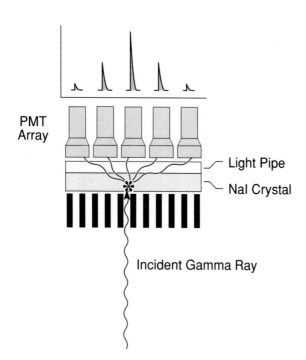

Figure 40–6. When a gamma ray photon excites the sodium iodide crystal, the amplitude of the voltage pulse produced by any photomultiplier tube (PMT) depends on its distance from the light burst. The position-logic circuit weighs the outputs of all the PMTs and estimates the most likely position, within the crystal, of the gamma ray interaction.

mode, and at the end of data acquisition, the image is already in a form suitable for immediate display.

> Whole-body scanning employs a variant of static frame mode. The patient's entire body is partitioned by means of, say, a 128×512 or 256×1024 grid. The body is moved past the gamma camera at constant speed, and the computer ensures that the addresses of scintillations correspond to voxels fixed in the body, rather than to positions on the face of the gamma camera.

If the temporal changes in an image are of interest, one can use the **dynamic frame mode** of data acquisition. The system counts into one frame for a preselected period, then closes out and stores that frame and begins on a fresh one. This procedure is repeated until the study is finished (Fig. 40–7C). The activities within a pair of kidneys were separately followed over time in Figure 39–9, for example, and the difference between them revealed the blockage of one ureter. But even much smaller effects may indicate an abnormality. This exemplifies the beauty of dynamic nuclear medicine: it allows the imaging of time-dependent physiologic processes, not merely anatomy.

A **multiple-gated (MUGA)** *cardiac study* employs a modification of the dynamic frame mode of data acquisition, and exploits the periodic, repetitive nature of the heart's pumping. Initiated by an R-wave trigger from an electrocardiogram (ECG) the first frame accumulates counts for a specified period, such as 40 milliseconds; after that, the second frame takes over, for the same time interval, and so on. This stepping procedure continues for 20 or 30 frames, long enough to cover one

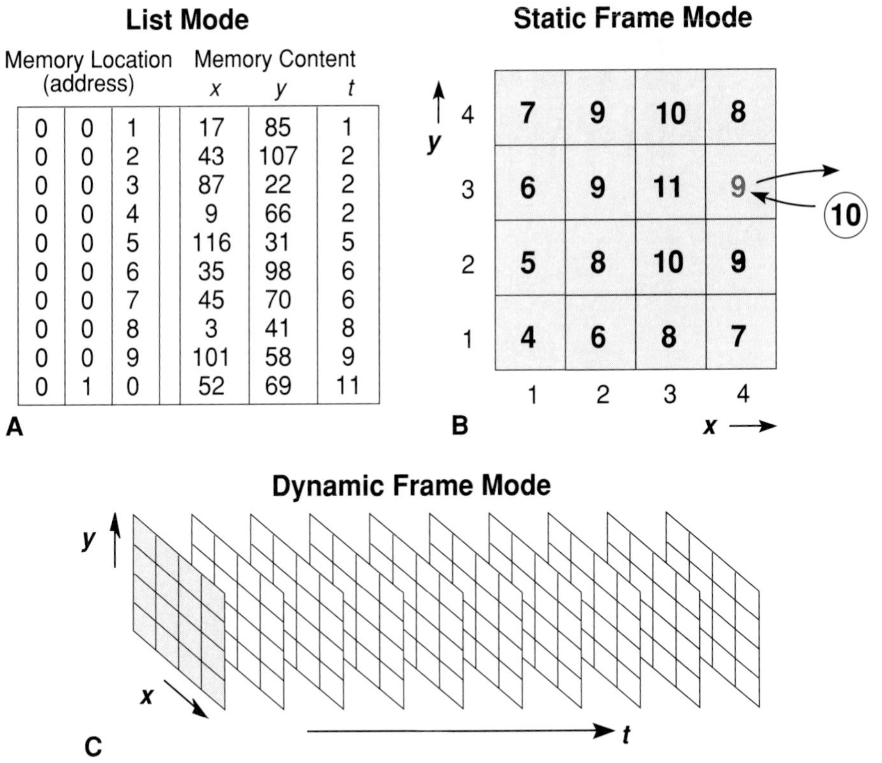

List Mode

Memory Location (address)			Memory Content		
			x	y	t
0	0	1	17	85	1
0	0	2	43	107	2
0	0	3	87	22	2
0	0	4	9	66	2
0	0	5	116	31	5
0	0	6	35	98	6
0	0	7	45	70	6
0	0	8	3	41	8
0	0	9	101	58	9
0	1	0	52	69	11

A

Static Frame Mode

B

Dynamic Frame Mode

C

Figure 40–7. Methods of storing scintillation information. **A.** With list mode, complete information (the spatial address and the time) for each event is stored in memory. **B.** Static frame mode stores image information by keeping track of the number of counts associated with each pixel in the frame. Here, the number of counts at the pixel with address $(x, y) = (4,3)$ is being incremented by 1. **C.** With dynamic frame mode, information is stored in a frame for a predetermined period, after which new data are directed to the next frame. Multiple-gated (MUGA) dynamic frame mode, a variant of this, cycles repeatedly through a set of several dozen different frames in synchrony with the cardiac cycle.

heartbeat, until the next ECG R-wave starts the whole business over again, back at frame 1. Special programs track and reject counts occurring during arrhythmia. And although few data are obtained over any one cycle, several hundred repetitions result in images with sufficient numbers of counts.

Once an image has been produced, the computer can enhance its quality in various ways. One standard technique for smoothing out naturally occurring, random fluctuations in the numbers of counts in pixels was discussed in Chapter 35, Section 7. The count in any pixel is replaced with a new value: a weighted average of the number in the pixel and in its neighbors as well. In a dynamic study, the number of counts in each pixel address can be averaged temporally, over several sequential frames. Spatial and temporal smoothing involves losses of high-frequency components of spatial information, but nonetheless may result in images more meaningful to the eye.

4. CONTRAST, SPATIAL RESOLUTION, AND SENSITIVITY

The achievable quality of a nuclear medicine image is determined by three separate factors: (1) the differential uptake of the radio-pharmaceutical in various tissues; (2) the amount of attenuation and scattering of gamma ray photons by overlying and adjacent tissues; (3) the characteristics of the equipment and the duration of the study (hence the number of counts recorded).

The *subject* or *object contrast* in a nuclear medicine image, which reflects only the first of these, is commonly expressed as the relative difference in radionuclide concentrations [Conc] existing in normal and pathologic tissues (Fig. 40–8)

$$C_{obj} = (\text{Conc}_{norm} - \text{Conc}_{path}) / \text{Conc}_{norm} \qquad (40.1a)$$

Subject contrast, attenuation by overlying tissues and scatter, and the machine characteristics and study duration together determine the *image contrast*, defined as the relative difference in the displayed number of counts, N, per unit area, A, in the region of interest:

$$C_{image} = [(N/A)_{norm} - (N/A)_{path}] / (N/A)_{norm} \qquad (40.1b)$$

As with radiography, scatter radiation degrades contrast, but energy windowing and the collimator (like an antiscatter grid) both remove much of the Compton radiation created within the patient. Nuclear medicine differs from radiography, however, in that C_{image} is strongly influenced by the depth within the body of the organ being imaged, because of both the loss of gamma rays in overlying tissues and the activity uptake by those tissues.

The *resolving power* of a gamma camera, R, may be taken to be the full width at half-maximum (FWHM) of the point spread function (PSF; see Chapter 18, Section 4),

$$R = \text{FWHM of PSF} \qquad (40.2)$$

(Fig. 40–9). With this convention, *larger* values of R indicate *worse* resolution. System resolution is determined by the detection system (i.e., the sodium iodide crystal plus the photomultiplier tube array) and by the collimator. The effects of these two components can be considered separately.

The **intrinsic resolution**, R_{intr}, is the FWHM of the PSF for the sodium iodide crystal, the photomultiplier tube network, and the position-logic circuit, in the *absence of any collimator*. The range of a photoelectron in NaI (hence, the dimensions of the volume from which a burst of light is emitted) is less than a millimeter, so *that* does not degrade resolution appreciably. The intrinsic spatial resolution is limited, rather, by the natural

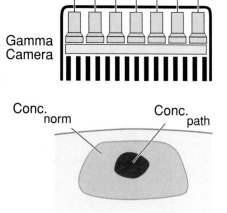

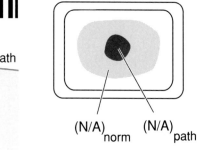

Subject Contrast   **Image Contrast**

Figure 40–8. Subject contrast expressed in terms of radionuclide concentrations in normal and pathologic tissues of the patient, and the corresponding image contrast in the display, shown as a difference in counts per unit area.

random variations in the heights of the voltage pulses coming out of the PMTs: Even if every gamma ray were absorbed at exactly the same point in the crystal, there would still be appreciable variations in the values of the x- and y-coordinate voltages, V_x and V_y, because of voltage fluctuations in the scintillation-location circuit and other sources of noise.

Intrinsic resolution improves (i.e., R_{intr} decreases) with in-

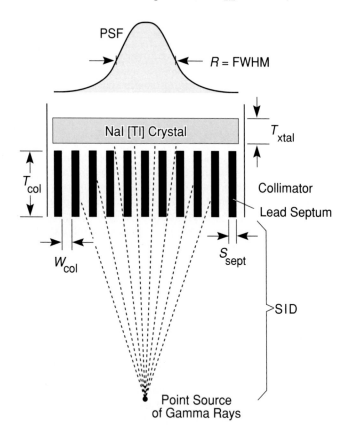

Figure 40–9. The resolving power of a gamma camera may be described in terms of the full width at half-maximum (FWHM) of the point spread function (PSF) or line spread function (LSF). It is determined by the characteristics of the collimator and by those of the scintillation-location system (consisting of NaI crystal, photomultiplier tube array, and position-logic circuit).

creasing photon energy, up to a point. Resolution worsens with greater detector crystal thickness because (as with radiographic screens) scintillation light can spread out more before reaching the photomultipliers. The intrinsic resolution of a modern gamma camera is such that it can make out the bars in a 3 to 6 lp/cm (note: cm, not mm) bar pattern.

The **collimator resolution** R_{col} of a parallel-hole collimator is a function of its thickness, T_{col}, and channel width, W_{col}, the thickness of the scintillation crystal, T_{xtal}, and the source-to-image receptor distance (SID) from the gamma ray source plane (within the patient's body) to the face of the collimator:

$$R_{col} = (W_{col}/T_{col})(T_{col} + SID + T_{xtal}) \qquad (40.3)$$

Equation 40.3 follows from the geometry of the situation: As with a radiographic grid, long and narrow channels lead to greater rejection of undesirable photons. The decline of resolution with distance of the camera face from the organ is illustrated in Figure 40–10A (which takes no account of attenuation by tissue) and also by the set of corresponding PSF curves (Fig. 40–10B) and modulation transfer functions (Fig. 40–10C). Resolution is halved, typically, as SID goes from 0 to 5 cm, and is of the order of 1 cm at a distance of 10 cm (Fig. 40–11). Diverging-hole collimators have somewhat worse resolutions than this; resolutions of converging-hole collimators are better.

As with the screen–film system of Equations 22.5 and 18.9c, the overall **system resolution** of the collimator/detector combination, R_{sys}, is determined by the capabilities of its constituent parts:

$$R_{sys} = \sqrt{(R_{intr}^2 + R_{col}^2)} \qquad (40.4)$$

The system resolution is worse than that of either detector or collimator alone, of course, but it is normally dominated by the latter. The best resolution actually achievable by a given camera depends on its design and physical condition (which may degrade over the years), on the object being imaged, and on the viewing conditions. A nice round figure frequently bandied about is 0.5 cm for a test object at the collimator face.

The *sensitivity* or *efficiency* of a gamma camera is also affected by both the detector and the collimator. The photopeak detection efficiency of the crystal/PMT system is nearly 100% for gamma ray energies up to 100 keV. At higher energies, it depends strongly on crystal thickness. The collimator sensitiv-

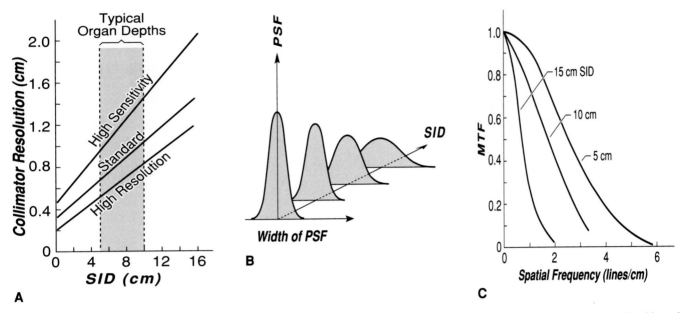

Figure 40–10. Three related ways of describing loss of detail as the source-to-image receptor distance (SID) increases, that is, as the object of interest moves further from the camera face. **A.** Resolution as a function of depth of the organ in the patient's body, for three parallel-hole collimators. Resolution can be determined from a bar pattern or as the full width at half-maximum (FWHM) of the point spread function (PSF) or line spread function (LSF). Resolution is defined here in cm, not lp/cm. **B.** PSF at different depths for the standard collimator. **C.** Modulation transfer function (MTF) for the standard collimator, for organs 5, 10, and 15 cm beneath the skin surface.

ity, S_{col}, a measure of the relative number of gamma rays that will make it through the collimator, is given approximately by

$$S_{col} = K \cdot [W_{col}^2 / (T_{col})(W_{col} + S_{sept})]^2 \qquad (40.5)$$

where S_{sept} is the thickness of the septa between collimator channels, and K is a constant (about $\frac{1}{4}$). The septal thickness needed for adequate resolution increases with gamma ray energy (and thus with its power of penetration).

There is a simple and useful, but approximate, quantitative relationship between the sensitivity and resolution of a gamma camera collimator. Equation 40.3 indicates that R_{col} increases approximately as W_{col}/T_{col}. But by Equation 40.5, sensitivity is nearly proportional to $(W_{col}/T_{col})^2$. Comparing these,

$$S_{col} \sim R_{col}^2 \qquad (40.6)$$

which indicates that for a fixed septal thickness, resolution improves only at the expense of diminished sensitivity. Larger collimator holes will allow through more gamma rays, but will decrease the ability to pinpoint their places of origin, as suggested by Figure 40–2.

Commercial collimators are specified by energy ("low-energy" collimators, with thin septa, may be used up to about 150 keV), or by reference to the resolution–sensitivity trade-off ("high resolution," "high sensitivity," or "general purpose").

_____ **EXERCISE 40–1.** _____

Why is sensitivity relatively independent of SID for a parallel-hole collimator?

SOLUTION: The number of holes through which gamma rays can pass increases roughly as SID². By the inverse square

effect, however, the number of photons that pass through any one of them decreases as 1/SID². The total number detected (proportional to the product of the two factors) remains about the same.

5. LESION DETECTABILITY IS ULTIMATELY DETERMINED BY INFORMATION DENSITY

With a correct setting of the display CRT's brightness control, the brightness and degree of mottle of a region are determined ultimately by the **information density (ID)**, or number of gamma rays detected and displayed per square centimeter of the object being imaged,

$$\text{information density} = \text{counts/subject area} \qquad (40.7a)$$

or, in the notation of Equation 40.1b,

$$\text{ID} = N/A \qquad (40.7b)$$

Gamma camera image quality tends to increase with number of counts—rapidly, at first, but then with diminishing returns. Patient throughput, on the other hand, declines with greater counting times. An average ID of the order of 1000 counts/cm² is commonly held to represent a good balance of the two factors.

Poisson statistics and the capabilities of the eye place lower bounds on possible combinations of lesion size, contrast, and ID for which an irregularity can be detected. Suppose that the area of the lesion is A and that the information density there is ID. The number of counts in that region is

$$N = A \cdot \text{ID} \qquad (40.8)$$

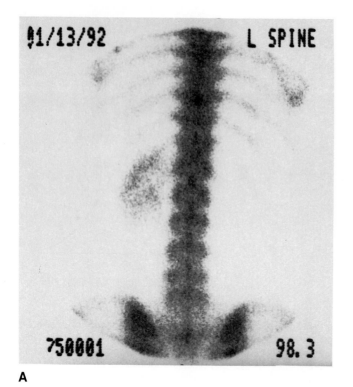

A

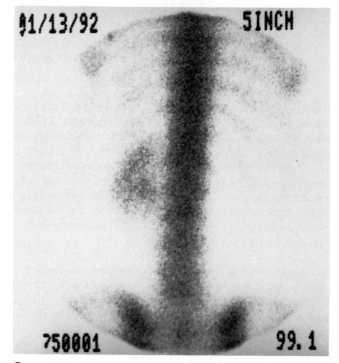

B

C

Figure 40–11. These three ^{99m}Tc bone scan images (750,000 counts each) demonstrate the dependence of image quality on source-to-image receptor distance. They were taken with the patient's back **(A)** touching the face of the gamma camera, **(B)** 2 in. from it, and **(C)** 5 in. from it.

The relative variation in that number (see Equation 18.4c), also known as the *noise contrast*, is

$$\text{noise contrast} = \sqrt{N}/N = 1/\sqrt{N} = 1/\sqrt{(A \cdot \text{ID})} \quad (40.9)$$

Humans are generally capable of visually detecting objects (that are not too large or small) amid noise when the contrast is at least two to five times the noise contrast. If the minimum detectable image contrast is denoted $C_{\min}$, then

$$C_{\min} = (2 \text{ to } 5) \cdot (\text{noise contrast}) = (2 \text{ to } 5)/\sqrt{(A \cdot \text{ID})}$$
$$(40.10a)$$

or

$$C_{\min} \cdot \sqrt{(A \cdot \text{ID})} = 2 \text{ to } 5 \quad (40.10b)$$

which has the general form of Equation 18.6. Thus, if a lesion is suspected to be small or of low contrast, the camera must accumulate a large number of counts to overcome the loss of image signal amid the statistical noise. This can be achieved either by imaging for a long time (increasing the likelihood of motion blurring) or with high radiopharmaceutical activity (and dose to the patient).

_____ **EXERCISE 40–2.** _____

There are 600 counts/cm² of healthy organ in the vicinity of a 5-cm² lesion. What is the minimum detectable contrast for the lesion? What if counts were accumulated for a period twice as long?

SOLUTION: Setting the constant on the right-hand side of Equation 40.10b equal to 2, then, with an ID = 600 counts/cm², $C_{min} = 2/\sqrt{(5\text{ cm}^2) \cdot (600\text{ cm}^{-2})} = 0.04 = 4\%$. With 5 on the right-hand side of Equation 40.10b, this becomes 9%. So the minimum contrast is somewhere in the range 4% to 9%. If the ID were doubled, the minimum detectable contrast would be lower by a factor of $\sqrt{2}$.

A related argument leads to a fourth-power relationship between information density and spatial resolution:

$$\text{ID} \sim 1/R_{sys}^4 \tag{40.11}$$

So to improve the system resolution by a factor of 2, you can switch to a collimator with twice the resolution. But then you have to compensate for lost sensitivity (and reduced capability of the eye to pick out the relevant visual patterns) by increasing the number of counts by a factor of about 16.

6. GAMMA CAMERA QUALITY ASSURANCE

In addition to the radiopharmaceutical quality assurance and radiation safety programs discussed in the preceding chapter, a nuclear medicine department must have a procedure for routinely monitoring the performance of imaging equipment.

Standard checks for a gamma camera and its computer system (some of which should be performed as often as daily) include tests of the following:

- Field *uniformity*, in which a planar *flood phantom* exposes the crystal uniformly, with the collimator both in place and removed. The sensitivities of the individual PMTs may drift over time, which will lead to dark areas, distortions, and loss of resolution if not corrected. Even when the flood image appears uniform, a computer-generated histogram of numbers of pixels versus numbers of counts (which should be consistent with Poisson statistics) may provide an early indication of the need for servicing. Modern gamma cameras have microprocessor circuits that adjust the PMTs or in other ways compensate for minor nonuniformities automatically; testing with the uniformity correction circuit disabled provides a more demanding test of the conditions of the PMTs.
- *Resolution*, as determined with a bar pattern between the camera and the flood phantom (Fig. 40–12). Alternatively, the image of a thin tube filled with radionuclide allows determination of the line spread function (LSF),

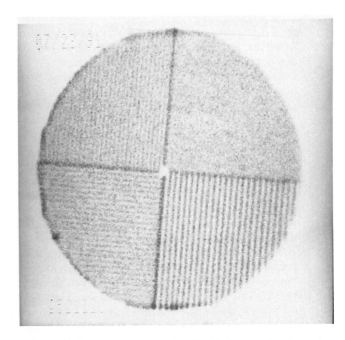

Figure 40–12. A bar pattern, interposed between a flood phantom and the camera face, provides information on resolution and linearity.

the FWHM of which is a good measure of resolution. If more complete information is needed, the Fourier transform of the LSF yields the modulation transfer function (MTF).
- *Linearity* and distortion, as seen in the image of a long, narrow tube filled with radionuclide.
- *Energy window* peaking, that is, centering the energy window on the photopeak of a reference radionuclide and selecting the window width for optimal signal-to-noise.
- *Counting efficiency* or sensitivity, as determined, for example, with a (relatively long-lived) cobalt-57 or cesium-137 sample of known activity.
- *Background* count, in which the camera is turned on with no patient or phantom present.
- Imaging capability of the camera/computer combination when operating at *high count rate*. The total dead-time per pulse, typically around 10 microseconds, depends on various electronic components of the system, some of which are paralyzable, some nonparalyzable. The system should be able to produce proper images at 75,000 counts per second or more.

7. SOME STANDARD IMAGING STUDIES

Here is a sampler of some commonly found clinical examinations. In general, an abnormally dark area within the image of an organ may indicate missing tissue, or a failure to take up the radiopharmaceutical, or the presence of an overlying growth or other irregular structure. A bright area, conversely, suggests tissue that for some reason has accumulated an unusually high concentration of the radiopharmaceutical. Note that, with some important exceptions, the radionuclide activities of most of these studies are in the range 40 to 400 MBq (about 1 to 10 mCi).

- *Liver*: 80 to 200 MBq (2 to 5 mCi) of ^{99m}Tc, bound to sulfur colloid particles averaging 0.5 μm in diameter, is injected into a vein. The particles are picked up by the reticuloendothelial cells that are distributed fairly evenly throughout the liver, spleen, and bone marrow. A region of reduced radionuclide take-up in any of these organs (Fig. 40–13) may indicate replacement of normal tissue by tumor.
- *Spleen*: 8 to 10 MBq (0.2 to 0.3 mCi) of chromium-51 attached to heat-damaged erythrocytes.
- *Lung*: Lung *ventilation* can be assessed following inhalation of technetium, in mist form, or xenon gas. A dark region indicates an inability of air to reach volumes it normally occupies, as with blockage of air passages, the presence of fluids, or the replacement of lung tissue with tumor. Similarly, lung *perfusion* is imaged minutes after 100 MBq (3 mCi) of technetium bound to macroaggregated serum albumin (MAA) is injected intravenously (see Figure 1–9). The microscopic lumps of MAA (15 to 75 μm in diameter) become lodged in about 0.1% of the capillaries of the lung (but are dissolved and flushed away within a few hours). A cold region indicates a region where the MAA does not reach the capillaries in the first place, as with a pulmonary embolism. Ventilation and perfusion studies are commonly carried out in tandem. This involves exploiting the separation of the photopeaks of ^{133}Xe at 80 keV (^{127}Xe, with a 203-keV gamma ray, is preferable for imaging, but harder to come by) and ^{99m}Tc at 140 keV.
- *Thyroid*: 40 to 80 MBq (1 to 2 mCi) of sodium pertechnetate. The behavior of the TcO_4^- ion mimics that of iodine.

Thyroid nodules, which may be cancerous, do not take up the technetium, and give rise to cold spots in the image.
- *Brain*: 400 MBq (10 mCi) of ^{99m}Tc-labeled diethyltriamine pentaacetic acid (DTPA). Damage to brain vascularity from injury or tumor and breakdown in the blood–brain barrier may show up as increased activity. It is somewhat ironic that although conventional nuclear medicine imaging for the brain has largely been supplanted by CT and magnetic resonance imaging (MRI), PET has found its most rewarding applications there.
- *Kidneys*: 400 MBq (10 mCi) of ^{99m}Tc glucoheptonate or DTPA. Renal trauma, a tumor, or a cyst may lead to a region of reduced uptake. A dynamic study of uptake (see Fig. 39–9) can provide an early indication of the success of a renal transplant.
- *Skeleton*: 400 to 800 MBq (10 to 20 mCi) of ^{99m}Tc-labeled methylene diphosphonate (MDP). The phosphate compound adsorbs to hydroxyapatite crystals, and half of what is injected is taken up by bone within 15 to 20 minutes (Fig. 40–14). Bone that is being broken down by a tumor may attempt to undo the damage by laying down new bone tissue, incorporating the technetium, and giving rise to a hot spot. But so, too, may arthritis and some other noncancerous diseases.
- *Pancreas*: 10 MBq (0.25 mCi) of selenium-75 methionine.

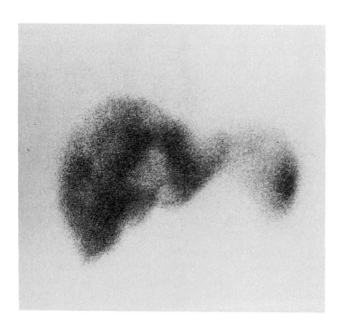

Figure 40–13. Five millicuries of technetium-99m sulfur colloid administered intravenously gave rise to this 500,000-count liver–spleen scan of a 60-year-old man. Multiple focal defects in the liver are due to metastatic colon cancer. Compare this with the three-dimensional rendering by SPECT in Figure 1–11. *(Courtesy of Patrick J. Peller.)*

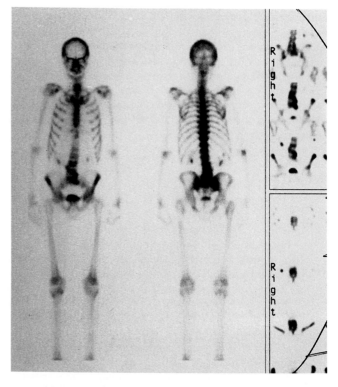

Figure 40–14. Whole-body bone scan, generated in 15 minutes by an imaging machine that can produce either conventional images, such as this, or SPECT. *(Courtesy of Picker International.)*

- *Tumor or abscess*: 200 MBq (5 mCi) of gallium-67 citrate. Also, tumor-specific, radiolabeled monoclonal antibodies are the subject of intense investigation, especially for use with SPECT or PET.
- *Heart*: Thallium acts as a potassium analog, and the rate of thallium uptake by myocardial cells may be significantly affected by coronary artery disease or myocardial infarction. 60 MBq (1.5 mCi) of thallous (^{201}Tl) chloride allows imaging of heart perfusion. Also, ^{99m}Tc-labeled red blood cells or serum albumin is commonly used for cardiac blood pool studies. Dynamic imaging of the heart depends heavily on the use of the computer, as will be discussed in the next section.

These are but a few examples of the many imaging procedures in common use. For each of the organs listed, other radiopharmaceuticals and activities have been used as well. The radiopharmaceuticals and activities noted here are typical, but are *not* necessarily what should be employed in any particular clinical situation.

8. NUCLEAR CARDIOLOGY: FIRST-PASS AND MULTIGATED STUDIES

Nuclear medicine offers noninvasive alternatives to some cardiac catheterization studies. It also provides nontraumatic ways of following the response of the heart to surgical or other kinds of therapy, both in the resting state and under stress. Studies are of two general kinds, and both reflect the heart's action as a reciprocating pump.

As noted in Section 3, information on different phases of the cardiac cycle can be obtained by means of ECG-driven, **multiple-gated (MUGA)** imaging. After the two dozen or so individual frames have all stored a sufficient number of counts, each may be examined separately (Figure 40–15). A cold region in a single frame (which is not blurred by cardiac motion) may indicate a region of ischemic or infarcted muscle. Alternatively, the frames can be displayed in rapid sequence, creating a cine of a pulsating heart. Quantification of wall thickness and motion, cardiac chamber size, ejection fraction, and other aspects of the image statics and dynamics can provide valuable information on cardiac pathology. And abnormal patterns of perfusion response to exercise may be suggestive of coronary artery disease.

A problem with multigated imaging, however, is that both ventricles contain radionuclide and, unless viewed from the left anterior oblique (LAO) angle, they overlap. But from the LAO angle, important portions of the myocardium are not clearly revealed. This difficulty does not arise with the second major category of cardiac imaging, the **first-pass cardiac study**. An intravenously injected, high-activity bolus of radionuclide is followed as it passes through the right ventricle and, subsequently, through the left. When seen from the right anterior oblique (RAO) angle, for example, the ventricles overlap, but by the time the bolus reaches the left ventricle, nearly all of the radionuclide will have already washed out of the right. The study is completed within 30 to 60 seconds and must be recorded at a high frame rate following sharp injection of the radionuclide. First-pass studies allow determination of the transit times of passage of the bolus through the various parts of the cardiovascular system,

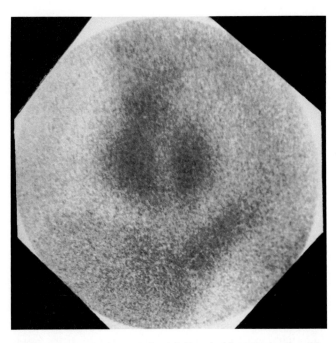

Figure 40–15. One frame of a left lateral oblique technetium-99*m* multiple-gated (MUGA) cardiac study. The photopenic halo that surrounds both ventricles indicates a pericardial effusion. *(Courtesy of Patrick J. Peller.)*

which are affected by valvular disease, abnormal ventricular function, and irregular pulmonary circulation. It also provides a means of quantifying left-to-right cardiac shunt.

9. SINGLE-PHOTON EMISSION COMPUTED TOMOGRAPHY

As with x-ray (transmission) imaging, a variety of attempts have been made to produce three-dimensional information via (emission) nuclear medicine. The "tomoscanner," like conventional x-ray tomography (not CT), uses motion of the detector relative to the patient to extract the image of a single, thin slab of tissue. The seven pinhole camera and the four-quadrant slant-hole collimator camera produce seven and four images, respectively, on different parts of a NaI[Tl] crystal at the same time; obtaining images from slightly different vantage points gives rise to a quasi three-dimensional perspective, somewhat like stereoscopy. A CT-like radionuclide imaging device appeared in 1964, but only in the past decade has single-photon emission computed tomography (SPECT) assumed the clinical role of the nuclear medicine counterpart to x-ray CT.

Between one and four fairly standard gamma camera heads (each with collimator, crystal, and PMT array), mounted on a supporting gantry (see Fig. 40–4A), are rotated slowly around the patient. Data are acquired at 32, 64, or 128 projection angles. Motion of the camera head is circular for some machines, but others provide for an elliptical orbit that allows closer approach to the patient at some angles and, hence, better overall resolution and sensitivity. The data are processed, most commonly by filtered back-projection (see Chapter 37, Section 6), so as to generate CT-like images. Reconstruction computations are more complicated and susceptible to artifacts than in CT, however, as the detected signal depends upon not only the three-dimensional spatial distribution of the attenuation tissues (as with CT), but also the distribution of the radionuclide. Algorithms that correct efficiently for tissue attenuation are still being developed.

The results of a SPECT study can be presented either as transverse slices or in three dimensions (see Fig. 1–11). The visual impact of three-dimensional display, and perhaps its clinical utility, can be enhanced by causing the patient (or at least the organ being imaged) to appear to rotate continuously about an axis.

SPECT is effective in imaging myocardial infarctions and ischemia, and shows promise in quantitating cerebral blood flow. It has proven to be more sensitive than conventional planar gamma camera imaging at detecting occult fractures and some other bone irregularities. It may also be useful in the detection of tumors, with radiotagged monoclonal antibodies as agents. Not surprisingly, when considering the purchase of a new gamma camera, growing numbers of nuclear medicine facilities are opting for a SPECT system instead.

Quality assurance and maintenance are more demanding than with either planar gamma camera imaging or CT. Field uniformity and the precise mechanical motion of the heads about the center of rotation are especially critical.

10. POSITRON EMISSION TOMOGRAPHY

A nucleus is held together by means of the *strong nuclear force* acting among its protons and neutrons. But the protons also repel one another electrically because of their charge. For a nucleus with a relatively high proton-to-neutron ratio, this electric repulsion, together with the *weak nuclear force,* may lead to nuclear instability. Such a nucleus will attempt to achieve stability by reducing its net positive charge. And one way to do that is to emit a **positron,** as with Equation 7.4a.

If released into tissue, such a positron loses most of its kinetic energy in ionizing atoms along its path. After traveling less than a millimeter, typically, it collides with an electron, and the two particles annihilate one another. Their masses are converted into electromagnetic energy, in the form of a pair of

511-keV photons that leave the site of the collision in nearly opposite directions (180 ± 0.25 degrees apart) (see Equation 7.6 and Exercise 7–3). The existence of this *annihilation radiation* makes possible another type of emission CT, very different from SPECT.

Several general types of positron emission tomography (PET) cameras have been built. One design makes use of a half-dozen or so adjacent rings of small, independent solid scintillation detectors that are separated from one another by lead septa. A ring might contain several hundred individual crystals of bismuth germanate (which has a higher sensitivity than NaI), each viewed by its own PMT. A **coincidence circuit** accepts only those events in which two opposing detectors (across from one another in either the same or different rings) are struck by 511-keV photons at virtually the same time (Fig. 40–16). PET cameras do not use collimators, but rather employ coincident detection as the sole means of emission localization.

Resolution within a transverse plane of the patient is determined primarily by the size of the individual scintillation crystals, which might be 0.5×1.2 cm in cross section (and 3 cm deep in the radial direction). The ultimate achievable resolution is inherently limited to about 2 mm or so, however, because of positron travel in the patient and because the 511-keV photons are not emitted in exactly opposite directions.

As with SPECT, reconstruction is complicated by the presence of attenuating tissues, but the problem is not quite so bad here. Gamma rays that register in a particular pair of detectors must originate from some point along the straight line connecting them (Fig. 40–16). The probability that one of the gamma rays will travel through x_1 of tissue and reach a detector is proportional to $e^{-\mu \cdot x_1}$. The corresponding odds for its partner annihilation photon go as $e^{-\mu \cdot x_2}$. The likelihood of a coincidence event, in which the two photons both arrive at their respective detectors without having been absorbed or scattered in tissue, is therefore proportional to

$$P_{\text{coin}} = (e^{-\mu \cdot x_1})(e^{-\mu \cdot x_2}) = e^{-\mu \cdot (x_1 + x_2)}$$

That is, the probability of a coincidence event depends on the total thickness $(x_1 + x_2)$ of the tissue along the line between the detectors, but not on the position of the positron-

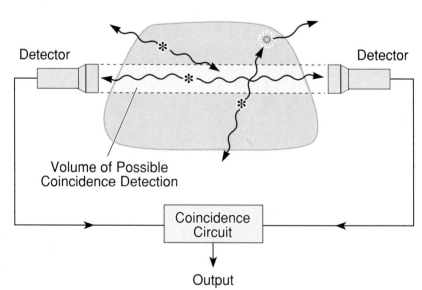

Figure 40–16. With positron emission tomography, a gamma ray event registers if two 511-keV annihilation photons are detected simultaneously. The positron-emitting nucleus lies somewhere along the line joining the two excited detectors.

emitting nucleus along that line. This is a valuable additional piece of information, not available with SPECT, that significantly ameliorates the reconstruction process.

Some positron-emitting radionuclides are listed in Table 40–1. Among these are isotopes of carbon, nitrogen, oxygen, and other elements of special biochemical relevance. These have been prepared as gaseous O_2, CO, CO_2, and NH_3 and incorporated into saccharides and amino acids for a wide variety of imaging uses in tracing biochemical pathways. O_2 containing one atom of ^{15}O has been used extensively to monitor both blood flow and oxygen metabolism.

Fluorodeoxyglucose (FDG), a glucose analog labeled with ^{18}F, can cross the blood–brain barrier. Its metabolic products differ from those of glucose, however, in that they are not highly mobile: the fluorine becomes trapped where the molecule is first used. FDG can therefore map glucose uptake in the brain, which can be affected by a variety of physical and mental stimuli and by diseases (see Fig. 1–12B). Again, the importance of PET is not in anatomic imaging, but rather in its ability to reveal subtle physiologic processes not accessible by other means.

The production of positron-emitting radionuclides generally requires complicated and expensive equipment. All but two items in Table 40–1 are created by bombarding stable nuclei with protons, deuterons (nuclei of hydrogen-2), or nuclei of ^3He or ^4He that have been accelerated to high velocity in a *cyclotron*. (^{68}Ga and ^{82}Ru come from generators.) And the radiopharmacology is difficult because of the short half-lives. A PET scanner is itself elaborate, a commercial device costing ten or so times more than a CT machine. And that does not account for the masters- or doctorate-level personnel required to operate and maintain the scanner and cyclotron continuously and to perform the radiopharmacology.

One clever means of producing ^{11}C-labeled glucose is to feed isotope-enriched CO_2 to plants that metabolize it quickly, then grind up the leaves and chemically extract the desired radiopharmaceutical.

At present, there are still only a few dozen centers with one or more PET scanners in North America and a comparable number in Europe and Japan. But several commercial systems are currently on the market, along with a wide variety of support services. Vendors can now even provide small and relatively inexpensive "tabletop" cyclotrons that produce protons

TABLE 40–1. SOME POSITRON-EMITTING RADIONUCLEI USED FOR PET IMAGING

Z	Nuclide	Half-life
6	Carbon-11	20.3 min
7	Nitrogen-13	10.0 min
8	Oxygen-15	2.1 min
9	Fluorine-18	110 min
29	Copper-64	12.7 h
31	Gallium-68	68 min
33	Arsenic-72	26 h
35	Bromine-76	16.1 h
37	Rubidium-82	1.3 min
53	Iodine-122	3.5 min

in the range 8 to 12 MeV, which is adequate for generating most clinical positron emitters. If costs drop significantly, as some are predicting, and if third-party reimbursements are made, PET may well find widespread use in the clinic.

11. RADIONUCLIDE DOSES FROM NUCLEAR MEDICINE PROCEDURES

One of the more challenging problems of medical radiation dosimetry is that of a radioactive substance taken up by an organ and irradiating the organ itself and other tissues. We shall illustrate the situation with a simple example—the calculation of dose to the liver from a nuclear medicine liver scan.

> Eighty megabecquerels (2 mCi) of sulfur colloid labeled with metastable technetium-99 is injected into a patient for a liver scan. Typically, 90% of the 2.5×10^{12} technetium atoms go to and decay in the liver, each with the emission of a 140-keV photon. The total energy released is therefore $(0.9)(2.5 \times 10^{12}$ decays)$(1.4 \times 10^5$ eV/decay)$(1.6 \times 10^{-19}$ J/eV) = 0.05 J. The liver of the average man is of 1.8-kg mass. Thus, *if* all the 140-keV photons were deposited uniformly and locally, the liver dose would be 0.05 J/1.8 kg = 0.028 Gy = 2.8 cGy. The Auger electrons, conversion electrons, and low-energy x-rays that accompany the 140-keV gamma rays contribute an additional 0.4 cGy.

EXERCISE 40–3.

Demonstrate that 80 MBq of ^{99m}Tc yields 2.5×10^{12} decays.

SOLUTION: By Equations 39.7 and 39.19, the total number of ^{99m}Tc nuclei in an 80-MBq sample is $A(0) \cdot t_{0.5}/0.693 = (80 \times 10^6$ decays/s)(6 hours)(3600 s/h)/0.693 = 2.5×10^{12}. All of these radionuclei eventually decay, with a 6-hour half-life.

The only difficulty with this calculation is that most of the gamma rays escape the liver without interacting with it. (Otherwise, ^{99m}Tc would not be very good for imaging!) In fact, only about 15% of the 140-keV photons deposit their energy locally, with a contribution to the liver dose of only 0.4 cGy. The energy of the Auger electrons, conversion electrons, and low-energy x-rays, on the other hand, does go to the liver, so the final liver dose ends up to be 0.8 cGy. The issue of critical importance is thus determining how much of the gamma ray energy emitted from one piece of tissue will be absorbed in any other (or the same) piece of tissue.

Much of this kind of information has been determined by gamma ray *Monte Carlo* calculations, and has been presented by the Medical Internal Radiation Dose (MIRD) Committee of the Society of Nuclear Medicine in the very simple and convenient form of *S factors* (Table 40–2). An *S* factor reveals the *dose* deposited in a target organ *for each nuclear disintegration* that takes place within a source organ. If all N_{source} radionuclei coming to the source do eventually disintegrate, the total dose laid down in the target is

$$D_{target} = S(T \leftarrow S) \cdot N_{source} \qquad (40.12a)$$

where the SI units for $S(T \leftarrow S)$ are Gy/Bq-s (the conventional units are rad/μCi-h), and

TABLE 40–2. S FACTORS FOR TECHNETIUM-99m (rad/μCi-h)

Target	Source				
	Bladder Content	**Kidneys**	**Liver**	**Lung**	**Thyroid**
Bladder wall	1.6×10^{-4}	2.8×10^{-7}	1.6×10^{-7}	3.6×10^{-8}	2.1×10^{-9}
Stomach wall	2.7×10^{-7}	3.6×10^{-6}	1.9×10^{-6}	1.8×10^{-6}	4.5×10^{-8}
Kidneys	2.6×10^{-7}	1.9×10^{-4}	3.9×10^{-6}	8.4×10^{-7}	3.4×10^{-8}
Liver	1.7×10^{-7}	3.9×10^{-6}	4.6×10^{-5}	2.5×10^{-6}	9.3×10^{-8}
Lungs	2.4×10^{-8}	8.5×10^{-7}	2.5×10^{-6}	5.2×10^{-5}	9.4×10^{-7}
Thyroid	2.1×10^{-9}	4.8×10^{-8}	1.5×10^{-7}	9.2×10^{-7}	2.3×10^{-3}
Ovaries	7.3×10^{-6}	1.1×10^{-6}	4.5×10^{-7}	9.4×10^{-8}	4.9×10^{-9}
Testes	4.7×10^{-6}	8.8×10^{-8}	6.2×10^{-8}	7.9×10^{-9}	5.0×10^{-10}

After Snyder WS, Ford MR, Warner GG, Watson SB: Absorbed Dose per Unit Cumulated Activity for Selected Radionuclides and Organs. *MIRD pamphlet no. 11. New York: Society of Nuclear Medicine, 1975.*

$$N_{\text{source}} = A_{\text{source}}(0) \cdot t_{0.5}/0.693 \qquad (40.12b)$$

The tabulated value of $S(\text{liver} \leftarrow \text{liver})$ for ^{99m}Tc, for example, is 3.45×10^{-15} Gy/Bq-s (or, in conventional units, 4.6×10^{-5} rad/μCi-h). This leads to good agreement with our earlier dose estimate for the liver.

_____ **EXERCISE 40–4.** _____

Confirm this.

SOLUTION: $S(\text{T} \leftarrow \text{S}) \cdot N_{\text{source}} = (3.45 \times 10^{-15}$ Gy/Bq-s$)(2.5 \times 10^{12}$ decays$) = 0.86$ cGy.

_____ **EXERCISE 40–5.** _____

Confirm that for $S(\text{liver} \leftarrow \text{liver})$, 3.45×10^{-15} Gy/Bq-s corresponds to 4.6×10^{-5} rad/μCi-h.

SOLUTION: $(4.6 \times 10^{-5}$ rad/μCi-h$)(0.01$ Gy/1 rad$)$ $(1$μCi$/ 3.7 \times 10^4$ decays/s$)(1$ h$/3600$ s$) = 3.45 \times 10^{-15}$ Gy/Bq-s.

Part 9

Magnetic Resonance Imaging

Chapter 41

Magnetic Resonance I: The Quantum View of Nuclear Magnetic Resonance

1. **Magnetic Resonance Imaging Versus Computed Tomography**
2. **The Nuclear Magnetic Dipole Field and the Nuclear Magnetic Moment, μ**
3. **Flipping Over a Nucleus in a Strong External Magnetic Field**
4. **The Quantum Mechanical View of Nuclear Magnetic Resonance: Transitions Within a Two-State System**
5. **The World's Simplest Nuclear Magnetic Resonance Experiment**
6. **One-Dimensional, Proton Density-Weighted Imaging**

This four-chapter introduction to magnetic resonance imaging (MRI) explores three fundamental, separate issues and then brings them together: the nuclear magnetic resonance (NMR) phenomenon; the nature of the primary biophysical information (on the tissue proton density and relaxation times T1 and T2) that NMR yields; and methods of mapping such NMR-generated biophysical information throughout the body. We shall consider the first of these topics in this chapter and the next. The two subsequent chapters cover the ways that NMR may be used to create anatomic maps that reflect regional variations or differences in proton density and T1 and T2. A road guide to our approach is provided in Figure 41–1.

The strong, steady main magnetic field used in most clinical MRI systems is aligned in the horizontal plane, and will be shown as such in Chapter 44. In this chapter and the next two, however, it simplifies matters for the principal field B_0 to be aligned vertically.

1. MAGNETIC RESONANCE IMAGING VERSUS COMPUTED TOMOGRAPHY

Magnetic resonance imaging (MRI) is among the most promising, and certainly the most celebrated, of the newer imaging modalities. It seems capable of doing nearly everything that computed tomography (CT) does, and much more. Like CT, it provides high-quality anatomic information, as evident from Figures 1–8 and 1–14. But it goes far beyond that and, like nuclear medicine, reveals information on the physiologic status of soft tissues. It may even allow the performance of certain kinds of noninvasive histopathology. And it carries out all its good deeds with apparently little risk to the patient. There are no x-rays and, unlike nuclear medicine, MRI involves only stable, nonradioactive nuclei. (MRI does make use of a very strong magnetic field, however, and this can pose hazards of a different sort, unless treated with appropriate respect.)

Recall that x-ray transmission imaging, of which CT is a variant, makes use of the partial transparency of the body to high-energy photon probes. Quanta of x-ray electromagnetic energy enter the patient and may, or may not, interact with the tissues. Nonuniformities in the spatial distribution of those materials give rise to variations in the intensity of the exiting beam. In this fashion, CT provides information on the *electron* density and on the effective atomic number of the tissues, that is, on the kinds and amounts of chemical elements present.

Ultraviolet, visible, infrared, and microwave energy generally cannot (with some exceptions, as in diaphanography) be used for imaging, because electromagnetic radiations of these wavelengths do not penetrate far into tissue. (They interact strongly with biologic matter, rather, by means of the mechanisms noted in Chapter 12, Section 1.)

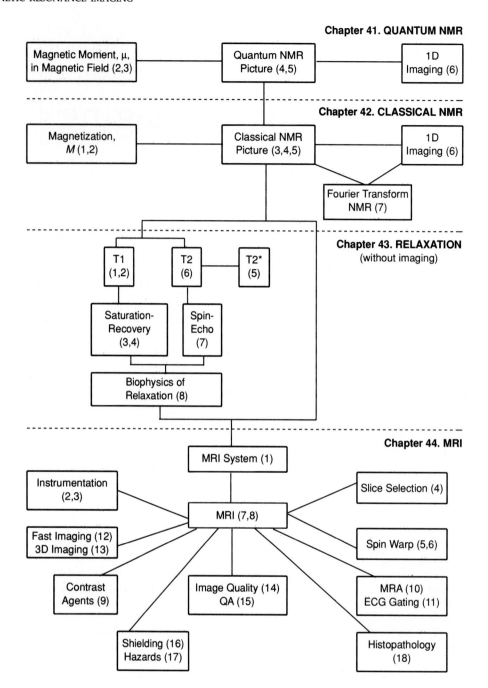

Figure 41–1.   Road map for the four chapters (Chapters 41 to 44) on magnetic resonance imaging. Section numbers are given in parentheses.

Below 60 MHz or so, however, there exists a low-energy window into the body through which *radio-frequency (rf)* radiation can readily pass. This rf radiation can, in highly special circumstances, be made to interact with atomic nuclei (in particular, the nuclei of hydrogen atoms, i.e., protons) by means of the **nuclear magnetic resonance** phenomenon. NMR can thereby reveal the relative **proton** densities (number of protons per unit volume) of different tissues.

Of far greater clinical interest, however, is the ability of NMR to provide information on the **nuclear spin relaxation times** of those protons. As we shall see, the values of the tissue parameters T1 and T2 are determined primarily by the precise manner in which water molecules are moving about and interacting with other molecules within the cell. And that, to some extent, is determined by the physiology of the tissues. Thus, by producing a map of the body that reflects differences in T1 or T2, MRI can provide valuable diagnostic information not only on anatomy, but also on cell physiology.

NMR, hence MRI, can take place only for certain nuclei in a magnetic field and only in the presence of rf energy with certain highly specific characteristics. We shall begin by considering the conditions under which NMR will occur.

2. THE NUCLEAR MAGNETIC DIPOLE FIELD AND THE NUCLEAR MAGNETIC MOMENT, μ

A magnetic field has both magnitude and direction. Like velocity and force (see Chapter 3, Section 1), the field, commonly called **B**, is a *vector* quantity, and can be represented by an arrow. The arrow's direction indicates that of the field, and its length is proportional to the field strength (Fig. 41–2). The arrows indicating the magnetic field of an external magnet run, by convention, from its North to its South pole.

In these four chapters on MRI, a vector quantity will be indicated with a **boldface** symbol. The *magnitude* of a vector (when its directionality is not of interest) will be represented by the same symbol, but in italic print. The strength of the magnetic field **B**, for example, is denoted B.

When several magnetic fields of interest are present, they will be distinguished by means of subscripts: $\mathbf{B}_0$ will refer to the strong, steady vertically aligned (in this chapter and the next two) "main" field, in particular, and $\mathbf{B}_1$ to a weak radio-frequency field lying within the horizontal plane.

The SI measure of magnetic field strength is the tesla* (T). The conventional unit, the gauss, is 10^4 times smaller:

$$1 \text{ tesla} = 10{,}000 \text{ gauss}$$

MRI is normally performed with the magnitude of the main external field $\mathbf{B}_0$ fixed at some value between 0.15 and 1.5 T (1500 and 15,000 gauss). The field strength at the surface of the small magnet that holds papers to your refrigerator door is 0.1 T or so, by comparison, and that of the Earth is of the order of 0.5×10^{-4} T (0.5 gauss).

Chapter 4, Section 4, indicated that there are two important connections between moving, electrically charged particles and magnetic fields: A moving charge (1) gives rise to a magnetic field and (2) experiences a force when moving within another magnetic field already in existence.

Both of these phenomena are relevant to nuclear magnetic resonance. A nucleus behaves somewhat like a spinning ball of charge, and will therefore generally do the following:

1. Create a *nuclear magnetic dipole field*, like that from the two (North and South) poles of a bar magnet or compass needle. The field varies throughout the space around the nucleus, but its presence may be indicated

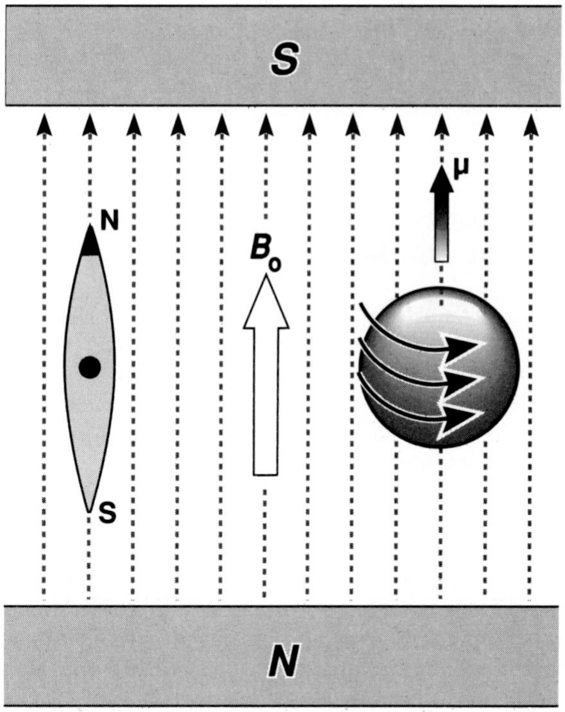

Figure 41–2. The lowest-energy alignment of a bar magnet (or compass needle), and of a spinning nucleus, in an external magnetic field, B_0.

by means of a single **nuclear magnetic moment** vector, μ, a measure of the *magnetic* potency of the nuclear field's source. The length of the arrow representing μ is proportional to the relative "magneticness" of the nucleus, and the convention for its direction may be expressed as a "right-hand" rule[†]: Wrap your right hand around the nucleus in the direction of its rotation, and your thumb will point along "the direction of the spin" and along μ (see Figure 41–2).

2. If the nucleus is placed in an external magnetic field, it will (like a compass needle) tend to find the alignment of lowest potential energy, in which the nuclear magnetic moment is *parallel* to the external field (see Figure 41–2).

The particular isotopes ^{12}C, ^{16}O, and ^{40}Ca are notable exceptions to all of this. In a nucleus composed of an even number of protons and an even number of neutrons, the protons

---

*Nikola Tesla, who was born in Yugoslavia in 1856 and emigrated to the United States 28 years later, invented much of the technology used in generating and harnessing electric power. According to the March 4, 1991, issue of the *New Yorker*, "He couldn't tolerate the sight of pearl earrings, the smell of camphor, the act of shaking hands, or close exposure to the hair of other people. He strongly favored numbers that were divisible by three. He seldom ate or drank anything without first calculating its volume. He counted his steps. He washed his hands compulsively. He never married, but he told a friend he had once loved a particular pigeon 'as a man loves a woman.'"

[†]The nuclear dipole magnetic field produced by a spinning, positively charged nucleus runs parallel to the direction of the spin. (This follows from the more basic convention that if your right thumb points in the direction of "conventional" [positive] charge flow through a wire [i.e., opposite to the direction of electron flow], then the direction in which your fingers curl around it defines the direction of the magnetic field produced around it; and a nucleus may be viewed as a stack of spinning, positively charged hoops.) The nuclear moment μ, in turn, is defined to point along the nuclear magnetic dipole field, hence also along the spin.

tend to pair up antiparallel to one another, in such a fashion that their magnetic dipole fields cancel out, and so also with the neutrons. Such a nucleus produces no net magnetic field and plays no active role in MRI.

3. FLIPPING OVER A NUCLEUS IN A STRONG EXTERNAL MAGNETIC FIELD

Once again: A nucleus creates its own dipole magnetic field; it also tends to orient its magnetic moment (and axis of rotation) along any strong external magnetic field present. It is the second of these two points that is of immediate interest here; the significance of the magnetic field produced by the nucleus itself will become apparent in the next chapters.

Imagine a nucleus sitting in a strong magnetic field, $\mathbf{B}_0$, with its magnetic moment μ aligned comfortably along (parallel to) the field (Fig. 41–3). NMR consists, in essence, of somehow grabbing the nucleus and twisting or flipping it through 180 degrees, so that it ends up rotating in the opposite direction, with its magnetic moment pointing antiparallel to the external field, instead. The stronger the magnetic field, the greater the amount of energy involved in doing this. Indeed, the energy required, ΔE_{flip}, is linear in (proportional to) field strength B_0:

$$\Delta E_{\text{flip}} \sim B_0 \qquad (41.1)$$

ΔE_{flip} also increases with the magnitude of the magnetic moment, μ, that is, with the "magnetness" of the nucleus: $\Delta E_{\text{flip}} \sim \mu$. This proportionality is expressed more commonly in terms of another measure of the strength of the nuclear magnetic dipole field, the **gyromagnetic ratio**, γ. The gyromagnetic ratio is proportional to the magnitude of the magnetic moment, $\gamma \sim \mu$, from which

$$\Delta E_{\text{flip}} \sim \gamma \qquad (41.2)$$

Except for those nuclei with zero nuclear moment (^{12}C, ^{16}O, ^{40}Ca, etc.), each isotope of every element has its own unique, characteristic γ, and values of $\gamma/2\pi$ (not of γ alone) are listed in Table 41–1. The justification for the indicated units of $\gamma/2\pi$, namely, megahertz per tesla, will soon become apparent.

In combining Equations 41.1 and 41.2 to obtain an overall expression for ΔE_{flip}, the constant of proportionality needed to get the units right is $h/2\pi$, where h is Planck's constant. The energy required to twist a nucleus through 180 degrees is thus

$$\Delta E_{\text{flip}} = (h/2\pi) \cdot \gamma \cdot B_0 \qquad (41.3)$$

ΔE_{flip} is shown as a function of magnetic field strength, B_0, in Figure 41–4 for ^{1}H and ^{31}P nuclei. As indicated along the right-hand border of the graph, ΔE_{flip} for NMR is typically in the range 0.01 to 0.6 μeV (10^{-6} eV). This is a dozen orders of magnitude (a factor of 10^{12}) less than the energies typically exchanged in x-ray photon–electron (i.e., Compton and photoelectric) interactions.

The nuclei that have been seriously considered for MRI are listed in Table 41–1. ^{12}C, ^{16}O, and ^{40}Ca are out of the picture

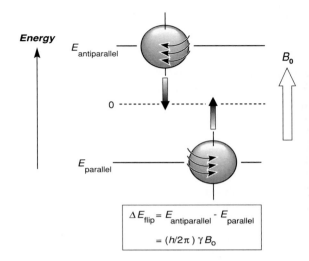

Figure 41–3. A nucleus of magnetic moment μ in an external magnetic field of magnitude B_0. Flipping the nucleus over (or twisting it through 180 degrees), from the ground state to the high-energy state, involves the transfer of ΔE_{flip} of energy. In this energy-level diagram for the nuclear spin states, the dashed line corresponds to the energy the nucleus would have if $B_0 = 0$.

altogether, as noted earlier. (Because calcium has no effect on NMR signals, moreover, tissues *within* bone, such as the contents of the posterior fossa and the vertebral bodies, can be examined without the beam-hardening effects that accompany imaging with x-rays.) That leaves the field of MRI open primarily to hydrogen, and to a lesser extent ^{31}P (some important work has been done using the phosphorus of metabolically relevant molecules), with research possibilities for ^{13}C-enriched metabolites and a few other nuclei.

—————— **EXERCISE 41–1.** ——————

What is the energy required to flip a proton through 180 degrees in a 1.0-T field? To what frequency photon does that correspond?

SOLUTION: By Equation 41.3, and with $\gamma = (2\pi)(\gamma/2\pi)$ from Table 41–1, $\Delta E_{\text{flip}} = (6.626 \times 10^{-34}$ J-s$/2\pi)(2\pi)(42.57 \times 10^6$ s$^{-1})$ $(1.0$ T$) = 2.82 \times 10^{-26}$ J $= 0.176$ μeV. By the Einstein relation

TABLE 41–1. PROPERTIES OF NUCLEI IMPORTANT IN CLINICAL MAGNETIC RESONANCE IMAGING[a]

Nucleus	$\gamma/2\pi$ (MHz/T) = f_{Larmor} at 1 T
^{1}H	42.57
^{31}P	17.23
^{18}C	No nuclear moment
^{16}O	No nuclear moment
^{40}Ca	No nuclear moment

[a]Also, ^{13}C, ^{14}N, ^{19}F, and ^{23}Na are of research interest.

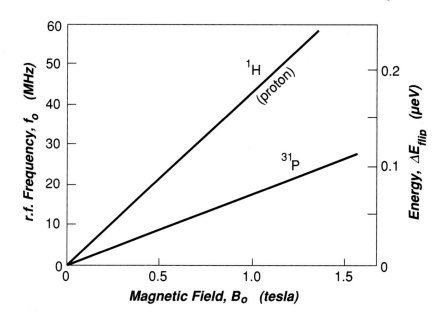

Figure 41–4. The energy required to cause a nuclear spin state transition (spin flip), ΔE_{flip}, is proportional both to the magnetic moment, μ (hence to the gyromagnetic ratio γ), of the nucleus and to the strength of the external magnetic field, B_0. ΔE_{flip} is plotted (in micro-electron volts) against B_0 for normal hydrogen (^{1}H) and for phosphorus (^{31}P). Also shown is the rf frequency, f_0 (in MHz), of a photon of the right energy for causing the transition.

Equation 6.1), this is the energy of a 42.57-MHz photon. Note the entry in Table 41–1 under f_{Larmor}.

_____ **EXERCISE 41–2.** _____

How much more energy is required to flip a proton than a ^{31}P nucleus in a 0.15-T field?

SOLUTION: At any field strength, the energies differ by a factor of $42.57/17.28 = 2.47$, the ratio of the γ values.

_____ **EXERCISE 41–3.** _____

Use the f_{Larmor} entry of Table 41–1 to find the energy, in electron volts, required to flip a proton in a 0.15-T field.

SOLUTION: A photon of frequency $(42.57 \text{ MHz/T})(0.15 \text{ T})$ = 6.4 MHz is required. From the Einstein relation (Equation 6.1), its energy is $(6.626 \times 10^{-34} \text{ J-s})(6.4 \times 10^6 \text{ s}^{-1})/(1.6 \times 10^{-19} \text{ eV/J}) = 2.7 \times 10^{-8} \text{ eV}$.

4. THE QUANTUM MECHANICAL VIEW OF NUCLEAR MAGNETIC RESONANCE: TRANSITIONS WITHIN A TWO-STATE SYSTEM

A nucleus that is in a strong external magnetic field and aligned in the low-energy orientation can be flipped over by supplying the right amount of energy (see Equation 41.3). In this sense, it behaves like an ordinary compass needle. It differs radically, however, in that although you can twist a compass needle through *any* angle whatsoever with your fingers and hold it there, Nature demands that nuclei be oriented along the field, or against it, but in *no other* directions. This **spatial quantization** is another example of the kinds of restrictions quantum mechanics places on atom-sized systems.

A nucleus in a magnetic field may thus be viewed as a

quantum mechanical system that can inhabit either of two, but only two, *spin states*, with its magnetic moment either parallel* (ground state) or antiparallel (high-energy state) to the external field (see Fig. 41–3). The splitting apart of (difference in energy between) the two states is proportional to B_0, in accord with Equation 41.3.

We have talked of flipping over nuclear spins, but have not said how actually to cause the transitions. One process by which a nucleus can be elevated from the lower-energy spin state to the higher state is through the absorption of a photon of the right energy. Recall that according to Equation 6.1, the energy, E, and frequency, f, of a photon are related through the Einstein relation, $E = hf$, where h is Planck's constant. In a magnetic field of strength B_0, a nucleus of gyromagnetic ratio γ requires a photon of frequency given by[†]

$$hf_0 = \Delta E_{flip} = (h/2\pi) \cdot \gamma \cdot B_0 \qquad (41.4)$$

The photon frequency at which this occurs, for a given type of nucleus and external field strength, is known as the **Larmor**

---

*It has been asserted, for simplicity, that a proton lines up either "along" or "against" an external magnetic field. A picture that is quantum mechanically slightly more correct would show the spin axis of a proton, in either spin state, canted off from the vertical by a small angle. The use of our simpler picture has no harmful effect on the discussion and may help to avoid some of the confusion that might otherwise arise.

^{23}Na and some other nuclei have more than two nuclear spin states, and are allowed more than two distinct alignments in an external field.

[†]Equation 41.4 may appear in the equivalent form

$$hf = g_n \cdot \beta_N \cdot H$$

The nucleus-specific parameter g_n is proportional to the gyromagnetic ratio, β_N is a constant known as the nuclear magneton, and H is the "magnetic intensity," which is practically the same as the magnetic field. In this book, we shall stay with Equation 41.4.

frequency and written f_{Larmor} or f_0. The Larmor frequencies for ^{1}H and ^{31}P are shown as functions of field strength in Figure 41–4, and the Larmor frequencies at 1 T for the nuclei of MRI interest are listed in Table 41–1. Radiation of these energies and frequencies falls in the radio-frequency portion of the electromagnetic spectrum.

From Equation 41.4, the Larmor frequency is given by

$$f_0 = (\gamma/2\pi) \cdot B_0 \qquad (41.5a)$$

Hence the usefulness of the values of $\gamma/2\pi$ listed in Table 41–1. The Larmor relationship is seen in the MRI literature much more commonly, however, in the completely equivalent form

$$\omega_0 = \gamma \cdot B_0 \qquad (41.5b)$$

The *angular frequency*, ω_0, is numerically equal to 2π times the ordinary frequency,

$$\omega_0 = (2\pi) \cdot f_0 \qquad (41.5c)$$

and is expressed in radians per second. Be careful with the units — although more compact than Equation 41.5a, Equation 41.5b suffers the disadvantage that you must multiply the ordinary frequency f_0 (in MHz) by 2π to get the angular frequency ω_0 (in radians per second); conversely, you must divide ω_0 by 2π to obtain f_0.

The NMR interaction between an rf photon and a nucleus sitting in a magnetic field is different, in a fundamental way, from the photon–electron interactions explored in earlier chapters. With photoelectric and Compton interactions, the *electric* field of the photon exerts a force on a (charged) atomic electron, resulting in a change in its quantum state. With NMR, it is the rapidly oscillating *magnetic* field of the electromagnetic radiation interacting with the magnetic moment of the nucleus that brings about a change in nuclear spin quantum state.

This suggests that *any* magnetic field (not only that of an rf photon) that varies at the Larmor frequency can induce nuclear spin state transitions. Indeed, spontaneously occurring local fluctuations in the magnetic fields produced and felt by hydrogen nuclei are primary determinants of the critically important tissue *relaxation times* T1 and T2, as will be seen.

Nearly all magnetic resonance imaging involves the nuclei of the hydrogen atoms of intracellular *water* and *lipids,* so hereafter the focus will be on proton NMR, for those two classes of materials.

5. THE WORLD'S SIMPLEST NUCLEAR MAGNETIC RESONANCE EXPERIMENT

Figure 41–5A illustrates the world's simplest (hypothetical) proton NMR experiment. A transmitter pumps monochromatic, fairly low frequency (1 MHz, say) rf energy into an antenna, which directs a beam of photons through the sample (a volume of water), to a second antenna, which is attached to a power meter. Pure water is transparent to 1-MHz energy.

An electromagnet is added and adjusted so that $\mathbf{B}_0$ within the water sample is uniform and exactly 1 T in strength. Nothing significant happens, and the amount of rf power reaching the meter does not change.

The frequency of the transmitted radiation is now slowly

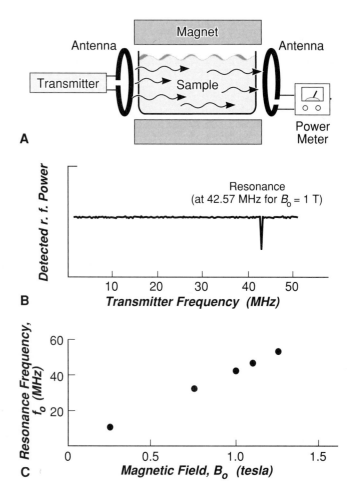

Figure 41–5. World's simplest nuclear magnetic resonance experiment. **A.** The equipment consists of a transmitter whose frequency can be slowly and continuously increased, and a receiver attached to a power meter. The sample under consideration sits within a uniform magnetic field of strength B_0, which is held fixed during a measurement. **B.** With some fixed setting of the magnetic field, such as 1.0 tesla (T), the frequency of the radio-frequency signal is increased slowly. At resonance, the sample absorbs power, and less energy reaches the detector. **C.** With increases in B_0, resonance occurs at correspondingly higher frequencies. See also Figure 41–4.

increased, with the transmitted power level held constant, and detected power is plotted as a function of this frequency in Figure 41–5B. The graph remains constant up to 42.57 kHz, at which point it dips sharply. This is the Larmor frequency, f_0, for protons in a 1-T field. Some Larmor frequency photons are absorbed in the process of exciting water hydrogen nuclei (protons) into the higher-energy spin state (see Equation 41.5), and less energy reaches the detector. (Where might the "lost" energy go?) As the transmitter frequency passes beyond 42.57 kHz, the detected power returns to its previous level.

If the whole experiment is repeated with various fixed settings of the magnetic field, this same phenomenon recurs (Fig. 41–5C), but in each case at the Larmor frequency corresponding to the current value of the field strength, as determined by Equation 41.5.

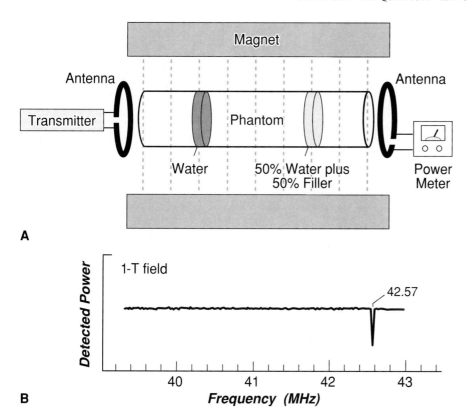

Figure 41–6. In our "phantom" for demonstrating one-dimensional magnetic resonance imaging. The lower sample chamber contains water, and the upper 50% water and 50% inert filler; the rest of the phantom is air. **(A)** When the phantom is in a uniform magnetic field, **(B)** all the water resonates at the same frequency.

This is somewhat different from what is done in a real laboratory NMR experiment. But it is a fairly good description of the workings of the closely related and valuable research tool, electron spin resonance (ESR). With ESR (also known as electron paramagnetic resonance [EPR]), it is an unpaired *electron* that can exist in either of two spin states split apart by a magnetic field. (An electron, like most nuclei, acts like a spinning charged particle, and aligns parallel or antiparallel to a strong magnetic field). If microwave (rather than rf) equipment were employed (as ESR frequencies tend to be about a thousand times higher than those for NMR), then Figure 41–5 would accurately represent a rudimentary ESR experiment. ESR is used, for example, in the study of radiation-produced free radicals (which carry unpaired electrons) which can attack DNA molecules and bring about changes that lead to carcinogenesis, as discussed in Chapter 32.

6. ONE-DIMENSIONAL, PROTON DENSITY-WEIGHTED IMAGING

The preceding experiment suggests a simple way of mapping the tissue proton density throughout a body, or at least a one-dimensional body. This section offers a brief, preliminary excursion into the realm of (one-dimensional) magnetic resonance imaging.

The plastic "phantom" in Figure 41–6 consists of a number of transverse, thin-slice hollow compartments. All of these are empty, except for two. One, located one fourth of the way up from the bottom, contains pure water. A second, three fourths of the way up, contains a half-and-half mixture of water and inert filler; that is, the average proton density is half that of

water. Our objective is to determine experimentally the proton density of the phantom as a function of position along it.

With the experimental setup of Section 5 and with a *uniform* 1-T main magnetic field (Fig. 41–6A), the water molecules in both compartments undergo resonance at the same radio frequency, 42.57 MHz (Fig. 41–6B). Not very interesting.

By canting the magnet pole faces slightly relative to one another, however, one can add a **magnetic field gradient** (Fig. 41–7A). The new field is everywhere still vertical, but its strength now increases linearly with the x-coordinate (Fig. 41–7B) (because of which this gradient is said to be an **x-gradient field**). Suppose the total field strength varies from 0.98 T at the bottom of the phantom to 1.02 T at the top. The field strength is 0.99 T at the lower water chamber and 1.01 T at the upper. When the NMR experiment is performed anew, one resonance signal occurs at 42.14 MHz, and a second, of half the amplitude, at 43.00 MHz (Fig. 41–7C).

The frequency of an NMR peak indicates, by Equation 41.5, the local field strength. But the local field strength is proportional to the x coordinate (Fig. 41–7A). Thus, the *water density*, as a function of *position* within the phantom, is revealed through the functional dependence of the *NMR signal amplitude* on *rf frequency* (Fig. 41–8). We have, in effect, found a way to differentiate the NMR signals that come from different parts of the body.

It is possible to produce a magnetic resonance image of a real, three-dimensional anatomic region of interest by performing the NMR experiment point by point throughout the region. This involves manipulating several magnetic field gradients and the rf radiation so that conditions are right for the NMR phenomenon to occur at one, and only one, place in the body.

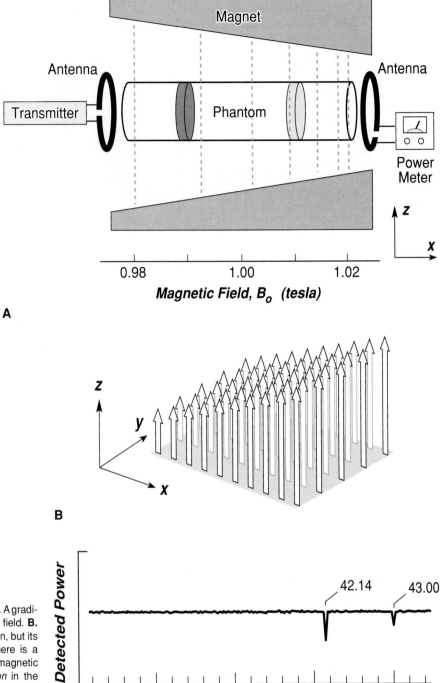

Figure 41–7. Our phantom in a field gradient. **A.** A gradient field is superimposed on the uniform external field. **B.** The magnetic field still points only in the *z*-direction, but its strength increases with the *x*-coordinate. **C.** There is a direct link between *field strength,* hence nuclear magnetic resonance (NMR) signal *frequency*, and *position* in the phantom. The strength of NMR signal at any frequency, moreover, is proportional to the amount of water at the corresponding point in the phantom.

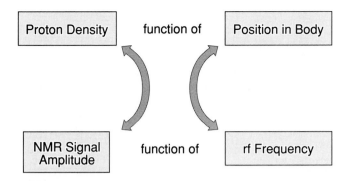

Figure 41–8. Representation of the relationship, in a nonuniform external field, between (1) the distribution of protons within the one-dimensional phantom and (2) the amplitudes of the corresponding nuclear magnetic resonance signals of different frequencies.

The magnetic fields are then altered slightly, and the NMR experiment is repeated at another, nearby location, and so on. Thus unlike the situation for CT, one can, in principle, obtain NMR-type information directly, by examining one voxel at a time, with no reconstruction calculations. Such an approach is not used in practice, however, and sophisticated, much more efficient reconstruction methods (some of which are similar to those of CT) are normally employed instead.

Chapter 42

Magnetic Resonance II: The Classical View of Nuclear Magnetic Resonance

1. Thermal Equilibrium of Nuclear Spins in a Strong Magnetic Field
2. The Net Magnetization, M
3. The Classical View of Nuclear Magnetic Resonance: Precession of the Net Magnetization at the Larmor Frequency
4. The "Resonance" in Nuclear Magnetic Resonance: Nutation of the Net Magnetization
5. Detection of Nuclear Magnetic Resonance: Induction by the Precessing Net Magnetization of a Voltage in a Pickup Coil
6. One-Dimensional Imaging, Again
7. Fourier Transform Nuclear Magnetic Resonance

In attempting to understand nuclear magnetic resonance (NMR), it helps to consider the behavior of a nucleus in a magnetic field from two quite different perspectives. A nucleus seems, in some ways, to act like a quantum compass needle, which can exist in only two quantum states; transitions between these states involve the absorption and emission of radio-frequency (rf) energy. This quantum picture offers the advantage of making the NMR phenomenon relatively easy to comprehend. Unfortunately, it is not very helpful in explaining NMR's imaging applications.

Less obvious, but of much greater utility for our purposes, is the *classical picture*, in which the net magnetization of a volume of tissue (rather than any particular nucleus) is viewed behaving in an external magnetic field like a gyroscope or a toy top spinning and precessing in a gravitational field.

The preceding chapter introduced the quantum picture. The present one explores the classical.

It will not be evident how these two models relate to one another. Indeed, such an understanding requires a rigorous quantum mechanical treatment. But if you are willing to accept that each of them provides only a partial picture of what is happening, it is possible to account for practically all aspects of NMR without having to work through the quantum theory.

1. THERMAL EQUILIBRIUM OF NUCLEAR SPINS IN A STRONG MAGNETIC FIELD

Let us return to ordinary (nonimaging) NMR in a uniform magnetic field.

We have argued that a proton in a strong and steady magnetic field can be excited from the ground spin state into the high-energy spin state by means of a second, much weaker

magnetic field oscillating at the Larmor frequency. It can be demonstrated experimentally, and shown theoretically with quantum mechanics, that such a Larmor frequency magnetic field is equally adept at tickling protons sitting in the higher-energy state down into the ground state.

But, as suggested at the end of Chapter 41, Section 4, the Larmor frequency magnetic fields that can raise a proton into the higher-energy state, or tickle it down to the lower state, do not have to be those of photons supplied by means of an rf antenna. Such fields occur naturally and spontaneously within any material. Thermal energy will cause an individual water molecule in a tissue, for example, to move about, vibrate, and rotate randomly. The weak magnetic fields generated by each of its protons (and sensed by the other) therefore fluctuate rapidly. Some of those fluctuations will happen to occur at the Larmor frequency.

Imagine a glass of water at body temperature and sitting in a steady field of strength B_0. The protons will all have a natural tendency to align in the low-energy configuration, with their magnetic moments parallel to the field. But the small amount of energy required to raise a proton into the higher-energy orientation (or to tickle it back down into the ground state) can easily be provided thermally, via spontaneously occurring Larmor frequency magnetic fields. There are two fundamental opposing processes at work here. Because of the main magnetic field, the spins would all prefer (energetically) to be in the lower-energy state (Fig. 42–1A). But the thermal jostling tends to distribute the protons randomly (and with equal numbers) in the two states, thereby maximizing the disorder (entropy) of the system (Fig. 42–1B).

The outcome of this battle between energy (trying to create order) and entropy (leading to disorder) is revealed by the *Boltzmann equation* of statistical mechanics. The result, which

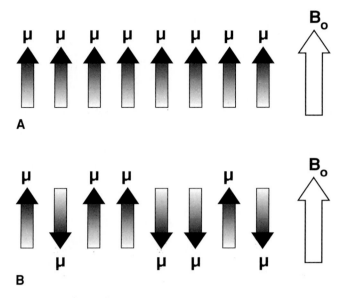

Figure 42–1. Spins in a magnetic field. **A.** Perfect alignment of the individual nuclear magnetic moments. **B.** The alignment is partially disrupted by thermal jostling.

we shall state without proof, is that for protons at body temperature,

$$(N_- - N_+) = 3 \times 10^{-6} N_p \cdot B_0 \qquad (42.1)$$

N_p is the proton density, and N_- and N_+ refer to the protons in the low- and high-energy spin states, respectively (where $N_+ + N_+ = N_p$). At any instant, slightly (but only slightly) more than half the nuclei are in the lower-energy spin state. In a 1-T magnetic field, for example, the relative excess of spins in the lower level, $(N_- - N_+)/N_p$, is only about three parts in one million—for every 500,000 protons in the lower-energy state, there will be something like 499,997, on average, in the upper. This situation, known as **thermal equilibrium**, is stable, in the sense that for every proton that drops from the high-energy to the low-energy state, one other proton, on average, will soon go the other way.

_____ EXERCISE 42–1. _____

What is the excess number of protons in the lower spin state in 1 mL (= 1 g) of water in a 1-T field?

SOLUTION: The molecular weight of water is 18. Eighteen grams of water contains Avogadro's number (6×10^{23}) of molecules, with two protons in each. One gram of water therefore contains 1/18th of Avogadro's number of molecules, and about 7×10^{22} protons. A relative excess of 3×10^{-6} implies that there is an absolute excess of 2×10^{18} protons per gram in the lower-energy state.

2. THE NET MAGNETIZATION, M

In a strong external magnetic field, the protons in a sample of water (or in soft tissue) at thermal equilibrium will be aligned with their magnetic moments either parallel or antiparallel to the field. In any small volume of water or tissue, there will be a

slight excess of protons in the lower-energy state; as a result, these particular protons will themselves give rise to a small communal magnetic field. The net magnetic moment per unit volume (a measure of the overall magnetic field that the protons in the volume collectively create) is called the net magnetic moment or **net magnetization.**

The net magnetization at thermal equilibrium is a vector quantity, and will be denoted in **boldface** type as $\mathbf{M}_0$. The magnitude of $\mathbf{M}_0$ is proportional to the relative excess number of protons aligned parallel to the external field* (Fig. 42–2A). In a 1-T field and at body temperature, according to Equation 42.1, this is about 0.0003%. The excess is proportional to the strength of the external magnetic field, by Equation 42.1, which is an important motivation for using strong fields in imaging. (It also increases as the temperature of the sample goes down, but that doesn't help much in the clinic.)

The net magnetization has just been introduced by way of the particular case of protons at thermal equilibrium. Thermal equilibrium is, however, quite special a situation. If the strength or direction of the external field $\mathbf{B}_0$ is abruptly changed, for example, a system of nuclear spins will be out of thermal equilibrium for a while.

But the concept of net magnetization is still meaningful, even in these more general circumstances. Whenever a collection of nuclei themselves give rise to a local magnetic field (whether or not there is thermal equilibrium), their net magnetic moment per unit volume (Fig. 42–2B) defines the net magnetization:

$$\mathbf{M} = (N_- - N_+)/\text{volume} \qquad (42.2)$$

In the general, nonequilibrium situation, the net magnetization is represented by an $\mathbf{M}$ without the subscript zero.

It may come as something of a surprise to learn that for protons in a strong magnetic field, $\mathbf{M}$ does not necessarily lie along or against the field; at times, it may be pointing off in any direction whatsoever, at least briefly. Likewise, its magnitude may be quite different from $\mathbf{M}_0$. In fact, over most of the time that a magnetic resonance image is being produced via the NMR process, $\mathbf{M}$ is nothing at all like $\mathbf{M}_0$. Read on.

3. THE CLASSICAL VIEW OF NUCLEAR MAGNETIC RESONANCE: PRECESSION OF THE NET MAGNETIZATION AT THE LARMOR FREQUENCY

NMR has been described, so far, employing simple pictures of compass needles and two-state quantum systems. Another approach overlaps these somewhat, but is inherently very different. It involves treating the net magnetization $\mathbf{M}$ as if it were itself a gyroscope.

According to Newton's First Law, (see Chapter 3, Section 3), the motion of an object will not change unless something is done to change it. If a wheel or a child's top is in outer

_____

*In case this is not obvious, imagine a charged spinning body, with its axis of rotation oriented along the external field. Doubling its charge will double the magnetic field it produces. So also will putting a second charge, spinning in the same direction, near the first, either behind or beside it. The magnetic fields of adjacent equal charges spinning in opposite directions, by contrast, will cancel one another.

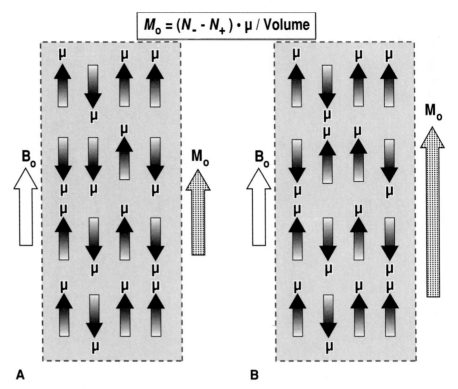

$$M_o = (N_- - N_+) \cdot \mu \: / \: \text{Volume}$$

Figire 42–2. The net magnetization, **M,** is defined as the net (vector sum) magnetic moment per unit volume. **A.** For the particular unit volume element at thermal equilibrium shown here, there is an excess of 2μ in the lower spin state, and the magnetization is represented by the upward pointing vector $\mathbf{M}_0$. **B.** For some reason (e.g., following emission of a Larmor frequency photon by a spin), there happens to be a 4μ excess in the lower state, and the magnitude of the magnetization, **M,** is now $2 \cdot \mathbf{M}_0$.

space and spinning freely about an axis, for example, neither the rate of rotation nor the orientation of the axis will change over time (Fig. 42–3A). The constancy of this motion exemplifies the Law of the Conservation of Angular Momentum (see Chapter 5, Section 12).

A top spinning on a table on Earth or a gyroscope that is supported at one end of its axle, however, is *not* in a state of unchanging motion: It *precesses* slowly about the vertical (Fig. 42–3B). The reason is that gravity (pulling downward) and the supporting force at its foot (pushing up) together apply a

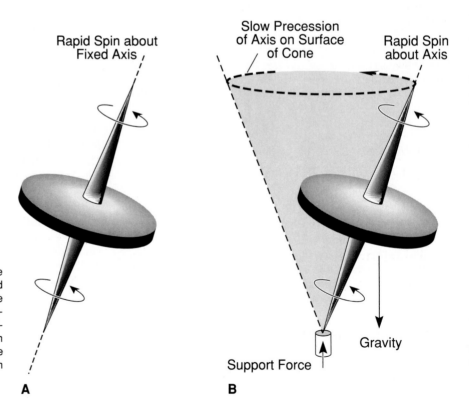

Figure 42–3. Frictionless top or gyroscope spinning rapidly. **A.** In outer space, the speed and orientation (i.e., the direction in which the axis points) remain constant. **B.** In a gravitational field, supported at the bottom, the resulting torque, or twisting force, causes the system to precess at a constant, slow (relative to the rate of spin) rate and at a fixed angle of tilt from the vertical.

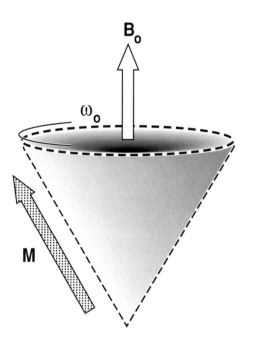

Figure 42–4. Precession of the net magnetization, **M**, in a constant magnetic field.

torque, or twisting force, to the gyroscope. This torque attempts to twist the gyroscope downward, but its spin (and Conservation of Angular Momentum) resist its toppling over. The resultant motion is a slow precession of the axis of rotation about the vertical, along the surface of a hypothetical vertical cone. This behavior is explained in elementary physics texts by extending Newton's Second Law, $F = ma$, so as to account for torques and rotations.

A proton acts like a spinning body. And because it has a magnetic moment, it experiences a torque in an external magnetic field. Although not much can be said about what any single proton may be doing without resorting to quantum mechanics, it is possible to describe classically the behavior of the net magnetization vector **M** for a population of protons. If the net magnetization happens to be tipped away from the vertical (and we shall soon see how that condition can occur), **M** will precess about a vertical magnetic field (Fig. 42–4), exactly like the gyroscope in the gravitational field. The angular frequency of precession, ω_0, depends on the magnetic moment of the nucleus, parameterized by the gyromagnetic ratio γ, and on the strength of the magnetic field, B_0. The constant of proportionality turns out to be 1, so

$$\omega_0 = \gamma \cdot B_0 \tag{42.3}$$

That is, **M** precesses about B_0 at the Larmor frequency.

The meaning of this is somewhat different from that of Equation 41.5b. Equations 41.4 and 41.5 revealed the energy and frequency of an rf photon capable of inducing a transition between the states of a two-level quantum mechanical spin system. Equation 42.3, by contrast, gives the natural precessional frequency (namely, the Larmor frequency) of a classically behaving vector quantity, namely, the net magnetization of a set of protons in a magnetic field. There is an important

link between these two pictures, and this is where the "resonance" of NMR comes in.

4. THE "RESONANCE" IN NUCLEAR MAGNETIC RESONANCE: NUTATION OF THE NET MAGNETIZATION

Many kinds of mechanical systems display one or more natural resonant frequencies. If applied at a natural **resonant frequency,** even a very weak external force can cause the eventual buildup of large-amplitude oscillations of the system. That is, energy is transferred to an oscillating system very efficiently through application of a periodic, resonance frequency force.

Pushing a child on a swing offers a fine example. If you apply many little pushes in rapid succession, the swing will barely move. If you apply pressure very slowly, the swing will simply move with your hand. But if applied at the natural *resonant frequency* of the child-plus-swing system, even very gentle shoves will cause the eventual buildup of large-amplitude oscillations of the swing, as in Figure 42–5.

The natural resonant frequency of a gyroscope is its frequency of precession. This depends on properties such as the mass, shape, and spin rate of the fly wheel of the gyroscope, and also on the strength of the gravitational field that produces the torque on it—a gyroscope would take six times longer to make a complete circuit around the vertical on the Moon than on Earth, because the Moon's gravitational field is that much weaker.

Resonant transfer of energy to a gyroscope can be demonstrated by pulling very lightly on a thread attached to it. A particular kind of pull is required: the tension in the thread should be constant, but tangential (parallel to the motion of precession), hence the direction from which the pull comes must move in a circle (Fig. 42–6A). If the pull direction changes too rapidly or too slowly, it will have small effect on the gyroscope's behavior. If, however, the pull direction circles

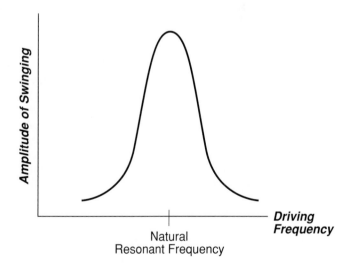

Figure 42–5. Resonance. The amplitude of oscillation passes through a peak when a system is driven, by an external force, at its natural resonant frequency.

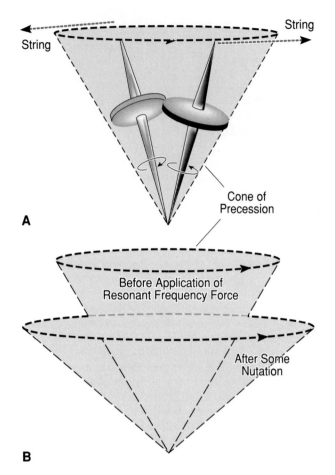

A

B

Figure 42–6. Resonance in the gyroscope. **A.** Applying a force to the tip of the axis—pulling with constant tension on a thread. **B.** When the direction of the pull changes at the natural precessional frequency in such a way that the pull is always tangential, the resonance condition is manifest as nutation.

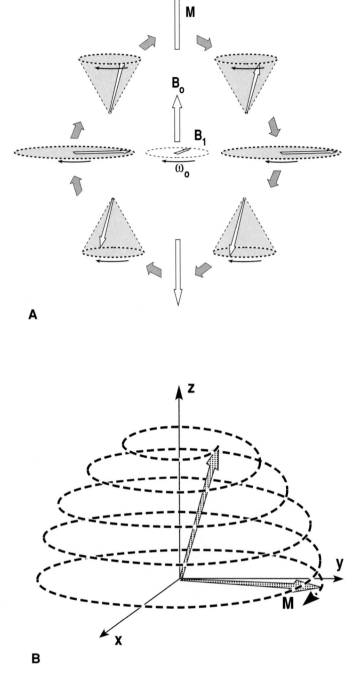

A

B

Figure 42–7. Nutation of the net magnetization, **M,** in a uniform magnetization, with no relaxation processes. **A.** Snapshots of the precessing magnetization at different times. The radio-frequency field $\mathbf{B}_1$ is designed to rotate, always perpendicular to $\mathbf{B}_0$, at the angular frequency ω_0. **B.** Motion of **M**, with the rate of nutation exaggerated.

at the resonant (processional) frequency and is of proper phase, the gyroscope will undergo *nutational* motion: Not only does the axis of rotation precess, but also it slowly (relative to the rate of precession) spirals down toward the horizontal (Fig. 42–6B). That is, the axis of rotation moves on the surface of an imaginary cone, but the cone itself slowly opens up.

The net magnetization of an ensemble of protons behaves in a similar fashion. In a strong and constant vertical magnetic field, $\mathbf{B}_0$, the net magnetization simply precesses about the field at the natural resonant (Larmor) frequency (see Fig. 42–4). Suppose, however, the protons are exposed to an additional, relatively weak magnetic field, $\mathbf{B}_1$, designed specifically to circle in the horizontal plane. If the frequency of $\mathbf{B}_1$ is significantly above or below the Larmor frequency, not much happens. But if $\mathbf{B}_1$ circles *at* the Larmor frequency, **M** undergoes nutation.

Figure 42–7A shows how this works for a system initially near thermal equilibrium, with **M** lying almost along $\mathbf{B}_0$. The hypothetical cone on which **M** precesses opens up slowly (relative to the Larmor frequency). At some point, the cone actually coincides briefly with the horizontal plane. After that, it begins to fold up again, but now below the horizontal plane. The nutation continues, with the magnetization eventually returning to where it started. Then the whole process repeats it-

self. The continuous motion of **M** corresponding to the early part of this cycle is indicated, in Figure 42–7B, with the rate of nutation greatly exaggerated relative to the rate of procession.

Figure 42–7 depicts the evolution of **M** as seen by an outside observer in a *fixed frame of reference* (also called the laboratory frame). But just as the motions of the horses of a carousel appear simpler to one actually standing on it (in the *rotating frame of reference*), so also the behavior of **M** over time is most readily followed by one who is in a frame of reference that rotates at the precessional frequency.

Before the weak rf field **B**$_1$ is turned on, for example, the net magnetization precesses at the Larmor frequency about the main field **B**$_0$, when viewed by a fixed-frame observer (Fig. 42–8A). When seen from within a reference frame that rotates at the same frequency, however, **M** does nothing at all; it just sits there, unchanging over time (Fig. 42–8B). It's as if the act of jumping into the rotating frame has the effect of switching off the main field **B**$_0$, just as jumping onto the carousel, in effect, cancels out its rotational motion. So when viewed from the rotating frame, **B**$_0$ apparently vanishes.

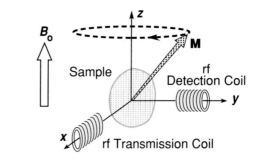

A

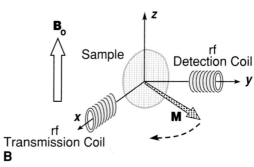

B

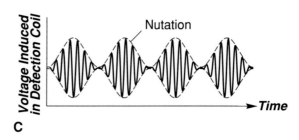

C

Figure 42–9. Detection of the NMR signal. **A.** Location of the radio-frequency transmission and detection coils, in the transverse (*x–y*) plane and outside the sample. **B.** When **M** precesses in or near the transverse plane, it induces a strong Larmor frequency voltage in the pickup coil. **C.** As **M** nutates from parallel to **B**$_0$ down into the transverse plane and beyond, as in Figure 42–7A, the amplitude of the Larmor frequency voltage it induces in the detection coil varies accordingly.

Now turn on **B**$_1$, which also circles at the Larmor frequency. As seen from the rotating frame, **B**$_1$ appears to be a fixed, constant field—in fact, the *only* such field present. **M** precesses about *it* (Fig. 42–8C) with a frequency of $f_1 = (\gamma/2\pi) \cdot B_1$, or with an angular frequency of

$$\omega_1 = \gamma \cdot B_1 \qquad (42.4)$$

The result, when observed from back in the *fixed* frame, is the nutational motion of Figure 42–7.

This section has sketched a simple version of the "classical" picture of the phenomenon of nuclear magnetic resonance. It ignores the critically important effects of spin relaxation mechanisms, and will have to be modified in the next chapter.

One aspect of all of this may have troubled you. The two-state picture of Chapter 41 allows individual spins to be aligned along or against the static magnetic field, but nothing else. Yet here we find collections of protons whose net magnetization can be at any angle relative to the external

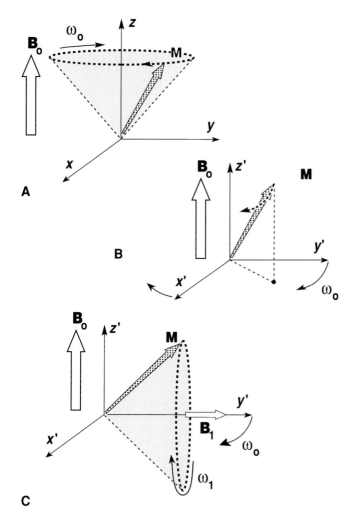

Figure 42–8. Advantage of viewing precession and resonance from a rotating frame of reference. **A.** Precession at frequency ω_0, as seen from a frame of reference *fixed* in space. **B.** When seen from a frame of reference (with *x′*, *y′*, and *z′* axes, where the *z′* axis is colinear with the *z*) that *rotates* at the precessional frequency, ω_0, the net magnetization seems to stand still. **C.** Nutation of **M** at the (relatively slow) rate ω_1 about the applied Larmor frequency magnetic field, which rotates with the *y′* axis, as seen from the rotating frame. (This is to be contrasted with Fig. 42–7B). Here, **M** happened not to be along the *z′* axis when the radio frequency power was turned on; how would the picture be different if **M** had been *along* the *z′* axis at that time?

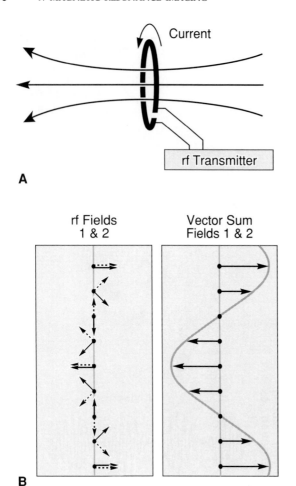

B

Figure 42–10. Generating the rotating radio-frequency field, **B**$_1$. **A.** Creation of a linearly polarized rf field from current in a loop of wire. **B.** The linearly polarized field is equivalent to the vector sum of a pair of fields in the X–Y plane (seen here from above) that rotate in opposite directions. The one that rotates in the direction of precession of **M** is **B**$_1$, and the other is irrelevant. Time steps downward.

field. **M** can even precess purely in the horizontal plane. The problem is that our elementary quantum treatment, although correct enough for some purposes, is not sufficiently refined to allow our avoidance of this apparent paradox.

The classical model of NMR can be fully presented (even including the effects of spin relaxation) by means of the *Bloch equations*, which describe the behavior of the net magnetization vector over time (Fig. 42–7 or 42–8). The Bloch equations, in turn, can be extracted from a rigorous, comprehensive quantum mechanical treatment, which we cannot pursue here. But unfortunately, that is the only route by which the spin paradox can be resolved.

5. DETECTION OF NUCLEAR MAGNETIC RESONANCE: INDUCTION BY THE PRECESSING NET MAGNETIZATION OF A VOLTAGE IN A PICKUP COIL

So much for causing NMR to occur, but how is it detected? How does one tell, for a particular static magnetic field, **B**$_0$, that the frequency of the rf power being pumped into a spin system

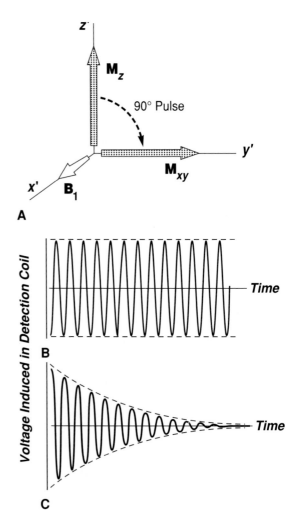

Figure 42–11. Especially important 90° ($\pi/2$) pulse. **A.** A 90° pulse drives the net magnetization from the vertical down into the transverse plane. (Shown here in the rotating coordinate frame.) **B. M**, now precessing in the transverse (x–y) plane, induces a Larmor frequency signal that will be of constant amplitude if no relaxation processes are present. **C.** With relaxation, however, the free induction decay (FID) signal falls off exponentially with time.

via **B**$_1$ is identical to the Larmor precessional frequency, so that **M** undergoes nutation? Nothing was said in the last section about the flipping over of protons with the absorption of rf power, or about photons not reaching the antenna of a receiver. That all related, rather, to the quantum nuclear spin state picture.

Suppose that **M** is precessing in a strong (e.g., 1 T) static vertical magnetic field, **B**$_0$, at the Larmor angular frequency, ω_0, of Equation 42.3. Now create a second, weak (10^{-3}-T) magnetic field, **B**$_1$, circling in the horizontal plane. Such a field can be generated by means of a wire **rf transmission coil** situated outside the sample and on the horizontal plane (Fig. 42–9A). If (and only if) **B**$_1$ happens to be of the correct (Larmor resonance) frequency, **M** will undergo nutation, as discussed in the last section.

Passing an rf current through a loop of wire will give rise to a "linearly polarized" oscillating magnetic field (Fig. 42–10A). This field may be viewed as the sum of two "circularly polarized" fields circling in opposite directions (Fig.

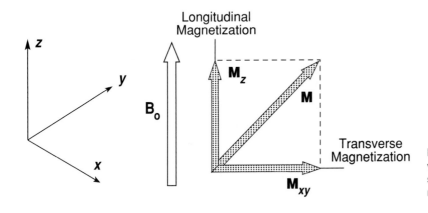

Figure 42–12. The components of the net magnetization vector **M** along **B**$_0$ and perpendicular to it are called, respectively, the longitudinal (**M**$_z$) and transverse (**M**$_{xy}$) magnetizations.

42–10B). (Their components in the y direction cancel, and those in the x direction add together, thereby producing the linear field.) One of these circularly polarized fields is our **B**$_1$, and the other is rotating in the wrong direction and of no significance.

This nuclear magnetic resonance condition may be detected by a means of a small **rf detection coil,** also located on the horizontal plane. Any changing magnetic field produces a voltage in the coils, by means of Faraday induction (see Chapter 4, Section 5). When the net magnetization happens to be pointing nearly up or down, almost along or against the main external field (Fig. 42–9A), the pickup coils are oblivious to it. But when **M** is precessing in or near the horizontal plane at the Larmor frequency (Fig. 42–9B), the detection coils experience a magnetic field that oscillates at that frequency. Thus, as **M** nutates through 360 degrees about **B**$_1$ (as seen in the rotating frame of reference), the amplitude of the rf voltage induced in the detection coils will slowly (relative to the Larmor frequency) vary (Fig. 42–9C). The presence of such a signal indicates the occurrence of NMR.

Suppose that the magnetization starts off aligned parallel to the external field, but that the Larmor frequency rf is left on only long enough for **M** to nutate through 90 degrees or $\pi/2$ radians, down to the horizontal plane (Fig. 42–11A). The rf is then switched off. The time that **B**$_1$ is to be applied, $t_{\pi/2}$, may be determined from Equation 42.4 and from the condition $f_1 \cdot t_{\pi/2} = 90°$, or

$$\omega_1 \cdot t_{\pi/2} = \pi/2 \qquad (42.5)$$

(Note that the stronger **B**$_1$ is, the shorter the time it has to be left on, and vice versa.) As the magnetization has nutated through 90 degrees, from the vertical down to the horizontal plane, this is called a **90° or $\pi/2$ rf pulse.** What signal will be induced in the pickup coil? One might think, from what has been said so far, that the magnetization would precess forever in the horizontal plane, generating a constant-amplitude, Larmor frequency signal (Fig. 42–11B). That would, indeed, be the case if there were no spin relaxation processes at play. But because, in fact, there is spin relaxation, the situation is much more interesting (Fig. 42–11C), as will be seen in the next chapter. In particular, the strength of the **free induction decay** (FID) signal falls off exponentially over time, and the characteristic decay time (which is closely related to the T2 of MRI) may be of clinical importance.

At any instant, the component of the net magnetization in the direction of the external field, in the z direction, is known as the **longitudinal magnetization** and is denoted **M**$_z$ (Fig.

42–12). The component in the x–y plane is the **transverse magnetization,** and denoted **M**$_{xy}$. Two particular situations are of special importance: At thermal equilibrium, the net magnetization points along the external field and is entirely longitudinal in nature, **M**$_z$ = **M**$_0$. When **M** is precessing in the x–y plane, on the other hand, as in Figures 42–9B and 42–11B, it is all transverse. More generally, **M** may have both longitudinal and transverse components, and these are likely to be changing over time.

6. ONE-DIMENSIONAL IMAGING, AGAIN

Let us now return briefly to the one-dimensional imaging example of Chapter 41, Section 6, but this time with a classical, rather than quantum, approach.

Recall that for our phantom, two thin pancake slices of water are situated in local magnetic environments that differ from one another because of an x-gradient field. Each slice gives rise to a net equilibrium magnetization, but because the proton density of the upper volume element is half that of the lower, its net magnetization is only about half as great.

We initiate the imaging process at time t_0 (Fig. 42–13A) by switching on the x-gradient field, and soon thereafter pump in a 90° pulse of rf (Fig. 42–13B). The Larmor frequencies for the two slices of water in the gradient are 42.14 and 43.00 MHz, respectively. To induce resonance in both water samples, the rf pulse can no longer be monochromatic; it must contain, rather, a band of frequencies ranging, at least, from below 42.14 MHz to above 43.00 MHz. That way, the magnetizations of both volumes of water will be caused, independently, to nutate down into the x–y plane. At the cessation of the pulse, the two magnetization vectors will be precessing at 42.14 and 43.00 MHz, respectively, inducing signals of these two frequencies in the pickup coil. Interference of the two components gives rise to a beating (see Fig. 4–9) in the detected composite NMR signal (Fig. 42–13C). The composite rf signal decays slowly over time because of relaxation processes.

The NMR signals from the two volume elements of water can be separated from one another and measured by the computer-based Fourier transform method described in the next section. The component at the higher frequency is found to have half the intensity of the other (Fig. 42–13D), which is consistent with Figure 41–7C.

Once again, we have found a way to distinguish NMR signals coming from different voxels: We have been able to pro-

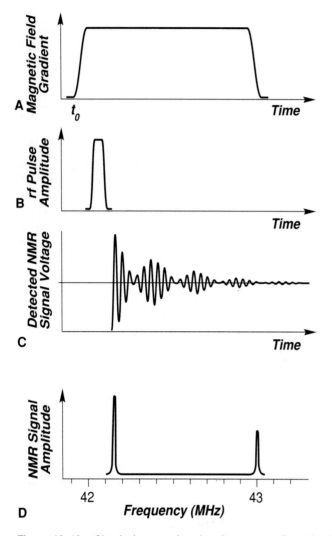

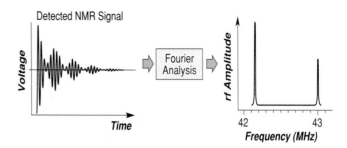

Figure 42–14. Spectral representation of the frequency components of a complex signal, brought about by Fourier analysis. Also called "transforming from the time domain to the frequency domain."

Figure 42–13. Classical approach to imaging our one-dimensional phantom (see also Fig. 41–7). With the x gradient on (**A**), a 90° pulse is pumped into the phantom (**B**), and the free induction decay (FID) signal is recorded (**C**). **D.** Fourier analysis of the FID signal reveals components at 42.15 and 43.01 MHz, with amplitudes proportional to the corresponding amounts of water present. Compare with Figure 41–7.

duce an image of proton density as a function of position, by plotting NMR signal intensity as a function of frequency (see Fig. 41–8). But this time, there is a new link between the two functions: the magnetization. The magnetization of a volume element depends on its proton density and, in turn, is a determinant of the intensity of the corresponding NMR signal. (**M** at any moment also depends, we shall see, on T1 and T2.) This link is fundamental to clinical MRI and will be explored further in Chapters 43 and 44.

7. FOURIER TRANSFORM NUCLEAR MAGNETIC RESONANCE

Unlike the swept rf method of Chapter 41, Sections 5 and 6, the pulsed rf approach just described does *not* carry out separate NMR measurements at many, slightly different frequencies.

Rather, it makes a single measurement, but uses one (or several) pulse(s) designed to contain a continuous band of frequencies, wide enough to include any and all resonances of interest. Every resonance that does occur will then give rise to an rf signal that contributes to the composite NMR signal induced in the detection coil. In the case of our one-dimensional phantom, the coil sees the beat signal (Fig. 42–13C) created by the superpositioning and interference of the separate signals coming from the two volumes of water, in which the magnetization vectors are precessing at two slightly different frequencies.

With respect to imaging, the pulsed rf NMR imaging method just described differs from the swept frequency method of Chapter 41, Section 6, in one critically important, practical regard: It is much faster. The time for data acquisition is only what is required for the magnetization to decay somewhat after one (or several) rf pulse(s). But the price that we must pay for that speed is a complicated NMR signal, generated simultaneously by the magnetizations in different volume elements precessing at different frequencies. That signal must somehow be untangled.

This difficult task is carried out by a **Fourier analyzer** (Fig. 42–14), an electronic instrument and/or computer program that performs a Fourier transform on the signal (see Chapter 24, Section 2). The output of the Fourier analyzer is a *Fourier decomposition* of the signal into the corresponding spectrum. For our phantom, the decomposition (Fig. 42–13D) is the same as the spectrum obtained the slow way, one frequency at a time, in Figure 41–7C. And again, because every frequency in Figure 42–13D is associated with a unique position along the phantom, the positions of the peaks within the spectrum provide a direct anatomic map of proton density.

_____ **EXERCISE 42–2.** _____

What do you get if you image our one-dimensional phantom with the gradient turned off, and with a uniform **B**₀ of 1.00 T?

SOLUTION: After the 90° pulse, all the water precesses at a frequency of 42.58 MHz. The NMR signal decays slowly because of relaxation effects. Fourier analysis yields a spectrum with a single peak, at the resonant frequency. The peak would have infinitesimal width (i.e., the signal would be monochromatic) were it not for the relaxation and signal decay.

Chapter 43

Magnetic Resonance III: Relaxation Times (T1 and T2), Pulse Sequences, and Image Contrast

When a system of nuclei in a magnetic field is disturbed from thermal equilibrium, the magnitude and direction of the net magnetization $\mathbf{M}(t)$ varies in time. For the protons of intracellular water, in particular, the parameters describing different aspects of the return to equilibrium (tissue T1 and T2) are determined in part by cellular physiology, and may be affected by some pathologic conditions.

A magnetic resonance image is generally not a direct, voxel-by-voxel map of any one of the three primary NMR tissue parameters (proton density, T1, or T2). It is, rather, something more subtle: a map of the relative strength of the nuclear magnetic resonance (NMR) signal originating in each voxel (hence of the magnitude of the magnetization there) at a special, particular instant of time. This magnetization, in turn, *does* depend on the three tissue parameters, and also on the choice of pulse sequence and other imaging machine settings. Thus, proton density, T1, and T2 have indirect but significant influences on image contrast. An image that is produced in such a fashion that the contrast reflects differences primarily in tissue T1 is said to be "T1-weighted." T1-, T2-, and proton density-weighted imaging is adequate for many clinical purposes.

This chapter focuses on the nature of the relaxation processes taking place in a voxel of tissue during magnetic resonance imaging (MRI) and on how those processes affect MRI image contrast. The way that the mapping program is actually carried out in two or three dimensions will be addressed in the next chapter.

1. A SPIN SYSTEM APPROACHES THERMAL EQUILIBRIUM EXPONENTIALLY WITH CHARACTERISTIC LONGITUDINAL (SPIN–LATTICE) RELAXATION TIME T1

The spins of the protons in a glass of water normally point randomly in all directions and give rise to zero net magnetization. Suppose, however, that you place the glass between the poles of a powerful electromagnet, and turn the field on abruptly at time $t = 0$. Because of spatial quantization (see Chapter 41, Section 4), all the protons will immediately snap into alignment either along or against the (vertical, z-directional) external field. During that initial moment of mass confusion, roughly equal numbers fall into the spin-up and spin-down (i.e., lower- and higher-energy) states, and the net magnetization is still of zero magnitude.

This is not, however, a situation of thermal equilibrium. The system therefore settles down, and the longitudinal magnetization $M_z(t)$ grows exponentially over time t toward its equilibrium value $\mathbf{M}_0$:

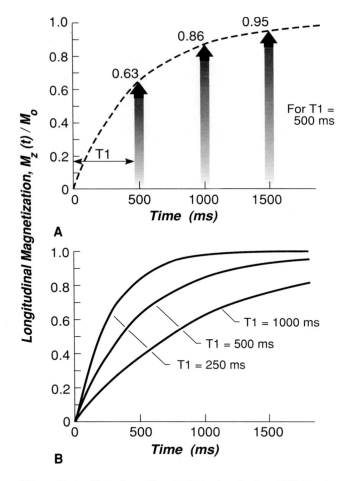

A

B

Figure 43–1. The return of longitudinal magnetization, $M_z(t)$, in water to the equilibrium value, M_0, after an external field is applied abruptly at $t = 0$. **A.** Exponential shape of $M_z(t)/M_0$ (Equation 43.1). **B.** Relaxation for systems with some different values of T1.

$$M_z(t) = M_0 \cdot [1 - e^{-t/T1}], \quad \text{longitudinal relaxation (43.1)}$$

(Fig. 43–1). The longitudinal magnetization (see Chapter 42, Section 5) will have reached 63% of its equilibrium value after time T1, 86% after 2 T1, 95% after 3 T1, and so on. Because it characterizes the regrowth of the longitudinal component of the magnetization, and involves transitions between the spin-up and spin-down states, T1 is commonly called the **longitudinal relaxation time.** Because it was first described in connection with the magnetic resonance properties of nuclei in solids, in which spin-state energy is transferred to and from a crystal lattice in the form of phonons (quanta of vibrational energy), T1 is also known as the **spin–lattice relaxation time.** We shall use the two terms interchangeably. The term 1/T1 describes the *rate* at which the system comes to thermal equilibrium.

A hand-waving argument, à la Chapter 15, on the exponential form of $M_z(t)$: The probability per unit time that any one proton will be flipped is independent of the time that it has already spent in the higher or lower energy state, and also of what has happened to its fellow protons. Therefore, in the notation of Equation 42.1, the rate of change of $(N_- - N_+)$ will

be proportional to how far $(N_- - N_+)$ is from its equilibrium value. Hence Equation 43.1.

The situation is actually somewhat more complicated than this, as a proton can re-enter the higher (or lower) energy state again after leaving it. But the system still does approach equilibrium exponentially.

EXERCISE 43–1.

Show that Equation 43.1 reduces to the correct forms at $t = 0$ and $t = \infty$, and behaves correctly inbetween.

SOLUTION: At $t = 0$, $M_z(t)$ becomes $M_z(0) = M_0[1 - 1] = 0$. For $t = \infty$ (infinity), $M_z(t)$ reduces to $M_z(\infty) = M_0$. Between $t = 0$ and $t = \infty$, $M_z(t)$ approaches M_0 exponentially.

---

2. LONGITUDINAL RELAXATION IS CAUSED BY WEAK MAGNETIC "NOISE" FLUCTUATING AT THE LARMOR FREQUENCY

The following discussion focuses on water, but similar arguments apply to protons in lipids and other biomolecules of relevance to MRI.

The characteristic time T1 for thermal equilibration of a system of protons depends on the effectiveness of the processes that can cause *spontaneous* spin flips (with no Larmor frequency rf power being pumped in intentionally from outside sources). The rate of equilibration, 1/T1, will be fast, and T1 will be short, if mechanisms are present by which a proton can interact readily with its surroundings in the necessary manner.

Longitudinal relaxation can be brought about by naturally occurring magnetic field "noise" that happens to be varying at the Larmor frequency. There are a number of ways by which protons of the water molecules in living cells, in particular, can experience such magnetic "noise." The most important of these involve *intra*molecular proton–proton magnetic dipole interactions that fluctuate over time because of random motions of the water molecules themselves.

As a water molecule undergoes translational, vibrational, and rotational motion in the presence of a strong, constant external magnetic field, each of its protons remains, nearly all of the time, independently aligned parallel or antiparallel to the field (Fig. 43–2). The dipole magnetic field that a proton itself produces in the vicinity of its partner proton ranges from nearly zero (when the two are one above the other, relative to the external field) to about 4×10^{-4} T (when they are side by side). Thus, as the molecule tumbles, each proton generates for its partner a magnetic field, with an amplitude of up to 4×10^{-4} T, that varies at the tumbling frequency. Since a dipole field falls off rapidly with distance, the varying magnetic fields produced by nuclei on other molecules are generally much weaker. (The fields from the molecules of paramagnetic contrast media are produced by unpaired *electrons*.)

Suppose a molecule of H_2O happens to be tumbling at the Larmor frequency. The dipole magnetic field produced by proton a and felt by its partner proton b will vary at the Larmor frequency and with an amplitude of something like 4×10^{-4} T. A Larmor frequency magnetic field of this amplitude can, like

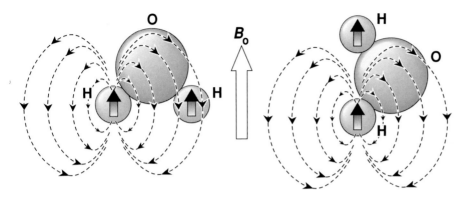

Figure 43–2. At any instant, the dipole magnetic field produced by one proton of a water molecule, as experienced by the other, depends strongly on their relative positions in the external magnetic field, and that changes rapidly as the molecule moves about.

a radio-frequency photon supplied by an external rf coil, cause proton spin-state transitions. So even in the absence of rf energy from the outside, a proton can be elevated into, or tickled out of, the higher-energy spin state by the randomly fluctuating dipole magnetic field produced by its partner proton.

> Other kinds of motions can generate the requisite Larmor frequency field. If the molecule is tumbling at half the Larmor frequency, say, then the time-varying magnetic fields it produces may contain a small component at the Larmor frequency itself (the first harmonic of the tumbling frequency), as can be shown by Fourier analysis (see Chapter 24, Section 2).

The proton longitudinal relaxation time T1 for water in cells is determined largely by the amplitude of Larmor frequency fluctuations in the local magnetic fields, hence by the nature of the rotations and other motions of the intracellular water molecules. It is influenced in subtle ways, as we shall see in Section 8, by any factors that affect this motion. Most importantly from a clinical perspective, it appears that T1 depends on the degree to which the water molecules within a cell are bound to intracellular macromolecules. The amount of water and the binding of water molecules, in turn, can depend on the cell type and physiologic status. Proton T1 for a tissue is thus affected by its histology and, significantly, by some pathologies. It is for this reason that one objective of MRI is to detect variations in the value of T1 for water protons, and related parameters, throughout the anatomic region of interest.

3. MEASURING T1 WITH THE SATURATION–RECOVERY PULSE SEQUENCE, 90°–TR–90°

It was just argued that abruptly turning on a magnetic field will leave a system of protons in a state of thermal nonequilibrium. Similarly, as seen in the preceding chapter, for a set of spins already at equilibrium, pumping in Larmor frequency rf energy (so that the net magnetization nutates away from the direction of the external field) also disturbs the thermal equilibrium. Here, too, the system returns to equilibrium exponentially, with characteristic time T1, once the rf power is turned off.

This suggests a method of measuring T1. You somehow drive the spin system away from its equilibrium state, and then monitor the recovery of the longitudinal magnetization over time. The behavior of **M** during the return to equilibrium and, in particular, the time it takes for the function $M_z(t)$ to level off will reveal the value of the spin–lattice time.

One way to do this is by means of the *saturation–recovery* pulse sequence. Saturation–recovery consists of three parts (Fig. 43–3A): (1) a 90° (or $\pi/2$) *saturation pulse* of Larmor frequency rf power that drives the spin system far from thermal equilibrium; (2) a quiet period of duration TR, the *repetition time*, during which the magnetization is allowed to relax part of the way back to its equilibrium state; and (3) a 90° interrogation or *detection pulse* at $t = $ TR, to reveal the magnitude of the longitudinal magnetization at that time, M_z(TR). Several repetitions of the sequence with different choices for TR indicate the shape of $M_z(t)$ of Equation 43.1 (Fig. 43–3B), hence the value of T1.

> The closely related *inversion–recovery* sequence begins with a 180° (inversion) pulse that turns the equilibrium magnetization upside down, rather than just through 90°. Both inversion–recovery and saturation–recovery find limited use in MRI; the standard clinical sequence is the *spin-echo* (see Section 7).

Let's go through this again, in a bit more detail. The objective is to keep track of the components of **M**(t), the magnetization vector, as functions of time. Suppose that a system of protons in an external magnetic field is at thermal equilibrium. The net magnetization lies along the direction of the field, and starts off with magnitude M_0. At time $t = 0$, a pulse of resonant frequency rf energy is pumped in with a combination of amplitude and duration that causes **M** to nutate through 90 degrees. Immediately following this saturation pulse, the net magnetization will be precessing freely in the transverse (x–y, or horizontal) plane, initially with magnitude $M(0) = M_0$. The voltage it induces in the detection coils at this time is *not* used or recorded.

Of interest here is the recovery of the longitudinal magnetization over time, that is, the regrowth of the component of **M** lying along the z axis (see Equation 43.1). We therefore let the system sit undisturbed for a period of duration TR, the repetition time. Precisely at $t = $ TR, we obtain the value of the (partially regrown) longitudinal magnetization: A 90° detection pulse swings the z component of **M**, now of magnitude M_z(TR), rapidly down into the x–y plane. This component of **M** precesses in the transverse plane, and produces in the pickup

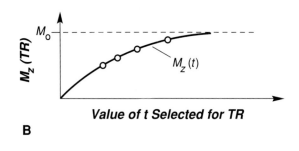

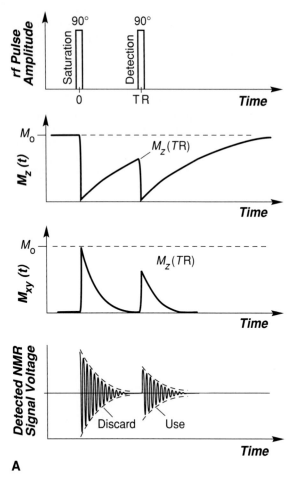

Figure 43–3. Saturation–recovery pulse sequence, being used here to determine T1. **A.** At $t = 0$, the first 90° pulse saturates the longitudinal magnetization. $M_z(t)$ is then allowed to recover along the z axis until $t = $ TR. At that time, a second 90° pulse drives the recovered component of magnetization back into the transverse plane, where its current magnitude, $M_z(TR)$, is read. **B.** Repetition of the procedure with different choices of TR yields the shape of $M_z(t)$, hence the value of T1.

coils a signal whose voltage is proportional, at first, to $M_z(TR)$. This is the data point we need.

Now the system is finally allowed to return to thermal equilibrium. The entire saturation–recovery pulse sequence is then repeated several times, with different choices of TR. T1 is obtained by fitting the resulting data to Equation 43.1. Four such data points are shown in Figure 43–3B.

4. WITH SATURATION–RECOVERY IMAGING, T1-WEIGHTED CONTRAST DEPENDS ON THE REPETITION TIME, TR

Repeating the 90°–TR–90° pulse sequence for a number of different values of TR and fitting the results to Equation 43.1 is good at providing a relatively accurate estimate of T1 for a sample in a test tube, but it does not lend itself to the efficient generation of images. It is possible, however, to produce, much more rapidly, a map of something that reflects T1 (or T2 or proton density) indirectly, namely, the local magnetization (albeit at a particular instant of time, and after that magnetization has been prepared by means of a special sequence of rf pulses).

Fortunately, such a magnetic resonance image turns out to be clinically very useful.

Let us make this important point another way: An MRI picture could be, but normally is not, an anatomic map of precise values of T1, T2, or proton density. Usually, however, it is something simpler and more readily created—a voxel-by-voxel map of the tissue net magnetization that results, at a specific instant, and from a specific imaging pulse sequence. (With the saturation–recovery pulse sequence, the special instant of time is $t = $ TR; for the spin-echo sequence, as we shall see, it is the moment that the echo signal appears.) This map is obtained (exactly as in the classical one-dimensional imaging example of Chapter 42, Section 6) by determining, at that instant, the relative amount of proton NMR signal that originates in each voxel. The greater the magnetization in a voxel, the stronger the NMR signal coming from it at the time of signal detection, and the brighter the pixel in the corresponding MRI image.

The strength of the signal from a voxel depends on the T1, T2, and proton density of its tissue, and also on the details of the pulse sequence and various other MRI instrument settings. One cannot readily alter the three physiologic parameters (except by means of a contrast agent), but one can optimize the operating parameters of the imaging machine. What is ulti-

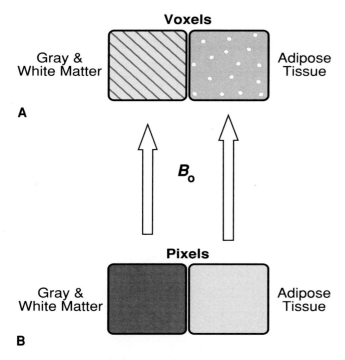

A

B

Figure 43–4. T1-weighted contrast 1-D example. **A.** Adjacent voxels containing different tissues and experiencing different local magnetic fields. **B.** $M_z(t)$ will have recovered more, at t = TR, for the voxel containing adipose tissue, because of the shorter T1, than for that with gray and white matter. The greater value of M_z(TR) for the adipose tissue at t = TR will be reflected, in the display, as a brighter pixel.

mately sought clinically is an image that somehow reflects, in a significant way, the *differences* in T1, T2, and/or proton density for the various healthy and pathologic tissues, and much of the skill and science of MRI therefore involves the selection of pulse sequences and other MRI instrument characteristics that most effectively enhance such contrasts.

Figure 43–4A explores this idea with a new, somewhat more realistic one-dimensional example. Two adjacent in-

tracranial voxels lie in magnetic fields that differ slightly because of the presence of a gradient. The voxel to the left contains largely white and gray matter, and the other, adipose tissue. Assume that the proton densities of the two are about the same. A saturation–recovery-type pulse sequence, consisting of a single pair of 90° pulses separated by TR, is applied. After the second 90° pulse, the NMR signal intensity from each voxel will be independently proportional to the value of M_z(TR) in the voxel, that is, to the magnitude of the recovered longitudinal component of magnetization at t = TR, the time it is driven down into the transverse plane by the 90° detection pulse. The signals from the two voxels are separated by means of a Fourier analysis. Figure 43–4B is a map obtained by, in effect, making the brightness of each pixel proportional to M_z(TR) for the corresponding voxel.

T1 for lipid (typically about 250 milliseconds for a 1-T magnetic field) is significantly less than T1 for white and gray matter (600 to 800 milliseconds). Thus, fatty material equilibrates more rapidly following the 90° saturation pulse than do white and gray matter (Fig. 43–5). The difference between the values of $M_z(t)$ for the two media is greatest at a time that is roughly midway between their respective T1 values. So a choice of TR of something like 500 to 600 milliseconds will maximize the image contrast. M_z(TR) is considerably greater for adipose tissue than for white and gray matter with such a choice of TR, and its pixel shows up much brighter in the image. In Figure 43–6, for example, the lipoma (a fatty tumor) seen displacing the pituitary appears bright. As the contrast in this case is attributable largely to differences in T1, the image is said to be **T1-weighted.**

5. PRECESSION OF M IN THE TRANSVERSE PLANE: FREE INDUCTION DECAY SIGNAL OF CHARACTERISTIC TIME T2*

Let us leave saturation–recovery now, and turn to the NMR signal produced when a single 90° pulse is applied to a system of spins at equilibrium in a uniform external magnetic field.

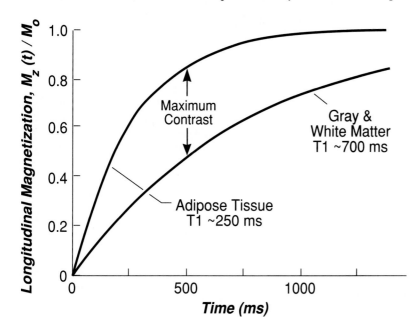

Figure 43–5. The difference in values of M_z(TR), hence the contrast for the two pixels, will be greatest with a TR roughly midway between the values of T1 for the two voxels. Here, T1 is about 700 milliseconds for white and gray matter and 250 milliseconds for adipose tissue.

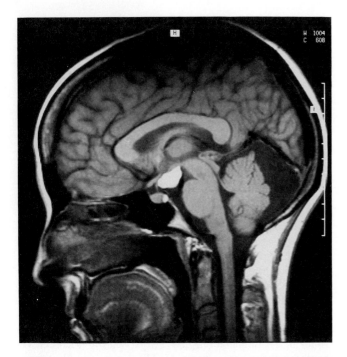

Figure 43–6. T1-weighted image of the brain. The lipoma displacing the pituitary shows up brightly because of the relatively short T1 of adipose tissue. *(Courtesy of Siemens Medical Systems, Inc.)*

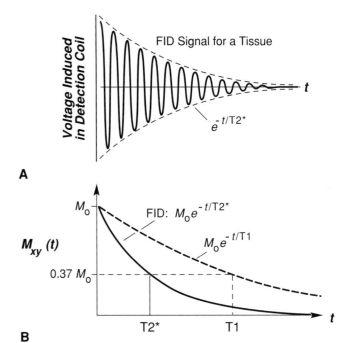

Figure 43–7. Free induction decay (FID). **A.** An FID signal falls off exponentially with characteristic time T2*. **B.** FID falls off much more rapidly than $e^{-t/T1}$, the rate that would be expected if the decay in M_{xy} were attributable only to the recovery in M_z.

The pulse drives the magnetization down into the transverse plane, where it undergoes *free precession*. The **free induction decay** (FID) signal generated in the pickup (detection) coils falls off exponentially with time (Fig. 43–7A) because of relaxation effects.

If the spin–lattice mechanism were the only relaxation process at work, then the transverse magnetization in the x–y plane (as indicated by the amplitude of the FID signal) would die out with the same characteristic time T1 that the longitudinal magnetization recovers. With nonviscous liquids, such as pure water, this is exactly what happens.

With solids, viscous fluids, or tissues, however, the FID signal vanishes much faster than would be caused by T1 relaxation alone (Fig. 43–7B). That is, the transverse magnetization is gone long before the longitudinal magnetization has regrown significantly. (You may have already noticed this in Figure 43–3 in comparison of the $M_z(t)$ and $M_{xy}(t)$ curves.) Thus, the transverse and longitudinal magnetizations are not just the two components of a single $\mathbf{M}(t)$ vector of constant length. The detected FID signal falls off exponentially, rather,

$$\text{FID signal} \sim e^{-t/T2^*}, \quad \text{transverse relaxation}$$
$$\text{(real magnet)} \quad (43.2)$$

with a characteristic FID time T2* (called "tee two star") which is found to be shorter (and in some cases *much* shorter) than T1: T2* < T1. Why, following a 90° pulse, should the transverse magnetization in a sample of tissue die out faster than $e^{-t/T1}$?

The answer must be that longitudinal relaxation is not the only mechanism that contributes to the decay of the transverse magnetization. It is, in fact, one of three.

A second such mechanism has to do with slight nonuniformities in the field produced by the external magnet. Sup-

pose, for the moment, that a 90° pulse causes the axes of rotations of individual protons to nutate down together into the x–y plane.[†] The protons precess separately in the transverse plane at the Larmor frequency. They are initially in phase and give rise to the precessing transverse net magnetization that produces the FID signal. The external magnetic field is not perfectly uniform, however, because of imperfect magnet design and manufacture. The individual protons therefore experience local magnetic fields that are slightly different from one another, and they precess at slightly different frequencies. At any instant, half the protons will be precessing a little faster than the median proton, and the others will go around more slowly. As a result, Figure 43–8A (left-hand side of the diagram), after a 90° pulse the spins will lose their initial phase coherence; that is, their *spin orientations will fan out*. Over a time, the proton orientations become evenly spread out in the transverse plane. The individual spins will end up pointing in all directions, like the spokes of a bicycle wheel, and their magnetic moments will cancel one another out. As a result, the net magnetic field they produce at the pickup coils drops to zero. Hence the decay of the FID in accordance with Equation 43.2. Figure 43–8B shows the spin dephasing as it would appear to an observer in a coordinate system that rotates at the average Larmor frequency.

The asterisk on the T2* in Equation 43.2 is meant to indicate that inhomogeneities in the external field contribute to the free induction decay process. The **transverse relaxation time** (also known as the **spin–spin relaxation time**) refers to the inherent effects that remain even when the external field in-

---

[†]This picture is inconsistent with the (overly simplistic) idea of all protons being always either spin-up or spin-down; but suppose it anyway.

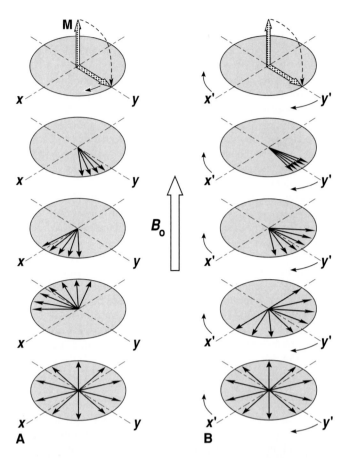

Figure 43–8. Spin dephasing caused by inhomogeneities in the external field is one of the mechanisms that determine T2*. **A.** The loss of phase coherence of spins is brought about by inhomogeneities in the external magnetic field. **B.** The same thing, as seen from a reference frame that rotates at the average Larmor frequency.

homogeneities are removed. It is a parameter of biologic interest, and is denoted simply T2. And 1/T2 is the rate at which a cohort of spins would dephase in the transverse plane, following a 90° pulse, in the field of a *perfect external magnet*,

$$\text{FID signal} \sim e^{-t/T2}, \quad \begin{array}{l}\text{transverse relaxation}\\ \text{(perfect magnet)}\end{array} \quad (43.3)$$

(Fig. 43–9). T2 is always a longer time than T2*,

$$\text{T2} > \text{T2*} \quad (43.4)$$

T2* becomes T2 only in the idealized case of spins in a perfect external field that contained no inhomogeneities.

_____ **EXERCISE 43–2.** _____

Demonstrate that T2 > T2*.

SOLUTION: 1/T2 is the rate at which a certain relaxation process occurs in a population of spins. Inhomogeneity in the field of the external magnet speeds up the fanning out process, and thereby increases the total relaxation rate from 1/T2 to 1/T2*. The result to be demonstrated follows from 1/T2* > 1/T2. The same argument applies to T1 > T2*, which followed Equation 43.2.

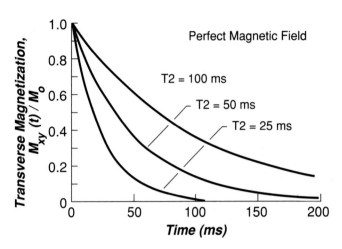

Figure 43–9. Decay in transverse magnetization, in a perfectly homogeneous external magnetic field, for various values of transverse relaxation time T2.

Figure 43–10 summarizes the relaxation story, so far. The FID signal decays with a characteristic time T2*. If the effect of external field inhomogeneities is removed from the picture (as can be made to happen with the spin-echo pulse sequence), then the transverse magnetization decays with the biologically meaningful transverse (spin–spin) relaxation time T2. This transverse relaxation time, in turn, is determined by two processes: the longitudinal (spin–lattice) transitions, which occur at the *rate* 1/T1, and the spin–spin interactions, which provide the "secular" contribution to 1/T2, and to which we shall now turn.

6. FREE INDUCTION DECAY IN A PERFECTLY HOMOGENEOUS EXTERNAL MAGNETIC FIELD: THE T1 AND SECULAR CONTRIBUTIONS TO THE TRANSVERSE (SPIN–SPIN) RELAXATION RATE, 1/T2

Static, high (Larmor)-frequency, and low-frequency magnetic fields all play roles in the transverse relaxation story. Static imperfections in the external magnetic field contribute to T2*, but

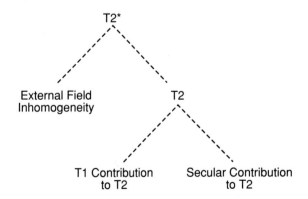

Figure 43–10. There are two components to the spin–spin rate 1/T2, namely, the 1/T1 and the secular contributions. T2 and inhomogeneities in the external magnetic field together determine T2*.

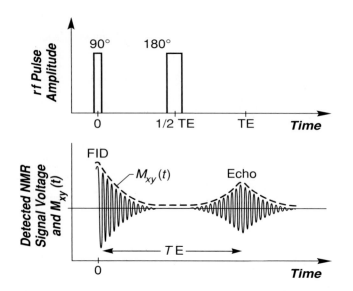

Figure 43–11. The spin-echo pulse sequence is used to eliminate the effects of inhomogeneities in the external magnetic field.

their effects can be removed adequately by means of the spin-echo rf pulse sequence, as will be seen in the next section, so we can forget about that problem for now. Spin–lattice transitions brought about by Larmor frequency magnetic fields provide the "*T1 contribution to T2.*" Measured values of T2 are usually shorter than T1, however, which means that there must be yet another possible transverse relaxation mechanism. That's where the slowly varying (low-frequency) fields come in—they are responsible for the "*secular* contribution to T2."

Every proton is exposed to the dipole magnetic fields produced by its neighbors and, in a water molecule, by its partner proton in particular. If the water molecule is tumbling and vi-

brating freely, as in pure water, such fields will be changing much too fast to have any appreciable effect on the proton's Larmor frequency of precession. But suppose that for some reason the water molecule's motions are significantly slowed down, or intermittently hindered. Each proton will be subject to a (relatively) slowly varying or static dipole field from its partner—sometimes adding to the external field and sometimes subtracting from it—over appreciable periods of time. As a result, the proton will intermittently precess faster or slower than the average Larmor frequency. Exactly as with a nonhomogeneous external field, this leads to loss of spin phase, hence to a decaying transverse magnetization. This mechanism provides the secular contribution to T2. Unlike the dephasing resulting from the totally static imperfections in the external magnetic field, however, it is characteristic of the proton spin system itself.

To reiterate: Longitudinal relaxation (involving transitions between the lower- and higher-energy spin states) is only one of the two processes responsible, in general, for the spin dephasing parameterized by T2 (the other being the secular contribution) (Fig. 43–10). So by the same argument as that of Exercise 43–2, the transverse relaxation process is always as fast as, or faster than, the longitudinal relaxation, $1/T2 \geq 1/T1$. Equivalently,

$$T2 \leq T1 \quad \text{(always)} \tag{43.5}$$

In solids, such as ice, there is relatively little motion of the nuclei, so that the slowly changing local field variations give the spins ample time to dephase. The secular relaxation mechanism is therefore very fast, and the transverse relaxation time is much shorter than the longitudinal:

$$T2 << T1 \quad \text{(solid)} \tag{43.6a}$$

In nonviscous liquids such as water, the molecular motions and the resulting fluctuations in the local fields are far too

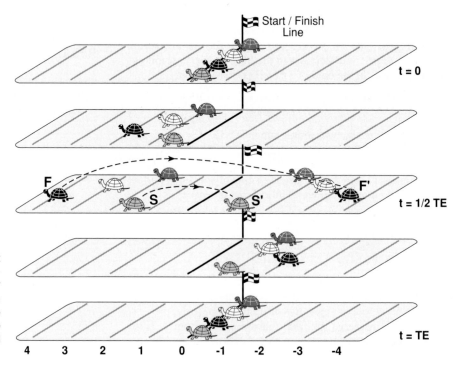

Figure 43–12. The First (Annual) Shall be Last Turtle Derby. Halfway through the race, precisely at $t = \frac{1}{2}$TE, all the participants are instantly teleported to the other side of the start/finish line. For each turtle, the distance from the line just after the move equals that just prior to it. The fastest (F) and slowest (S) are noted. All will cross the finish line together at $t = $ TE.

rapid to be effective in causing secular spin dephasing. In this special case, T2 is nearly all attributable to T1-type transitions (spin flips), so that

$$T2 = T1 \quad \text{(liquid)} \qquad (43.6b)$$

Soft tissues lie somewhere inbetween:

$$T2 = 0.1 \cdot T1 \text{ to } 0.3 \cdot T1 \quad \text{(tissue)} \qquad (43.6c)$$

With a static field of 1 T, T1 in soft tissue is typically between 200 milliseconds and 1 second (Table 43–1). It should be emphasized that these numbers are very rough, at best, and each represents a near midpoint for a wide range of reported values. T2 for a tissue is commonly one third to one tenth of its T1, suggesting the dominance of the secular contribution to T2.

7. DETERMINING T2 WITH THE SPIN-ECHO PULSE SEQUENCE, $90°-\frac{1}{2}TE-180°-\frac{1}{2}TE$

We have argued that the decay time T2* for free induction decay following a 90° pulse consists of a part that is physiologically relevant (T2) and another that is a nuisance caused by the equipment (an imperfect external field). Fortunately, the **spin-echo pulse sequence** allows us to get rid of the latter.

Before the spin-echo pulse sequence begins, the net magnetization lies along the z axis. The sequence starts off with a 90° *excitation pulse*. Immediately thereafter, the magnetization, still of magnitude M_0, is precessing in the transverse plane. A time $\frac{1}{2}TE$ later, where TE is known as the **echo time**, a 180° **refocusing** or echo-generating pulse is applied. The NMR (echo) signal appears and is detected $\frac{1}{2}TE$ later yet, which is to say, a full TE after the excitation pulse. The sequence goes $90°-\frac{1}{2}TE-180°-\frac{1}{2}TE$, or $\frac{1}{2}\pi-\frac{1}{2}TE-\pi-\frac{1}{2}TE$ (Fig. 43–11).

Spin echo works just like the First (Annual) Shall be Last Turtle Derby (Fig. 43–12). At the sound of the 90° pulse, the noble beasts bolt from the start/finish line in a fury of dust and flying hooves. By time $t = \frac{1}{2}TE$, the fastest turtle will have traveled 4 m, say, and the slowest, a little less than 2 m, with the rest inbetween. In a flash, precisely at $t = \frac{1}{2}TE$, a 180° pulse teleports the lead turtle to a point 4 m on the other side of the start/finish line, but it leaves her or him galloping full tilt in the original direction. At the same time, the slowest one is put down a bit less than 2 m from the line, and so on. Over the next $\frac{1}{2}TE$, each turtle has exactly the right amount of time needed to reach the line, so they all cross it together.

TABLE 43–1. TYPICAL VALUES OF THE RELAXATION TIMES T1 AND T2 FOR VARIOUS TISSUES AND FIELD STRENGTHS

Tissue	T1 (0.5 T) (ms)	T1 (1.5 T) (ms)	T2 (ms)
Adipose	210	260	80
Liver	350	500	40
Muscle	550	870	45
White matter	500	780	90
Gray matter	650	920	100
Cerebrospinal fluid	1800	2400	160

After Sprawls, P Jr: Physical Principles of Medical Imaging. Rockville, MD: Aspen, 1987 (Table 27–1).

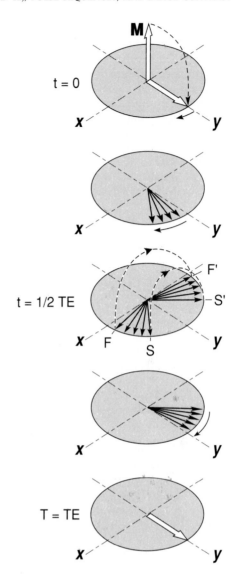

Figure 43–13. Spin-echo process. (1) At time $t = 0$, a 90° pulse swings the magnetization **M** into the transverse plane, along the y axis. (2) The spins "fan out" and lose phase coherence, in part because of inhomogeneities in the external magnetic field. (3) At $t = \frac{1}{2}TE$, a 180° pulse flips each spin to its mirror-image orientation on the other side of the y axis. (4) The spins continue to precess in the same direction, but now are *de*fanning. (5) At $t = TE$, all converge along the y axis.

Exactly the same thing happens with protons and spin echo, except that it is the spin orientation of each nucleus that is transformed at $\frac{1}{2}TE$, rather than its location.

Spin echo involves reversing and canceling out that part, but only that part, of the spin dephasing that is caused by the inhomogeneities in the external magnet's field. Suppose, for the moment, that the fanning out of individual spins occurs *only* because of static field inhomogeneities. That is, we assume the absence of any spin–lattice or spin–spin relaxation. Immediately following the 90° excitation pulse at $t = 0$, all the spins point along the y axis (Fig. 43–13). They will dephase (because of the constant external field inhomogeneities) over the next $\frac{1}{2}TE$. For any proton that happens to be in an above-average local field, the spin axis precesses slightly faster (hence further away from the y axis) than the average proton.

At $t = \frac{1}{2}$TE, the 180° pulse transforms every proton orientation into its mirror-image orientation (relative to the y axis), but leaves each proton with the same direction of precession. It then takes a period of exactly $\frac{1}{2}$TE for each spin to precess back to the y axis. All the spins will have come back together again, and crossed the y axis in unison, at the end of the second $\frac{1}{2}$TE period, that is, at $t =$ TE. Since (we are still assuming) the spin dephasing is all caused by constant inhomogeneities in the magnetic field, the amplitude of the echo FID signal at $t =$ TE will be the same as the initial FID value. For a brief instant at $t =$ TE, the dephasing caused by external magnetic field non-uniformities is completely reversed, and its effect is eliminated from the FID signal.

The situation is totally different for the irreversible dephasing of spins that is brought about by T1-type transitions, or by slow fluctuations in the magnetic fields resulting from the random motions of nearby protons. A 180° pulse cannot reverse *this* fanning out, so it causes the FID to fall off exponentially, with a characteristic time of T2.

Combining the two arguments: With the spin-echo pulse sequence, the echo of the FID signal will appear briefly at the particular time $t =$ TE, but its amplitude will be diminished by a factor of

$$\text{FID echo amplitude} \sim e^{-TE/T2}, \quad \text{pulse echo} \quad (43.7)$$

relative to its amplitude at $t = 0$. (This is clearly apparent with the Carr–Purcell pulse sequence, or its variant the Carr–Purcell–Meiboom–Gill sequence, in which a chain of 180° pulses leads to the appearance of multiple echoes.) The loss of echo signal is attributable to T2-type relaxation and none to imperfections in the field of the magnet.

As noted in connection with T1 and the saturation–recovery pulse sequence, the objective in MRI normally is not to *measure* T2, but rather to create images in which contrast indirectly reflects differences in T2 among tissues. As will be seen in the next chapter, the spin-echo technique is amenable to that task.

Spin echo is a highly flexible approach, in fact, that can produce not only T2-weighted images, but T1-weighted and proton density-weighted ones, as well. For these and other reasons, it is the pulse sequence most widely used in the clinic.

8. THE BIOPHYSICS OF RELAXATION TIMES

T1 is a measure of the rate at which naturally occurring, Larmor frequency magnetic field fluctuations bring about proton spin flips. T2 is affected, in addition, by slight differences in the Larmor precession frequencies of individual protons, and their resultant spin dephasing, and those differences arise from static and relatively low-frequency variations in the local magnetic fields. The amount of either Larmor frequency or low-frequency magnetic field experienced by a proton in a water molecule depends, in turn, on the molecule's motions. The effect of molecular motions on the relaxation times may be illustrated with this fact: When ice melts, T2 jumps from 10^{-5} second to about 1 second.

The simplest situation is that of pure water. An H_2O molecule will rotate briefly about some axis, collide with another water molecule, rotate at a different rate about another axis, collide again, and so on. There will be a wide range of motions that the individual water molecules are undergoing, and a correspondingly broad spectrum of local magnetic field frequencies for the sample as a whole (Fig. 43–14, curve a). The amplitudes of the fluctuating magnetic field, both at the Larmor frequency and at low frequency, in particular, will be small, so both T1 and T2 will be long (Fig. 43–15, point a).

Relaxation within a living cell is more complex. A water molecule can bind to a medium-sized biomolecule, which may be either free-floating or part of a membrane or organelle. When water is attached, either permanently or intermittently, to a macromolecule that is itself rotating more slowly than free water (because of its greater mass, and because of frictionlike forces dragging on it), the Larmor frequency and/or low-frequency components of the noise magnetic field may be of sig-

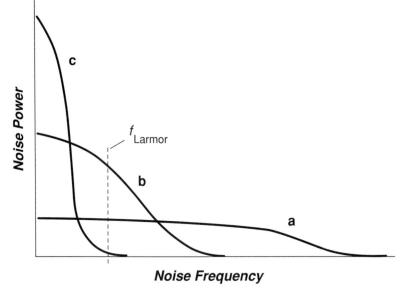

Figure 43–14. The motions of a small, free molecule will be much faster, in general, than the Larmor frequency; the resulting contribution to the noise spectrum at the Larmor frequency will be small (curve a). Likewise, the slow motions of a large molecule, or of water bound tightly to a large molecule, will produce little Larmor frequency noise (curve c). But if many of a molecule's movements occur at the Larmor frequency (curve b), the resulting noise power can induce spin–lattice transitions at a significant rate, by the mechanism suggested in Figure 43–2. In that case, T1 is short.

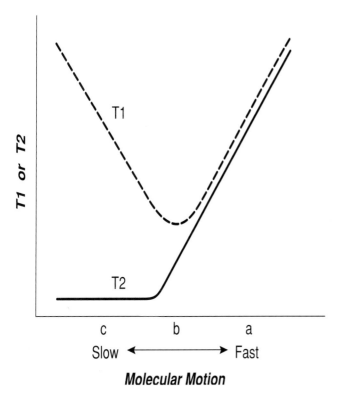

Figure 43–15. Dependence of T1 and T2 on molecular motion. T1 is shortest (relaxation occurs most rapidly) when the frequencies of rotations, vibrations, collisions, and so on, of the water molecules are comparable to the Larmor frequency. A short T1, in turn, causes T2 to be short. T2 is short for large, slow molecules because low-frequency motions give spins time to dephase.

nificantly greater amplitude than for free water (Fig. 43–14, curve b, and Fig. 43–15, point b). T1 and T2 may then be much shorter than for pure water.

The case of a water molecule that is tightly bound to a very large macromolecule is indicated by curve c in Figure 43–14 and point c in Figure 43–15. As with a solid (see Equation

43.6a), the paucity of Larmor frequency fields causes T1 to be long, but the abundance of low-frequency fields leads to short T2. Protons in solidlike situations undergo such fast spin–spin relaxation, in fact, that their transverse magnetization decays away before it can be detected for the construction of an image, in effect, removing these protons from the image altogether.

To complicate the issue further, T1 is a function of field strength B_0. As the field strength increases, for example, so also does the Larmor frequency. For curve b in Figure 43–14, this leads to a reduction in the strength of the magnetic noise at f_{Larmor} and an increase in T1. Thus, it is not enough to state T1; one must know the field strength at which the measurement was made, as indicated by differences in the two T1 columns in Table 43–1. In a tissue, T2 is determined primarily by the low-frequency fields and the secular contribution, so it is much less sensitive to external field strength.

We have focused attention, so far, on the protons of water molecules. Protons on other kinds of molecules may produce their own proton NMR signals, and this is particularly significant in cells with high lipid concentrations. Such molecules undergo motions that are typically very different from those of free water, and display correspondingly different relaxation times. Proton relaxation times for cerebral white matter, for example, tend to be shorter than those for gray matter, because of the relatively greater number of fast-relaxing lipid protons.

To summarize a very complex situation in simple terms: The protons in any voxel of tissue inhabit a broad range of environmental conditions and may take part in a wide variety of spin relaxation processes, each with its own characteristic time. The tightness of the binding of a water molecule to a macromolecule and the extent to which its rotations might be hindered depend on the macromolecule's chemical makeup and three-dimensional structure and on the thickness of the layer of water of hydration surrounding it. It is possible to correlate much of this, albeit crudely, with the single pair of "effective" relaxation parameters, T1 and T2. Fortunately, the relaxation times are sufficiently tissue sensitive and specific for T1- and T2-weighted MRI patterns to be clinically useful.

Chapter 44

Magnetic Resonance IV: Imaging

Here we consider the most common (spin-echo spin-warp) means by which nuclear magnetic resonance (NMR) may be used to generate an image that reflects the spatial distribution of proton density, T1, and/or T2 within a slice of tissue. This involves creating conditions such that the NMR signal from every voxel of protons carries information that allows its localization within in the body.

In the first three magnetic resonance imaging (MRI) chapters (Chapters 41–43), the strong, uniform magnetic field was oriented vertically. In most MRI machines, the main field points horizontally and will be shown as such hereafter. The (now horizontal) orientation of the principal field will still define the z axis of our coordinate system, and x and y coordinates will refer to points on a transverse plane within the patient. For simplicity, we shall focus attention on imaging computed tomography (CT)-like transverse slices of tissue, even though MRI (unlike CT) can just as easily image other planes. Indeed, for some clinical studies, such as of the brain or spine, it may be the ability to produce high-resolution coronal or sagittal display that makes MRI the modality of choice.

Resolution in commercial imagers is of the order of a millimeter. Contrast among soft tissues of interest can be, in some situations, orders of magnitude greater than with CT.

1. A COMPLETE MAGNETIC RESONANCE IMAGING SYSTEM

Figure 44–1 is the block diagram of a complete MRI system.

A critical and expensive component is the **magnet.** The magnet must have a **bore** large enough to accommodate the patient comfortably, and yet be capable of providing a field that is strong (typically between 0.1 and 1.5 T), *stable,* and *highly uniform* over the region being imaged.

The three sets of **gradient magnetic field coils** must be exactly positioned within the bore. The gradient coils are intermittently energized by the *gradient drivers*, which are, in effect, highly specialized audio amplifiers.

The radio-frequency (rf) fields are produced by **rf coils**, also within the bore. Precisely sculpted bursts of rf energy are generated by the *pulse shaper*, and amplified and delivered to the coils via the **rf transmitter.** The weak resonance signals produced within the patient's body are picked up by the same or other rf coils. After being amplified and demodulated by the **rf receiver**, the NMR signals are sampled, digitized, and entered into the *computer*.

The timing and other characteristics of the gradient fields and rf pulses are determined by the **pulse programmer**, which

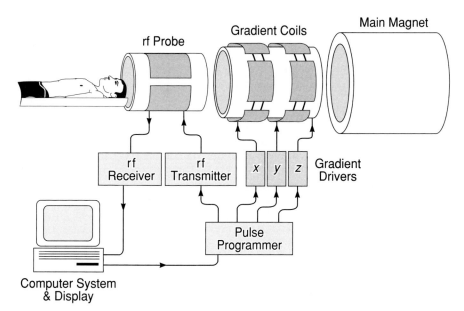

Figure 44–1. Block diagram of the principal components of a magnetic resonance imaging system.

itself is under computer control. When not running the procedures involved in generating and acquiring the resonance data, the computer performs the separate tasks of analyzing the data and reconstructing and processing images for display.

2. INSTRUMENTATION: PRINCIPAL AND GRADIENT MAGNETIC FIELDS

Three types of magnets have found use in imaging: permanent magnets, electromagnets, and superconducting magnets.

Some MRI systems employ a **permanent magnet,** in which magnetic fields are frozen into large blocks of ferrous metal. Unlike the situation of electromagnets and superconducting magnets, with a permanent magnet the main field is aligned vertically. Permanent magnets are largely maintenance-free and consume no electric power or cryogens (i.e., liquid helium and liquid nitrogen), but they are capable of producing only relatively low fields (0.35 T). Despite a certain bias that has grown up in favor of high fields, the lower acquisition and operating costs of lower-field, permanent magnet systems may make them highly cost-effective in some clinical settings.

Most MRI systems are built around a superconducting magnet or an electromagnet, either of which uses electrical current to generate a uniform field. An adequate field can be produced by several pairs of large-diameter coils of wire, known as *Helmholtz coils* (Fig. 44–2). The primary field is made as homogeneous as possible both by moving about *shim plates* of steel and by adjusting the small currents in various additional *shim coils*, which produce slight field corrections.

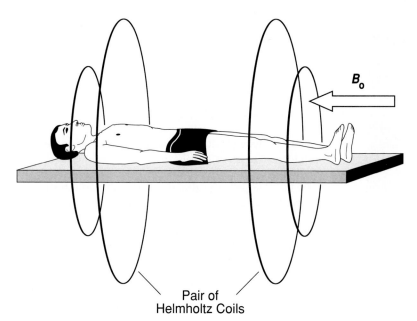

Figure 44–2. Two pairs of Helmholtz coils can produce a main external field that (with adequate shimming) is sufficiently uniform, over a large enough region, for body imaging. Note that the *z* axis is now horizontal.

The main coil of an MRI air-core, room-temperature *resistive* or **electromagnet** might consist of copper or aluminum conductor wound on an aluminum frame with a 1-m-diameter bore, within which are fitted the gradient field coils and the rf coils. An inner *clear bore*, 60 cm or more in diameter, is left free for the patient. Resistive heating of the conductor may consume 50 kW of electrical power, and requires the removal of heat at that rate. The conductor may be a hollow tube through which cooling water is pumped at 50 L/min or so. The maximum achievable field strength within the bore rarely exceeds about 0.15 T.

Most modern machines employ a **superconducting magnet,** which exploits the disappearance of electrical resistance in some materials at very low temperatures (see Chapter 7, Section 3). A wire of superconducting material, such as niobium–titanium alloy, conducts electricity with absolutely no resistive losses below –253°C or so ("absolute zero" occurs at –273°C, or 0°K). Once the current is initiated, there is no further need for power input, nor is heat given off.

To achieve and maintain the superconducting condition, however, the entire coil must be immersed in **liquid helium** (at –269°C, or 4°K) contained within a **cryostat** (helium dewar vessel) (Fig. 44–3). The helium dewar, in turn, is commonly surrounded by a bath of *liquid nitrogen* (with a boiling point of –196°C, or 77°K). (Some cryogenic systems use a *refrigerator* instead of the liquid nitrogen outer bath.) The slowly boiling off liquid helium must be replenished every few months, and the liquid nitrogen (which is much more readily obtained), more frequently. The precision manufacture of the magnet/cryostat assembly accounts for a large part of the high initial cost of an MRI device. But only superconducting magnets are capable of achieving large-volume fields much above 0.3 T.

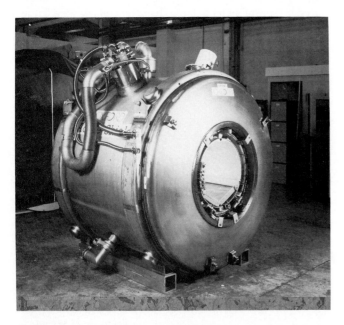

Figure 44–3. A superconducting magnetic resonance imaging magnet is sealed within a stainless-steel, vacuum-insulated cryostat, which will be filled with liquid helium. The liquid helium (boiling point –269°C) maintains the magnet at a few degrees above absolute zero, and the surrounding refrigerator helps to prevent warming of the helium by the outside world. *(Courtesy of Oxford Magnet Technology Limited.)*

Intense research activity is under way to find substances that remain superconducting above liquid nitrogen temperature or, ideally, even at room temperature. But the materials created to date become superconducting only at temperatures that are still way below 77°C, and have tended to lose their superconductivity in the presence of a strong magnetic field. Also, they have been brittle and difficult to produce in the form of wire.

Aside from field strength and patient access, the critical issues in magnet design are field stability and homogeneity. The first of these is no problem for a superconducting magnet, where a **stability** of better than 0.1 part per million (ppm) per hour is easily achieved. **Homogeneity** is another matter. If the field strength, B, is plotted at a number of points within the bore, then the homogeneity might be defined as

$$\text{homogeneity} = (B_{\max} - B_{\min})/B_{\text{central}} \qquad (44.1)$$

where $B_{\max}$ is the largest reading, and so on. A homogeneity of 10 ppm may be achievable over a spherical imaging region 50 cm in diameter, but an acceptable value for this parameter depends on magnet design and field strength. Excessive inhomogeneity of the static field can lead to image distortion, and diminish spatial resolution.

Gradient coils situated within the bore (Fig. 44–4) and the associated electronics generate three independent, orthogonal (mutually perpendicular) gradient fields, which must be superimposed intermittently on the principal, homogeneous static field. These gradient fields are much weaker than the principal field, and the gradients range from about 1 to 10 millitesla/meter (0.1 to 1.0 gauss/cm) for normal body imaging. Although gradient fields do not receive the attention from sales people that the main magnetic field does, gradient field strength and rise time may prove to have as significant an effect on instrument flexibility and performance.

NMR microscopy, in which the region of interest is much smaller than usual and the resolution correspondingly finer, employs gradients as much as a thousand times greater than those used in clinical MRI. Despite the much weaker NMR signals involved (because voxel dimensions are typically 100 times smaller, and there are a factor of 10^6 or so fewer spins in a each), studies on small experimental animals have achieved 10-µm (0.01-mm) resolution.

3. INSTRUMENTATION: RADIO-FREQUENCY TRANSMISSION AND RECEPTION

The other principal MRI hardware component, aside from the computer, is the rf coils and electronics that generate and apply the pulses of Larmor frequency energy and then detect the resultant NMR signal. The situation is like that of transmitting and receiving amplitude modulation (AM) radio signals.

A brief aside on AM radio, as background for MRI: Transmission of an AM radio signal involves producing and detecting rf electromagnetic radiation that falls within a very narrow band of frequencies. In that way, the transmission of interest can be received and isolated, with electromagnetic signals and noise at all other frequencies filtered out and rejected. As the initial step, a transmitter generates a nearly

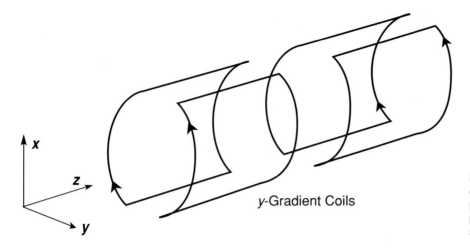

Figure 44–4. The arrows indicate the flow of direct current through the *y*-gradient coils, which produces a relatively weak magnetic field that points in the *z* direction, but increases in strength with the *y* coordinate.

monochromatic rf *carrier* signal (for commercial AM broadcasting in the United States, somewhere in the range 535 to 1605 kHz) (Fig. 44–5). Audio information of much lower frequencies (typically 30 Hz to 10 KHz), is introduced by *modulating* the amplitude of the carrier. If the carrier is at 1 MHz and the information signal happens to be an audible, pure 4000-Hz tone, for example, then the amplitude of the carrier is made to vary at that frequency.

Fourier analysis of a modulated (e.g., at 4 kHz) rf signal would reveal a spectrum consisting of components at the (1-MHz) carrier frequency and also close to it (4 kHz above and below). For undistorted transmission of the signal, the *bandwidth* of the transmitter and receiver must be sufficiently broad to cover the carrier frequency and its information-bearing sidebands. With our 1-MHz carrier modulated at 4 kHz, the bandwidth of the equipment must be great enough to process a carrier-plus-sidebands signal that extends at least from 996 to 1004 kHz.

Detection of the radio signal by the receiver involves tuning to (selecting out a narrow band of frequencies around) the correct carrier frequency, then *demodulating* (rectifying and smoothing) the audio-modulated rf signal. The result is a replica of the original audio signal, which is amplified and sent to the loudspeaker. This concludes the aside on AM radio.

A similar situation exists for MRI. Instead of audio modulation, a *pulse shaper* is used to form 90- or 180-degree or any other needed pulses, of precise and highly specialized shapes, out of carrier rf, typically in the range 10 to 60 MHz. When a magnetic field gradient is being applied, the carrier cannot be strictly monochromatic, but rather must contain a band of frequencies partially (sometimes) or fully as wide as the gradient-induced spread in proton Larmor frequencies. The bandwidth of the rf generator, amplifiers, and other electronic equipment

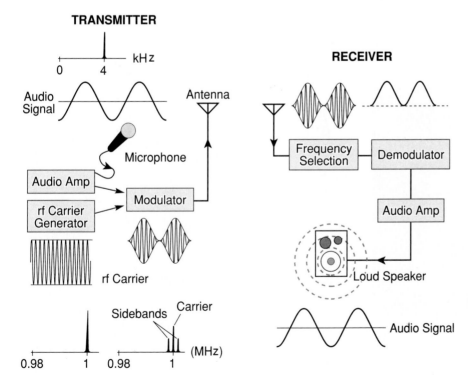

Figure 44–5. The radio-frequency (rf) instrumentation of MRI is similar to that of AM radio. In this example, a 1-MHz carrier signal is amplitude modulated with a 4-kHz audio signal; the transmitted radio signal consists of carrier plus sidebands at 996 and 1004 kHz. The receiver demodulates the radio signal and extracts a replica of the original audio signal.

must be sufficiently broad to accommodate this range of Larmor frequencies, but narrow enough to exclude most extraneous signals and noise. Finally, the detection process for the NMR signal is more complicated than the simple rectification and smoothing of the rf used with AM radio, and allows the retention of information on the phase, as well as on the frequency and amplitude, of the NMR signal.

Magnetic resonance normally occurs only if the magnetic field of the exciting rf signal is perpendicular to the principal magnetic field. The *rf probe coil* (Fig. 44–6) produces such a transverse field. As detection of an NMR signal comes only after the transmission of the excitation rf pulse is completed, a single coil may be used in MRI for both the production and the subsequent detection of resonance. But the objective of pulse transmission (the creation of an intense and uniform rf field) differs from that of pulse reception (sensitivity to weak signals emanating from precessing protons within the patient's body, with low noise generation), so separate and differently designed coils are used for some applications. In examination of tissues near the surface of the patient's body, for example, signal-to-noise can be enhanced significantly through the use of *surface* rf detection coils that lie close to the skin.

4. PLANAR METHODS BEGIN WITH THE SELECTION OF A SLICE OF TISSUE

In principle, magnetic resonance imaging, unlike CT, can be performed without any reconstruction calculations. We could, for example, cause the external "static" magnetic field to fluctuate wildly at all but one point in the patient's body; as with conventional tomography, the NMR condition would be blurred out of existence everywhere else. The image could thereby be acquired point by point.

Such an approach works, but other techniques are much more efficient. Of the many that have been developed, the most widely used is the *two-dimensional Fourier* method, of which the **spin-warp** method is the principal variety. Also, some machines have employed *projection reconstruction*, which

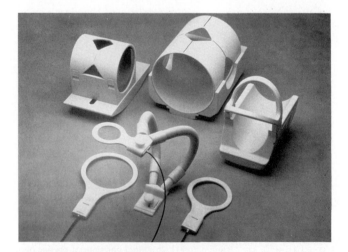

Figure 44–6. Typical radio-frequency volume imaging coils, which can be either transmit-receive or receive-only, and receive-only surface coils used for high-resolution examination of the vertebra, orbit, joints, etc. *(Courtesy of Toshiba America Medical Systems.)*

is similar to the CT approach of the same name. Both of these are **planar** methods that map one entire slice of tissue at a time.

Planar imaging begins with the isolation of the slice of tissue to be mapped, by means of **selective excitation.** Suppose, for example, that with a spin-warp system, we choose to image a transverse slice. (Similar arguments pertain for coronal, sagittal, or other image planes.)

Spin-warp, in its simplest form, employs the spin-echo pulse sequence, but with a z-gradient magnetic field (to select a *transverse* slice) turned on during application of the 90° rf pulse. (The field points only in the z direction, and gradually increases in strength as one moves along it. A z-gradient field may be produced by a colinear pair of coils that generate weak fields pointing in opposite directions.) The rf pulse must be of narrow bandwidth; it is designed to contain frequencies that

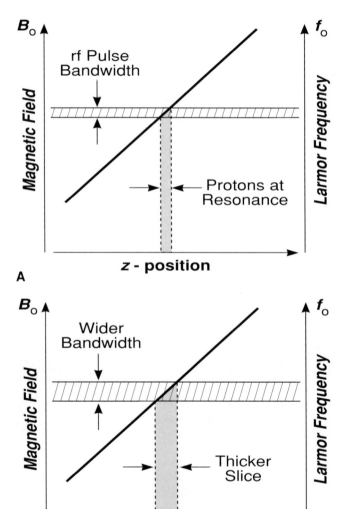

Figure 44–7. Determinants of slice thickness. **A.** With a z gradient, a narrow band of radio frequency (rf) can cause protons in a narrow slice of tissue to resonate. **B.** Either a wider band of radio frequency (shown) or a less steep z gradient will result in a thicker slice of tissue. There will be more spins in each voxel, which leads to improved signal-to-noise ratio, but resolution decreases.

will cause the resonance of protons for a corresponding narrow range of magnetic fields, which occurs only in our particular thin transverse slice of tissue (Fig. 44–7A). The protons in this slice are thus singled out—they, and only they, end up precessing in the x–y plane, all with nearly the same frequency—and prepared for subsequent two-dimensional mapping.

The thickness of a slice selected is determined both by the bandwidth of rf frequencies included in the 90° pulse and the steepness of the gradient field. Either a wider band of rf frequencies in the pulse (Fig. 44–7B) or a flatter field gradient will result in a thicker tissue slice. Current MRI machines can provide a choice of slice thicknesses ranging typically from 0.5 to 10 mm. As with CT, a thicker slice means better signal-to-noise and perhaps contrast, but reduced spatial resolution.

After one transverse slice within the patient has been selected, the system turns off the z gradient and proceeds with the x–y mapping within the slice. After completion of the mapping within the slice, the next slice is selected: The main field remains the same, as does the steepness of the z-directional gradient, but the center frequency of the rf pulse is shifted slightly. A new cohort of protons is thereby made ready for mapping.

5. SPIN-WARP IMAGE RECONSTRUCTION: PHASE-FREQUENCY ENCODING OF TWO-DIMENSIONAL INFORMATION

Now that a single transverse slice of tissues has been selected by means of the 90° pulse (with the z-gradient on) of a spin-echo pulse sequence, we can focus attention on what then happens in the x–y plane of that slice. Our objective is to determine the magnitude of the magnetization vectors for the various voxels precisely at $t = TE$, the time that the echo signal appears. Spin warp achieves this through the sequential application of y-gradient and x-gradient magnetic fields (Fig. 44–8). (Recall that an x-gradient field points only in the z direction, but its strength is proportional to the x coordinate.)

Soon after the slice-selection z gradient is removed, a y

gradient, G_y, is turned on for a precisely specified span of time, called the **phase-encoding period.** The magnetization of a voxel located higher up in the selected plane is now in a stronger local magnetic field than one with a lower y position. It therefore precesses faster, and will pass through a greater total angle during the time that G_y is on. The *accumulated phase angle* of the magnetization vectors for a particular row of voxels is thus *proportional to,* and can later reveal, its *y position* (Fig. 44–9A). After completion of this period of phase evolution, the y gradient is removed.

The 180° echo-generating pulse is applied at time $t = \frac{1}{2} TE$, and the system is left alone for nearly another $\frac{1}{2}$ TE. Then, just before the echo is due to appear (i.e., just before $t = TE$), the x gradient is turned on. Because the x gradient is present while the echo is being read, the *frequency* of a voxel's contribution to the echo signal will be *proportional to its x coordinate* (Fig. 44–9B).

All of this is summarized in Figure 44–10. The slice (z coordinate) was selected with a 90° pulse while G_z was on. The relative *phase* of a voxel's magnetization vector at $t = TE$ was set when the y gradient was being applied, and corresponds to its y coordinate, its row in the voxel matrix. The *frequency* of its contribution to the echo signal corresponds to its x coordinate, the column in the voxel matrix. But the (previously encoded) phase still remains significant, and has a detectable effect, at the time that the echo signal is being read, as should be apparent from Figure 24–20.

Unfortunately, it is not possible simply to route the detected NMR signal into a black box that generates a spectrum in which the amplitude is a (two-dimensional) function of both phase and frequency. It is necessary, rather, to repeat the above procedure a number of times, each time with a different amount of y gradient (hence a different amount of accumulated phase at each value of the y coordinate in the patient), and then perform a computer-based Fourier analysis of the totality of the information thus obtained.

For a square image of n^2 pixels, separate echo signals must be detected with n different settings of the steepness, of the y

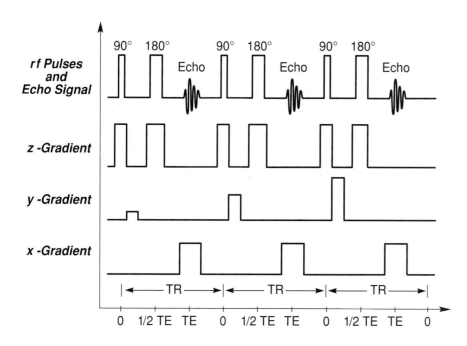

Figure 44–8. Simplified version of the spin-warp pulse and field gradient sequence. The magnitude of the y gradient increases after each spin-echo pair of pulses.

G_y ON DURING PHASE ENCODING

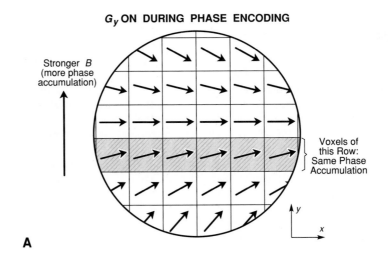

Stronger B (more phase accumulation)

Voxels of this Row: Same Phase Accumulation

A

G_x ON DURING ECHO READOUT

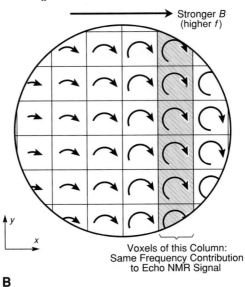

Stronger B (higher f)

Voxels of this Column: Same Frequency Contribution to Echo NMR Signal

B

Figure 44–9. What is happening to the tissue magnetizations in the voxels during spin-warp imaging. **A.** When the y gradient is on (but with no radio frequency present), phase accumulates in a voxel at a rate proportional to its y coordinate within the body. The phase accumulated now will affect the nuclear magnetic resonance signal detected later. **B.** Because the x gradient is on during nuclear magnetic resonance signal detection, the x coordinate of a voxel determines the frequency of its contribution to the signal.

gradient, G_y (see Fig. 44–8). The finer the desired mesh of pixels (and resolution) and/or the larger the region of interest, the greater the number of measurements that must be made with different values of the y gradient. A commercial MRI machine will provide a selection of possible values of n, ranging typically from 128 to 512 or more.

6. A SIMPLE SPIN-WARP EXAMPLE

This is all a bit tricky, so let's illustrate it with a simple example: the spin-echo, spin-warp imaging of a body that consists of only four voxels ($n = 2$) in a plane. The voxels and field gradients are indicated in Figure 44–11. The magnitude of the net magnetization from voxel 1 at the instant that the echo signal appears (at $t =$ TE) will be denoted M_1; the voxel-1 contribution to the echo signal will, in turn, be proportional to M_1. The full

sequence of rf pulses and field gradients to be used will consist of the first two spin-echo sequences in Figure 44–8, with special choices for the values of G_y.

Suppose our plane of interest has just been selected with a 90° pulse, and is now sitting in a uniform field. The magnetization vectors for all four voxels are precessing in the transverse plane at the same Larmor frequency and in phase (Fig. 44–12A).

We begin the spin-warp process itself by turning on the y gradient, G_y. To simplify our example, we cleverly choose the value for G_y that will cause the magnetization vectors in voxels 1 and 3 (in the same local magnetic field, as determined by the y coordinate) to precess, during the phase-encoding period, exactly 180° more than those in voxels 2 and 4 (which are in a slightly lower local field) (Fig. 44–12B). (This has nothing to do with the 180° pulse about to be applied.) At the end of the phase-encoding period, G_y is turned off. The magnetization from the voxel 1 protons ends up pointing opposite that from

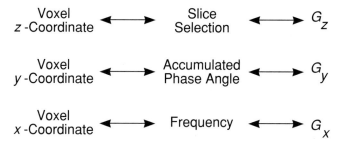

Figure 44–10. Voxel position coordinates, field gradients, and a voxel's contribution to the nuclear magnetic resonance signal for spin-warp generation of a transverse slice.

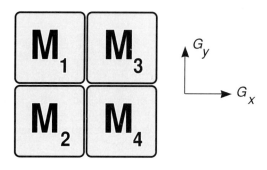

Figure 44–11. The four voxels that constitute the "body" in the simplified spin-warp example in Section 6.

voxel 2, at any instant, and so also for voxels 3 and 4. The four magnetization vectors are again precessing at the same rate, but there is a new phase relationship among them.

The 180° rf pulse is applied at $t = \frac{1}{2}$TE, and the system is then left alone for another $\frac{1}{2}$TE.

Just before the echo signal appears at TE, the x gradient is turned on and is left on as the echo signal is read (Fig. 44–12C). Voxels 1 and 2 are now in the same local field, but their respective magnetizations happen to be 180 degrees out of phase (because of the prior phase encoding). The net magnetization they together produce as they precess (at the same frequency) is therefore the *difference* of their separate magnetizations. The strength $S_{180}(1,2)$ of their combined contribution to the echo signal is proportional to that difference:

$$S_{180}(1,2) \sim M_1 - M_2 \qquad (44.2)$$

The subscript 180 is a reminder that there happens to be a 180-degree phase difference between the voxel 1 and voxel 2 magnetization vectors, encoded earlier.

Likewise, the protons in voxels 3 and 4 are precessing at a slightly different frequency. Their contribution to the echo signal is proportional to $M_3 - M_4$:

$$S_{180}(3,4) \sim M_3 - M_4 \qquad (44.3)$$

$S_{180}(1,2)$ and $S_{180}(3,4)$ are contributions of different frequencies to the measured total NMR signal, $S_{NMR} = S_{180}(1,2) + S_{180}(3,4)$. They can be separated from one another by means of a Fourier transformation (Fig. 44–12D).

Equations 44.2 and 44.3 are two equations in four unknowns. To learn the values of the four unknowns M_1 through M_4, we need a total of four independent relationships among them. So we perform a second spin-echo measurement. This time, again to simplify things, we choose to set G_y equal to zero during the phase-encoding period. By the end of the phase-encoding period, with this particular setting of G_y, zero degrees of phase difference will have accumulated between the magnetizations in voxels 1 and 2, and so also for those in 3 and 4. Now turn on G_x. The strength of the contribution to the echo signal from the protons in voxels 1 and 2 together is now proportional to the *sum* in their magnetizations, as they are in phase:

$$S_0(1,2) \sim M_1 + M_2 \qquad (44.4)$$

So also for voxels 3 and 4:

$$S_0(3,4) \sim M_3 + M_4 \qquad (44.5)$$

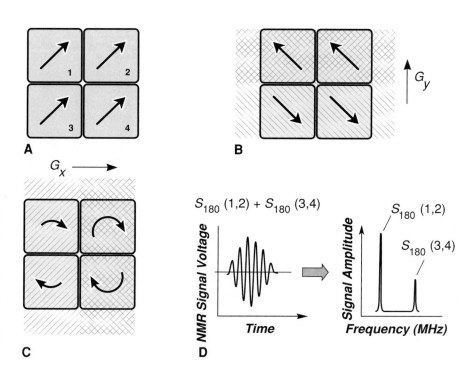

Figure 44–12. Our spin-warp example. **A.** Immediately after a 90° pulse, in a uniform external field the magnetizations of the four voxels precess at the same rate and in phase. **B.** A y gradient is turned on for a precisely specified period of time; for some particular value of G_y, during that time the magnetization vectors in voxels 1 and 3 will precess through exactly 180° more than those in 2 and 4. **C.** An x gradient is turned on during nuclear magnetic resonance signal readout, and the contributions from voxels 3 and 4 are of higher frequency than are those from 1 and 2. The detected composite signal depends both on the accumulate phase (determined earlier by the value of G_y) and on the present value of G_x. **D.** The composite nuclear magnetic resonance signal can be separated into components of two different frequencies by means of Fourier analysis.

Fourier analysis provides separate values for $S_0(1,2)$ and $S_0(3,4)$.

Equations 44.2 through 44.5 are independent, and can be solved unambiguously. In this four-pixel case, a total of two sets of measurements, with different amounts of phase encoding, were adequate to generate the map of the voxel magnetizations existing at the time of echo formation. The particular choice of values of TR and TE for the pulse-echo sequences determines, as we shall see, whether the resulting image is T1-, T2-, or proton density (PD)-weighted.

_____ **EXERCISE 44–1.** _____

The following signal amplitudes result from the Fourier analysis: $S_0(1,2) = 5$; $S_0(3,4) = 2$; $S_{180}(1,2) = -3$; and $S_{180}(3,4) = 2$. Find the map of voxel magnetizations at $t = TE$.

SOLUTION: Figure 44–13. Compare this procedure with the CT example of Chapter 37, Section 5.

7. SPIN-ECHO SPIN-WARP MAGNETIC RESONANCE IMAGING AGAIN, IN MORE DETAIL

Here we shall again walk through, but in more detail, the entire process of creating MRI images by means of the spin-echo, spin-warp method. Our maps will be 128 × 256 voxels in dimension. There is great variety in the sequences and timing of rf pulses and gradient fields used in commercial MRI systems, but the following one is (aside from several simplifications we shall make) fairly typical.

The rf pulses and gradient fields, as determined by the pulse programmer and applied to the patient, are presented in Figure 44–14. Also shown are the NMR echo signal detected by the rf pickup coil and the demodulated echo signal about to be digitized and entered into the computer for image reconstruction.

The sequence begins with the selection of the transverse slice. The z gradient is turned on at time $t = 0$ millisecond, and achieves the value appropriate for the desired slice with a *gradient switching time* of 2 milliseconds. As soon as the gradient field has stabilized, the 90° rf saturation pulse is applied. Its shape is carefully designed in an effort to optimize the balance among signal-to-noise and the other parameters that affect

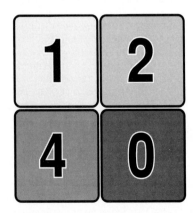

Figure 44–13. Proton densities of the four voxels in Exercise 44–1. Compare the meaning of this with that of Figure 37–5B.

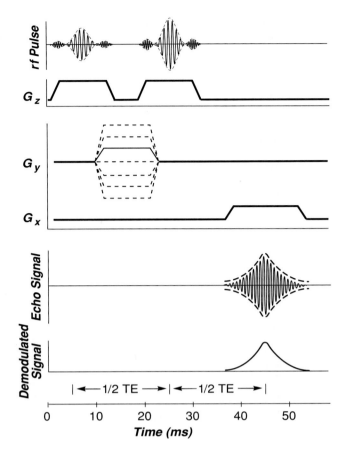

Figure 44–14. The (simplified) spin-warp spin-echo sequence again, in more detail. See also Figure 44–8.

image utility. The pulse is of a duration and amplitude that will cause the net magnetization for all the protons in one thin slice of tissue to swing down into the x–y plane, where it continues to precess after cessation of the rf (at $t = 10$ milliseconds).

As the z gradient switches off, the phase-encoding y gradient comes on. Within the selected slice, the rate of precession (and the accumulated phase angle) of the magnetization of the protons in any narrow strip of tissue lying parallel to the x axis will be determined by its y coordinate, by the steepness of the y gradient, and by the time that the y gradient remains on. At the end of the phase-encoding period, the y gradient is removed.

The 180° pulse is applied a time $t = \frac{1}{2}TE$ (here, 20 milliseconds) after the 90° pulse. It has roughly the same shape and duration as its predecessor, but twice the amplitude. This creates the conditions that will give rise to an echo pulse a time $\frac{1}{2}TE$ later. The z gradient is on again briefly, so that the 180° pulse affects only the original slice of protons; this second application of G_z is not essential, but it helps when several slices are being imaged simultaneously (see below).

Just before the NMR echo signal makes its appearance, the readout x gradient field is switched on. This, in effect, allows the separation the NMR signal into 256 different component signals, each occurring at a slightly different Larmor frequency (corresponding to 256 different values of x). The echo signal is detected by the pickup coil, amplified, demodulated, digitized, and sent to the computer for Fourier analysis.

The next sequence begins TR (the repetition time) after the

first 90° pulse appeared. The entire pulse and gradient sequence will have to be repeated 128 times, each with a different value (but the same duration) of the y gradient, to produce a single-slice image. Real clinical pulse and gradient sequences are more elaborate than this, but most of the important points are covered in Figure 44–14.

> y gradients are imposed intentionally in spin-warp imaging, to impart different amounts of spin phase accumulation to voxels with different values of y coordinate. But *unwanted* phase accumulation occurs whenever the z- and x-gradient magnetic fields are on, and compensatory gradient fields are imposed at various times to undo that damage.
>
> Also, gradients are employed in the gradient echo pulse sequence in place of the 180° pulse, as described in more advanced texts.

A run of several *identical* pulse/gradient sequences (rather than only one, as implied above) may be applied in rapid succession. By an argument like that in Chapter 35, Section 7, the signal-to-noise ratio (SNR) of the data improves as

$$\text{SNR} \sim \sqrt{N_{EX}} \qquad (44.6)$$

where the *number of excitations* (N_{EX}) is the number of measurements made under completely identical operating conditions (i.e., same TE and TR and same rf pulses and gradient magnetic fields) and averaged together. A resulting improvement of even $\sqrt{2}$ can make the difference between a clinically useful image and one in which the necessary contrast or resolution is lost in noise.

8. T1-, T2-, AND PROTON DENSITY-WEIGHTED IMAGES

As you would expect, the nature of the information obtained in spin-echo spin-warp MRI is a function of the echo time, TE, and repetition time, TR, of the pulse sequence.

A spin-echo sequence chosen with a TE comparable to the T2 values of the tissues of interest emphasizes T2 contrast (Fig. 44–15). A relatively long TR largely removes T1 effects. Such a combination of choices for TE and TR therefore yields a T2-weighted image (Fig. 44–16A). As the transverse magnetization of a tissue in a voxel with a *longer T2* will have decayed less at the time the echo signal materializes, it appears as a *brighter* pixel. Differences among tissues in proton density may obscure (or augment) T2 contrast.

Similarly, a relatively short TE together with a TR chosen to be comparable to the T1 values of the tissues of interest (see Chapter 43, Section 4) gives a T1-weighted image (Fig. 44–16B), emphasizing differences in T1 among them. And a long TR and short TE produces images that reveal primarily proton density (PD) (Fig. 44–16C). Under other sets of operating conditions, an image reflects some hybrid of T1, T2, and PD weighting that may, or may not, be clinically useful. This is all summarized in Figure 44–17.

The main problem with a long TR or TE is the extended data acquisition time. This contributes to slow patient throughput, and sometimes to motional blurring. Efforts to minimize these times, on the other hand—by reducing the gradient switching time, for example, or by shortening gradient field

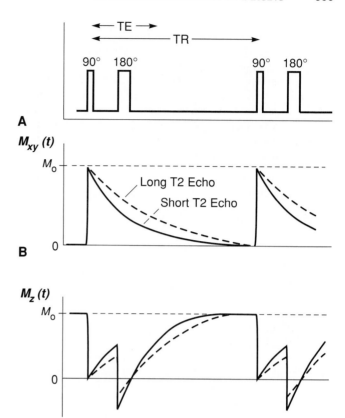

Figure 44–15. T2-weighted spin-echo imaging. **A.** The pulse sequence. **B.** Decay curves $M_{xy}(t)$ for the transverse magnetization for two tissues. The vertical separation between the two curves is greatest at the time t that is about midway between the T2 values for the two tissues. Selecting a TE time comparable to the tissue T2 values enhances T2 contrast. **C.** A long TR, with time for nearly complete equilibration of the longitudinal magnetization, reduces the influence of tissue T1 values on the image. The result of high T2 contrast and little T1 influence is a T2-weighted image. *(After Smith H-J, Ranallo FN. A Non-Mathematical Approach to Basic MRI. Madison, WI: Medical Physics Publishing, 1989 (Fig. 14–3).)*

and rf pulse duration (but increasing their amplitudes correspondingly)—eventually run into a number of technical problems. The *fast-imaging* techniques that have been developed to circumvent these difficulties will be discussed in Section 12.

9. PARAMAGNETIC CONTRAST AGENTS SHORTEN RELAXATION TIMES

Two factors that can radically alter real or apparent relaxation times for a voxel of tissue are the presence of **paramagnetic contrast agent** and, if the voxel contains blood, *blood flow*.

An MRI contrast agent exploits the dipole magnetic field that an electron produces (see Chapter 41, Section 5). Most electrons in atoms and molecules are spin-paired, in the sense that the magnetic field generated by one electron is effectively canceled out by that from another one (on the same atom or molecule) spinning in the opposite direction. (Recall that protons are also spin-paired in a nucleus, as are neutrons.) But an atom

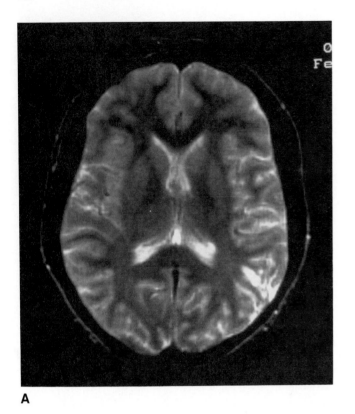

A

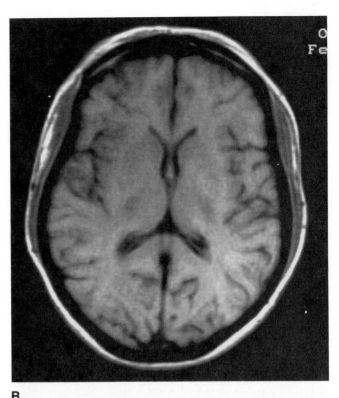

B

Figure 44–16. With judicious choices for TE and TR, one can produce spin-echo images that emphasize different physiologic aspects of various tissues. **A.** A T2-weighted transverse slice of the brain. B_0 = 0.3 T (permanent magnet), TE = 85 milliseconds, TR = 3000 milliseconds. **B.** T1-weighted image of the same slice. TE = 20 milliseconds, TR = 585 milliseconds. **C.** Proton density (PD)-weighted image of the same slice. TE = 30 milliseconds, TR = 1800 milliseconds. *(Courtesy of Fonar Corporation.)*

C

or molecule containing one (or more) unpaired electron(s) may give rise to a field a thousand times stronger than that of a proton, and is said to be *paramagnetic*. The fluctuating magnetic field from a paramagnetic molecule can strongly influence relaxation rates of nearby protons and modify measured relaxation

times. Unlike the situation of radiographic contrast agents, which themselves absorb x-ray photons, MRI contrast agents work indirectly, by affecting the T1 and T2 of water protons.

As with the radionuclide and carrier agent of a nuclear medicine radiopharmaceutical, the paramagnetic contrast

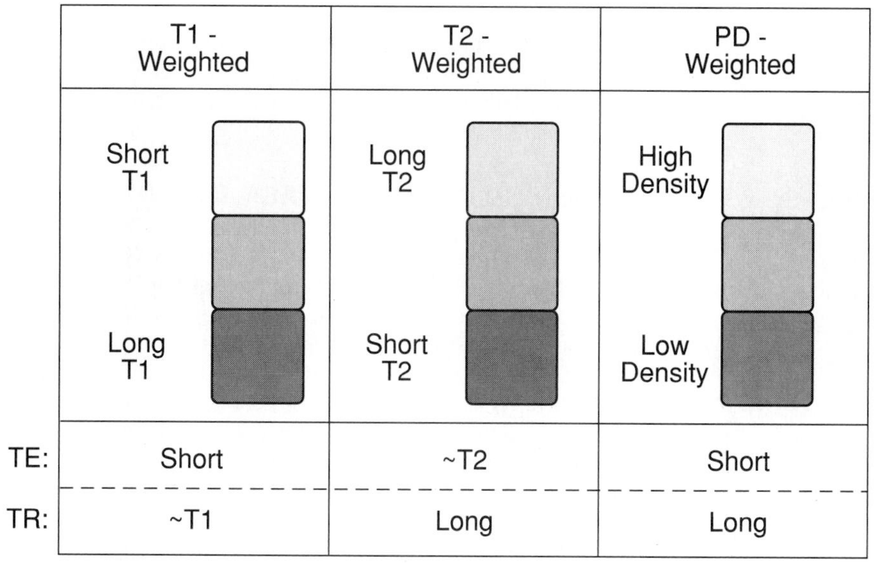

T1 - Weighted	T2 - Weighted	PD - Weighted
Short T1 ... Long T1	Long T2 ... Short T2	High Density ... Low Density

	T1 - Weighted	T2 - Weighted	PD - Weighted
TE:	Short	~T2	Short
TR:	~T1	Long	Long

Figure 44–17. Summary table for the parameters TE and TR that yield T1-, T2-, and proton density-weighted spin-echo images.

agent must be tissue specific and safe at concentrations that are high enough to have an appreciable effect. Most widely explored, so far, have been complexes involving transition metal and rare earth elements such as iron, manganese, and gadolinium. Clinical trials have already demonstrated the efficacy of gadolinium–DTPA (diethylenetriaminepentacetic acid) in imaging breakdown of the blood–brain barrier, renal lesions, myocardial infarctions, and other pathologic conditions (Fig. 44–18).

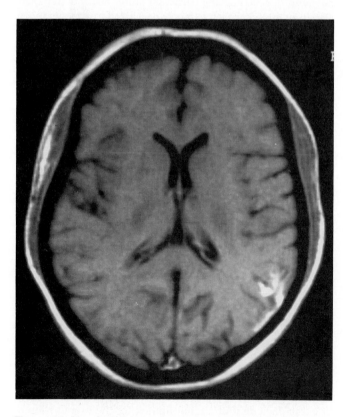

Figure 44–18. Gadolinium-enhanced T1-weighted image of the same slice as in Figure 44–16. *(Courtesy of Fonar Corporation.)*

10. BLOOD FLOW AND MAGNETIC RESONANCE ANGIOGRAPHY

Motivated in part by the complications that may arise with intraarterial contrast angiography (e.g., vascular injury, reactions to contrast agent, stroke), noninvasive MRI angiography is undergoing rapid development.

Flow or diffusion can alter the measured NMR relaxation times of any fluid. As a simple spin-echo example, suppose that the 90° pulse is delivered to the arterial blood in some voxel in the selected plane. By the time the echo pulse is detected, this particular cohort of blood protons will have flowed into (and perhaps beyond) the adjacent plane, and the blood originally in the voxel be replaced with fresh blood. The apparent relaxation time that determines the pixel brightness will therefore be different from that of static blood, and the shift in apparent relaxation time will increase with the flow rate. Flow of blood thus has an effect similar to that of adding contrast agent to it (the bringing about of a contrast enhancement of vasculature) and forms the basis for **magnetic resonance angiography (MRA)** (Fig. 44–19). A pair of separate images are produced, one with flow image effects enhanced and the other with such effects largely suppressed, by techniques known as *flow compensation*; the difference image reveals the flow.

The process just described is known as *time-of-flight* MRA. There are at least three other mechanisms that have been exploited in MRA, involving phenomena such as the changes of phase that occur when blood flows through a magnetic field gradient. Each MRA approach has its advantages and limitations, and it is not yet clear which (if any) will become dominant.

11. CARDIAC GATING

As with nuclear medicine and computerized tomography, an electrocardiogram signal can be used to gate pulse sequences. This can yield images (for any planar section) of the heart in different phases of the cardiac cycle. Likewise, gating can be

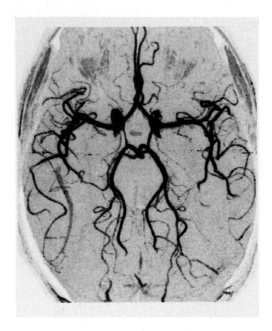

Figure 44–19. Magnetic resonance angiography of the intracranial vessels, in which the flow of blood acts, in effect, like a contrast agent. *(Courtesy of Siemens Medical Systems, Inc.)*

coupled with MRA, revealing the time dependence of blood flow through the major vessels. These techniques require the use of highly specialized, fast pulse and gradient sequences.

12. FAST IMAGING

Much recent research has focused on ways of reducing data acquisition time. Fast MRI approaches employ combinations of *small flip angle* (pulses significantly shorter than 90°), *gradient echo* (rather than 180-degree pulse) refocusing, reduced numbers of phase-encoding steps, pulse repetition times much less than tissue T1 values, and $N_{EX} = 1$. The different techniques involved, going by acronyms such as EPI (echoplanar imaging), FISP (Fast Imaging with Steady-State Processing), FLASH (Fast Low-Angle Shot), GRASE (Gradient and Spin Echo), GRASS (Gradient Recalled Acquisition in the Steady State), and RARE (rapid acquisition relaxation enhancement), can reduce the scan time to a fraction of a second per slice, and are described in more advanced or specialized texts.

13. MULTIPLE SLICES AND THREE-DIMENSIONAL IMAGING

As with CT, a number of different planar images are usually obtained in a clinical examination. Imaging time is reduced if work on several slices is interwoven; data acquisition occurs for one slice, for example, while another slice is moving toward thermal equilibrium.

Alternatively, two-dimensional Fourier imaging can be expanded into truly three-dimensional (as opposed to multiple two-dimensional slice) imaging by means of methods in which each NMR signal contains contributions from an entire volume

of tissue. The pulse and gradient sequences involved are more complex, requiring, for example, phase encoding in two separate (z and y) dimensions, rather than slice selection (for the z dimension) followed by one (y)-dimensional phase encoding.

14. DETERMINANTS OF IMAGE QUALITY

By now it is doubtless well apparent that the quality and clinical utility of an MRI image depend strongly on a number of parameters. While some of these are difficult or impossible to alter, as with the strength of the principal magnetic field, others are under the immediate control of the operator. The latter include the types (spin-echo, inversion–recovery, saturation–recovery) and timing (TE, TR) of pulses for a sequence, the slice thickness and interslice separation, the dimensions of the voxel matrix and the size of the field of view (which together determine voxel size and resolution), the number of excitations (N_{EX}), the use of contrast agent or of physiologic (such as electrocardiogram) gating, and the employment of surface coils to detect the echo rf pulses.

As with any other imaging modality, the selection of MRI operating parameters involves trade-offs that influence contrast, resolution, noise level, and image acquisition time. Perhaps what most distinguishes MRI, from the operator's perspective, is the vast number of possible combinations of operating parameters and the extent to which the nature of the information revealed is sensitive to the particular combination of parameters chosen.

Parameter selection is a complex (and still evolving) business and depends on the particular study being undertaken. Details of this will be left to more specialized treatments and to hands-on experience in the clinic.

Equations 42.1 and 42.2 indicate that the magnetization in any voxel depends on the strength of the principal magnetic field. As a result, the signal-to-noise in an MRI image improves roughly in proportion to B_0, which is one significant motivation for the use of high fields, up to 1.5 or 2.0 T. The cost of the magnet, however, increases with field strength much more rapidly.

The problem of cost has led to attempts to construct an ultralow-field (0.02-T) imaging system. For several reasons (including the field strength dependence of relaxation times), signal-to-noise and contrast are significantly better at 0.02 T than one would expect from magnetization considerations alone. Construction and operation expenses, moreover, are significantly less than for a 1.5-T machine. Although it is unlikely that ultralow-field systems will find widespread use in developed countries, in the Third World they could make accessible nearly state-of-the-art diagnostic imaging capabilities.

15. QUALITY ASSURANCE

Standard quality assurance (QA) procedures address the same sorts of issues (contrast, resolution, noise, geometric distortions, artifacts, etc.) as do those for CT and other modalities. QA tests include (but are not limited to) the examination of slice thickness; spatial resolution; image uniformity and linearity; image signal-to-noise ratio; rf pulse parameters; contrast in

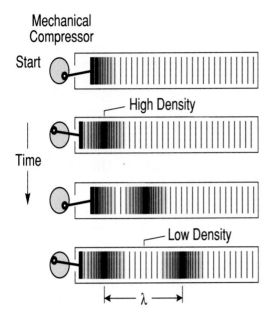

Figure 45–3. Sound can be created by a piston, membrane, etc., that alternately compresses and rarefies a medium. The greater the displacement of the medium, the greater the corresponding sound intensity.

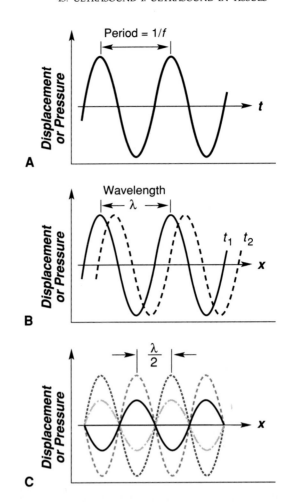

Figure 45–4. Representations of wave motion. **A.** At a fixed point in space, displacement of the medium and the local pressure vary sinusoidally as functions of time. **B.** A traveling wave at two instants of time as a function of position in space, as might be produced by a pair of snapshots, one taken right after the other. **C.** A standing wave at five different instants of time.

where f is the frequency of the wave. For diagnostic US in soft tissue, the amplitude of this motion, X (*displacement amplitude*), is typically less than 0.1 μm, one tenth of a micron. Equation 45.1a and Figure 45–4A could just as easily illustrate the variation in the local pressure within the medium.

The disturbance travels as a wave through the tissue with a speed typically of about 1540 m/s. Figure 45–4B shows two snapshots of such a *traveling wave,* one taken immediately after the other. The shape of the wave at the first instant may be described as

$$X(x) = X \cdot \sin 2\pi x / \lambda \qquad (45.1b)$$

and that of the other differs from it by a phase angle that is proportional to the time lapse between the two. Both waves are of wavelength λ. (Some kinds of vibration, such as that of a piano string, form *standing waves* [Fig. 45–4C]. For the most part, we shall be concerned, rather, with traveling waves.)

Sound or US in air, water, or tissue, in which the wave propagates along the direction of the back-and-forth motions of the medium (hereafter designated the x direction), is said to consist of **longitudinal** oscillations. In solid (but not within fluid or gaseous) media, a local disturbance can also involve motion perpendicular to the direction of propagation; such transverse waves play no role in medical US imaging. (What kind are the waves moving along the surface of the ocean?)

Any *single point source* of a mechanical disturbance, such as a pebble dropped into a smooth lake, creates *spherical waves* (Fig. 45–5) that diminish in intensity as they radiate outward from their place of origin.

A set of closely spaced point sources distributed on a plane surface (such as a loudspeaker's diaphragm) will all produce spherical waves that immediately combine (undergo interference) in such as fashion as to form a plane wave (Fig. 45–5B). By this means, a flat piezoelectric crystal of an US

transducer produces disturbances that are planar and parallel to the face of the crystal source. An array of small, independent piezoelectric elements will, if activated simultaneously, produce the same sort of plane wave. (This is an example of the phenomenon known as *Huygens' principle.*) If independent piezoelectric elements are fired in a rapid, evenly spaced sequence, rather than simultaneously, the resultant wavefront leaves the source at an angle (Fig. 45–5C).

3. FREQUENCY SPECTRUM OF PULSED ULTRASOUND IS CONTINUOUS

Audible sounds involve oscillations in the range 20 Hz to 20 kHz. The middle C string of a piano resonates with a **fundamental frequency** of 261.6 Hz (for the equally tempered scale) and gives rise to local disturbances of the air primarily of this frequency. (It also produces **harmonics** at integer multiples of the fundamental, but generally of much lower amplitudes.) Clinical ultrasound involves much higher frequency oscilla-

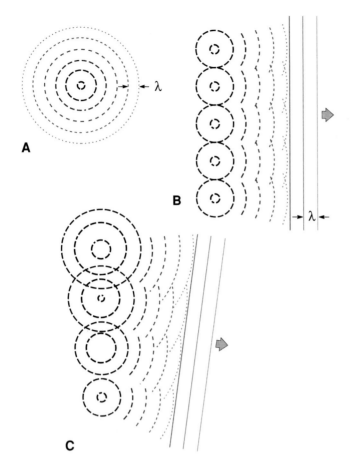

Figure 45–5. Creation of waves. **A.** Spherical waves from a point source. **B.** Plane waves produced by a straight row of closely spaced point sources moving periodically and in phase. **C.** A row of independent point sources. Each is triggered a short time after its neighbor to the left, and the resulting beam angles off to the right.

tions, 1 to 10 MHz, propagating through soft tissues and fluids. Sound waves at these frequencies and in these media are of much shorter wavelength than audible sound in air, and tend to be attenuated much more rapidly.

Clinical pulsed US differs from audible sound in another important way. Much of what you hear is made up of combinations of distinct, monochromatic tones that last for hundreds or thousands of cycles or more. The corresponding spectra consist (at least briefly) of numbers of distinct, discrete peaks. The disturbances used in pulsed US, by contrast, are a microsecond or so in duration and last only a few cycles (Fig. 45–6A). As revealed by Fourier analysis (see Chapter 24, Section 2), the spectrum is then continuous, rather than discrete, and spans a finite range of frequencies (Fig. 45–6B). That is, to create such a pulse out of monochromatic waves, a continuum of frequencies centered on the central frequency, f_0, of the pulse would be required. It is a characteristic of *any* kind of wave disturbance that the uncertainties in its duration, Δt, and its frequency bandwidth, Δf, are related approximately as

$$\Delta f \cdot \Delta t \geq 1/2\pi \qquad (45.2)$$

(This fundamental relationship even underlies Heisenberg's uncertainty principle of Chapter 6, Section 5, as there is a

wavelike aspect to moving electrons and other very small particles.) The shorter the pulse, the wider the band of frequencies it must contain. For most audible sounds, on the other hand, or for continuous-wave (as opposed to pulsed) clinical ultrasound, Δt is relatively long. As a result, Δf for each component can be negligibly small, and the spectrum can be practically discrete.

4. THE VELOCITY OF SOUND IN A MEDIUM IS NEARLY INDEPENDENT OF THE FREQUENCY AND WAVELENGTH

As with any other wave motion, the wavelength, frequency, and velocity of sound are interconnected through

$$\lambda \cdot f = c \qquad (45.3)$$

seen earlier as Equation 4.4. Note that the symbol, c, is also used for the speed of *light* in a vacuum.

It is found that the speed of sound depends on the nature of the medium through which it is traveling, but hardly at all on the frequency (or wavelength). That is, c is practically a constant for any particular material, and, by Equation 45.3, λ and f are related inversely to one another (Fig. 45–7). The velocities of sound for a number of media of clinical interest are listed in Table 45–1 and Figure 45–8.

The reason for the near constancy of c is not obvious. The speed of sound for a material is determined by its density, ρ, and its compressibility, K, according to

$$c = 1/(K \cdot \rho)^{1/2} \qquad (45.4)$$

(Compressibility refers to the fractional change in volume, $\Delta V/V$, of a material per unit increase in the pressure acting on it, ΔP: $K = -\Delta V/V \cdot \Delta P$. The easier it is to squeeze something, the greater its compressibility.) But the compressibility depends only very weakly on the λ and f of any US passing through it. And the average density of a material is totally unrelated to the wavelength or frequency. As a result, the speed of propagation of sound in soft tissue varies by less than 1% over the range of frequencies used in medical ultrasonography. The speed of visible light in a medium, by contrast, *does* depend strongly on λ, which is why prisms and raindrops refract sunlight into its constituent colors.

The fact that c is *nearly independent of frequency* is important for pulse-echo US. The last section showed that an US pulse is made up of components of a range of frequencies. If some of these traveled faster than others, the pulse would spread out over time, resulting in a loss of image resolution and a reduction of peak echo intensity. Because c is nearly constant for any material, this pulse blurring is rarely a major problem.

_____ **EXERCISE 45–1.** _____

What is the wavelength in air of a piano's middle C?

SOLUTION: $\lambda = (331 \text{ m/s})/(261.6 \text{ s}^{-1}) = 1.3$ m.

_____ **EXERCISE 45–2.** _____

What is the wavelength of 1 MHz US in soft tissue?

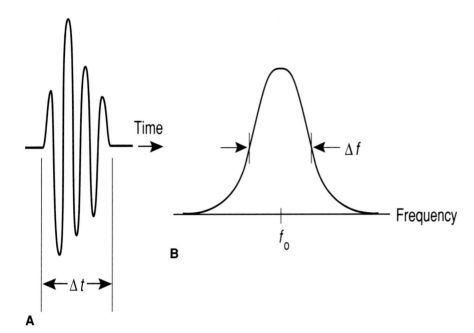

Figure 45–6. An ultrasound pulse. **A**. A localized, propagating disturbance of central frequency f_0, width Δf, and duration Δt. **B**. Its frequency spectrum.

SOLUTION: By Equation 45.3 and Table 45–1, and assuming an average c of 1540 m/s, $\lambda = c/f = (1540 \text{ m/s})/(10^6 \text{ s}^{-1}) = 1.5$ mm for 1 MHz US.

Exercise 45–2 provides a number that is useful to bear in mind for quick comparisons: $\lambda = 1.5$ mm at 1 MHz in soft tissue. According to Equation 45.3, the wavelength is an order of magnitude shorter at 10 MHz.

5. INTENSITY OF SOUND: THE DECIBEL

Because US imaging involves the processing of echoes that range widely in amplitude, it is convenient to compress that range by introducing a logarithmic measure of sound intensity. As with the optical density (OD), the logarithm is taken to the base 10.

The **intensity** of sound (like that of light or of an x-ray beam) refers to the rate at which energy passes through a unit area, and may be measured in SI units in watts per square

1.0 MHz

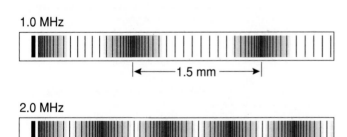

2.0 MHz

Figure 45–7. The velocity, c, of ultrasound in a medium is nearly independent of the ultrasound frequency, f. By Equation 45.3, the wavelength, λ, and frequency are therefore inversely proportional to one another.

meter (W/m²). A person with normal hearing can barely make out a 1-kHz signal of 10^{-12} W/m² intensity.

For purposes of US imaging, the **decibel (dB)** serves as the standard *relative* (rather than absolute) measure for comparing the intensities of two signals. If the intensity of a pulse originally transmitted is I_1 and that of its echo is I_2, the *ratio* of their intensities can be expressed in decibels as

$$\text{intensity ratio (dB)} = 10 \cdot \log_{10}(I_2/I_1) \quad (45.5)$$

(Fig. 45–9 and Table 45–2). By convention, this definition contains a multiplicative factor of 10. So, to report a difference or change in intensity in decibels, you take the logarithm of the ratio I_2/I_1 of the intensities involved, and multiply the logarithm by 10. (Equivalently, express the ratio as a power of 10; the exponent, multiplied by 10, is the intensity ratio, in decibels.)

The threshold of audibility of a 1000-Hz tone occurs at an intensity of about 10^{-12} W/m². A whisper might be 100 times louder than that, or 20 dB higher in intensity. Ordinary conversation across a distance of a meter or so involves sound intensities about 60 dB above the threshold level (Table 45–2).

_____ **EXERCISE 45–3.** _____

The intensity of a beam falls by a factor of 1000 in passing through tissue. Express this drop in decibels.

SOLUTION: The ratio of intensities is 1/1000, the logarithm of which is –3. (Equivalently, 1/1000 may be expressed as a power of 10 as 10^{-3}, the exponent of which is –3.) Multiplying this logarithm (or the exponent) by 10, as called for by Equation 45.5, yields the intensity ratio, –30 dB.

_____ **EXERCISE 45–4.** _____

Two signals differ in intensity by 20 dB. What is the ratio of their intensities?

TABLE 45–1. ACOUSTIC PROPERTIES OF TISSUES AND OTHER MATERIALS OF IMPORTANCE IN CLINICAL ULTRASOUND

Material	Speed of Sound, c (m/s)	Acoustic Impedance $Z = \rho c$ (10^6 kg/m²–s)	Attenuation Coefficient at 1 MHz (dB/cm)
Blood	1575 ± 11	1.62 ± 0.02	0.15 ± 0.04
Bone	3183 ± 618	4.8 ± 0.99	14.2 – 25.2
Brain	1565 ± 10	1.54 ± 0.05	0.75 ± 0.17
Breast	1430 – 1570		0.3 – 0.6
Fat	(1450)	[1.38]	(0.63)
peritoneal	1490		2.1
subcutaneous	1478 ± 9		0.6
Heart	1571 ± 19	1.64	2.0 ± 0.4
Liver	1604 ± 14	1.63 – 1.75	1.2
Lung			[40]
Muscle		(1.70)	
Perpendicular	1581 ± 8		0.96 ± 0.35
Parallel	1581 ± 19		1.4
Soft tissue (mean)	[1540]	[1.63]	[1]
Air	[331]	[0.0004]	(12)
Castor oil	(1500)	(1.4)	(0.95)
PZT*	(4000)	(30)	
Water	[1498]	[1.50]	(0.0022)

*Lead zirconate titanate.

Numbers not in brackets or parentheses are from NCRP Report No. 74, 1983 (Table 2.3). Tabulated values of acoustic impedance are in units of 10^6 kg/m²–s; that is, Z for blood is 1.62×10^6 kg/m²–s. Attenuation coefficients in dB/cm were obtained by multiplying the "phase-dependent" entries in NCRP Report 74, 1983 (Table 2.3) (given in Np/cm), by 8.686. Entries in square brackets are from Hendee WR, ed, 1985 (Tables 20–2, 20–3, and 20–4). Those in parentheses are from Curry TS III, et al, 1990 (Tables 25–1, 25–4, and 25–6).

SOLUTION: Use Equation 45.5 the other way around. 20 dB = $10 \cdot \log_{10}(I_2/I_1)$; $\log_{10}(I_2/I_1) = 2$, which means $I_2/I_1 = 10^2 = 100$.

_____ **EXERCISE 45–5.** _____

An echo signal is half as intense as the original signal. Express the drop in intensity in decibels.

SOLUTION: $I_2/I_1 = 0.5$. Taking the logarithm, $\log_{10}(0.5) = -0.3$. (Equivalently, $0.5 = 10^{-0.3}$.) In decibels, the intensity ratio is therefore $-(10)(0.3) = -3$ dB. That is, reducing a signal by 3 dB amounts to cutting its intensity in half.

_____ **EXERCISE 45–6.** _____

A reflected signal is 3 dB weaker than the original. By how much has its intensity changed?

SOLUTION: The change in intensity is –3 dB. By Equation 45.5, -3 dB = $10 \cdot \log_{10}(I_2/I_1)$. Therefore $-0.3 = \log_{10} I_2/I_1$, which means $I_2/I_1 = 10^{-0.3}$. But $10^{-0.3} = 0.5$.

_____ **EXERCISE 45–7.** _____

According to Table 45–1, a 1-MHz US beam is attenuated at the rate of about 1 dB/cm (i.e., changes by –1 dB in passing

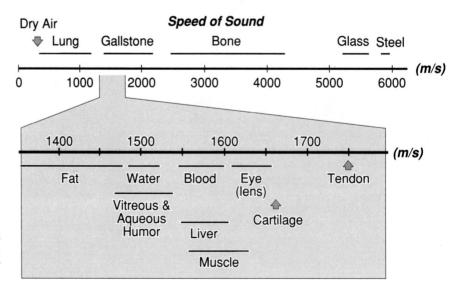

Figure 45–8. Velocities of ultrasound in a number of media. *(After Webb S, ed. The Physics of Medical Imaging.* Philadelphia: Adam Hilger, 1988 [Fig. 7.1].)*

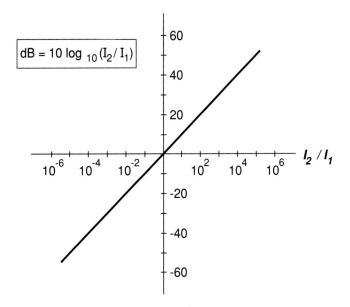

Figure 45–9. The decibel (dB) is a convenient measure of the relative intensities of two ultrasound signals.

through each centimeter) in soft tissue. By how much is the intensity reduced in transiting 1 cm of the tissue?

SOLUTION: In 1 cm of tissue, the intensity of the signal decreases by a factor of $(-1 \text{ dB/cm})(1 \text{ cm}) = -1$ dB. By Equation 45–5, $10 \cdot \log_{10} (I_2/I_1) = -1$, from which $I_2/I_1 = 0.79$. Thus, the signal decreases by 21%, to 0.79 of its original value, in 1 cm of tissue.

6. EXPONENTIAL ATTENUATION OF ULTRASOUND WITH DEPTH IN A HOMOGENEOUS MEDIUM

Ultrasound energy is absorbed by any tissue through which it passes, and it is reflected and refracted at boundaries between different kinds of tissues. Reflection at interfaces is the process

TABLE 45–2. EXPRESSING THE RATIO OF INTENSITIES OF TWO ULTRASOUND SIGNALS IN TERMS OF DECIBELS (dB)

dB	I_2/I_1	Relative to Hearing Threshhold
−40	1/10,000	
−30	1/1000	
−20	1/100	
−10	1/10	
−6.0	0.25	
−3.0	0.50	
−1	0.79	
0	1	Threshold of hearing
3.0	2.00	
20	100	Whisper
60	10^6	Conversation
80	10^8	Loud city noises
120	10^{12}	Painful to ear

that makes possible US image formation. Refraction causes image distortions. Absorption normally plays little useful role in US imaging, but it must nonetheless be taken properly into account.

When a pulse of US passes through relatively homogeneous tissue (i.e., in which the dimensions of any non-uniformities are much less than the wavelength of the US, and no significant echoes are created), its intensity diminishes exponentially with the distance it travels, x,

$$I(x) = I_0 \cdot e^{-2\mu \cdot x} \qquad (45.6)$$

(see Figure 45–2A) by arguments like those in Chapter 15. Some of the energy of the beam is absorbed by the tissue and transformed into heat, and some is scattered diffusely out of the beam by small irregularities. The factor of 2 in the exponent has to do with the formal definition of the attenuation coefficient for sound, μ, and with the details of the relationship between displacement amplitude and intensity.

The attenuation coefficient μ in Equation 45.6 is a perfectly respectable parameter. But it is common practice, instead, to characterize attenuation of US in terms of decibels of intensity loss per centimeter of tissue (dB/cm) (see Table 45–1) and the amount of tissue traversed, x:

$$dB = (dB/cm) \cdot x \qquad (45.7)$$

As shown in the footnote* and in Exercise 45–8, the use of dB/cm in calculations is fully equivalent to (but simpler than) working with the exponential form.

EXERCISE 45–8.

By how much is a 1-MHz US signal attenuated in passing one way through 3 cm of soft tissue?

SOLUTION: By Table 45–1, soft tissue attenuates 1 MHz US at about 1 dB/cm. Over 3 cm, the decrease is $(-1 \text{ dB/cm})(3 \text{ cm}) = -3$ dB, corresponding to an intensity reduction of 0.5.

Alternatively, by Exercise 45–7, 1 dB/cm means an intensity reduction by a factor of 0.79 in 1 cm. Signal intensity is diminished by a second factor of 0.79 over the next centimeter, and by yet another 0.79 over the third. The final intensity is down by $(0.79)^3 = 0.5$ over 3 cm. This agrees with what we just found, and illustrates the legitimacy and ease of determining the exponential attenuation of US in matter directly from the decibels per centimeter.

EXERCISE 45–9.

What is the attenuation of 1 MHz US in passing one way through 2 cm of liver and then along 3 cm of muscle?

---

*Equation 45.7 is easily obtained from Equation 45.6. Take the logarithm of Equation 45.6 to the base 10 and multiply by 10:

$$dB = 10 \cdot \log_{10} (I/I_0) = 10 \cdot \log_{10} (e^{-2\mu \cdot x})$$

By the definition of decibel and by Exercise 14–6, it follows that the attenuation over the distance x is

$$dB = (8.686 \, \mu) \cdot x$$

This is equivalent to Equation 45.7, and even relates decibels per centimeter to μ. The HVL is another measure of attenuation.

SOLUTION: Attenuation in the liver is (1.2 dB/cm)(2 cm) = 2.4 dB, and that in muscle is (1.4 dB/cm)(3 cm) = 4.2 dB, for a total drop in intensity of 6.6 dB. In addition, some of the energy will be reflected at the interface and never reach the muscle, as will be seen in Section 8.

The rate of attenuation of US by homogeneous tissue, unlike its speed of propagation, does depend strongly on the frequency (and wavelength) (Fig 45–10). Energy is removed from the beam by frictionlike forces that act at the molecular level. The rate at which energy is dissipated depends on the viscosity of the medium and on the natural *relaxation processes* that allow the medium to settle back down to an equilibrium condition after the passage of an US wave. For muscle, blood, and most soft tissues, the rate of energy attenuation, in decibels per centimeter, is approximately linearly proportional to the frequency:

$$dB/cm(f) \sim dB/cm(\text{at 1 MHz}) \cdot f \qquad (45.8a)$$

This frequency dependence is sometimes explicitly noted by writing the attenuation coefficient as dB/cm-MHz or dB/cm/MHz.

In water, bone, and a few other materials, the rate of attenuation increases more nearly with the square of the frequency,

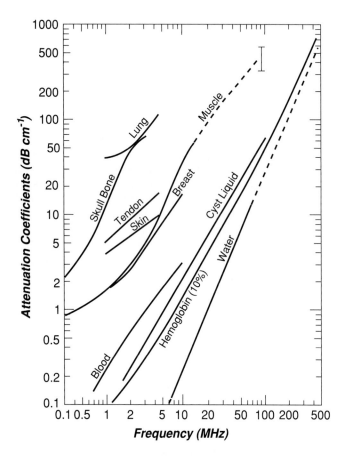

Figure 45–10. The attenuation coefficient (in dB/cm) for a medium increases with the ultrasound frequency. *(After Webb S, ed.* The Physics of Medical Imaging, *Philadelphia: Adam Hilger, 1988 [Fig. 7.2].)*

$$dB/cm(f) \sim dB/cm(\text{1 MHz}) \cdot f^2 \qquad (45.8b)$$

The attenuation rates at 1 MHz for a number of materials are listed in Table 45–1, and in Figure 45–10 at other frequencies as well.

_____ **EXERCISE 45–10.** _____

By how much is 3.5 MHz US attenuated in passing one way through 3 cm of soft tissue?

SOLUTION: At 3.5 MHz, by Equation 45.8a, dB/cm = (1 dB/cm/MHz)(3.5 MHz) = 3.5 dB/cm. The US is attenuated by 10.5 dB, or by a factor of 0.09, in 3 cm of soft tissue.

Frequencies commonly used for medical imaging are 1, 2.25, 3.5, 5, 7, and 10 MHz. The specific frequency chosen for any particular examination is determined largely by optimizing the trade-off between beam penetration and resolution requirements, as will be seen in Chapter 47.

7. REFRACTION OF ULTRASOUND AT AN INTERFACE BETWEEN MEDIA WITH DIFFERENT VELOCITIES OF SOUND

When a beam of ultrasound energy passes from one medium, in which the speed of sound is c_1, into another with speed of sound c_2, the direction of propagation of the beam generally (but not always) changes (Fig. 45–11A). This phenomenon of **refraction**, which occurs also with light entering and leaving glass lenses, is an inevitable consequence of the wave nature of US and of the geometry of the situation.

Consider first the special case of a beam of US that is "normally incident" on (i.e., the direction of propagation is perpendicular to) the interface (Fig. 45–11B). There is nothing that alters the frequency of a pulse as it crosses the boundary; a small mass on the far side of the interface is being pushed and pulled back and forth at the same frequency as a small mass on the near side. But if the velocity of sound is lower, by Equation 45.3 the wavelength must be less, where

$$\lambda_2/\lambda_1 = c_2/c_1 \qquad (45.9)$$

The left–right symmetry of Figure 45–11B suggests that for normal incidence on an interface, there will be no change in the direction of propagation of the beam. For if it *were* to change, would it go to the left or to the right? There is nothing to favor one possibility over the other, so neither occurs.

The story is different, however, when the beam approaches the interface at an angle. Consider the wavefronts that are partly in the new medium but still partly in the old, in Figure 45–11A. The wave crests must be separated by the distance λ_1 in the first medium, but by λ_2 in the second. The only way that can happen is if a discontinuity in direction of propagation occurs at the interface. Working through the trigonometry will convince you that the angle θ_2 of the refracted (transmitted) beam in the second medium is related to the angle θ_1 of incidence in the first by *Snell's Law* (Fig. 45–12)

$$\sin \theta_2/\sin \theta_1 = c_2/c_1 \qquad (45.10)$$

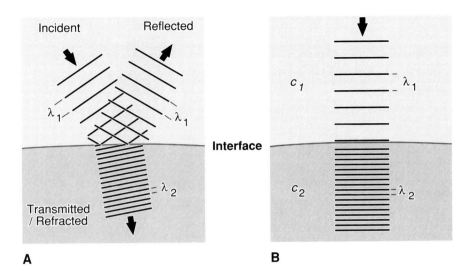

Figure 45–11. Reflection and transmission/refraction at a tissue interface. **A.** The frequency of a refracted beam will not change, but its wavelength and direction of propagation will. **B.** Change in the wavelength of the refracted beam for the special case of "normal" (perpendicular) incidence.

This relationship works regardless of whether the US is passing into a region of higher or lower velocity of sound. The same expression describes the bending of a beam of light in entering glass or water.

Refraction can cause distortions in US images, apparent displacements of objects from where they really are, and some loss of resolution. Unfortunately, not much can be done about it at present.

8. REFLECTION OF ULTRASOUND AT AN INTERFACE BETWEEN MEDIA WITH DIFFERENT ACOUSTIC IMPEDANCES

Sharp ultrasound echoes will be produced at a sizable and relatively flat boundary between two materials with different physical characteristics.

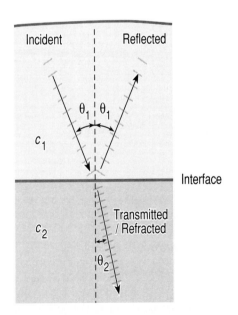

Figure 45–12. Snell's Law, relating the angles of incidence, θ_1, and refraction, θ_2, as sound or light passes from one medium into another.

As with a bouncing ball or a beam of light reflecting from a flat mirror, the angle of *specular reflection* of an US beam is equal to the angle of incidence (see Fig. 45–12). In US imaging, the same transducer is usually used to produce and detect pulses. As a consequence, only those tissue interfaces that happen to lie nearly perpendicular to the direction of propagation of the beam will give rise to echoes that return to the probe and contribute to an image. Figure 45–13 shows what happens when such is *not* the case.

The amount of reflection of sound that occurs at an interface depends on the **acoustic impedances** of the two media involved. The acoustic impedance of a material, denoted Z (not to be confused with atomic number), is determined by its density, ρ, and compressibility, and may be expressed in terms of the speed of sound, c, as

$$Z = \rho \cdot c \qquad (45.11a)$$

The acoustic impedances of some materials of interest in imaging are recorded in Table 45–1. From the units of ρ and c in Equation 45.11a, it may be seen that the SI unit for Z is the kg/m^2–s, also called the *Rayl*.

_____ **EXERCISE 45–11.** _____

Estimate Z for water from its density ($1\ g/cm^3 = 10^3\ kg/m^3$) and the velocity of sound in it (1500 m/s).

SOLUTION: From Equation 45.11a, $Z = 1.5 \times 10^6\ kg/m^2$–s.

_____ **EXERCISE 45–12.** _____

Using Equation 45.4, express Z in terms of density and compressibility.

SOLUTION: $Z = \rho \cdot c = (\rho/K)^{1/2}$. $\qquad$ (45.11b)

Chapter 12, Section 3, and Chapter 14, Section 7, implied that the dynamics of the collisions of billiard balls, and of photons with electrons, must be consistent with the Laws of Con-

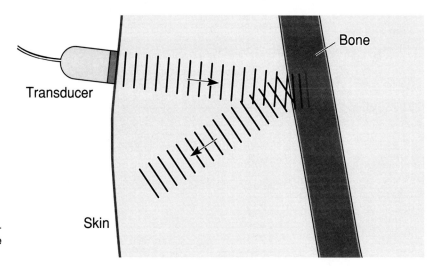

Figure 45–13. Generally, only those waves that reflect back through about 180 degrees can contribute to an ultrasound image.

servation of Energy and Conservation of Momentum. These two separate requirements together determine the energies and angles with which billiard balls, electrons, and photons leave the scene of an interaction. In a similar fashion, the **reflection coefficient,** R (the fraction of the energy or intensity of incoming US that is reflected at an interface), is determined by the relationships among the amounts of compression within the incident, transmitted, and reflected waves and among the corresponding flows of energy. For normal incidence on a large, flat interface surface, R may be expressed in terms of the acoustic impedances of the materials on the two sides of it:

$$R = (Z_2 - Z_1)^2 / (Z_2 + Z_1)^2 \qquad (45.12)$$

The rest of the energy, of relative intensity $1 - R$, is transmitted across the interface and into the second tissue.

Thus, the greater the difference, or mismatch, between the density, compressibility, or speed of sound for the media on the two sides of an interface, the greater the fraction of incident US that is reflected there. If the two materials have the same value for Z, all the US energy will pass from one to the other.

An analogy may be helpful. Imagine giving one end of a wire coil a shake, causing a ripple to run along it (Fig. 45–14). The weight per unit length and the elasticity (or "springiness") of the coil determine its "acoustic impedance." If the far end of the coil is attached to a much heavier grade of coil, a ripple will reflect at the juncture and head back toward you (and another wave will continue on along the second coil). Likewise, there will be a reflection if the far end is attached to a much lighter weight coil. But if the coil interfaces with another of the same type, the wave just keeps on going. So also for US energy coming to a tissue interface.

The acoustic impedance of a medium, and the consequent reflection coefficient at an interface between two media, depend only weakly on US frequency: As noted in Section 4, a material's density is unrelated to the frequency of any US passing through it, and the material's compressibility and speed of US propagation are nearly independent of the frequency. By Equations 45.11 and 45.12, then, Z and R vary little with f and λ.

EXERCISE 45–13.

Does the relative amount of US power reflected at an interface depend on which way the US is traveling across it?

SOLUTION: No. R in Equation 45.12 is symmetric under (unaffected by) an interchange of Z_1 and Z_2.

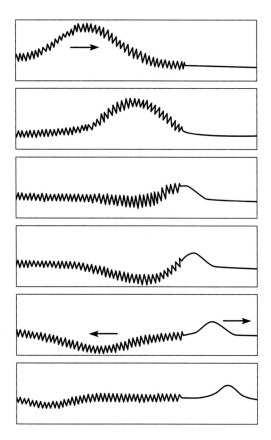

Figure 45–14. Reflection that occurs when a wave moving along a wire coil comes to an interface with a heavier grade of coil. *(Redrawn from Alonso M, Finn E.* Fundamental University Physics. *Reading, MA: Addison-Wesley, 1967: Fig. 20–16.)*

_____ **EXERCISE 45–14.** _____

How much of the energy of an US pulse is reflected as the beam passes from muscle to fat? What fraction is transmitted into the fat?

SOLUTION: From Table 45–1, the acoustic impedances of muscle and fat are, respectively, 1.70×10^6 and 1.38×10^6 kg/m²–s. The powers of 10 cancel in Equation 45.12, and

$$R = [(1.70 - 1.38)/(1.70 + 1.38)]^2 = 0.01$$

This amount of reflection may be large enough to be detected. The fraction *transmitted* into the fat is $1 - R = 0.99$.

_____ **EXERCISE 45–15.** _____

How much of the energy of an US pulse is reflected as the beam passes from fat to muscle?

SOLUTION: Application of Equation 45.12 leads to exactly the same result as for US entering fat from muscle.

9. PHYSICAL/BIOLOGIC SOURCES OF MEDICALLY RELEVANT ULTRASOUND INFORMATION

The amounts of energy reflection occurring at several important kinds of tissue interface are presented in Table 45–3. As would be expected from the large differences in density and compressibility, ultrasound energy does not pass readily across tissue/bone or tissue/air boundaries. Although the modality can be of value for obstetric and gynecologic and abdominal imaging, it is of limited use in the study of the lung or adult intracranium. In imaging the abdomen, moreover, the strongest signals may be from air bubbles.

Soft tissues other than fat all have nearly the same density. Variations in acoustic impedance among soft tissues are thus due primarily to differences in elasticity and/or compressibility (see Equation 45.11b). The elasticity/compressibility, in turn, is largely determined by the nature of the stroma of collagenous material that binds the parenchymal cells of the tissue together. Thus, much of the ability to differentiate normal organs with US is attributable to differences in their stromal collagen content. Diseases that significantly alter the distribution of collagenous material within an organ (e.g., cirrhosis of the liver and some malignancies) may give rise to diagnostically useful image patterns.

Some organs, such as the kidneys, pancreas, spleen, and liver, comprise many small subregions of dissimilar tissues,

TABLE 45–3. FRACTIONS OF POWER/INTENSITY REFLECTED AND TRANSMITTED AT SOME CLINICALLY IMPORTANT TISSUE INTERFACES

Interface	Reflected Fraction, *R*	Transmitted Fraction
Muscle/fat	0.01	0.99
Muscle/bone	0.23	0.77
Muscle/air	0.999	0.001

and *scattering* at the interfaces among them gives rise to characteristic US image *textures*. Structures containing fluid, such as the bladder, cysts, the common bile duct, and the aorta and other large blood vessels, have no internal structures, and the US images of their interiors are blank. The lungs also appear blank, but for a different reason: some of the US energy is reflected at the tissue–air interface, and the rest is rapidly attenuated out of existence.

10. CASE STUDY: ECHOES FROM A BONE EMBEDDED IN TISSUE

We shall tie together some of the main points of this chapter by working through a simple example. Suppose that a flat bone is covered by 3 cm of muscle, which in turn is under 1 cm of fat (Fig. 45–15). If a 1-MHz US beam of time-averaged intensity 0.05 W/cm² is directed in toward the bone, what will be the echo strength?

The calculation is summarized in Table 45–4, which shows the factor by which the beam is reduced at each stage of its journey and the remaining intensity, relative to the initial value. (The numbers are kept to three significant figures not

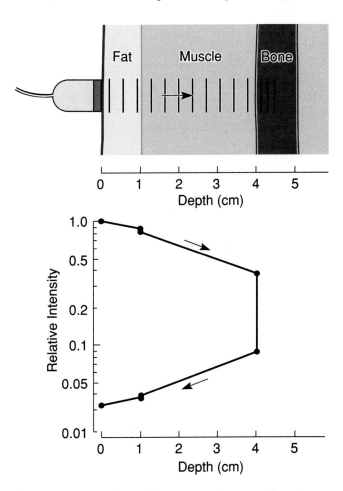

Figure 45–15. An ultrasound beam enters fat, passes through muscle, and is reflected by bone. By the time it returns to the transducer, its intensity will have fallen by 14.9 dB (i.e., it will possess only 3% of its original power).

TABLE 45–4. LOSS OF INTENSITY AND REMAINING BEAM INTENSITY FOR THE EXAMPLE ILLUSTRATED IN FIGURE 45–15

Tissue or Interface	Distance (cm)	Intensity Reduction Factor	Remaining Relative Intensity
			1
Fat	1	0.865	0.865
Fat/muscle	—	0.99	0.856
Muscle	3	0.437	0.374
Muscle/bone	—	0.23	0.0861
Muscle	3	0.437	0.0376
Muscle/fat	—	0.99	0.0372
Fat	1	0.865	0.0322

because such accuracy can realistically be expected, but rather to help you follow the argument.) Reflections occurring at the transducer–skin interface have not been considered. (Should they be?)

In passing through the centimeter of fat, by Table 45–1 the attenuation is –0.63 dB, which translates to a reduction in intensity by a factor of 0.865. At the fat/muscle interface, accord-ing to Table 45–3 the transmitted beam is reduced by a further factor of 0.99, so that the relative intensity of the remaining beam is now 0.856. (The reflected beam is not of concern in this example.) Averaging the attenuation coefficients for US propagation parallel and perpendicular to the muscle fibers yields 1.2 dB/cm; attenuation over 3 cm therefore diminishes the beam intensity by a factor of 0.437. At the muscle/bone interface, it is now the reflected intensity that is of interest, and that is down by 0.23. The loss factors in muscle and fat are the same on the way out as they were coming in. The end result is that the echo intensity is only about 3% of that of the original beam, or 1.5 mW/cm^2.

EXERCISE 45–16.

Run through this exercise using decibels rather than loss factors.

SOLUTION: The losses in the fat and muscle are –0.63 and –3.6 dB, respectively, each time the beam passes through. At the fat/muscle and muscle/bone interfaces, they are –0.04 and –6.4 dB. The total loss in the round trip is –14.9 dB, which corresponds to a 97% intensity loss.

Chapter 46

Ultrasound II: Creating the Ultrasound Beam

1. **An Ultrasound Transducer Creates High-Frequency Mechanical Oscillations Out of an Electrical Signal, and Vice Versa**
2. **Resonance of the Piezoelectric Crystal**
3. **Impedance Matching the Piezoelectric Crystal to the Damping Material and to the Patient's Body**
4. **The Fresnel Zone of an Unfocused Beam**
5. **Focusing the Beam Improves Beam Penetration, Echo Strength, and Lateral Resolution**
6. **Sweeping the Beam (for B-Mode)**
7. **Creating a Swept, Focused Beam with an Electronic Phased Array**
8. **Measures of Beam Intensity**

A beam of ultrasound (US) energy is created, and US echoes are detected, by means of a transducer. The heart of a transducer is a piece of piezoelectric material, or many such elements, that transform electric signals into mechanical vibrations, and vice versa. This chapter explores the ways in which a transducer produces an US beam focused to a particular point in tissue and/or swept back and forth in a plane within the patient.

1. AN ULTRASOUND TRANSDUCER CREATES HIGH-FREQUENCY MECHANICAL OSCILLATIONS OUT OF AN ELECTRICAL SIGNAL, AND VICE VERSA

The heart of an **US transducer** is one carefully sculpted piece of **piezoelectric** material (from the Greek *piezo*, meaning "to press") (Fig. 46–1) or an array of such pieces. Piezoelectric materials used for US include the natural crystal quartz, lead zirconate titanate (PZT), which is a ceramic, and the plastic polyvinylidine difluoride (PVDF). A single *crystal* might be a disk or rectangle 1 cm or so across; an element in an array is much smaller. In either case, it is a fraction of a millimeter thick. Its two faces are coated with thin veneers of conductor, such as silver, to which wires are attached for the application and detection of voltages.

A piezoelectric material displays two characteristic properties, both of which are essential for ultrasonography:

- Application of a voltage across a piece of the material will cause it to deform slightly. Its thickness, in particular, may change by an amount proportional to the voltage.
- Conversely, compression of the piece, thereby slightly reducing its thickness, gives rise to a voltage across it. And the voltage generated will be proportional to the amount of pressure and the resulting strain.

A piezoelectric substance might be made up of polar molecules, each with a small, permanent excess of electron charge at one end and a deficiency at the other (Fig. 46–2). When an electric field is applied across the crystal, the molecules twist around a little, trying to align along it, and this results in small changes in its physical dimensions. Conversely, forcing a rotation of the molecules by compressing the piece alters the electric status quo within it, resulting in the appearance of a voltage across it. Other mechanisms of piezoelectricity exist, as well.

2. RESONANCE OF THE PIEZOELECTRIC CRYSTAL

If an external periodic force is applied to a mechanical system that can undergo oscillation, the amplitude of the resulting motion will depend on the frequency of the force, as was discussed in Chapter 42, Section 4. If the driving frequency is too high or too low, the oscillations will be small. But when the frequency of the force is the same as the natural resonant frequency of the system, the amplitude of the oscillations goes through a maximum (see Fig. 42–5).

A *resonance* can take place in a piezoelectric crystal in response to an applied oscillating mechanical force or alternating-current voltage of the appropriate frequency. For a piezoelectric crystal at resonance, the thickness of the crystal becomes, alternately, slightly greater and less than its resting thickness (Fig. 46–3A). A standing wave is established within the crystal, with a wavelength that is twice the crystal thickness:

$$\lambda_{res} = 2 \cdot T_{xtal} \qquad (46.1)$$

(With a piano string pinned at both ends, by comparison, the wavelength of the fundamental standing wave mode of vibration is twice the string length [Fig. 46–3B].)

419

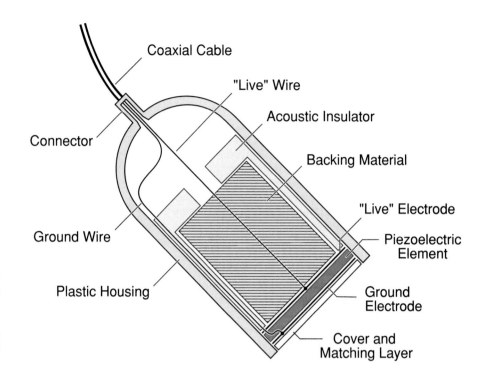

Figure 46–1. Medical ultrasound transducer consisting of a single piezoelectric element sandwiched between a pair (live and grounded) of electrodes. The backing material is designed to absorb all ultrasound energy initially heading away from the patient. Such a transducer might be used for A-mode imaging.

_____ **EXERCISE 46–1.** _____

What is the thickness of a PZT crystal that will generate 1 MHz US?

SOLUTION: With the aid of Equation 45.3, express the resonance condition (Equation 46.1) in terms of the frequency and the speed of sound in the piezoelectric material. By Table 45–1, the speed of sound in the crystal material, c_{PZT}, is 4000 m/s. The wavelength corresponding to a 1-MHz acoustic wave in PZT is $\lambda = 4$ mm. The thickness of a PZT crystal resonant at that frequency is half the resonance wavelength, or 2 mm.

A piezoelectric crystal is not a perfectly monochromatic resonator. The relative amplitude of oscillation of a typical crystal is shown as a function of the frequency of the applied voltage as the dashed line in Figure 46–4A. (Alternatively, this curve shows the amplitude of the voltage signal resulting from a sinusoidal mechanical driving force, as a function of its frequency.) The sharpness of the resonance is commonly expressed in terms of its Q, defined as the ratio of the resonant frequency, f_{res}, to the full width at half-maximum (FWHM) of the resonance curve:

$$Q = f_{res}/\text{FWHM} \qquad (46.2)$$

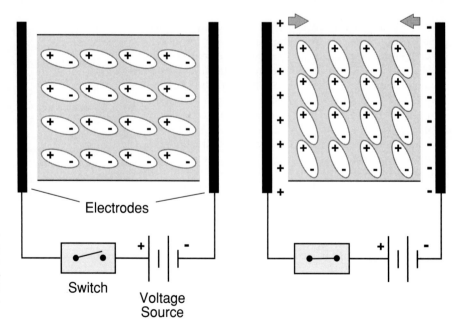

Figure 46–2. One mechanism of piezoelectricity. When a voltage is applied across the crystal, the resulting realignment of the permanently polarized molecules leads to a change in crystal thickness. Conversely, mechanical stresses on the crystal can cause the generation of a voltage.

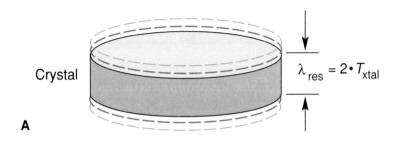

Crystal

$\lambda_{res} = 2 \cdot T_{xtal}$

A

$\lambda_{res} = 2 \cdot \text{Length}$

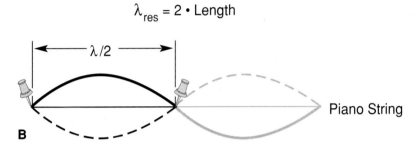

$\lambda/2$

Piano String

B

Figure 46–3. Two examples of resonance. **A.** A standing wave resonance can exist in an ultrasound piezoelectric crystal if the thickness of the crystal, T_{xtal}, is half the wavelength of sound in the material. **B.** The *fundamental* standing wave resonance in a string pinned at both ends. The wavelength is twice the length of the string, but the resonant frequency depends also on the tautness of the string.

The narrower the band of frequencies that will cause large oscillations (and the smaller the FWHM), the higher the Q. The Q of a piece of quartz may be in the tens of thousands, and that of a piece of PZT in the tens or hundreds.

SOLUTION: The resonant frequency is 1000 kHz. The amplitude of the oscillations falls to half its maximum value at about 992 and 1008 kHz, which are separated by 16 kHz. By Equation 46.2, Q is about 60.

_____ **EXERCISE 46–2.** _____

What is the Q of the system whose (dashed) resonance curve is marked "low Q" in Figure 46–4A?

When the frequency of an applied voltage coincides with the natural resonant frequency of a piezoelectric crystal, especially large vibrations arise. But just as a swing can be set in large-amplitude motion by one good shove (rather than by

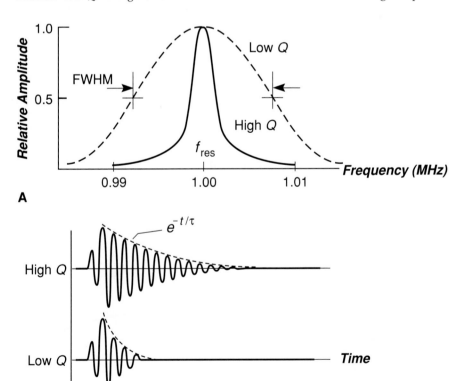

A

B

Figure 46–4. The Q of a system is a measure of the sharpness of its resonance. **A.** The Q of the high-Q system in this figure (solid line) is, by Equation 46.2, 1000 kHz/3 kHz = 333. **B.** The sharper the resonance of a system, and the higher its Q, the longer it will ring. FWHM, full width at half-maximum.

many gentle pushes at the resonant frequency), so also a transducer crystal can be made to resonate by a sudden voltage impulse. Like the ringing of a bell following a sharp blow, the amplitude of the resulting mechanical and voltage oscillations decays with a characteristic time, τ (Fig. 46–4B):

$$V(t) = V_0 \cdot e^{-t/\tau} \cdot (\sin 2\pi f_{res} t) \qquad (46.3)$$

Some fancy Fourier footwork related to Equation 45.2 reveals that the decay time τ is related to the crystal Q as

$$\tau = Q/2\pi f_{res} \qquad (46.4)$$

The sharper the resonance and the higher the Q, the slower the decay.

Pulses of US can be produced by driving the transducer briefly at its resonant frequency. More commonly in practice, the crystal is rung with an abrupt change (typically by 100 V or so) in the applied voltage. Either way, the pulses of US energy emitted from the transducer must be short. This is necessary, as will be seen in the next chapter, so that echoes returning promptly from shallow tissue interfaces can be detected, and also to achieve good spatial resolution. One way to limit the duration of a pulse is to cement a *damping material,* such as tungsten powder embedded in epoxy, to the back of the crystal (see Fig. 46–1). (The backing block also provides mechanical support for the crystal.) Alternatively, with *dynamic damping,* a second pulse is generated soon after the first but 180 degrees out of phase with it. Either approach can artificially shorten the pulse decay time τ (and lower the Q) of a crystal.

A *caveat*: Transducers are delicate instruments, and should be handled with care. It is possible to erase the piezoelectricity irreversibly by taking a crystal above its Curie temperature, which may be only several hundred degrees centigrade. A transducer should therefore never be autoclaved, but only gas or liquid sterilized. Also, one must not bring it into contact with sources of excessive voltage or submerge it in water or other fluids unless it is watertight.

3. IMPEDANCE MATCHING THE PIEZOELECTRIC CRYSTAL TO THE DAMPING MATERIAL AND TO THE PATIENT'S BODY

Extraneous echoes should be prevented from arising within the transducer itself, to the extent possible, and the power transmitted into and from the body should be maximized. These objectives can be largely achieved by minimizing the mismatches in acoustic impedance between the piezoelectric crystal and its damping material, on the one side of the crystal, and between the crystal and the patient, on the other (see Fig. 46–1).

Transducer manufacturers address the first problem by constructing the damping block out of material with the same acoustic impedance as that of the crystal. Ideally, all the US energy heading off into the damping block will be absorbed, and none reflected.

The effects of the difference in Z between the transducer crystal and the patient can be diminished by means of **impedance matching.** This involves covering the front of the transducer with a *matching layer* of material, the acoustic impedance of which is the geometric mean of that of the piezoelectric material and that of soft tissue:

$$Z_{match} = \sqrt{Z_{piezo} \cdot Z_{soft\ tissue}} \qquad (46.5)$$

The optimal matching layer is generally a quarter-wavelength in thickness, and the approach is known as *quarter-wave matching*. In addition, all air pockets between probe and patient

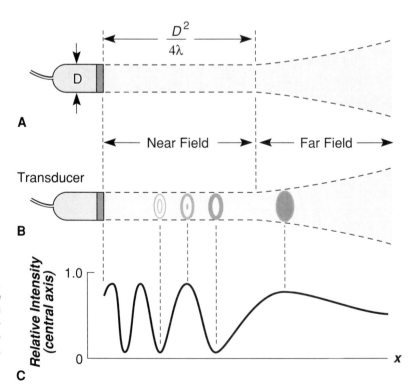

Figure 46–5. Typical medical ultrasound beam. **A.** "Near" (the source) and "far" zones (fields). **B.** The intensity across the beam face at several distances from the transducer, showing wave interference effects. **C.** Intensity along the central axis, also revealing wave interference effects. Side lobes surrounding the primary beam, another consequence of interference, are not shown.

should be eliminated, and good physical contact ensured, with a layer of coupling gel or mineral oil.

_____ **EXERCISE 46–3.** _____

What should be the acoustic impedance and thickness of the matching layer for a PZT transducer operating at 1.5 MHz? Assume c = 2000 m/s for the matching material.

SOLUTION: The acoustic impedances of PZT and soft tissue are 30×10^6 and 1.63×10^6 kg/m²s. By Equation 46.5, Z_{match} = 7×10^6 kg/m²s. The quarter-wave thickness of a 1.5-MHz signal in the matching material (c = 2000 m/s) can be determined from Equation 45.3: $\lambda = c/f = (2000 \text{ m/s})/(1.5 \times 10^6 \text{ s}^{-1}) = 1.33$ mm; from this, the quarter-wavelength thickness is 0.33 mm.

4. THE FRESNEL ZONE OF AN UNFOCUSED BEAM

An US beam produced by a simple, flat piezoelectric crystal starts out with a cross-sectional area comparable to that of the crystal itself (Fig. 46–5A). The region over which the beam retains this form is called the **Fresnel** or **near zone.** It can be shown that the Fresnel zone extends to a depth of

$$x' = D^2/4\lambda \qquad (46.6)$$

where D is the diameter of the transducer. As suggested by Figures 46–5B and 46–5C, wave interference effects may be considerable in the near zone and give rise to *intensity peaks* at various places within the beam. They are also responsible for *lobes* of US energy coming off in directions other than that of the beam.

Beyond the Fresnel zone, in the "Fraunhofer" or "far" zone, the beam diverges with the angle φ, for which sin φ = 1.2λ/D. In the far zone, the intensity of the beam falls off with distance from the source because of both attenuation (as is the case within the Fresnel zone) and the inverse square effect.

It is possible to construct images from echoes only if one knows the direction from which the echoes come. Hence for the unfocused beam just described, only anatomic features that lie within or near the Fresnel zone can be resolved. And that requirement is problematic.

_____ **EXERCISE 46–4.** _____

What is the length of the Fresnel zone for 3.5 MHz US in soft tissue produced by a 6-mm-diameter crystal?

SOLUTION: With US traveling 1540 m/s through soft tissue, the wavelength is $(1540 \text{ m/s})/(3.5 \times 10^6 \text{ s}^{-1}) = 0.044$ cm. By Equation 46.6, the depth of the Fresnel zone is $(0.6 \text{ cm})^2/(4)(0.044 \text{ cm}) = 2$ cm.

5. FOCUSING THE BEAM IMPROVES BEAM PENETRATION, ECHO STRENGTH, AND LATERAL RESOLUTION

Normally a clinical US beam is **focused** (Fig. 46–6) for three reasons:

- Focusing the beam energy partially overcomes the problem of inadequate *beam penetration.*
- The *lateral resolution* (in the scan plane, perpendicular to

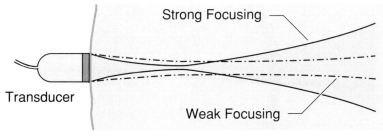

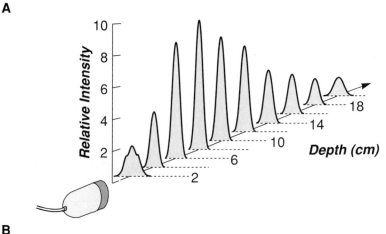

Figure 46–6. Two representations of how focusing reduces the cross-sectional area of an ultrasound beam in the focal region and concentrates the sound energy there. **A.** Isointensity lines. **B.** Intensity profiles at various depths: 19-mm-diameter, 2.25-MHz source with an 8-cm-deep focus. *(After National Council on Radiation Protection and Measurements (NCRP): Biological Effects of Ultrasound: Mechanisms and Clinical Implications (Report No. 74), [Fig. 3.9]. Bethesda, MD: NCRP, 1983.)*

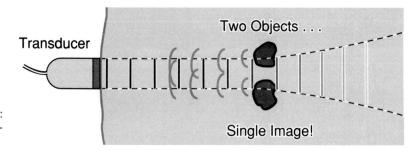

Figure 46–7. An important reason to focus the beam: Lateral resolution can be no better than the beam dimensions.

the direction of beam propagation) is comparable to the beam width. Two objects that are both covered by (and therefore not resolvable with) a large-diameter beam (Fig. 46–7) may be separately distinguishable by a narrower focused beam. With a focused beam, lateral resolution may be of the order of a few millimeters.

- Constricting the beam diameter concentrates its intensity (by as much as a factor of 100) over the region where it runs into reflecting objects. The echoes produced there will be accordingly stronger.

The region over which the beam is most narrowed, and can be used for imaging, is called the **focal zone.** The distance from the crystal to the center of the focal zone is the transducer's *focal length*, and the distance over which the beam is in reasonable focus is the *depth of focus*.

There are several ways of producing focused beams. One is to employ a suitably curved (rather than flat) piezoelectric crystal (Fig. 46–8A). The geometry of such a crystal should satisfy two conditions: The plane wavelets originating from all

points on the crystal surface should move toward a single *focal point*. And the phase relationships of the wavelets should be such that the interference that occurs at the focal point is predominantly constructive, rather than destructive. A crystal with a spherical curvature satisfies these criteria approximately.

An US *lens* composed of epoxy resins and plastics positioned in front of a flat crystal (Fig. 46–8B) can achieve the same end. Because US generally travels faster in a lens than in tissue, a lens that focuses to a point is concave (as opposed to a focusing lens for light, which is convex).

The production of a focused beam electronically, by means of an electronic phased array of piezoelectric elements, will be discussed in Section 7.

6. SWEEPING THE BEAM (FOR B-MODE)

The creation of a tomographic, or "slice"-type, B-mode US image involves sweeping the beam repeatedly back and forth through the patient's body. In the early days of B-mode, a

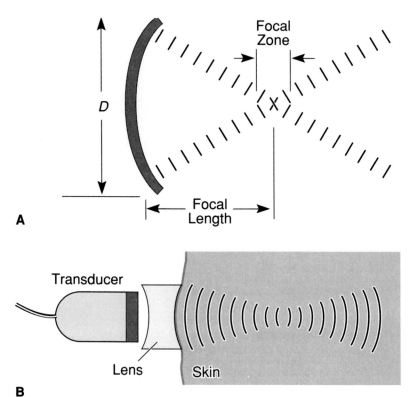

Figure 46–8. Focusing an ultrasound beam by mechanical (as opposed to electronic) means. **A.** With a curved piezoelectric crystal. **B.** With an acoustic lens.

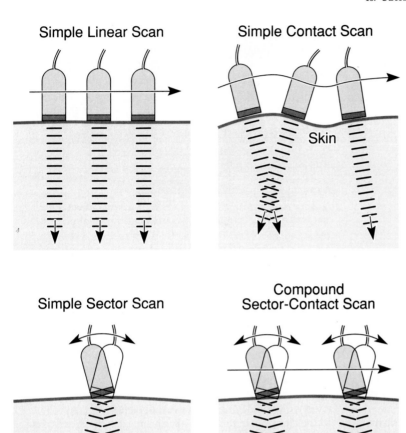

Simple Linear Scan

Simple Contact Scan

Skin

Simple Sector Scan

Compound
Sector-Contact Scan

Figure 46–9. Standard patterns of manual or mechanical beam sweep for B-mode.

transducer would contain a single, rigidly held piezoelectric crystal, which would have to be rocked back and forth manually and/or moved across the body. Several standard patterns of sweep were developed, and a few of the most commonly used of these are shown in Figure 46–9.

Some transducers perform the beam sweep themselves *mechanically*, either by rocking the crystal or by rotating a wheel that holds several independent crystals (of which only the one closest to the output window functions at any time). More modern transducers create a swept US beam for B-mode imaging *electronically*, by phasing the pulses from an array of independent, small piezoelectric elements.

7. CREATING A SWEPT, FOCUSED BEAM WITH AN ELECTRONIC PHASED ARRAY

It is possible to produce a swept, focused beam electronically, by means of an *array* of independent piezoelectric *elements*. A *linear array* might consist of several tens (or even hundreds) of separate elements, each 2 mm (or less) by 10 mm, say, aligned side by side (Fig. 46–10A) and electrically insulated from one another. An *annular array* consists of perhaps a half-dozen concentric ring elements (Fig. 46–10B). Either kind of array can

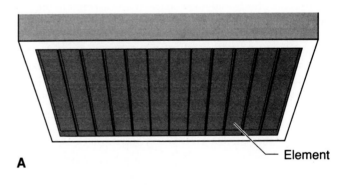

A

Element

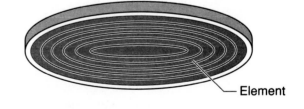

B

Element

Figure 46–10. A "crystal" made up of independent piezoelectric elements can electronically direct and focus a beam. **A.** Linear array of elements. **B.** Annular array.

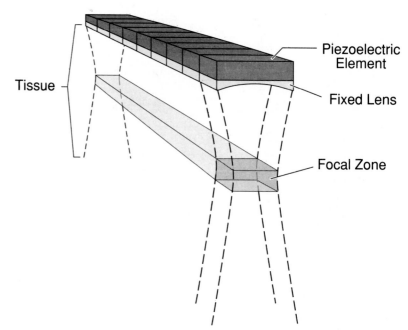

Figure 46–11. A phased array plus a fixed acoustic lens for sweeping out a narrow tomographic slice of tissue.

generate US beams with a variety of different characteristics, simply by varying the timing and amplitudes of the excitations of its individual constituent elements.

If a single element in a linear array is excited, the disturbance will radiate out through the nearby soft tissue with a nearly spherical wavefront (see Fig. 45–5). But if all the separate elements of the array fire simultaneously and with the same amplitude, the separate wavelets will combine to form a single, flat wavefront parallel to the array, in accord with Huygens' Principle. (An array of small elements acts somewhat like an optical grating, however, and gives rise also to interference effects that must be taken into account in the design of a transducer.)

The electrical independence of the elements of an array endows it with great beam-generating flexibility. Suppose that element 2 is excited a small fraction of a microsecond after element 1 (much less than the duration of an US pulse), and element 3 is delayed by the same amount after element 2, and so

on. An unfocused plane wave will be produced that comes away from the array at an angle that depends on the amount of interelement delay between excitations (see Fig. 45–5C). After all the elements in the array have been excited, one can change the amount of the interelement delay a little and produce a new beam propagating in a different direction. By generating a sequence of such beams one after another, a *phased* or *steered array*, in effect, *electronically sweeps* the US beam back and forth. By adding a fixed concave acoustic lens, moreover, the swept beam may be confined to a thin slice of tissue (Fig. 46–11), known as a *tomographic slice*.

Alternatively, the US from an array can be *electronically focused* within the plane of the tomographic slice. Suppose the two outermost elements, on either end of the array, are excited simultaneously. After a brief delay, the two next-to-outermost elements are excited, and so on (Fig. 46–12). With proper timing, the effect is like that of exciting the single, curved crystal of Figure 46–8A. But that's not the end of the story. The amounts

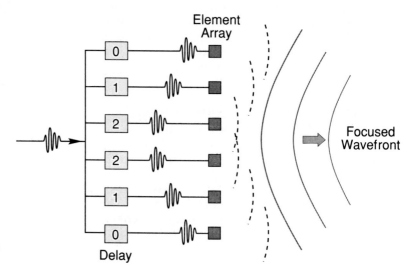

Figure 46–12. Phased array for lateral focusing within a tomographic slice.

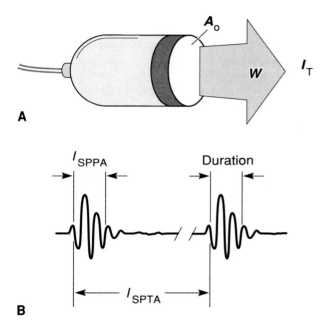

A

B

Figure 46–13. Measures of intensity. **A.** Average power per unit area at the source, I_T. **B.** Beam intensity averaged only over the pulse itself, I_{SPPA}, and averaged over a long period of time, I_{SPTA}.

of the delays between the excitations of adjacent crystals determine the focal length. The timing of these excitations can be varied slowly (relative to the pulse repetition rate), shifting the focal zone toward and away from the transducer array. By means of a focal zone that moves in and out within the body, this technique of *dynamic focusing* extends significantly the length of the effective focal zone.

With complex timing plus a fixed lens, a phased array can generate a focused US beam that sweeps back and forth within a tomographic slice of tissue, and in and out at the same time. Such an arrangement can be used in generating real-time B-mode images of thin slices of tissue, as will be discussed in the next chapter.

Another approach involves firing elements 1 through 5 together, say, then elements 3 through 7, and so on. This progression is designed to create a set of independent, but partially overlapping, side-stepping parallel beams. With suitable modification of the timing, focusing and directionality of the beams can be introduced.

8. MEASURES OF BEAM INTENSITY

Howsoever produced, the US energy in the vicinity of a transducer is a complex function of position, even within the beam (see Fig. 46–5). For pulsed US, it also depends on time. All of this precludes our finding a single number that can serve as a comprehensive measure of intensity.

Several entities have been defined, however, to provide useful partial information on the beam. The following examples (and there are others) employ the notation adopted by the American Institute of Ultrasound in Medicine (AIUM) and the National Council on Radiation Protection and Measurements (NCRP):

- A simple but coarse measure of beam strength is the I_T *intensity*, defined as the ratio W/A_0 of the time-average power output of a transducer, W, to the effective area of its radiation surface, A_0 (Fig. 46–13A).
- The *spatial-peak, temporal-averaged intensity*, I_{SPTA}, refers to the value of the intensity (energy flow through a unit area per unit time) at a point of peak intensity within the beam (see Fig. 46–5) as averaged over a relatively long period of time (Fig. 46–13B).

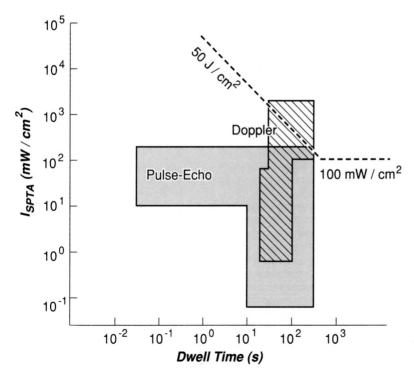

Figure 46–14. Typical combinations of I_{SPTA} and dwell time for pulse-echo (shaded) and Doppler (hatched) systems. There have been no independently confirmed significant biologic effects in mammalian tissues exposed in vitro with parameters in the region below the broken line. *(After National Council on Radiation Protection and Measurements (NCRP): Biological Effects of Ultrasound: Mechanisms and Clinical Implications (Report No. 74), [Figs. 3.12, 9.1, and 9.2]. Bethesda MD: NCRP, 1983.)*

- With pulsed US, it is important also to know (both for imaging purposes and for the consideration of bioeffects) the intensity at a point during the time that a single pulse is actually passing by. Hence the need for a *spatial-peak, pulse-averaged intensity,* I_{SPPA} (Fig. 46–13B). It is a simple exercise to demonstrate that the product of the I_{SPPA}, the *pulse duration* time, and the pulse repetition frequency equals the I_{SPTA}. (Pulse duration is to be distinguished from the *dwell time*, which is the total time that the focal zone of the beam covers a specific part of the patient's body.) Values of I_{SPTA} and dwell time commonly employed in pulse-echo imaging are shown in Figure 46–14.

When determined for a given transducer in a homogeneous material with no reflecting surfaces, such as a deep water bath, these and related intensities are known as *exposure* or *free field* parameters. A half-dozen or so methods have been devised for assessing free field intensities, three of them being measurement with an accurately calibrated piezoelectric sensor, calorimetry (sensing the slight rise in temperature brought about by pumping in the US power), and assessment and interpretation (from their motions) of the US radiation force acting on small test objects. The corresponding in situ intensities generated by the transducer within a patient cannot be measured directly, and can be estimated with only some degree of accuracy from a knowledge of the beam and tissue characteristics.

Ultrasound III: Imaging

The last two chapters discussed the propagation of ultrasound energy through tissues, the reflection of ultrasound (US) pulses at tissue interfaces, and the generation and detection of an US beam by a piezoelectric element or array of elements. Now we can consider the technologies by which US images are created (A-mode, M-mode, and B-mode) and the velocity of blood flow estimated (Doppler).

1. ULTRASOUND CAN IMAGE OBJECTS LARGE COMPARED WITH THE WAVELENGTH

Ultrasound images of the body can be created from the echoes produced when pulses of US energy strike the interfaces between different tissues. The nature of an echo formed at a particular interface, in turn, depends strongly on the properties of the media on both sides of it and on its dimensions (Fig. 47–1).

If all irregularities and nonuniformities (hence all interfaces) within a tissue are of dimensions d much smaller than the wavelength of the sound,

$$d \ll \lambda \qquad (47.1a)$$

then the tissue will appear to an US beam to be relatively smooth and homogeneous. Some sound energy may undergo nearly isotropic (by equal amounts in all directions) *diffuse* scattering from small tissue inclusions, like the scattering of long-wavelength ocean waves passing through the pilings of a pier. This phenomenon may manifest as tissue *speckle*, or fine *texture*, which can be of considerable diagnostic usefulness.

If the surface features of an organ are of dimensions generally much greater than the US wavelength,

$$d \gg \lambda \qquad (47.1b)$$

significant *specular* reflection may occur. The nature of the echo depends on the physical properties of the materials inside and outside the organ, on the characteristics of the interface (gradual versus sharp changes and smooth versus rough surface), and on the geometry of the situation (the angle with which the beam strikes the interface). Objects suitable for US imaging fall primarily into this category.

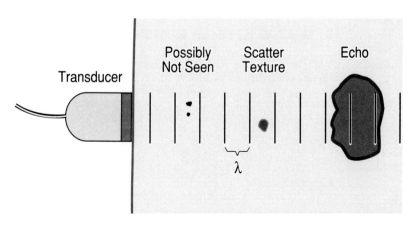

Figure 47–1. Objects of dimensions larger than a wavelength can give echo images; tissue inclusions much smaller than λ may still produce image texture.

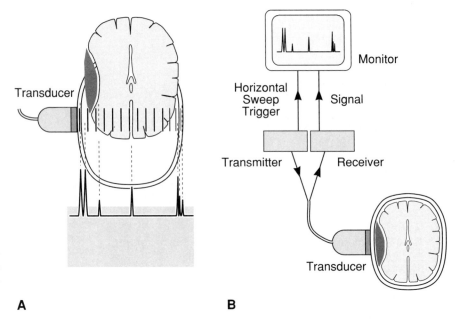

A   **B**

Figure 47–2. A-Mode, the simplest form of US imaging. **A.** It provides one-dimensional (i.e., along the line of sight of the beam) information on anatomy. **B.** At the instant of pulse transmission, the transmitter triggers the start of the horizontal sweep of a point of light across the monitor screen. Any detected echo signal produces a spike on the screen.

Between these two extremes are tissues that contain inclusions of sizes comparable to the wavelength of the sound,

$$d \sim \lambda \quad \text{(coarse texture)} \qquad (47.1c)$$

Scatter from these contributes coarse graininess and small-scale structure to the apparent texture of the tissue in an image.

2. CALCULATING THE DEPTH OF A TISSUE INTERFACE FROM THE ARRIVAL TIME OF AN ECHO: A-MODE

The earliest, and conceptually simplest, form of US is *A-mode* (Fig. 47–2A), in which the reflection from a tissue interface is displayed as a voltage amplitude spike on the screen of an oscilloscope.

A-Mode imaging begins with the transmission of a pulse of US energy into the body (Fig. 47–2B). At the instant of US transmission, a point of light begins sweeping horizontally across the screen of the oscilloscope. If and when the transducer detects an echo signal, it generates a voltage spike, which is applied to the scope's vertical displacement plates (see Chapter 8, Section 10). The position along the x axis of the spike corresponds to the time of the echo return, hence to the depth beneath the surface of the responsible tissue interface. The amplitude of the spike is determined by (among other things) the mismatch in impedances of the two tissues. More than one spike occurring along the x axis indicates the presence of several reflecting surfaces at different depths.

The transducer produces a pulse perhaps 1 microsecond in duration, and then listens quietly for any echo that might arrive over the next millisecond or so, before transmitting the next pulse. The transducer puts out 1000 pulses per second, typically, but still manages to spend more than 99% of its time acting as a receiver.

Over time t, US passing through tissue at an average velocity c will travel the distance $c \cdot t$. If an echo is detected a time

t_{echo} after pulse transmission, then the interface that caused it lies at a depth of

$$\text{depth} = \tfrac{1}{2}c \cdot t_{echo} \qquad (47.2)$$

The factor of $\tfrac{1}{2}$ arises because the sound has to complete both halves of a round trip before arriving back at the transducer.

A-Mode is still sometimes used in the study of the eye and of the brain (echoencephalography), primarily to reveal midline displacement. But it provides information only on the interfaces along the line of sight of the transducer, and has largely been superseded by B-mode, which generates two-dimensional images.

_____ **EXERCISE 47–1.** _____

A pulse passes through soft tissue and reflects off an interface, and an echo is heard 96 microseconds later. At how great a depth does the reflecting surface lie?

SOLUTION: The velocity of sound in soft tissue is about 1540 m/s, so the US must have traveled a total distance of $(1.54 \times 10^4 \text{ cm/s})(96 \times 10^{-6} \text{ s}) = 14.8$ cm. By Equation 47.2, the depth of the reflecting layer is half of that, or 7.4 cm.

3. M-MODE REVEALS MOTION

With **M-mode**, for motion (also called TM-mode, time–motion), the transducer looks only along a single line through the body, as with A-mode. M-Mode, however, provides a display of the motions of the tissues situated along that line.

As with A-mode, the electron beam of an oscilloscope sweeps once for each transmitted pulse of US. The display for M-mode is rotated 90 degrees from that of A-mode, however, so that the sweep is *vertical*. With M-mode, an echo modulates the point of light's brightness (rather than deflecting it from its vertical sweep). A dot of light appears on the screen only when an echo is being detected, in fact, and is suppressed the rest of the time (i.e., a dot appears in M-mode where a spike would have occurred in A-mode, and the brightness of the dot increases with the amplitude of the spike). Also, instead of retracing exactly over itself, the electron beam steps slightly to the right between consecutive pulses, with a television-like raster pattern. Immobile structures give rise to straight, horizontal lines of closely spaced bright dots. Periodic motions of interfaces are readily revealed as horizontal lines with repetitive vertical displacements (Fig. 47–3).

M-mode has been displaced by real-time B-mode for most applications, but can be of value in the study of processes that vary more rapidly than the B-mode frame rate. It still finds use, in particular, in cardiac studies.

4. AXIAL RESOLUTION IS COMPARABLE TO HALF THE PULSE LENGTH

The spatial resolution achievable with an US beam is determined by the dimensions of the volume occupied by a single pulse.

Axial resolution (along the direction of propagation of the beam) for any pulse-echo mode of US is comparable to half the spatial extent of a pulse:

$$\text{axial resolution} = \text{pulse length}/2 \qquad (47.3)$$

Pulse echoes from surfaces further apart than that will not overlap (Fig. 47–4A) and can be resolved. If the surfaces are separated by less than half a pulse length, on the other hand, the echoes overlap (Fig. 47–4B) and cannot be distinguished. The pulse length, in turn (Fig. 47–5) is determined by the number of cycles in the pulse and the wavelength, λ (of a single cycle),

$$\text{pulse length} = (\text{cycles}/\text{pulse}) \cdot \lambda = f \cdot \Delta t \cdot \lambda \qquad (47.4)$$

where f and Δt are the pulse frequency and duration.

To maximize axial resolution, a brief pulse of short wave-

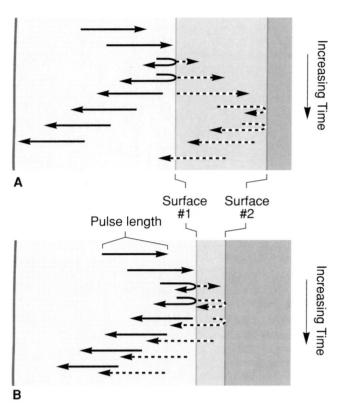

Figure 47–4. Resolution and pulse length. **A.** Echoes from two surfaces do not overlap, and can be resolved, if the depths of the surfaces differ by more than half a pulse length. **B.** But not if the surfaces are closer together than that.

length and high frequency is called for. But most tissues attenuate US at a rate roughly proportional to the frequency (see Equation 45.8a). A short wavelength means rapid attenuation and poor beam penetration into the patient's body. The selection of frequency and transducer for a specific clinical study on a particular patient depends largely on this fundamental trade-off. The need to visualize an organ deep within a large patient requires a low frequency; a requirement for high resolution means using a short wavelength.

EXERCISE 47–2.

Suppose a pulse of 5-MHz US energy is about three wavelengths long. What axial resolution is achievable?

SOLUTION: By Equation 45.3, $\lambda = 0.31$ mm in soft tissue. The pulse length is thus 1 mm, and the resolution is about 0.5 mm.

5. B-MODE DISPLAY PRODUCES A PICTURE OF A SLICE

B-mode has long been the most commonly employed form of ultrasound. Like CT, B-mode uses the two dimensions of display plus a gray scale of light intensity to image a two-dimensional slice of anatomy.

With a modern, **real-time B-mode** system, the relative ori-

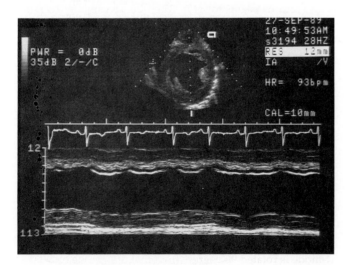

Figure 47–3. B-Mode echocardiogram (parasternal short-axis view of the left ventricle). (**Bottom**) M-Mode image as obtained along the vertical grid of dots in the B-mode image. *(Courtesy of Acuson Corporation.)*

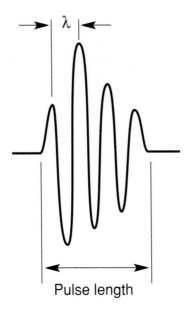

Figure 47–5. Pulse length is determined by the number of cycles ($f \cdot \Delta t$) and the wavelength (λ).

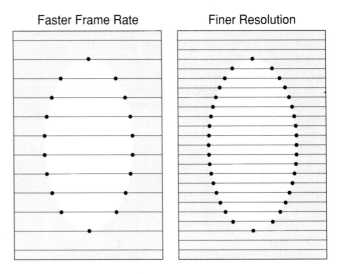

Figure 47–7. Trade-off between resolution and frame rate, as determined by scan line density (beam entering from left).

entation of the US beam within the patient's body is under electronic control (see Chapter 46, Section 7). The beam is swept back and forth perhaps several tens of times per second (which is slow, relative to the pulse repetition rate). Wherever the beam may be at any instant, the system calculates and generates an associated line on the display monitor (Fig. 47–6). The brightness at a point along a display line is proportional to the amount of reflection occurring at the corresponding point in the body: Relatively strong reflections and echoes give rise to bright spots on the line. As the US beam cuts a thin plane through the body, a two-dimensional tomographic image is generated by the brightness-modulated lines of display.

With a sufficiently rapid pulsing sequence and beam sweep, it is possible to produce up to 30 or so frames per second. This *frame rate* is fast enough to follow, for example, the

operation of mitral and tricuspid valves throughout the cardiac cycle.

Lateral resolution is determined by the tomographic thickness of the slice being imaged and by the width of the focused beam within the slice (see Chapter 46, Section 5). Resolutions of the order of a few millimeters are commonly achieved. The axial resolution, on the other hand, depends on the pulse frequency and duration (see Equation 47.3).

There is an inverse relationship between the frame rate of real-time B-mode and spatial resolution. The argument is exactly the same as the one involved in choosing a television raster scan pattern (see Chapter 28, Section 5). A B-mode image is constructed out of a number of individual line traces (Fig. 47–7). The resolution improves (up to a point) with an increase in the number of lines per frame, or *line density*, which typically is somewhere around 100 lines per frame. (The law of diminishing returns begins to set in when the spacing between the

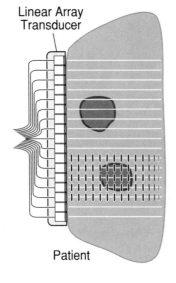

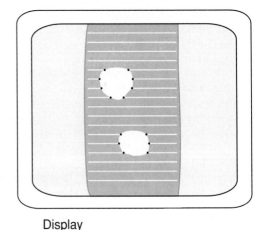

Figure 47–6. One beam-sweep pattern for generating B-mode images. Several adjacent elements in the linear array transducer are, at this instant, producing one tooth of a sideways-stepping comb beam.

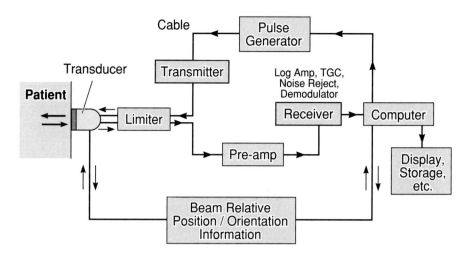

Figure 47–8. Schematic of a computer-controlled B-mode US system, in more detail than Figure 1–15. TGC, time-gain compensation.

lines is made less than the width of the focused beam.) But the same amount of time is required to produce each line trace. So more lines per frame means fewer frames per second.

_____ **EXERCISE 47–3.** _____

You desire to view a region 20 cm deep with 80-line-per-frame resolution. What is the maximum real-time frame rate?

SOLUTION: By Equation 47.2, with a soft tissue velocity of 1540 m/s, it takes 0.00026 second to create one line. The time to generate 80 lines, or 1 frame, is 0.02 second. The maximum frame rate is therefore 50 frames/s.

6. PROCESSING THE ECHO SIGNAL

Figure 47–8 outlines a computer-controlled B-mode US system with somewhat more detail than Figure 1–15.

Appropriately shaped electrical pulses are produced by the *pulse generator* and *transmitter* and sent to the transducer. A *limiter* (also known as a transmit/receive, or TR, switch) prevents high-intensity voltage spikes from entering the sensitive receiver during the pulse transmission phase.

The returning echoes are picked up by the transducer, and, at the limiter, the resulting voltage signal is directed into the *receiver*. A preamplifier may be attached physically close to the transducer and limiter, to eliminate the disruptive effects on weak echo signals caused by the capacitance of the cable linking the transducer to the receiver.

The various echoes that eventually reach the transducer after transmission of a single pulse may differ among themselves in intensity by as much as 100 dB. As with digital angiography, it is advantageous to send the detected signal into a *logarithmic amplifier* stage of the receiver before processing it further. The output voltage from a log amp is proportional to the logarithm of the input voltage (see Fig. 36–4), rather than linearly proportional to the input voltage itself. The amount of signal amplification is greatest for the weakest input signals, and decreases with increasing signal strength. This greatly compresses the range of possible voltages that must be handled by the electronic circuits that follow. Echo pulses that dif-

fer in intensity by the same ratio (regardless of their absolute magnitudes) will give rise to output signals that differ in amplitude by the same voltage. Subtle differences among weak signals are therefore less likely to be lost amidst the much larger variations in the stronger signals (see Chapter 36, Section 2).

The amplitude of a signal returning to the transducer depends not only on the reflection coefficient, R, at the interface where the echo was created, but also on the extent to which the pulse was attenuated during its travels. This is illustrated most easily with A-mode (Fig. 47–9). By the time it returns to the transducer, an echo signal is typically 60 dB (a factor of 10^6) weaker in intensity than the original transmitted pulse, solely because of attenuation (Fig. 47–9B), in addition to losses that occur at tissue boundaries. Unlike the situation in radiography, such attenuation does not contribute to the formation of an image. Indeed, it disguises the value of R, and it makes image construction more difficult.

It is possible, however, to compensate for the reduction in signal intensity caused by attenuation. The electronic system that carries out this task is known variously as **time-gain compensation (TGC)**, *depth-gain compensation (DGC)*, *time-varied gain (TVG)*, or *swept gain*. For each US pulse, the TGC circuit turns up the gain (amount of amplification) of the receiver by an amount that increases continuously with the time elapsed since pulse transmission (Fig. 47–9C). Echoes that are reflected from deeper interfaces and have traveled farther (hence for a longer time) are treated to a correspondingly greater amount of amplification. Although this process cannot compensate exactly for the effects of US attenuation (Fig. 47–9D), it can come close if the speed of sound and the rate of attenuation do not vary too much along the beam path. The *TGC delay control* determines the time at which the gain begins ramping up (Fig. 47–9C) and can be adjusted for optimal image quality. While a default attenuation correction of 1 dB/cm/MHz is generally adopted for all tissues, and 1540 m/s for the speed of sound, availability of a computer allows patient-specific adjustments.

Noise occurs in US echo signals because of reverberations occurring within both the patient's body and the transducer (Fig. 47–10A). It is also produced by the preamplifier. Either way, the signal-to-noise ratio decreases as the echo signal strength goes down, and increasing the *gain* can do nothing to

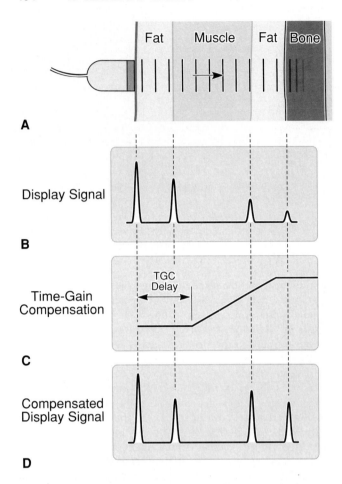

A

Display Signal

B

Time-Gain Compensation

C

Compensated Display Signal

D

Figure 47–9. Time-gain compensation (TGC) accounts for the attenuation of the US beam by the tissues through which it passes. **A.** Echoes as received by a transducer. **B.** The amount of compensation increases with time since pulse transmission, following a (adjustable) delay period. **C.** Compensated echo signals.

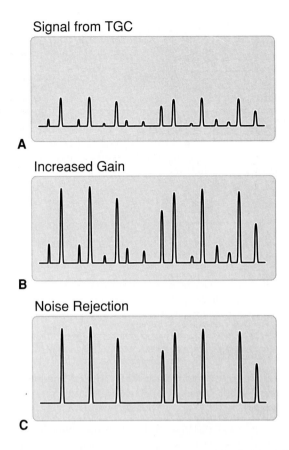

Signal from TGC

A

Increased Gain

B

Noise Rejection

C

Figure 47–10. Processing the echo signals. Echo signals, following (**A**) time-gain compensation (TGC) and (**B**) some amplification. Noise is amplified as well. **C.** Noise rejection eliminates some distracting interference, but possibly some weak, meaningful signals as well.

remedy that situation (Fig. 47–10B). (That is why, despite the TGC, the signal-to-noise may deteriorate with tissue interface depth in the body.) But the *noise reject control* can be adjusted to filter out weak noise signals, with some improvement in image quality (Fig. 47–10C). The danger, of course, is the inadvertent rejection of weak real signals as well.

Now back to B-mode. After passing through the log amp and the TGC and noise reject circuits, the high-frequency echo signal enters the computer (or the digital scan converter if there is no computer). The computer controls everything: It is responsible for the shaping and timing of US pulses; it continually monitors the beam's point of entry into the body and its orientation and, when appropriate, the depth of the focal region; it keeps track of the echo pulses and prepares the image and relevant alphanumeric information for display. Display is typically of a 512 × 512 matrix, 8 bits deep, on a standard, 525-line TV monitor.

Computers are not used as widely with commercial US systems, at present, as with gamma cameras. But computers will doubtless prove effective in enhancing US images through data smoothing and other filtering activities, windowing of the display gray scale, color coding of images, and by other means. It is to be expected, moreover, that ways will be found to ex-

ploit echoes scattered in all directions, not only those reflected straight backward—reconstruction algorithms similar to those of computerized tomography and magnetic resonance imaging might be needed to extract the maximum possible information from such complexities of echo signals.

Most tantalizingly, it also appears that recently developed pattern recognition programs can determine certain pathologic conditions, from statistical studies of tissue image textures, with a reliability comparable to that of experienced diagnosticians.

7. SOME STANDARD IMAGING STUDIES

US has found a broad range of applications. These include (but are not restricted to) studies of the following:

- *Abdomen.* Transabdominal B-mode, typically in the range 3.5 to 5 MHz, is used for a variety of abdominal examinations. Hepatomegaly and changes in US image texture commonly accompany liver diseases (Fig. 47–11). Gallstones and kidney stones larger than 1 mm show up clearly. US is effective in managing acute and chronic pancreatitis and trauma of the pancreas, spleen, and kidneys. B-Mode may reveal bladder tumors, and real-time US may be used in guiding biopsy needles for diagnosis of malignancies of a number of organs.

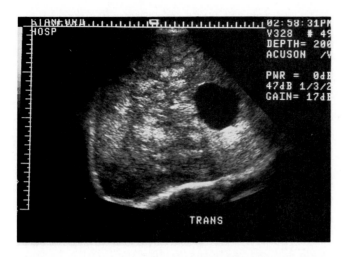

Figure 47–11. B-Mode ultrasound image revealing hepatic metastases, with an adjacent fluid-filled cyst. Note the absence of any structure within the latter. *(Courtesy of Acuson Corporation.)*

- *Breast.* Although not suitable for cancer screening, US has proven capable of differentiating cysts from solid masses found in the breast by physical examination or mammography. Sonography can also provide guidance of a fine needle during biopsy.
- *Fetus* (see Fig. 1–16). US is commonly used to confirm pregnancy, to direct the placement of the aspiration needle during amniocentesis, and to monitor the general development of the fetus. Abnormalities such as microcephaly, hydrocephaly, spina bifida, and some fetal malignancies are readily detectable. Real-time B-mode may reveal irregular fetal movement, and Doppler studies can assess fetal cardiac activity.
- *Eye.* Specialized high-resolution, shallow-penetration (8- to 20-MHz) systems have been developed to measure the thicknesses of the cornea and the lens, to detect intraocular tumors and foreign bodies (some of which may not show up with x-rays), and to diagnose retinal detachment.
- *Brain.* Echoencephalography may indicate a displacement of midline intracerebral structures by various lesions. Although the cranial bone precludes imaging of the adult brain, 3.5- to 7-MHz US can detect cerebral hemorrhaging and other disorders in infants.
- *Cardiovascular system.* In assessing the functioning of the heart, real-time B-mode can map the spatial relations of its constituent parts in two dimensions and locate a valve or wall of interest; after that, M-mode can provide more precise information on the amplitudes and velocities of its motions (see Fig. 47–3). Doppler studies can reveal various abnormalities in the arteries and veins, including cerebrovascular disease, as we shall soon see.

US transducers have been designed for a variety of special purposes (Fig. 47–12). These include endovaginal (for imaging the pelvis and fetus), endorectal (prostate and rectal wall),

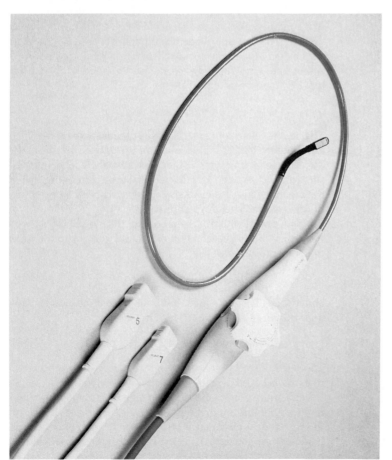

Figure 47–12. Some specialized transducers. The transducer on the long stem, at the top, contains two separate arrays of piezoelectric elements, for biplane (transverse and longitudinal viewing planes) transesophageal echocardiology. It can operate with center frequencies of 7.0, 5.0, and 3.5 MHz, providing a choice of three combinations of beam penetration and resolution. It can also be used for Doppler operation. The middle and lower transducers, which are significantly smaller than standard size, are designed for neonates and pediatrics, respectively. *(Courtesy of Acuson Corporation.)*

and transesophageal (echocardiography) probes. Transducers have also been developed with attached needle assemblies for performing directly guided biopsies. The number of such devices, designed for US guidance during invasive procedures, is bound to grow.

8. DOPPLER TECHNIQUES REVEAL MOTION AND BLOOD FLOW

Know how the whistle of an oncoming train drops in pitch as the engine rushes by you? This is an example of the **Doppler effect.** The same phenomenon can be exploited to reveal information about the flow of blood within the body.

The Doppler effect is a direct consequence of the wave nature of sound. The heart of the issue is the fundamental, geometrically based relationship

$$\lambda \cdot f = v \qquad (47.5)$$

among the wavelength, frequency, and velocity of propagation of any kind of wave.

Imagine that a *stationary source* in a medium produces continuous (not pulsed) monochromatic sound of frequency f_{source} (Fig. 47–13A). The wavefront will radiate outwardly through the medium with speed c, and, according to Equation 47.5, a *stationary observer* nearby will experience a signal of frequency f_{source} and wavelength

$$\lambda = c/f_{source} \qquad \text{(stationary observer)} \qquad (47.6a)$$

But suppose that the *observer* is *moving* toward the station-

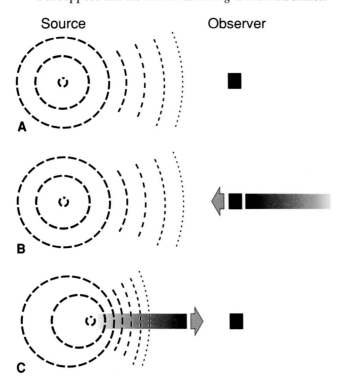

Source   Observer

Figure 47–13. Doppler effect: A shift occurs in the detected frequency when the source and receiver are moving relative to one another. **A.** The source and the observer experience the same frequency when they are not moving relative to one another. But there will appear to be a frequency shift when (**B**) the observer moves or (**C**) the source moves.

ary source with velocity v_{obs} (Fig. 47–13B). He will encounter waves oncoming with an apparent velocity of $(c + v_{obs})$. Nothing changes the wavelength of the US from its original value of λ, however, and, in accordance with Equation 47.5, wave crests strike at the rate

$$f_{obs} = (c + v_{obs})/\lambda \qquad \text{(moving observer)} \qquad (47.6b)$$

per second. That is, the frequency sensed by an observer who is moving toward the source, f_{obs}, is higher than f_{source} by an amount that increases with the observer's speed. (Likewise, if you are in a small boat and move toward oncoming waves, you bob up and down more rapidly than if you stay in one place.) Equation 47.6b can be expressed, with the aid of Equation 47.6a, in terms of f_{source}:

$$f_{obs} = f_{source} \cdot (1 + v_{obs}/c) \qquad (47.7)$$

If the observer is moving away from the source, the apparent frequency, f_{obs}, is shifted downward from f_{source}, and the + in Equation 47.7 is replaced by a minus sign.

The situation in which the *source* (rather than the observer) *moves* is similar. A disturbance produced by the point source at any instant radiates outward, with velocity c, as a spherical wavefront centered at the point, regardless of the motion of the source. But if the source itself shifts position between the generation of consecutive crests, the distance between them (i.e., the wavelength) is less, in the direction of motion, than what would be produced by a stationary source (Fig. 47–13C). Here, too, the frequency sensed by the observer is shifted upward.

All of this applies directly to Doppler blood flow measurement. Focus your attention on a small volume element of fluid that contains cells that can reflect US (Fig. 47–14). Suppose, for now, that the volume element is moving at speed v_{blood} toward a transducer that is producing US of frequency f_{trans}. The blood, acting like a moving "observer" (see Equation 47.7), encounters US wave crests at the rate

$$f_{obs} = f_{trans} \cdot (1 + v_{blood}/c) \qquad (47.8)$$

That is, the cells in our small volume of blood experience US of a frequency that is higher than that produced by the transducer. In reflecting this US, the blood cells themselves now become an US "source." But this new "source" is moving, so that the frequency of the echo signal detected back at the transducer is shifted even further upward.

The overall effect of the motion of the blood is to raise the frequency of the US echo that eventually returns to the transducer by the amount

$$\Delta f = 2 \cdot f_{trans} \cdot (v_{blood}/c) \qquad (47.9a)$$

above f_{trans}. (The frequency shift is negative if the blood is moving away from the transducer.) Equivalently,

$$\Delta f/f_{trans} = \pm 2 \cdot (v_{blood}/c) \qquad (47.9b)$$

The relative shift in frequency thus equals two times the relative (to the speed of sound) velocity of the blood.

The transmitted and reflected signals may undergo interference with one another (see Chapter 4, Section 6). The resulting *beat signal*, of frequency Δf (for blood flowing either toward or away from the transducer), commonly falls within the audible range, and may be detected by ear.

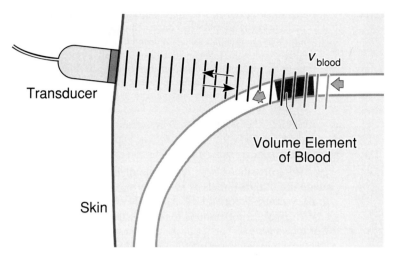

Figure 47–14. Reflection of ultrasound from a small volume element of flowing blood.

EXERCISE 47–4.

Blood flows through a portion of an artery away from a transducer at 15 cm/s. By how much is the frequency of an echo of a 4-MHz signal shifted?

SOLUTION: Inserting $v_{\text{blood}} = 0.15$ m/s, $c = 1540$ m/s, and $f_{\text{trans}} = 4 \times 10^6$ second^{-1} into Equation 47.9a yields $\Delta f_{\text{trans}} = -780$ Hz. Since the blood is moving away from the transducer, the frequency shift is downward.

EXERCISE 47–5.

A 3.2-kHz beat signal is heard from flowing blood with a 5-MHz Doppler system. What is the blood velocity?

SOLUTION: By Equation 47.9a, $v_{\text{blood}} = 0.5$ m/s.

In general, echoes are caused by blood moving through a vessel at an angle θ to the US beam, rather than directly toward it. Equation 47.9b then becomes

$$\Delta f / f_{\text{trans}} = 2 \cdot (v_{\text{blood}}/c) \cdot \cos \theta$$

Signals may come from different volumes of blood flowing in a number of directions, which clearly complicates things. Instead of a single beat frequency, a complex of echo signals are produced.

Medical *Doppler US* systems are of two general kinds, **continuous wave (CW)** and **pulsed.** With CW Doppler, the transducer consists of two separate piezoelectric crystals. One of these transmits a continuous, fairly narrow band (nearly monochromatic) signal, and the other continuously monitors the reflected signal. As there is no pulsing, there can be no depth resolution, but measurements of velocity are fairly accurate. The range and distribution of flow velocities occurring within a selected (under B-mode) volume of fluid can be displayed as a spectrum.

Pulsed Doppler allows for some axial resolution, but at a price. The shorter a pulse, the greater the spread of frequencies of the waves that go into its makeup (see Chapter 45, Section 3). Therefore, there is more imprecision in f_{trans} in Equation 47.9 than with CW Doppler. *Color-flow US* is a recent hybrid in which blood flow information is encoded in color and superimposed on a B-mode gray scale image, and perhaps accompanied by a spectral analysis.

The Doppler effect occurs not only with sound waves, but also with electromagnetic radiation. It is responsible for the *red shift* (to lower frequencies) of the light emitted from stars that are moving away from the solar system. And Doppler *radar* can determine the velocities of cars or planes.

9. QUALITY ASSURANCE

It is important, of course, to maintain image quality and ensure patient safety with a proper ultrasound quality assurance program. A variety of beam, receiver, display, and other parameters should be tested with the purchase of new equipment and routinely thereafter, to confirm that contrast, resolution, signal-to-noise, and general clinical performance are optimal (Fig. 47–15).

Protocols of checks and measurements have been established to that end, perhaps the most widely cited of these being that of the American Institute of Ultrasound in Medicine (AIUM). The interested reader is referred to the AIUM's publication *Quality Assurance in Diagnostic Ultrasound* for details.

10. PATIENT SAFETY

Early in the development of SONAR (sound navigation and ranging) for antisubmarine warfare, it was discovered that intense bursts of sound energy are capable of killing fish and other small animals. Since that time, the effects of US on all sorts of living organisms have been studied extensively, in vivo and in vitro, and at least three distinct mechanisms have been found that are capable of causing harm.

At the high levels of power employed in industry (in the search for faults in metal castings, for example), US can cause *cavitation* in a fluid (the creation and immediate, violent implosion of microscopic vacuum bubbles). Although cavitation can be destructive of tissues, it is believed not to occur in humans at the intensities employed medically.

The *heating* of tissues by US may cause a significant in-

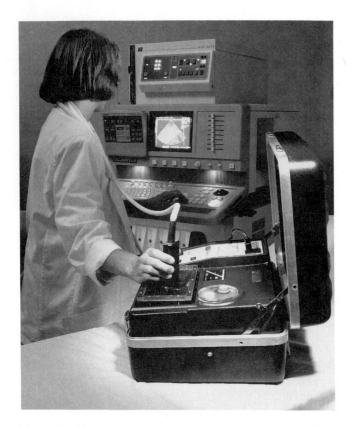

Figure 47–15. This Doppler quality assurance phantom and fluid control system can mimic the constant (venous) and pulsed (arterial) flow of blood through soft tissue. *(Courtesy of RMI.)*

crease in the local tissue temperature. Indeed, this phenomenon underlies the use of US in physical therapy for various joint and soft-tissue ailments and in the hyperthermia treatment of cancer. The temperature rise is potentially dangerous if not properly controlled. The degree to which US heating can be a problem with imaging is an issue of concern to some workers in the field.

Finally, US is capable of exerting significant sheering and twisting forces on small exposed objects. The spinning of intracellular particles and the *acoustic streaming* of cellular contents in ultrasound fields have been observed. These findings (together with some indications of US-induced increased incidence of fetal abnormalities and other effects in test mammals) suggest that there *might* be mechanisms capable of causing harm in humans even at low levels of exposure. There is no strong evidence, however, suggesting that harmful mechanisms such as these, or others yet unknown, actually *do* exist at diagnostic levels.

Following a review of bioeffects data, in 1987 the AIUM concluded:

In the low megahertz frequency range there have been (as of this date) no independently confirmed significant biological effects in mammalian tissues exposed in vivo to unfocused ultrasound with intensities[a] below 100 mW/cm^2, or to focused[b] ultrasound with intensities below 1 W/cm^2. Furthermore, for exposure times[c] greater than 1 second and less than 500 seconds for unfocused ultrasound or 50 seconds for focused ultrasound, such effects have not been demonstrated even at higher intensities, when the product of intensity and exposure time is less than 50 joules/cm^2.*

The intensities below which biologic effects are believed not to occur in mammals exposed in vivo are those beneath the broken line in Figure 46–14. Also indicated are typical intensity/duration combinations for both pulse-echo imaging and Doppler systems. The I_{STPA}/dwell time combination exceeds 50 J/cm^2 with some peripheral vascular Doppler methods.

Epidemiologic studies involving the accumulated clinical experience point to the safety of the modality. Over half of all pregnant women in the United States undergo at least one ultrasound examination during the pregnancy, and there is no firm evidence of any clinically induced adverse effects. But long delayed effects, genetic effects that would be expressed only in future generations, and certain subtle effects may well have been missed.

Having carefully examined the experimental and epidemiologic evidence, in 1988 the AIUM issued the following Official Statement on Clinical Safety:*

No confirmed biological effects on patients or instrument operators caused by exposure at intensities typical of present diagnostic ultrasound instruments have ever been reported. Although the possibility exists that such biological effects may be identified in the future, current data indicate that the benefits to patients of the prudent use of diagnostic ultrasound outweigh the risks, if any, that may be present.

To summarize: Although it is extremely difficult to prove such a thing beyond the shadow of a doubt, diagnostic US is widely held to be biologically safe. Further epidemiologic studies of US imaging (in particular, of the unborn) are currently underway, and it is hoped that these will support our faith in the modality. But still, as with any other clinical procedure, it would be prudent to employ US imaging (especially of the fetus) only if there are good medical reasons to do so.

---

*American Institute of Ultrasound in Medicine, Bioeffects Committee: Bioeffects considerations for the safety of diagnostic ultrasound. *J Ultrasound Med.* 1988; 2(suppl), Tables 1.4 and 1.5. Footnote *a* defines the intensity as the free-field I_{SPTA} for CW exposures and for pulsed operation with a pulse repetition frequency greater than 100 Hz. Footnote *b* specifies the width of a focused beam. Footnote *c* notes that exposure time is to include power-off time for pulsed US.

Part 11

Computer-Based Image Handling Networks

Chapter 48

PACS, IMACs, and the Totally Digital Department

1. **The Move Toward PACS**
2. **Organization of a PACS and of an IMAC System**
3. **Artificial Intelligence and Computer-Assisted Diagnosis**
4. **To IMAC or Not to IMAC?**

A picture archiving and communication system (PACS) increases the speed and reliability with which images can be stored, retrieved from storage, displayed, and moved from place to place. And a complete image management and communication (IMAC) system provides ready access to all pertinent patient information, not only images, that may enhance significantly the diagnostic value of the images themselves.

Many heads of radiology departments and hospital administrators have decided, despite the significant complexity and cost, and the rapid evolution of the technology, that they should go digital. They are less certain about how, how much, and when.

1. THE MOVE TOWARD PACS

An imaging department exists primarily to provide a critically important, highly specialized service to other physicians and patients.

Referring physicians may tend to view radiology as something of a black box: In goes the patient, and out comes a report or diagnosis and some film. They generally have little understanding of, or interest in, the sophisticated technology by which the image information is produced and processed. What they care about is diagnostic accuracy and speed, and perhaps they would like to glance at the final pictures. What makes a strong impression on them is the time taken to get to the radiology viewing area and then, after a considerable delay, the embarrassed admission that the films are signed out to Dr. Jones, who is in Burkina Faso for the next 3 weeks. It helps little to point out that the department produces a million images a year, and that

the logistics of keeping track of such volumes of information can be horrendous.

In the early 1980s, it became apparent to researchers and hospital administrators in the United States, Europe, and Japan that computer-based **picture archiving and communications systems (PACS),** also known as digital imaging networks (DIN), could turn that kind of ugly situation around. A digital image can be stored in a compact memory device from which, barring a major catastrophe, it cannot be lost. The image file for a patient can be retrieved in a matter of seconds (as, perhaps, could the files for all patients exhibiting specific characteristics, for research purposes). Images can be transmitted rapidly to different locations within the hospital, such as viewing terminals in the intensive care unit, physicians' offices, and classrooms, or over long distances. And unlike hard copy, digital images can be windowed by the viewer to emphasize particular clinical aspects, and in other ways massaged.

But despite the obvious need for and apparent feasibility of PACS, some of the early enthusiasm gave way to a sense that it simply does not do enough to justify the effort and expense (typically $5 million dollars for a 500-hundred-bed center) involved in setting it up. In particular, in many situations an image is fully useful only if other information on the patient's clinical condition is present, as well. And in the early days, it proved difficult to couple a system that deals primarily with image data with one that handles clinical records, such as a radiology information system (RIS) or a hospital information system (HIS). Early PACS processed pictures, but not much else, and that wasn't enough. At the same time, there were serious problems with management of the sheer volumes of data produced and required by a busy department and with limited access speed.

Finally, there arose (and remains) the concern that if images are widely accessible, they will be interpreted by physicians with less than adequate training and experience in the art.

But the needed technology has matured. And standards and conventions for interfacing data acquisition and other devices to a computer network, and for storage and communication of all files, are under development. The American Association of Physicists in Medicine (AAPM), the American College of Radiology and the National Electrical Manufacturers Association (ACR/NEMA), the authors of the Integrated Services Digital Network (ISDN), and other groups have been constructing standardized systems of electrical signals and hardware to allow for the **connectivity** of all kinds of imaging devices and database management systems. It is to be expected that eventually, one of these systems will become universally accepted.

As a result, the end of the 1980s saw a renaissance in efforts to bring clinically useful and cost-effective **image management and communication (IMAC)** systems on line. Known also as *I&IM* or *I2M (information and image management)* systems and by other such acronyms, these are intended to provide the referring physician or specialist with instantaneous access to all patient information—not only pictures from every imaging modality, but also a patient's complete record.

2. ORGANIZATION OF A PACS AND OF AN IMAC SYSTEM

The fundamental balance to be struck in the design of IMAC architecture, as with many political and social systems, is between central control and local independence. There is need both for universal access to a central computer system, on the one hand, and for decentralized, stand-alone data acquisition devices and their local workstations and computers, on the other. There are various of ways of achieving this (Fig. 48–1).

A typical *star* configuration is shown in greater detail in Figure 48–2. At the center of the star is a large computer and database management system. A rudimentary PACS (which handles pictures alone, and only locally) comprises, in addition, the individual image acquisition devices and their display and manipulation workstations, each under the control of its own dedicated personal computer (PC); the long-term archive, that is, permanent memory; hard-copy devices; and perhaps some capability for image communication within or near the hospital. A complete IMAC would include, above and beyond that, more sophisticated physician workstations; more flexible teleradiology channels; direct tie-ins to and from the radiology department's RIS and the hospital's HIS; remote (from radiol-

ogy) viewing stations within or near the hospital; and perhaps artificial intelligence (AI) programs that can be applied to all components of the PACS.

The initial generation of images occurs at *acquisition nodes* or *modules*. Digital imaging begins with the generation of an analog voltage signal by a signal receptor. In digital angiography, the detection system might consist of an image intensifier coupled to a TV camera; in computed tomography, it is an array of xenon or fluorescent detectors; in magnetic resonance imaging, a radio-frequency pickup coil. In each case, the voltage output is a radiation-induced signal that reflects on tissue characteristics along a line, on a plane, or within a volume within the patient. The analog detector signal must be digitized, and the speed of analog-to-digital (A/D) conversion is a critically important issue. The image is reconstructed or otherwise processed, typically with the aid of an array processor, and transformed into a matrix of pixel values directly corresponding to tissue parameters at different points in the body. The digital image feeds into an interactive display and manipulation workstation, under the control of its own dedicated local computer, with its own disk storage. Thus, an acquisition node, like the other components of a PACS, has its own processing and storage capability and should continue to operate even when disconnected from rest of the system, such as when the central computer is down.

The *central computer* and *database management system* are housed typically in the radiology department. They contain on-line archiving—moderate-volume magnetic hard-disk storage—that allows rapid access to the files of patients currently under examination. In essence, this replaces the view box alternator of the nondigital department. Access time is limited by the speed with which vast volumes of digital information (of the order of a million bytes per image) can be communicated between memory and the workstation. The development of such systems may be influenced by advances in general computer science, such as the development of much faster semiconductor or optical computer circuits, and the reduction in the cost of *supercomputers*, which can perform a billion or more arithmetic operations per second.

Long-term storage for most clinical computer systems consists of film *hard copy* and of magnetic tape and floppy devices to back up the magnetic disks. *Optical disks* and optical tape are relative newcomers and involve technologies that are still evolving at a fast pace, but they have considerably greater capacity than their magnetic counterparts. Typical amounts of storage required per image and per study by the standard digital imaging modalities are sketched in Table 48–1; the storage capabilities of archiving devices were listed in Table 35–4.

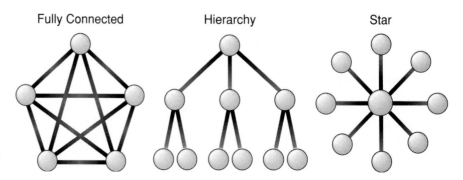

Fully Connected   Hierarchy   Star

Figure 48–1. Three of the ways in which information can be made to flow in a local area network (LAN).

Rudimentary PACS

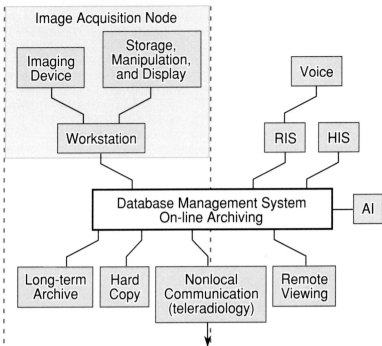

Figure 48–2. An image management and communication (IMAC) system in the "star" configuration. The imaging devices and workstations (each of which is under minicomputer control) and the other components all connect to a central computer.

Digital *communication* is incomparably faster and safer than mailing or carrying a film, and relatively immune to electrical noise. Within a hospital, digital signals are most commonly sent *on-line* by coaxial cable. (They can also be carried around *off-line* in the form of floppy disks.) For communication over greater distances, *modems* (modulate–demodulate) may be used (with acoustic or direct electronic coupling) to transmit over normal telephone lines, typically at rates of 2400 or 9600 "baud" (bits per second). Substantially higher transmission rates (up to 2 Mbit/s) can be achieved with special "T1" telephone lines and with microwave (plus geosynchronous Earth satellite, if needed) channels. Fiberoptic transmission has a carrying capacity much greater yet and other desirable features as well, and its use is growing rapidly.

The attractiveness of a PACS increases greatly when its *local area network* (*LAN*) ties in with the radiology department's RIS or the hospital's HIS, creating an IMAC system. This makes immediately available, along with any images, the patient's complete medical record, including dictated notes, graphs of clinical parameters, lab results, pathology images (perhaps obtained with a television camera attached to a microscope), heart sounds, electrocardiogram, etc. When the file of an inpatient is called up, the system might provide a report

on current medical status and draw attention to unusual clinical considerations. It could present the current differential diagnosis or, at the proposal of a drug or treatment, provide appropriate warnings.

It is helpful to situate *remote viewing stations* in critical care units, outpatient clinics, offices, classrooms, and other places where referring physicians and others can easily get to them. Users would be able, from a single workstation, to display and manipulate images acquired at any node. Although they would have no control over image acquisition parameters (of especial importance in magnetic resonance imaging), they would have access to user-friendly window level and width adjustments, zoom control, distance, and other quantitative measurement capabilities.

3. ARTIFICIAL INTELLIGENCE AND COMPUTER-ASSISTED DIAGNOSIS

The primary contribution of an IMAC will probably be, at least for a while, to increase greatly the speed and flexibility with which a radiology department can acquire, store, transmit, and display information. It will thereby allow radiologists to spend

TABLE 48–1. TYPICAL MEMORY REQUIREMENTS FOR THE VARIOUS DIGITAL IMAGING MODALITIES

Imaging Modality	Matrix (bits)	Depth (bits)	Mbyte/Image	Mbyte/Study
Computed tomography	512 × 512	11	0.4	8
Magnetic resonance imaging	512 × 512	8	0.3	5
Nuclear medicine	128 × 128	8	0.02	0.4
Ultrasound	512 × 512	8	0.3	10
Digital subtraction angiography	1024 × 1024	12	1.5	20
Digital radiography	2048 × 2048	12	6	20

more time and energy in their proper roles of image interpretation and consultation. But it can, and eventually will, do much more than that.

An IMAC system can link together different kinds of data acquisition nodes and make possible the integration of different forms of image information for composite display. Positron emission tomography (PET) images, for example, are low in resolution but potentially rich in revealed physiology and pathology; the diagnostic utility of PET may be enhanced when its images can be readily and routinely displayed superimposed on high-resolution anatomic maps generated by computed tomography or magnetic resonance imaging. An important aspect of this is the computer's causing the images from the two sources to be properly registered in three dimensions.

IMAC systems can also incorporate various types of computer-based "knowledge" support. *Artificial intelligence* (*AI*) and a variety of related computer-based analytical technologies are still in early stages of development. It is not unreasonable to assume, however, that their eventual impact on imaging (indeed, on all of medicine) over the next few decades will be profound.

Spoken words are signals that are functions of only one variable, time. And, as with electrocardiograms, considerable progress has been made in computer recognition of patterns in such one-dimensional "images." Commercial speech-processing computer systems are already available. As radiologists in the United States generate some 130 million reports annually, the ability of a computer to transcribe dictation could have a tremendous economic impact. Also, a voice is as distinctive as a fingerprint, and voice identification may greatly enhance patient file security. This is of growing importance, because concern about the confidentiality of medical information and the possibility of unauthorized access to it are both on the rise.

Searching for clinically significant patterns in two- or three-dimensional images is much more difficult. But computer programs already in existence can perform statistical analyses of the distribution of shapes and sizes of entities within a region, such as of the apparent texture of a tissue. Comparison with previously stored characteristics of normal and pathologic tissues can then, in some situations, provide a tentative diagnosis automatically. Programs have been developed that recognize, with fairly high reliability, the characteristic spatial patterns in radiographs of some lung and breast pathologies. Ultrasound of the liver has had similar successes. But the subtlety of many of the clinically significant variations in detail and contrast, together with the great range in normal and abnormal patterns occurring among different individuals, makes the general problem of automated diagnosis extremely challenging. It is unlikely that much of it will be seen in the clinic in the near future.

Other programs, the so-called *expert systems*, attempt to mimic the actual thought processes employed by physicians in decision making: They consider the implications of the evidence at hand, weigh the probability of correctness of each possible explanation, demand from the physician more information to reduce the range of possibilities, and generally propose and test hypotheses.

But although computers are ideally suited for carrying out some of the higher mental activities that we learn later on in life, such as logic and mathematics, they have a much harder time with the more intuitive commonsense and visual skills that play so important a role in radiologic diagnosis. Computers are not clever at coping with situations where "if–then" rules and tests do not clearly apply. We have little understanding of the thought processes involved in acquiring and drawing on a holistic knowledge of the world, and just as little ability to model and mimic those processes with an expert system program.

Still, what has been achieved since the 1970s, when AI programs first appeared on the scene, is impressive. And recent developments such as *neural networks*, which are programs that use feedback information from humans to "learn" decision rules from their own mistakes (without "understanding" the reasons for them) are enticing and promising. Pattern recognition and computer-based diagnosis in general are among the most demanding but exciting areas of research to be found in medicine. And where it all will lead should be of interest to every physician.

4. TO IMAC OR NOT TO IMAC?

The advocates of PACS and IMAC systems assert that their current and potential flexibility, speed, and efficiency will lead (if not now, then soon) to greater clinical accuracy and better overall health care, to greater accountability, and to reduced physician frustration. Such systems help to make the patient well in less time and possibly at less cost. An investment in an IMAC system offers payoffs, they feel, both to the patient and to the hospital.

But acquisition of an IMAC system involves not only direct costs, but also a certain element of risk. If the system is inadequate, or so complicated as to discourage its use, or lacking in technical support personnel, it may fail to do its appointed job. And that could lead to a significant financial burden and loss of credibility. So many heads of radiology departments and hospital administrators are wrestling mightily with the question of whether or not to invest in an IMAC system and, if so, what kind.

There is no correct system that satisfies all needs. What works well for a large consortium of medical institutions will be quite different from what is suited for the small clinic or local hospital. Indeed, as with any other major purchase, it is critical to know one's needs and what one really could use effectively. Only then is it meaningful to consider the price (in dollars, new personnel, and the psychological stress from a radically new and perhaps threatening technology) one is willing to pay to accrue those benefits.

If the prospect of acquiring a whole IMAC system is appealing but somewhat daunting, a good strategy might be a phased-in conversion to digital. Start small and add on a few blocks at a time. Indeed, one of the characteristic strengths of a modern IMAC system is the *modularity* of its constituent parts. Bits and pieces that individually contribute somewhat will, over time, come together to form a system whose potential may eventually far exceed that of the sum of its parts.

References

American Association of Physicists in Medicine (AAPM), New York.
—Monograph No. 10: The physics of nuclear medicine, recent advances. Rao D, Chandra R, Graham, M (eds); 1984.
—Monograph No. 11: Electronic imaging in medicine. Fullerton GD, Hendee W, Lasher J, et al. (eds); 1984.
—Monograph No. 12: Recent developments in digital imaging. Doi K, Lanzl L, Lin P (eds); 1984.
—Monograph No. 14: NMR in medicine—The instrumentation and clinical applications. Thomas SR, Dixon RL (eds); 1986.
—Monograph No. 18: Expanding the role of medical physics in nuclear medicine. Frey GD, Yester MV (eds); 1989.
—Monograph No. 20: Specification, acceptance testing and quality control of diagnostic x-ray imaging equipment. Seibert JA, Barnes GT, Gould GG (eds); 1992.
—Report No. 14: Performance specifications and acceptance testing for x-ray generators and automatic exposure control devices; 1985.
—Report No. 15: Performance evaluation and quality assurance in digital subtraction angiography; 1985.
—Report No. 18: A primer on low-level ionizing radiation and its biological effects; 1986.
—Report No. 20: Site planning for magnetic resonance imaging systems; 1987.
—Report No. 22: Rotation scintillation camera SPECT acceptance testing and quality control; 1987.
—Report No. 25: Protocols for the radiation safety surveys of diagnostic radiological equipment; 1988.
—Report No. 28: Quality assurance methods and phantoms for magnetic resonance imaging; 1990.
—Report No. 29: Equipment requirements and quality control for mammography; 1990.
—Report No. 31: Standardized methods for measuring diagnostic x-ray exposures; 1990.
—Report No. 33: Staffing levels and responsibilities in diagnostic radiology; 1991.
American College of Medical Physics (ACMP), Reston, VA.
—ACMP Report No. 1: Radiation control and quality assurance surveys—Diagnostic radiology. A suggested protocol; 1986.
—ACMP Report No. 3: Radiation control and quality assurance surveys—Nuclear medicine. A suggested protocol; 1986.
American College of Radiology (ACR) Reston, VA, and American Association of Physicists in Medicine (AAPM), New York.
—The physics of diagnostic radiology—Syllabus and study guide, 4th ed. 1987.

American Institute of Ultrasound in Medicine (AIUM).
—Goldstein A: Quality assurance in diagnostic ultrasound—A quality assurance manual for the clinical user; 1980.
—Safety considerations for diagnostic ultrasound; 1984.
—Bioeffects considerations for the safety of diagnostic ultrasound, *J Ultrasound*, Vol 7 (supplement); 1988.
Anderson, DW: *Absorption of Ionizing Radiation*. Baltimore, MD: University Park Press; 1984.
Attix FH: *Introduction to Radiological Physics and Radiation Dosimetry*. New York: Wiley; 1986.
Barrett H, Swindell W: *Radiological Imaging—The Theory of Image Formation, Detection, and Processing*, 2 Vols. New York: Academic; 1981.
Cameron JR, Skofronick JG: *Medical Physics*. New York: Wiley; 1978.
Carrington A, McLachlan AD: *Introduction to Magnetic Resonance—with Applications to Chemistry and Chemical Physics*. New York: Harper & Row; 1987.
Chandra R: *Introductory Physics of Nuclear Medicine*, 2nd ed. Philadelphia, PA: Lea & Febiger; 1982.
Chen C-N, Hoult DI: *Biomedical Magnetic Resonance Technology*. New York: Adam Hilger; 1989.
Conference of Radiation Control Program Directors (CRCPD).
—CRCPD Publication 87-4: Mammography Screening Guide; 1987.
—CRCPD Publication 88-5: Average Patient Exposure Guides; 1988.
—CRCPD Publication 92-4: Average Patient Exposure/Dose Guides; 1992.
—Suggested State Regulations for the Control of Radiation (SSRCR).
Curry TS III, Dowdey JE, Murry RC Jr: *Christensen's Physics of Diagnostic Radiology*, 4th ed. Philadelphia, PA: Lea & Febiger; 1990.
Dainty JC, Shaw R: *Image Science*. New York: Academic; 1975.
Eisberg, R., Resnick, R: *Quantum Physics—Of Atoms, Molecules, Solids, Nuclei, and Particles*, 2nd ed. New York: Wiley; 1985.
Farrar TC: *An Introduction to Pulse NMR Spectroscopy*, Revised ed. Washington, DC: Farragut Press; 1989.
Gray JE, Winkler NT, Stears J, Frank ED: *Quality Control in Diagnostic Imaging*. Baltimore, MD: University Park Press; 1983.
Hall EJ: *Radiology for the Radiologist*, 2nd ed. Hagerstown, MD: Harper & Row; 1978.
Hendee WR, Ritenour ER: *Medical Imaging Physics*—3rd ed. St. Louis: Mosby Year Book; 1992.
Hendee WR, (ed). *The Selection and Performance of Radiologic Equipment*. Baltimore, MD: Williams and Wilkins; 1985.

Hunter TB: *The Computer in Radiology.* Rockville, MD: Aspen; 1986.

International Commission on Radiation Units and Measurements (ICRU), Bethesda, MD.

—ICRU Report 33: Radiation quantities and units; 1980.

—ICRU Report 41: Modulation transfer function of screen–film systems; 1986.

International Commission on Radiological Protection (ICRP). New York: Pergamon.

—ICRP Publication 26: Recommendations of the ICRP; 1977.

—ICRP Publication 57: Summary of the Current ICRP Principles for Protection of the Patient in Diagnostic Radiology; 1989.

—ICRP Publication 60: Recommendations of the ICRP; 1991.

Johns HE, Cunningham JR. *The Physics of Radiology,* 4th ed. Springfield, IL. Charles C. Thomas; 1983.

Joint Commission on Accreditation of Health Care Organizations (JCAHO), Oak Brook, IL.

—Standards of the Joint Commission on Accreditation of Health Care Organizations relating to diagnostic radiographic services; 1990.

Knoll GF: *Radiation Detection and Measurement.* New York: Wiley; 1979.

Kruger RA, Riederer SJ: *Basic Concepts of Digital Subtraction Angiography.* Boston: G.K. Hall; 1984.

Kuni CC: *Introduction to Computers & Digital Processing in Medical Imaging.* St. Louis: Yearbook Medical Publishers; 1988.

National Academy of Sciences, National Research Council (NAS/NRC), Washington, DC.

—Report of the Advisory Committee on the Biological Effects of Ionizing Radiations (BEIR V); 1990.

National Council on Radiation Protection and Measurements (NCRP), Bethesda, MD.

—NCRP Report No. 74: Biological effects of ultrasound: Mechanisms and clinical implications; 1983.

—NCRP Report No. 85: Mammography: A user's guide; 1986.

—NCRP Report No. 91: Recommendations on limits for exposure to ionizing radiation; 1987.

—NCRP Report No. 93: Ionizing radiation exposure of the population of the United States; 1987.

—NCRP Report No. 99: Quality assurance for diagnostic imaging equipment; 1988.

—NCRP Report No. 100: Exposure of the U.S. population from diagnostic medical radiation; 1989.

—NCRP Report No. 102: Medical x-ray, electron beam, and gamma-ray protection for energies up to 50 MeV (Equipment design, performance, and use); 1989.

—NCRP Report No. 105: Radiation protection for medical and allied health personnel; 1989.

National Electrical Manufacturer's Association (NEMA), Washington, DC.

—Standards Publication No. XR 8-1979: Test methods for diagnostic x-ray machines for use during initial installation; 1979.

—Standards Publication No. NU1: Performance measurements of scintillation cameras; 1986.

Osborne A, Bunnell D: *An Introduction to Microcomputers, Volume 0—The Beginner's Book,* 3rd ed. Berkeley, CA: Osborne/McGraw-Hill; 1982.

Osborne A: *An Introduction to Microcomputers, Volume 1—Basic Concepts,* 2nd ed. Berkeley, CA: Osborne/McGraw-Hill; 1980.

Parker JA: Image Reconstruction in Radiology. Boca Raton, FL: CRC Press; 1990.

Schultz RJ: *Diagnostic X-ray Physics.* Vista, CA: GAF; 1977.

Sears FW, Zemansky MW, Young HD: *University Physics,* 6th ed. Redding, MA: Addison-Wesley; 1982.

Segre E. *From X-rays to Quarks—Modern Physicists and Their Discoveries.* New York: W.H. Freeman; 1980.

Shapiro J: *Radiation Protection: A Guide for Scientists and Physicians,* 2nd ed. Cambridge, MA: Harvard; 1981.

Smith H-J, Ranallo FN: *A Nonmathematical Approach to Basic MRI.* Madison, WI: Medical Physics Publishing; 1989.

Sorenson JA, Phelps ME: *Physics in Nuclear Medicine.* Philadelphia: Grune & Stratton; 1980.

Sprawls P, Jr: *Physical Principles of Medical Imaging.* Rockville, MD: Aspen; 1987.

Thompson TT: *A Practical Approach to Modern Imaging Equipment,* 2nd ed. Boston: Little, Brown; 1985.

Trevert E: *Something About X-rays for Everybody* (1896). Reprinted by Medical Physics Publishing Co, Madison, WI; 1988.

United Nations Scientific Committee on the Effects of Atomic Radiation (UNSCEAR), New York: United Nations.

—Sources, effects, and risks of ionizing radiation; 1988.

U.S. Department of Health and Human Services, Food and Drug Administration (FDA), Washington, DC.

—Organ doses in diagnostic radiology, by Rosenstein M. HEW Publication (FDA) 76-8030; 1976.

—Procedures to minimize diagnostic x-ray exposure of the human embryo and fetus. HHS Publication (FDA) 81-8178; 1981.

—An overview of ultrasound: Theory, measurement, medical applications, and biological effects, by Stewart HF, Stratmeyer ME (eds). HHS Publication (FDA) 82-8190; 1982.

—A basic quality assurance program for small diagnostic radiological facilities, by Burkhart RL. HHS Publication (FDA) 83-8218; 1983.

—Handbook of selected tissue doses for projections common in diagnostic radiology, by Rosenstein M. HHS Publication (FDA) 89-8031; 1988.

—Regulations published in the *Federal Register,* and compiled in the Code of Federal Regulations at 21 CFR 1000 and 21 CFR 1020; Washington, DC: Government Printing Office; 1989.

U.S. Nuclear Regulatory Commission (NRC) Washington, DC: Government Printing Office.

—Regulations published in the *Federal Register,* and compiled in the Code of Federal Regulations at 10 CFR 20 (1991).

Webb S (ed): *The Physics of Medical Imaging.* Philadelphia, PA: Adam Hilger; 1988.

Webster JG (ed): *Encyclopedia of Medical Devices and Instrumentation,* 4 Vols. New York: Wiley; 1988.

Wells PNT: *Biomedical Ultrasonics.* New York: Academic; 1977.

Some Symbols and Units

A	Ampere (electric current) (45)	
Å	Angstrom (length) (52)	
A	area (158)	
A	attenuation factor (radiation safety) (260)	
Al	aluminum (X-ray beam filtration, quality) (93)	
A(t)	activity (338)	
a	acceleration (30)	
B	Bucky factor (174)	
B	magnetic field (364)	
Bq	becquerel (activity) (337)	
C	coulomb (charge) (31)	
C	capacitance (72)	
C	contrast (149)	
°C	degree centigrade (temperature) (31)	
c-	centi- (10^{-2})	
c	speed of light (39)	
c	speed of sound (410)	
c	specific heat (47)	
cGy	centigray (dose, kerma)	
Ci	curie (activity) (337)	
D	dose (49)	
D	diameter (234)	
d	voxel dimension (320)	
dB	decibel (411)	
E	energy (42)	
EDE	effective dose equivalent (288)	
ESE	entrance skin exposure (269)	
e	2.718 . . . (119)	
e	charge on electron (36)	
eV	electron volt (energy) (44)	
F	force (31)	
F	focal spot size (196)	
FWHM	full width at half maximum (152)	
FOV	field of view (320)	
f	frequency (39)	
f_{med}	exposure-to-dose factor (267)	
g	acceleration due to gravity (32)	
Gy	gray (dose, kerma) (49)	
H	dose equivalent (279)	
H	Hounsfield (CT) number (321)	
HU	heat unit (90)	
Hz	Hertz (frequency) (39)	
h	Planck's constant (51)	
I	electric current (45)	
I	intensity (95)	

ID	information density (353)	
J	Joule (energy) (42)	
K	Kelvin (temperature) (21)	
K-	electron shell closest to nucleus (55)	
K	kerma (96)	
K	compressibility (410)	
k-	kilo- (10^3)	
keV	kilo-electron volt	
kg	kilogram (mass) (31)	
HVL	half value layer thickness (123)	
kVp	peak kilovoltage (71)	
L	light intensity (141)	
LET	linear energy transfer (278)	
log	common logarithm (base 10) (121)	
ln	natural logarithm (base e) (120)	
lp/mm	resolution (line pairs per millimeter) (150)	
M-	mega- (10^6)	
M	magnification (193)	
M	matrix size (320)	
M	magnetization (371)	
MTF	modulation transfer function (209)	
m-	milli- (10^{-3})	
m	meter (length, distance) (31)	
m	mass (31)	
mA	milliampere (electric current)	
mA	current through x-ray tube (71)	
mm	millimeter	
ms	millisecond (time)	
mSv	millisievert (dose equivalent)	
m_e	electron mass (36)	
N	newton (force) (31)	
N	number of counts, spins, etc. (153)	
N_a	Avogadro's number (36)	
N_{EX}	number of excitations (399)	
n	principal quantum number (52)	
n	number of photons (107)	
OD	optical density (141)	
P(A)	probability (111)	
p(A)	ray sum (323)	
PDD	percent depth dose (131)	
PSF	point spread function (152)	
Q	radiation quality factor (279)	

Q	sharpness of resonance (420)	
q	electric charge (35)	
R	electrical resistance (60)	
R	roentgen (exposure) (96)	
R	resolution (332)	
R	acoustic reflection coefficient (416)	
R_t	true count rate (340)	
RBE	relative biological effectiveness (279)	
rad	(dose) (49)	
rem	(dose equivalent) (279)	
rms	root mean square (68)	
S	survival probability (159)	
S	sensitivity (353)	
SID	source-to-image receptor distance (193)	
SOD	source-to-object distance (193)	
Sv	sievert (dose equivalent) (279)	
SNR	signal-to-noise ratio (156)	
s	second (time) (31)	
sin	sine function (217)	
T	temperature (47)	
T	occupancy factor (radiation safety) (260)	
T	tesla (363)	
T1, T2	nuclear spin relaxation times (379)	
TE, TR	NMR echo, repetition time (388)	
TAR	tissue air ratio (273)	
T/W	grid ratio (175)	
t	time	
$t_{0.5}$	half-life (344)	
V	voltage, electric potential (44)	
V	volt (unit of voltage) (44)	
v	velocity (29)	
U	unsharpness (195)	
U	use factor (radiation safety) (260)	
W	watt (power) (46)	
W	workload (radiation safety) (260)	
W	energy per ion pair (266)	
X	exposure (96)	
x	position, thickness, depth	
y	position, coordinate axis	
Z	atomic number (54)	
Z	acoustic impedance (415)	
z	position, coordinate axis	

Γ (Gamma)	film gamma (182)	μ (mu)	mean value (159)	σ (sigma)	standard deviation (160)
γ (gamma)	gyromagnetic ratio (364)	μ (mu)	linear attenuation coefficient (107)	σ (sigma)	Compton linear attenuation coefficient (113)
Δ (Delta)	small change, difference (29)	$[\mu/\rho]$	mass attenuation coefficient (109)	τ (tau)	photoelectric linear attenuation coefficient (113)
ε (epsilon)	electric field (35)	$[\mu/\rho]_{ab}$	mass energy absorption coefficient (264)	τ (tau)	detector dead time (340)
θ (theta)	angle (105)	π (pi)	3.14159; 180 degrees (217)	Ψ (Psi)	photon energy fluence (263)
λ (lambda)	wavelength (39)	ρ (rho)	density (109)	Ω (Omega)	ohm (60)
λ (lambda)	transformation constant (126)	Σ (Sigma)	summation symbol (159)	ω (omega)	angular frequency (218)
μ (mu)	micro- (10^{-6})				

Index

Page numbers followed by f and t indicate figures and tables, respectively.